Neurodegeneration: Molecular and Cellular Mechanisms

Neurodegeneration: Molecular and Cellular Mechanisms

Edited by Elena Poole

hayle
medical

New York

Hayle Medical,
750 Third Avenue, 9th Floor,
New York, NY 10017, USA

Visit us on the World Wide Web at:
www.haylemedical.com

ISBN: 978-1-63241-679-7

Cataloging-in-Publication Data

Neurodegeneration : molecular and cellular mechanisms / edited by Elena Poole.
     p. cm.
Includes bibliographical references and index.
ISBN 978-1-63241-679-7
1. Nervous system--Degeneration. 2. Nervous system--Degeneration--Molecular aspects.
3. Molecular neurobiology. 4. Nerves--Cytology. I. Poole, Elena.
RC394.D35 N48 2019
616.804 7--dc23

Table of Contents

Preface

The main aim of this book is to educate learners and enhance their research focus by presenting diverse topics covering this vast field. This is an advanced book which compiles significant studies by distinguished experts in the area of analysis. This book addresses successive solutions to the challenges arising in the area of application, along with it; the book provides scope for future developments.

The process of neurodegeneration is a progressive degeneration of neuron cells. It can be categorized into varied levels of neuronal circuitry ranging from molecular to systemic levels. Aging is the primary contributor to neurodegeneration. Neurodegenerative diseases are caused due to genetic mutations. Protein misfolding is another characteristic that is common in such conditions. Intracellular mechanisms such as protein degradation pathways, mitochondrial dysfunction, membrane damage, axonal transport, DNA damage, etc. along with programmed cell death mechanisms are other pathways of neurodegeneration. This book presents researches and studies performed by experts across the globe on the molecular and cellular mechanisms of neurodegeneration. While understanding the long-term perspectives of the topics, this book makes an effort in highlighting its impact as a modern tool for the understanding of neurodegenerative disorders. With state-of-the-art inputs by acclaimed experts of this field, this book targets students and professionals.

It was a great honour to edit this book, though there were challenges, as it involved a lot of communication and networking between me and the editorial team. However, the end result was this all-inclusive book covering diverse themes in the field.

Finally, it is important to acknowledge the efforts of the contributors for their excellent chapters, through which a wide variety of issues have been addressed. I would also like to thank my colleagues for their valuable feedback during the making of this book.

Editor

Differential induction of mutant SOD1 misfolding and aggregation by tau and α-synuclein pathology

Michael C. Pace[1†], Guilian Xu[1†], Susan Fromholt[1], John Howard[1], Benoit I. Giasson[1], Jada Lewis[1*] and David R. Borchelt[1,2*]

Abstract

Background: Prior studies in *C. elegans* demonstrated that the expression of aggregation-prone polyglutamine proteins in muscle wall cells compromised the folding of co-expressed temperature-sensitive proteins, prompting interest in whether the accumulation of a misfolded protein in pathologic features of human neurodegenerative disease burdens cellular proteostatic machinery in a manner that impairs the folding of other cellular proteins.

Methods: Mice expressing high levels of mutant forms of tau and α-synuclein (αSyn), which develop inclusion pathologies of the mutant protein in brain and spinal cord, were crossed to mice expressing low levels of mutant superoxide dismutase 1 fused to yellow fluorescent protein (G85R-SOD1:YFP) for aging and neuropathological evaluation.

Results: Mice expressing low levels of G85R-SOD1:YFP, alone, lived normal lifespans and were free of evidence of inclusion pathology, setting the stage to use this protein as a reporter of proteostatic function. We observed robust induction of G85R-SOD1:YFP inclusion pathology in the neuropil of spinal cord and brainstem of bigenic mice that co-express high levels of mutant tau in the spinal axis and develop robust spinal tau pathology (JNPL3 mice). In contrast, in crosses of the G85R-SOD1:YFP mice with mice that model spinal α-synucleinopathy (the M83 model of αSyn pathology), we observed no G85R-SOD1:YFP inclusion formation. Similarly, in crosses of the G85R-SOD1:YFP mice to mice that model cortical tau pathology (rTg4510 mice), we did not observe induction of G85R-SOD1:YFP inclusions.

Conclusion: Despite robust burdens of neurodegenerative pathology in M83 and rTg4510 mice, the introduction of the G85R-SOD1:YFP protein was induced to aggregate only in the context of spinal tau pathology present in the JNPL3 model. These findings suggest unexpected specificity, mediated by both the primary protein pathology and cellular context, in the induced "secondary aggregation" of a mutant form of SOD1 that could be viewed as a reporter of proteostatic function.

Keywords: Proteostasis, Protein misfolding, Tau, α-Synuclein, SOD1, Proteinopathy

Background

Neurodegenerative diseases such as Alzheimer's disease (AD), Parkinson's disease (PD), frontotemporal dementia (FTD), amyotrophic lateral sclerosis (ALS) and Huntington's disease are often defined pathologically by the accumulation of misfolded proteins that become aggregated to form intracellular and/or extracellular inclusions [1–4]. This underlying theme across these diseases has suggested that a similar pathogenic mechanism contributes, at least in part, to the development and/or progression of these disorders. To date, defects in many cellular pathways have been implicated in the pathogenesis of these diseases [5, 6]. Some of these suspected pathways are critical in cellular protein quality control such as the ubiquitin-proteasome system (UPS) (reviewed in [7]) and autophagy (reviewed in [8]). Indeed, it has been previously demonstrated that pathological forms of tau (associated with Alzheimer's disease and various tauopathies) and αSyn (associated with Parkinson's disease and other synucleinopathies) can

* Correspondence: jada.lewis@ufl.edu; drb1@ufl.edu
†Equal contributors
[1]Department of Neuroscience, Center for Translational Research in Neurodegenerative Disease, McKnight Brain Institute, University of Florida, 1275 Center Drive, BMS Building J-491, PO Box, Gainesville, FL 32610-0244, USA
Full list of author information is available at the end of the article

hinder the efficacy of the proteasome [9–16]. This finding is further supported by the accumulation of ubiquitin-positive inclusions in the cases of many neurodegenerative disorders [17–19]. Hence, one hypothesis that has gained traction is that protein aggregation in these neurodegenerative disorders is a biomarker of underlying dysfunction in protein quality control systems (reviewed in [20]).

Protein homeostasis (proteostasis) is maintained by a network of factors (reviewed in [21–23]) that primarily fall into three main components at the cytosolic level: molecular chaperones responsible for folding newly synthesized proteins and refolding misfolded proteins [24], the UPS which is responsible for the degradation of misfolded and inherently short-lived proteins (reviewed in [25, 26]), and the autophagy-lysosomal pathway which is necessary for the removal of large insoluble protein aggregates that cannot otherwise be degraded [27]. The implications of this systemic malfunction in proteostasis could be widespread at the cellular level, and one particular idea that has emerged is the concept of "secondary" protein misfolding, where the accumulation of one misfolded protein imposes a burden on the proteostasis network that leaves other vulnerable proteins with insufficient support to fold correctly [28, 29]. Disruption of the proteostasis network could potentially explain the origin of mixed pathologies in human neurodegenerative diseases, which are relatively common [30–34]. Accordingly, we have previously shown the aggregation of phosphorylated TDP-43 protein as a secondary event to the aggregation of phosphorylated tau in two independent transgenic models [35]. These instances of mixed pathologies could, however, have been a result of cross-seeding, which has been demonstrated for many proteins pathologically associated with neurodegeneration [36–41].

The original concept of secondary misfolding was characterized in the invertebrate *C. elegans*. In this study, it was found that the expression of an aggregation-prone protein could impair the folding integrity of other proteins, or "bystander" proteins [28]. Specifically, a fragment of (exon 1) mutant human huntingtin (*HTT*) gene containing a polyglutamine (polyQ) expansion was co-expressed with temperature-sensitive (TS) mutant forms of paramyosin and dynamin-1. Both proteins achieve functional conformations at lower temperatures (15 °C), but are inactive at 25 °C. Mutant huntingtin exon-1 fragments are very prone to aggregate [42] and, when expressed in the muscle wall of *C. elegans* concomitantly with these TS mutants, the TS proteins failed to achieve active conformations at 15 °C [28]. This outcome was thought to be due to the stress placed upon the proteostasis network by mutant huntingtin, overwhelming the system and preventing proteins that are particularly dependent upon the proteostasis network (e.g. TS mutant proteins) from achieving active conformations [28]. Interestingly, the added burden of co-expressed

TS mutant proteins exacerbated the aggregation of mutant huntingtin, supporting the argument that the capacity of the cellular protein folding machinery of *C. elegans* is limited and easily over-burdened.

In the present study, we asked whether the deposition of human tau or αSyn aggregates in the central nervous system (CNS) of mouse models might impose a burden on proteostatic function using a mutant form of SOD1 fused to YFP as a reporter in a paradigm akin to the foregoing *C. elegans* studies. We have been using a mouse model that expresses the G85R variant of SOD1 fused to YFP as model in studies of prion-like propagation of misfolded SOD1 [43–45]. Hemizygous mice expressing G85R-SOD1:YFP do not intrinsically develop ALS symptoms or show inclusion pathology, while homozygous G85R-SOD1:YFP mice develop paralysis from 6 months onward with spinal cords that contain fluorescent inclusions and detergent-insoluble G85R-SOD1:YFP [46]. Thus, the hemizygous G85R-SOD1:YFP mouse could be viewed as model that is sub-threshold for induction of disease. In such a setting, any perturbation that diminished proteostatic function could then lead to a breach of threshold to induce mutant SOD1 aggregation. Importantly, the YFP tag on the G85R-SOD1 protein allows for simple detection and visualization of aggregation and inclusion formation, and we use this feature as a readout to assess secondary misfolding in mice that develop tau and αSyn pathology. We crossed the G85R-SOD1:YFP mice to three different models of proteinopathies: 1) a model of spinal tau pathology expressing human P301L tau (termed JNPL3 [47]), 2) a model of spinal αSyn pathology expressing human A53T αSyn (termed M83 [48]), and 3) a model of cortical tau pathology expressing human P301L tau (termed rTg4510 [49, 50]). Despite abundant proteinopathy in these models, only bigenic mice from the cross with JNPL3 mice caused robust G85R-SOD1:YFP pathology to develop. Our findings demonstrate complex interactions between pathologically misfolded tau, αSyn and the proteostatic network in triggering the "secondary aggregation" of our mutant SOD1 reporter.

Methods

Transgenic mice

To model tauopathy, we utilized both the JNPL3 and rTg4510 mouse models. Briefly, JNPL3 mice (maintained on the Swiss Webster background from Taconic) express mutant human tau (P301L, 4R0N) under the mouse prion promoter which leads to mutant tau pathology primarily in the spinal cord and brainstem (though other regions are more modestly affected) [47]. rTg4510 mice (maintained on a hybrid 129S6/FVB background) are bigenic mice that express both human tau with the P301L mutation (4R0N) behind by a disrupted minimal

CMV promoter and the tet-transactivator (tTA) driven by a Ca²⁺ calmodulin kinase II (CaMKII) promoter (forebrain-specific). The tTA protein binds to the disrupted promoter to drive mutant tau expression at high levels, primarily within the hippocampus and neocortex [49, 50]. To model α-synucleinopathy, we used the M83 mouse model (maintained on the hybrid C3H/B6 background). This model overexpresses mutant (A53T) human αSyn under the mouse prion promoter [48], and develops αSyn pathology primarily within the spinal cord, brainstem midbrain, hypothalamus, thalamus and peri-aqueductal gray regions (with other brain regions also somewhat affected), resulting in a severe motor phenotype and paralysis. This pathology and phenotype occurs between 8 and 16 months of age in homozygous M83 mice, but later than 21 months in hemizygous M83 mice [48]. Lastly, hemizygous mice (maintained on the FVB background) expressing the G85R mutant of SOD1 tagged to YFP under the human SOD1 promoter were used for all crossing experiments [46].

All mice were kept in specific pathogen free cages prior to harvesting and histology procedures. All animals were handled and processed according to approved protocols by the University of Florida Institutional Animal Care and Use Committee (IACUC). All applicable international, national, and/or institutional guidelines for the care and use of animals were followed.

Breeding scheme to generate mice co-expressing G85R-SOD1:YFP and mutant proteins associated with human proteinopathies

Mice heterozygous for the G85R-SOD1:YFP transgene were bred to mice transgenic for either mutant tau or αSyn. In order to generate JNPL3-G85R-SOD1:YFP animals, we first bred heterozygous JNPL3 mice to heterozygous G85R-SOD1:YFP mice to produce male animals expressing both the JNPL3 tau and SOD1 transgenes. These were bred to a homozygous JNPL3 female mice to produce offspring that were then bred to generate a large cohort of mice, some of which expressed both mutant tau and our reporter G85R-SOD1:YFP transgene. A subset of these mice were expected to be homozygous for the tau transgene and to develop early onset tauopathy, with a subset of these mice being transgenic for the G85R-SOD1:YFP transgene. To generate mice expressing both mutant αSyn and our G85R-SOD1:YFP reporter, homozygous M83 mice were bred to mice heterozygous for the G85R-SOD1:YFP transgene. Mice expressing G85R-SOD1:YFP as well as the transgenes associated with the rTg4510 line are triple transgenic animals, which were generated by first crossing mice transgenic for P301L mutant tau to mice transgenic for G85R-SOD1:YFP. The double transgenic mice generated from this cross were then crossed to mice transgenic for tTA under the CaMKII promoter in order to generate rTg4510 mice (tau/tTA) expressing G85R-SOD1:YFP.

Intramuscular human αSyn fibril injections into hemizygous M83 and bigenic M83-G85R-SOD1:YFP transgenic mice to seed αSyn pathology

As has been previously described [51], sonicated wild type human αSyn fibrils (2 mg/mL) were injected at a volume of 5 µL into hemizygous M83xG85R-SOD1:YFP mice once they reached 8 weeks of age. Injections were conducted using a Hamilton 10 µL syringe (Reno, NV) along with a 25-gauge needle. The needle was injected ~ 1 mm deep into the gastrocnemius muscle bilaterally in each animal. Mice were anesthetized with isoflurane during the procedure.

Tissue processing, immunohistochemistry and image microscopy

Mice were euthanized by isoflurane anesthesia overdose with exsanguination and transcardial perfusion with cold PBS. The harvested brains were bisected sagittally and for a subset of animals, one hemi-brain was frozen on dry ice (stored at – 80 °C) and the other was drop fixed in 4% paraformaldehyde for 48 h. For a subset of the animals, both hemi-brains were drop-fixed with one used for cryostat sections (10 µm) to directly visualize fluorescence and the other was embedded in paraffin for sectioning (5 µm). The harvested spinal cords were divided into 4 equivalent segments. For two of the segments, the spinal column was drop-fixed in 4% paraformaldehyde for 48 h before embedding in paraffin for sectioning. In a subset of animals, spinal segments were flash frozen on dry ice and then stored at – 80 °C. For a subset of animals, all 4 segments of spinal column were drop-fixed in 4% paraformaldehyde so that 2 of the segments could be sectioned by cryostat with 2 segments embedded in paraffin for sectioning. All sections were attached to Superfrost Plus microscope slides (Fisher Scientific, Hampton, NH) for imaging. To prepare paraffin-embedded tissue for histology, sections first were de-paraffinized and rehydrated through immersion in serial dilutions of ethanol. For sections used for direct fluorescence microscopy, the frozen section or rehydrated paraffin section was coverslipped with Vectashield (Vector Laboratories, Burlingame, CA) mounting medium. Tissue sections used for immunohistochemistry were rinsed in water, followed by antigen retrieval via a 30-min incubation in a steamer containing citrate buffer (10 mM sodium citrate with 0.05% Tween-20, pH 6.0). The citrate antigen retrieval procedure quenches the fluorescence of the G85R-SOD1:YFP, requiring the use of a primary antibody to GFP/YFP for visualization. Tissue sections were blocked using a PBS solution containing 3% normal goat serum and 0.1% Triton X-100. Primary antibodies in 3% normal goat serum in PBS-T were incubated overnight at 4 °C. For DAB-mediated immunostaining, endogenous peroxidases were blocked using a solution of 0.3% H_2O_2 in PBS. An ABC kit (Vector Laboratories, Burlingame, CA) was used with a DAB reagent set (KPL, Gaithersburg, MD) to detect signal. Sections were then counterstained with hematoxylin prior to dehydration in ethanol and coverslipping. Primary antibodies used included AT8 (1:500, mouse monoclonal, Thermo Fisher, Waltham, MA), MC1 (1:125, mouse monoclonal, Peter Davies), PHF1 (1:500, mouse monoclonal, Peter Davies), GFP (green fluorescent protein)/YFP (1:200, rabbit polyclonal, Invitrogen, Waltham, MA) and JL-8 GFP/YFP (1:200, mouse monoclonal, Clontech, Mountain View, CA, USA). Secondary fluorescent antibodies used for immunofluorescence staining included goat anti-rabbit IgG (1:1000, Alexa Fluor 488, Invitrogen, Waltham, MA) and goat anti-mouse IgG (1:1000, Alexa Fluor 568, Invitrogen, Waltham, MA). Biotinylated secondary antibodies (Vector Laboratories, Burlingame, CA) were used for DAB-mediated staining for 30 min at room temperature (1:500). Tissue sections were imaged using an Olympus DSU-IX81 spinning disc confocal microscope (Tokyo, Japan) or scanned using the Scanscope FL image scanner (Aperio, Vista, CA).

Fluorescence quantification and statistical analysis

Fluorescence quantification, when necessary, was conducted using ImageJ (version 1.51 g). Statistical analyses were conducted using GraphPad PRISM (version 7.0 h, La Jolla, CA), as indicated in applicable figures.

Preparation of brain and spinal cord tissues for immunoblot analysis

To assess the levels of G85R-SOD1:YFP in the brains of trigenic rTg4510 x G85R-SOD1:YFP mice, one hemi-forebrain was homogenized in PBS (10% weight/volume) with 1% protease inhibitor cocktail P8340 in DMSO (Sigma Aldrich, St. Louis, MO). Protein concentrations were measured by the BCA (bicinchoninic) assay (Fisher Scientific, Hampton, NH) and 20 μg of protein from each brain homogenate was adjusted to 1 x Laemmli buffer, boiled, loaded onto a 4–20% Tris-glycine gel (Invitrogen, Waltham, MA) and subjected to SDS-PAGE (120 V for 90 min). Proteins were then transferred to nitrocellulose membranes overnight at 100 mA.

To generate detergent insoluble fractions from JNPL3/ G85R-SOD1:YFP mice, G85R-SOD1:YFP mice, JNPL3 mice, and nontransgenic control mice, we used a method used to fractionate insoluble SOD1 aggregates that has been previously described [52, 53]. Briefly, spinal cord tissues were dissected from the frozen spinal columns after a brief thaw and homogenized in 1× TEN (10 mM Tris-HCl pH 7.5/1 mM EDTA/100 mM NaCl)

at a 10:1 volume to weight ratio. This homogenate was then mixed 1:1 with a second buffer containing 1× TEN with 1% NP40 and 1% protease inhibitor cocktail P8340 (Sigma Aldrich, St. Louis, MO). This mixture was sonicated and centrifuged at > 1,000,000 g in an airfuge (Beckman Coulter, Brea, CA) for 10 min to separate soluble from insoluble protein fractions. The pellet fraction was then washed in a buffer containing 1× TEN with 0.5% NP40, sonicated, and spun down to obtain the final pellet fraction which was resuspended in 30 μL of buffer containing 1× TEN with 0.5% NP40, 0.25% SDS, 0.5% deoxycholate and 1% protease inhibitor cocktail. Protein concentrations in each fraction were measured by BCA (bicinchoninic) assay (Fisher Scientific, Hampton, NH). 20 μg of protein from each fraction, suspended in 1× Laemmli buffer, was boiled and then electrophoresed into 16% Tris-glycine gels before transfer to nitrocellulose membranes overnight at 100 mA. The membranes were then analyzed with antibodies to SOD1 as described below.

To examine the levels of insoluble αSyn and SOD1 in M83/G85R-SOD1:YFP mice, the protocol used for detergent extraction and sedimentation differed slightly, following a previously described method [54]. Briefly, the tissue was initially homogenized in PBS containing 1% protease inhibitor cocktail and then centrifuged at 100,000 x g for 30 min. The supernatant was collected and saved as the PBS-soluble fraction. The pellet was resuspended in 1× TEN buffer containing 0.5% NP40 by brief sonication and then centrifuged at 100,000 x g (Optima L100 K Ultracentrifuge [Beckman Coulter, Brea, CA] using a 70.1 Ti rotor at 35,000 RPM) for 30 min to produce NP-40 soluble and insoluble fractions. The NP-40 insoluble pellet was then resuspended in a volume of TEN with 2% sodium deoxycholate equal to the original homogenization volume by brief sonication. 30 μL of either PBS-soluble or NP40-insoluble protein fractions were mixed with 4 x Laemmli buffer, boiled, and loaded onto a 16% Tris-glycine gel. After transfer to nitrocellulose at 300 mA for 1 h, the membranes were probed with antibodies to SOD1 and αSyn as described below.

Immunoblotting and western blot quantification

Nitrocellulose membranes were blocked in a 5% powdered milk (Nestle Carnation, Glendale, CA) solution in PBS-T. The membrane was then incubated in primary antibody in the blocking solution overnight, followed by three 10-min washes in PBS-T. Primary antibodies included GAPDH (1:5000, Meridian Life Science, Memphis, TN), Tau13 (1:1000, BioLegend, San Diego, CA), mouse/human SOD1 (1:4000, generated in-house) and human SOD1 (1:2500, generated in-house [55]). Horseradish peroxidase-conjugated secondary anti-mouse or anti-rabbit antibody (Vector Laboratories, Burlingame, CA) was used in order to visualize proteins by chemiluminescence using the Pierce ECL Western Blot Substrate Kit (Thermo Scientific, Waltham, MA). Western blot quantification was conducted using GeneTools by Syngene (in correlation with the GeneSys imager, Daly City, CA).

Results

Mutant tau induces G85R-SOD1:YFP inclusion pathology in the spinal cord and brainstem

In order to determine whether tau pathology could induce G85R-SOD1:YFP to aggregate, we analyzed the JNPL3 transgenic mice model of spinal tau pathology on the hemizygous G85R-SOD1:YFP background. For this study, only female bigenic JNPL3/G85R-SOD1:YFP mice were analyzed due to the differences in tau transgene expression between males and females that we previously reported in the JNPL3 mice (specifically that females express mutant tau at much higher levels than their male counterparts) [56]. JNPL3/G85R-SOD1:YFP and JNPL3 transgenic animals were harvested at humane endpoints (ranging from 7 to 15.5 months of age), characterized by paralysis in at least one limb (usually a hind limb).

Compared to littermates that were transgenic only for tau, JNPL3/G85R-SOD1:YFP mice showed a statistically significant, but modest acceleration of the paralysis phenotype (Additional file 1: Figure S1).

We hypothesized that the presence of tau pathology in the JNPL3/G85R-SOD1:YFP animals could act as a stressor upon cellular proteostasis that could cause bystander aggregation of G85R-SOD1:YFP and the formation of fluorescent inclusions. In contrast to the soluble and diffuse distribution of G85R-SOD1:YFP seen in hemizygous animals (Fig. 1a and b), JNPL3/G85R-SOD1:YFP bigenic mice exhibited robust inclusion pathology in the form of widespread punctate aggregates in the gray matter visible by direct fluorescence (Fig. 1c and d). This pathology was predominantly observed in the spinal cord and brainstem (Fig. 1, Additional file 2: Figure S2), the same regions that are subject to heavy tau burden in the JNPL3 model (Additional file 3: Figure S3, spinal tauopathy shown) [47]. The abundant fluorescent neuropil aggregates with granular/punctate pathology in the cell body was

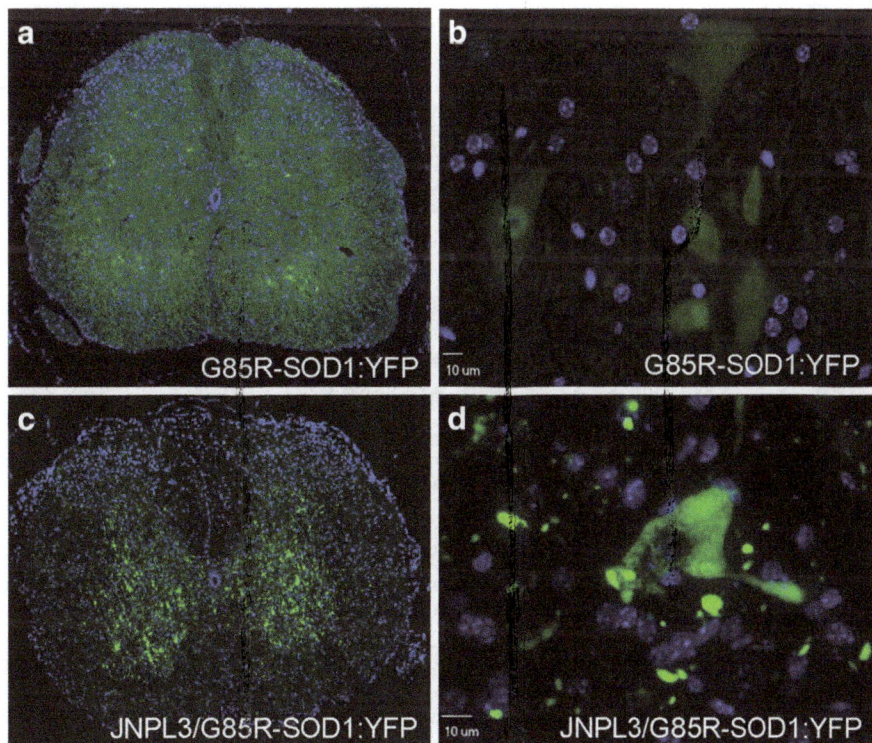

Fig. 1 G85R-SOD1:YFP aggregation into punctate inclusions within the spinal cord of JNPL3/G85R-SOD1:YFP mice. Compared to the diffuse distribution of G85R-SOD1:YFP in spinal motor neurons of single transgenic animals (a and b), the fluorescence is organized into large neuropil inclusions with granular/punctate accumulation in the cell bodies of spinal motor neurons of bigenic JNPL3/G85R-SOD1:YFP mice (c and d). Exposure times were kept consistent across images and set to capture images of the inclusions in the bigenic mice at optimal exposure. Nuclei were stained with DAPI (blue). All animals analyzed were female. Representative images (40× magnification) of the ventral horn within the spinal cord are shown for 8 JNPL3-G85R-SOD1:YFP double transgenic mice and 3 G85R-SOD1:YFP single transgenic mice (aged 7 to 15.5 months). An additional low power image of the spinal ventral horn bigenic JNPL3/G85R-SOD1:YFP mice is provided in Additional file 2: Figure S2a

similar in appearance to what has been described for the homozygous G85-SOD1:YFP mice that develop paralysis [46] and for G85R-SOD1:YFP mice induced to develop paralysis by prion-like transmission experiments [44].

To further confirm that G85R-SOD1:YFP in the bigenic tau/SOD1 mice was aggregated, we conducted detergent extraction and sedimentation of spinal cords from these mice to determine changes in protein solubility. In previous study, we have demonstrated that the aggregates formed by mutant SOD1 become aberrantly crosslinked through disulfide oxidation and to visual these aggregates the SDS-PAGE was performed in the absence of reducing agent [53]. As expected from this prior study, soluble G85R-SOD1:YFP was detected in spinal cord extracts from bigenic tau/SOD1 mice and mice expressing G85R-SOD1:YFP alone, but NP40-insoluble, highly crosslinked, G85R-SOD1:YFP was only detected in the tau/SOD1 bigenic mice that showed inclusion pathology (Additional file 4: Figure S4a and b). Collectively, these data demonstrate that the G85R-SOD1:YFP protein was induced to misfold and aggregate in the spinal cords of mice with abundant spinal tau pathology.

Localization of SOD1 pathology relative to tau pathology

We next sought to determine whether the G85R-SOD1:YFP inclusions were simply co-depositing with aggregating tau. To our knowledge, no interaction between these two proteins has been reported, nor has SOD1 pathology been described as a secondary event to tauopathy. We performed double immunostaining of brain and spinal cord tissues with three well-characterized tau antibodies (MC1, PHF1, or AT8) in conjunction with a primary antibody to YFP to assess tau and SOD1 pathology (Figs. 2 and 3, Additional file 5: Figure S5). Both end-stage JNPL3 mice and JNPL3/G85R-SOD1:YFP mice had extensive tau pathology (Figs. 2a-b, 3a-b; Additional files 3 and 5: Figures S3, S5a-b). Consistent with our original reports on the pathology of JNPL3 mice, both hyperphosphorylated tau as detected by AT8 and PHF1 immunostaining, and tau of an abnormal conformation as detected by MC1 immunostaining were present [47, 56]. We observed limited co-localization between the tau and SOD1 aggregates in the spinal cord of JNPL3/G85R-SOD1:YFP bigenic animals (Figs. 2d and 3d; Additional file 5: Figure S5d). Overall, bigenic animals exhibit both robust tau and SOD1 pathology, but with no obvious direct evidence for co-aggregation occurring between the two proteins.

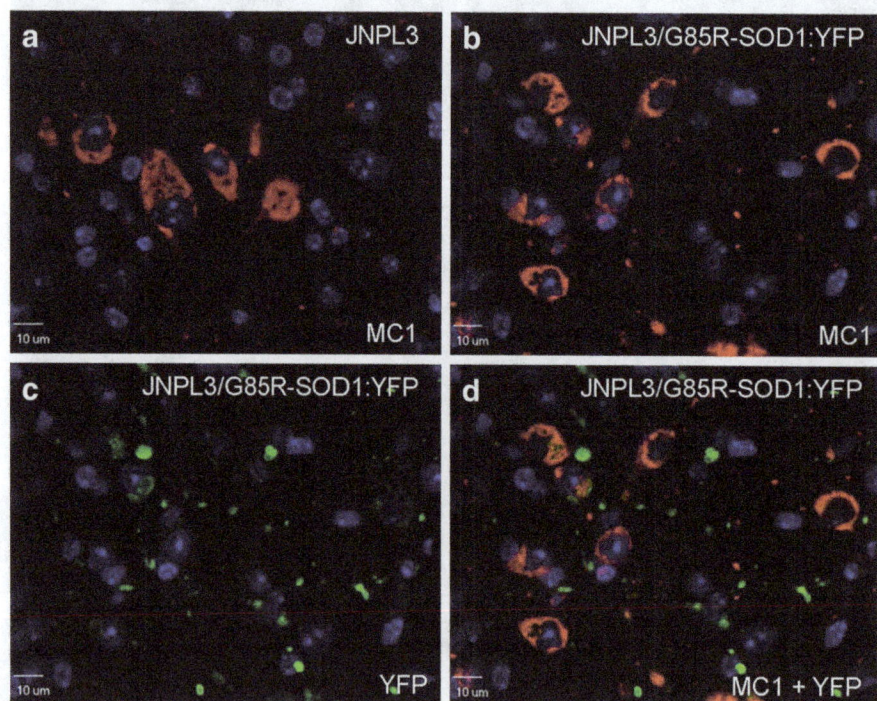

Fig. 2 Localization of tau MC1 immunoreactivity versus G85R-SOD1:YFP pathology in bigenic JNPL3/G85R-SOD1:YFP mice. Misfolded human tau recognized by the MC1 antibody (red) appears similar in JNPL3 tau-transgenic versus JNPL3/G85R-SOD1:YFP bigenic animals (**a**, **b**). G85R-SOD1:YFP pathology, detected by an YFP antibody (green) (**c**), does not robustly co-localize with tau pathology in double transgenic animals (**d**). Nuclei were stained with DAPI (blue). Representative images (60× magnification) are shown within the ventral horn of the spinal cord of 8 JNPL3 and 8 JNPL3/G85R-SOD1:YFP animals. All animals analyzed were female aged 7 to 15.5 months

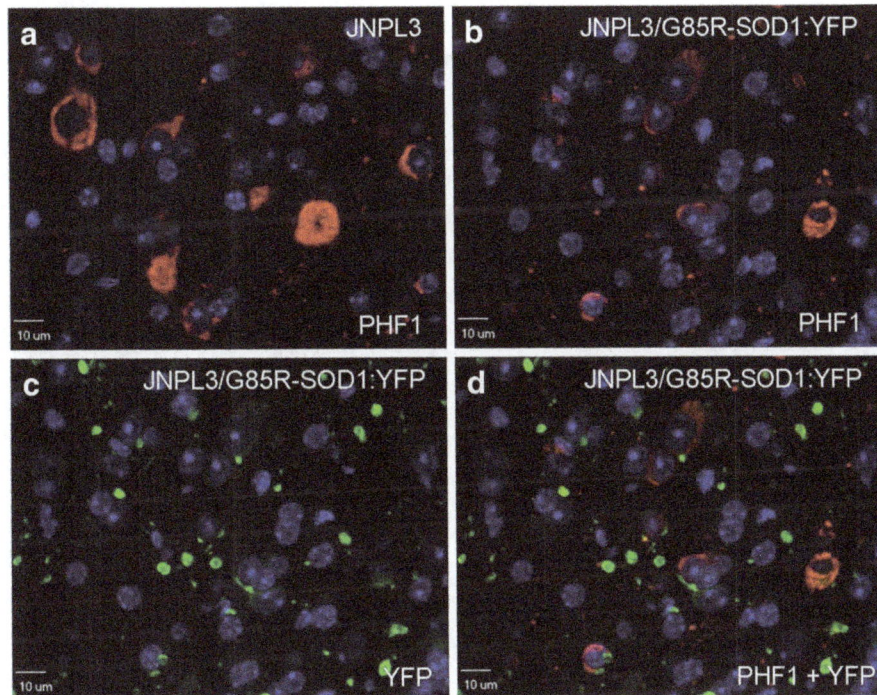

Fig. 3 Localization of phosphotau immunoreactivity versus G85R-SOD1:YFP pathology in bigenic JNPL3/G85R-SOD1:YFP animals. Hyperphosphorylated human tau pathology recognized by the PHF1 (Ser396/Ser404; red) antibody appears similar in JNPL3 tau-transgenic versus JNPL3/G85R-SOD1:YFP bigenic mice (**a, b**). G85R-SOD1:YFP pathology, detected using an YFP antibody (green) (**c**), does not robustly co-localize with tau pathology in double transgenic animals (**d**). Nuclei were stained with DAPI (blue). Images are of 60× magnification within the ventral horn of the spinal cord of JNPL3 and JNPL3/G85R-SOD1:YFP mice. The images shown are representative of 8 JNPL3 and 8 JNPL3/G85R-SOD1:YFP female animals aged 7 to 15.5 months

Lack of G85R-SOD1:YFP inclusion pathology induction in the rTg4510 model of cortical and hippocampal tauopathy

Neither homozygous nor hemizygous G85R-SOD1:YFP mice typically develop inclusion pathology in the forebrain (cortex, hippocampus, striatum) similar to the degree that is seen in the spinal cord [46]. To assess whether cortical/hippocampal tau pathology could also induce secondary aggregation of G85R-SOD1:YFP, we used the rTg4510 model that develops robust cortical tau pathology by 5.5 months of age (Fig. 4a-b; Additional file 6: Figure S6) [49, 50]. The introduction of G85R-SOD1:YFP expression in rTg4510 mice yielded no noticeable motor phenotype and despite very robust tau pathology, there was no clear formation of widespread fluorescent inclusions in rTg4510/G85R-SOD1:YFP mice (Fig. 4d, cortex shown). In these trigenic mice, there was a general increase in overall fluorescence intensity throughout the cortex and hippocampus with occasional cells that were intensely fluorescent (Fig. 4d; for quantification of direct fluorescence see Additional file 7: Figure S7) as compared to single transgenic G85R-SOD1:YFP controls (Fig. 4c-d). However, we could not attribute the increased fluorescence to increased levels of G85R-SOD1:YFP protein in immunoblot analysis of forebrains in the trigenic mice

compared to G85R-SOD1:YFP alone (Additional file 7: Figure S7) and thus the basis for the heightened fluorescence intensity is unknown. In any case, there was no evidence of fluorescent inclusions as was observed in the JNPL3/G85R-SOD1:YFP bigenic mice.

Paucity of induced G85R-SOD1:YFP aggregation in the M83 model of αSynucleinopathy

Given our observation of aggregated SOD1:YFP reporter in the JNPL3 model of spinal tauopathy, we next sought to determine whether the effects we observed were specific to tau or could be extended to a different type of spinal proteinopathy. We utilized the M83 model of αSyn-opathy that expresses mutant (A53T) αSyn under the mouse prion promoter [48], which is the same vector that was used to create the JNPL3 tauopathy model. The two models show very similar anatomical pathological burden (compare Additional file 3: Figure S3 to Additional file 8: Figure S8) and both develop paralytic phenotypes. To induce the αSyn pathology, bigenic M83/G85R-SOD1:YFP mice were injected intramuscularly with fibrillized human αSyn protein as previously described [51]. This seeded induction of αSyn pathology produces a predictably accelerated robust spinal pathology that is accompanied by a paralytic motor

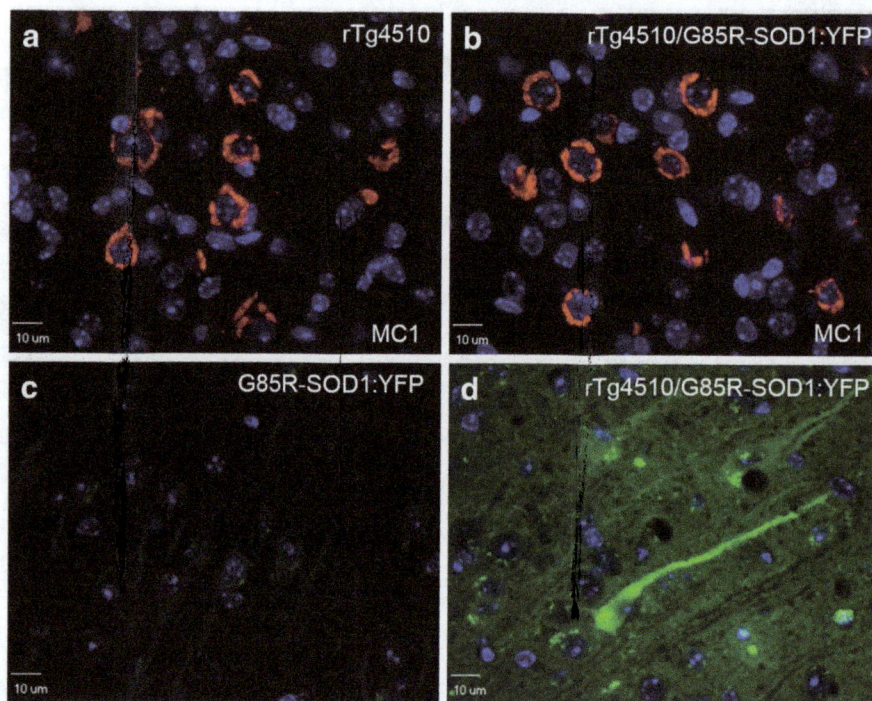

Fig. 4 G85R-SOD1:YFP does not form inclusions in the forebrain of rTg4510/G85R-SOD1:YFP bigenic. The severity of neurofibrillary tangle pathology in the hippocampus and cortex (**a**, cortex shown immunostained with the MC1 antibody, red) in rTg4510 mice is similar to that of rTg4510/G85R-SOD1:YFP bigenic mice (**b**). Although the intensity of YFP fluorescence in the trigenic P301L/G85R-SOD1:YFP mice was higher than that of mice expressing G85R-SOD1:YFP alone, but there was no evidence of organization into inclusion structures (**c** and **d**; see Additional file 6: Figure S6). There were isolated cells that were hyperfluorescent (**d**), but the fluorescence in these cells did not appear to be organized into fibrils. All images were taken at 60X magnification of 5 μm paraffin-embedded sections. Nuclei were stained with DAPI (blue). Exposure time and specifications were kept consistent across all images, optimized to the rTg4510/G85R-SOD1:YFP tissue sections. Representative images are shown for 5 rTg4510/G85R-SOD1:YFP mice (1 male, 4 female) and 4 G85R-SOD1:YFP mice (4 males) between 8 and 9 months of age

phenotype (between 3 and 4 months post-IM-injection) compared to uninjected hemizygous M83 mice, which acquire this phenotype later than 21 months of age [48, 51]. Unexpectedly, the spinal cords and brainstems of paralyzed bigenic M83/G85R-SOD1:YFP lacked any evidence of G85R-SOD1:YFP inclusions (Fig. 5). There was no significant difference observed in motor phenotype for mice expressing only αSyn versus double transgenic animals expressing both αSyn and G85R-SOD1:YFP (Additional file 9: Figure S9). The level of αSyn pathology in these bigenic mice was not obviously different from that of M83 littermates that also were IM injected with αSyn fibrils (see Additional file 8: Figure S8). Thus, in stark contrast to tau pathology, we do not observe secondary G85R-SOD1:YFP pathology in the presence of αSyn pathology.

To confirm the pathological findings, we assessed the levels of soluble and insoluble αSyn and G85R-SOD1:YFP in the mice resulting from this cross. For this study, we used a slightly different fractionation protocol (see Methods) that enabled detection both soluble and insoluble αSyn in the fractionated lysates of these mice (Additional file 10: Figure S10a and b). By contrast, and in agreement with the histological findings, we could only detect G85R-SOD1:YFP in the soluble fraction from the double transgenic mice (Additional file 10: Figure S10c and d). Collectively, these data indicate that despite robust αSyn pathology and aggregation in spinal cord, the G85R-SOD1:YFP protein remains soluble.

Discussion

In the current study, we crossed mouse models of tau and αSyn pathologies to mice that express a mutant form of SOD1 that we hypothesized could be vulnerable to proteostasis stress (in this case, the G85R-SOD1:YFP) to provide a reporter of secondary aggregation. Our study is the first that we are aware of to use a fluorescent reporter (e.g., a protein tagged to YFP) to investigate bystander misfolding in a mammalian system in vivo. We observed robust induction of G85R-SOD1:YFP inclusion pathology throughout the neuropil only when the protein was expressed in the JNPL3 model of spinal tauopathy. Importantly, with this model we demonstrate that G85R-SOD1:YFP pathology did not significantly co-localize with tau pathology in the spinal cord of JNPL3-G85R-SOD1:YFP animals, providing evidence against simple co-aggregation of the two proteins. Although it is possible that misfolded mutant tau

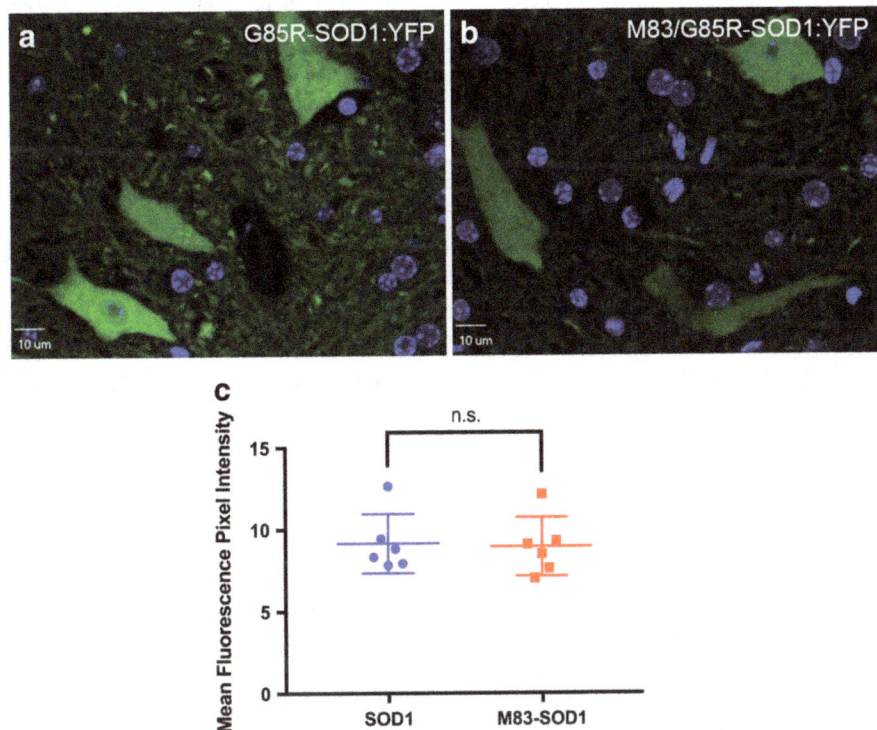

Fig. 5 Lack of G85R-SOD1:YFP inclusion pathology in the spinal cord of M83/G85R-SOD1:YFP mice. Mice were IM injected to induce αSyn pathology at 2 months of age and then euthanized at a humane endpoint (both hind limbs paralyzed). Compared to the diffuse distribution of G85R-SOD1:YFP in single transgenic animals (**a**), M83 mice expressing the G85R-SOD1:YFP reporter protein have a similar distribution of the protein (**b**), visible by direct fluorescence. Exposure times were kept consistent across images. Nuclei were stained with DAPI (blue). Representative images (60× magnification) of the ventral horn within the spinal cord are shown for 8 M83/G85R-SOD1:YFP double transgenic mice (5 female, 3 male) and 6 G85R-SOD1:YFP single transgenic mice (2 female, 4 male). Mean fluorescence intensity was not statistically significant between M83 mice expressing G85R-SOD1:YFP (abbreviated M83-SOD1) and those expressing G85R-SOD1:YFP alone (abbreviated SOD1) (**c**). Statistical analysis was conducted using GraphPad Prism (version 7.0 h). Error bars show mean ± S.D.; unpaired T-test

cross-seeded mutant SOD1 aggregation when co-expressed, we have previously reported that we could not cross-seed G85R-SOD1:YFP aggregation by injecting the spinal cords of these mice with spinal homogenates of paralyzed JNPL3 mice containing pathological tau aggregates [45]. Despite robust burdens of neurodegenerative pathology, we did not observe induced aggregation of G85R-SOD1:YFP in crosses to the spinal model of α-synucleinopathy or the cortical model of tauopathy. Our results suggest a model in which there are cell-type differences in the vulnerability of proteins to bystander misfolding, and a degree of specificity in terms of which proteins succumb to bystander misfold in response to the primary protein pathology.

Evidence of secondary protein misfolding in vivo is relatively scarce. Reports in *C. elegans* were some of the first described instances of secondary misfolding; these made use of temperature-sensitive mutants of paramyosin, dynamin, and ras that failed to achieve active conformations in the presence of aggregation-prone proteins (huntingtin and SOD1) [28, 29]. This finding was originally thought to occur because the expression of the

aggregation-prone protein overwhelmed the cellular protein folding machinery, thus leaving TS mutant proteins with too little support to fold correctly. We argue that the G85R-SOD1:YFP construct that is expressed at low levels in the transgenic model used here is a reasonable parallel to the study in *C. elegans* with TS mutant protein. Although we cannot assert that the mutant SOD1 protein is ever completely natively folded, in hemizygous mice the mutant SOD1 protein displays a diffuse cytoplasmic distribution and these mice do not develop evidence of motor neuron disease or the accompanying pathology (astrogliosis or microglosis [43]). However it is clear that the G85R-SOD1:YFP protein is vulnerable to the misfolding associated with aggregation, because it can easily be induced to do so by injecting small amounts of tissues containing aggregates of mutant SOD1 [43–45] or by raising the levels of the protein by generating homozygous mice as was described in the original model [46]. We have also previously observed induction of G85R-SOD1:YFP aggregation in bigenic mice generated by crosses to a transgenic G93A SOD1 animal [43]. Notably, the location and appearance of the fluorescent inclusion pathology we have observed here in bigenic JNPL3/G85R-SOD1:YFP animals is very similar to what we observed in bigenic G93A/G85R-SOD1:YFP mice and G85R-SOD1:YFP mice injected with tissue homogenates containing G93A SOD1 aggregates [43]. Importantly, intraspinal injection of tissue homogenates from paralyzed JNPL3 mice does not induce aggregation of G85R-SOD1:YFP [45]. Thus, in the case of the JNPL3 cross to the G85R-SOD1:YFP mice, we argue that the induced aggregation of the fusion protein is not likely to be due to direct cross seeding, but to an alternative mechanism.

One of the goals of using the G85R-SOD1:YFP mice as a reporter was to identify which cell types were experiencing proteostatic stress to induce secondary misfolding associated with aggregation. Our analysis of the JNPL3 cross to G85R-SOD1:YFP mice revealed the presence of inclusions in the cell bodies of a subset of large motor neurons. However, most of the inclusions were in the neuropil where it is very difficult to ascertain which cell type contains the inclusion. Additionally, as mentioned above, in the interim between when the studies were first initiated and the present we learned that some form of misfolded G85R-SOD1:YFP has the potential to propagate throughout the central nervous system [44]. Thus, it is difficult to decisively conclude whether a cell with a fluorescent inclusion was originally under proteostatic stress or if the inclusion was generated by intracellular spread of aggregate-inducing conformers of G85R-SOD1:YFP originating elsewhere in the CNS [44]. Moreover, the ability of some form of misfolded G85R-SOD1:YFP to mediate cell-to-cell propagation, coupled with the fact that raising expression levels of the protein can induce it to aggregate, makes it very difficult to rule out a scenario in which the presence of tau pathology caused a focal change in expression at some location that created "seeds" of aggregation-prone SOD1 that propagated throughout the spinal axis. Recent transcriptomic studies of mouse models of tauopathy, including the JNPL3 and rTg4510, and transcriptomic studies of human tauopathies (Alzheimer's Disease [AD] and progressive supranuclear palsy [PSP]), however, have demonstrated that SOD1 expression is not induced in any of these disease settings (Additional file 11; Table S1). The transgene construct used to produce the G85R-SOD1:YFP animals is an engineered fragment of human genomic DNA, which would be expected to be regulated as endogenous SOD1 in humans. Thus, there is little evidence to suspect that the induced misfolding of G85R-SOD1:YFP in the bigenic crosses with JNPL3 mice is due to an induction of the SOD1 transgene expression. The available data suggest that the more likely scenario is that loss of proteostatic function within the spinal axis of the JNPL3/G85R-SOD1:YFP mice led to the induced misfolding and aggregation of the mutant SOD1 reporter.

Our findings in the crosses of G85R-SOD1:YFP mice to JNPL3 mice were in contrast to findings in crosses with mice that develop cortical tau pathology (rTg4510 mice). These findings also contrast to previous observations of what appears to be "secondary induction" of cytoplasmic TDP-43 pathology (a protein that has been pathologically associated with both ALS and FTD) in response to tauopathy in both the JNPL3 and rTg4510 mouse models [35, 57]. In these models, tau pathology usually preceded TDP-43 pathology, suggesting that TDP-43 pathology may largely occur due to the presence of the pathological tau. The lack of G85R-SOD1:YFP inclusion formation in the rTg4510 cross is also remarkable given the fact that SOD1 aggregation is induced by relatively low levels of tau expression in JNPL3 mice (2X endogenous [47]); whereas, the rTg4510 mice produce much higher levels of mutant tau (13X endogenous [49, 50]). Notably, cortical pathology is generally not seen in mice that express mutant SOD1 including the homozygous G85R-SOD1:YFP mice [46]. The expression level of the G85R-SOD1:YFP protein in forebrain is about 2-fold lower than in spinal cord (Additional file 12: Figure S11), which could partially explain the lack of induced mutant SOD1 aggregation in the cross with the rTg4510 mice. However, the rTg4510 mice exhibit profound neurodegenerative changes by 5.5 months of age [50], and it is difficult to accept that the levels of G85R-SOD1:YFP are the sole determinate of whether or not it misfolds and aggregates. Alternatively, it is possible that cortical neurons express unique proteostatic factors that effectively limit the coalescence of misfolded mutant SOD1 into inclusions even in the setting of severe proteostatic distress (see hypothetical model in Additional file 13: Figure S12). Alternatively, there may be differences in the expression levels of one or more proteostatic factors (chaperones, ubiquitin ligases, etc.) between forebrain and spinal cord, such that spinal cord is more vulnerable (Additional file 13: Figure S12). One such factor that has previously been identified by Israelson and colleagues as potentially being responsible for tissue specificity of SOD1 misfolding is macrophage migration inhibitory factor (MIF) [58]. Cells that exhibited MIF localization to the cell bodies were protected from mutant SOD1 aggregation. However, the commercially available antibodies used to study MIF by Israelson in the foregoing study have been discontinued, and antibodies we obtained from other sources did not produce the same staining pattern. Therefore, we were not able to determine the levels or subcellular distribution of MIF in the cortex of the rTg4510 mice might explain our findings. Additionally, it has been shown that spinal motor neurons exhibit a higher threshold for the induction of the protective heat-shock response, specifically regarding a hindered ability in the activation of the transcription factor HSF1 [59]. HSF1 activation leads to the upregulation of the chaperones Hsp70 and Hsp90 which, when induced in mice expressing the G93A mutant SOD1 variant, leads to slower progression of disease [60]. This naturally lower threshold for the heat-shock response could contribute to a higher propensity for mutant SOD1 aggregation in the spinal cord compared to other regions.

Our results from the cross of M83 mice to G85R-SOD1:YFP mice strongly contrasted to the results from the cross with the JNPL3 model. Despite both the JNPL3 and M83 exhibiting robust spinal cord and brainstem pathology, the impact of tau versus αSyn pathology upon our G85R-SOD1:YFP aggregation was dramatically different. This was especially interesting given recent reports suggesting that αSyn and SOD1 interact, leading to increased SOD1 oligomerization [36, 61]. We postulate that our findings reveal the differential effects that tau and αSyn have upon proteostasis and the maintenance of protein folding. More specifically, the proteostatic factors (chaperones, ubiquitin ligases, deubiquitinating enzymes, etc.) that maintain the folding state of tau, αSyn and SOD1 could differ in a manner that leaves mutant SOD1 vulnerable to aggregation in the presence of severe tau pathology, but not in the presence of αSyn pathology (Additional file 13: Figure S12).

Unfortunately, the chaperone subnetworks that are critical in preventing mutant SOD1 aggregation or that are engaged by tau and αSyn pathology remain unclear. Mutant SOD1 has been shown to associate with Hsc70, Hsp70, Hsp27, Hsp25, αB-crystallin and Hsp110 subfamily chaperones [46, 62, 63]. Hsp70 has been shown to bind to the microtubule binding repeats of tau [64], regulating and stabilizing its association with microtubules [65, 66]. Complexes containing the carboxy-terminal Hsp70-interacting protein (CHIP) and either Hsp70 or Hsp90 have been found to promote tau degradation [67–69]. The interactions of tau with small Hsps are slightly less clear; however, Hsp27 has been shown to interact with hyperphosphorylated tau in human AD brain tissue [70]. Hsp70/CHIP have also been found to contribute to αSyn maintenance and combat fibril formation [71–75]. Additionally, the small Hsps (αB-crystallin, Hsp27, Hsp20, HspB8, and HspB2B3) all appear to interact with αSyn (both wild-type and mutant), working to prevent the development of fibrils [76]. Finally, Hsp90 is known to modulate αSyn aggregation, binding to oligomeric species to increase their stability and attenuate toxicity [77, 78]. Deciphering whether there are specific chaperones, or other proteostatic factors, that become engaged in attempting to mitigate misfolded tau in spinal neurons, leaving mutant SOD1 with inadequate access to factors that mitigate its aggregation and will require further study to confirm.

Conclusions

In conclusion, we have used the co-expression of G85R-SOD1:YFP, a protein that is inherently prone to misfolding,

to visualize and investigate "secondary misfolding" in settings of tau and αSyn pathology. The induced aggregation of G85R-SOD1:YFP in the presence of robust spinal tauopathy (as seen in the JNPL3 model) is an outcome consistent with bystander aggregation caused by proteostatic stress. Unexpectedly, the presence of either robust tau pathology in cortical neurons or αSyn pathology in the spinal cord, which in both cases causes severe degenerative changes, did not induce G85R-SOD1:YFP aggregation. One hypothesis that could explain this outcome is that tau and SOD1 have overlapping demands for proteostatic factors that are in limited supply in the spinal axis, such that the presence of the misfolded tau essentially competes for a factor, or factors, that are critical in preventing the aggregation of mutant SOD1 in spinal cord (Additional file 13: Figure S12). Further studies will be required to understand the molecular basis for selective induction of G85R-SOD1:YFP aggregation in these models. That being said, the G85R-SOD1:YFP model has nonetheless proved useful in clearly demonstrating that induced misfolding of one protein by another in neurodegenerative conditions is more complex than simple proteostatic failure. The complexity of bystander misfolding in response to proteinopathies could provide a basis for distinctive clinical symptoms associated with these disorders.

Additional files

Additional file 1: Figure S1. Kaplan-Meier survival curves in JNPL3/G85R-SOD1:YFP mice relative to single transgenic JNPL3 controls. JNPL3 mice expressing the G85R-SOD1:YFP reporter protein ($n = 8$) that exhibited SOD1 inclusion pathology reached an end-stage phenotype significantly faster than JNPL3 transgenic mice ($n = 7$) ($p < 0.05$, Mantel-Cox test). The graphed data originated from six bigenic JNPL3/G85R-SOD1:YFP mice and seven tau-only transgenic JNPL3 mice that were littermate controls. All mice were female. Figure generated using GraphPad Prism (version 7.0 h).

Additional file 2: Figure S2. Low power views of G85R-SOD1:YFP pathology in the spinal cord of bigenic JNPL3-G85R-SOD1:YFP mice (**a**). The box marks the position of the image shown in Fig. 1d of the main text. Low power view of fluorescence in mice expressing G85R-SOD1:YFP alone (**c**). Images shows midsagittal brain section (**b**). Nuclei were stained with DAPI (blue). The left and right arrows are drawn to magnified regions that are shown in the top left and top right of (**b**), respectively. Images shown are representative of 8 JNPL3-G85R-SOD1:YFP mice and 3 G85R-SOD1:YFP mice.

Additional file 3: Figure S3. Primary pathology burden in the JNPL3 spinal cord relative to those crossed to G85R-SOD1:YFP mice. JNPL3 mice (**a**) and those on the G85R-SOD1:YFP background (**b**) were stained with the MC1 antibody (misfolded human tau). Lumbar spinal cord sections are shown. Scale bar; 900 μm.

Additional file 4: Figure S4. Solubility of SOD1 in JNPL3/G85R-SOD1:YFP mice. For these immunoblots, we used a previously described method of detergent extraction and sedimentation (see Methods). To observe aberrant disulfide cross-links that form as mutant SOD1 aggregates, we performed the SDS-PAGE in the absence of reducing agent (**a** and **b**). In JNPL3/G85R-SOD1:YFP mice versus G85R-SOD1:YFP mice, soluble G85R-SOD1:YFP exists predominantly in higher molecular weight states in double transgenic mice versus single transgenic controls (**a**). However, aggregates of G85R-SOD1:YFP were detected in NP40-insoluble fractions only in the bigenic, paralyzed, mice (**b**). 20 µg protein loaded for all samples. Mouse/human SOD1 was detected using an in-house generated antibody. $n = 3$ per genotype.

Additional file 5: Figure S5. Localization of phosphotau immunoreactivity versus G85R-SOD1:YFP pathology in bigenic JNPL3-G85R-SOD1:YFP mice. Hyperphosphorylated human tau pathology recognized by the AT8 (Ser202/Thr205) antibody appears similar in JNPL3 single transgenic versus JNPL3- 85R-SOD1:YFP bigenic mice (**a, b**). G85R-SOD1:YFP pathology, detected by an YFP antibody (**c**), does not robustly co-localize with tau pathology in double transgenic mice (**d**). Nuclei were stained with DAPI (blue). Images are of 60× magnification within the ventral horn of the spinal cord of JNPL3 and JNPL3-G85R-SOD1:YFP mice.

Additional file 6: Figure S6. Primary pathology burden in the rTg4510 transgenic mouse cortex relative to those crossed to the G85R-SOD1:YFP mouse. rTg4510 mice (**a**) compared to trigenic rTg4510/G85R-SOD1:YFP mice (b) after immunostaining with the MC1 antibody (misfolded human tau). Scale bar; 300 µm.

Additional file 7: Figure S7. Quantification of G85R-SOD1:YFP levels between G85R-SOD1:YFP and rTg4510/G85R-SOD1:YFP mice using direct fluorescence and immunoblot densitometric analysis. Quantification of fluorescence intensity reveals a significantly more intense YFP fluorescence in rTg4510/G85R-SOD1:YFP mice (abbreviated rTg4510-SOD1) compared to G85R-SOD1:YFP controls (abbreviated SOD1) ($n = 4$) (**a**). However, immunoblot analysis using an antibody to both mouse and human SOD1 demonstrates no statistical difference between levels of G85R-SOD1:YFP in the two mouse groups (**b, c**) (n = 3 per genotype). Endogenous mouse SOD1 (mSOD1) was used as a loading control, and was detected on the same blot shown. Statistical analysis was conducted using GraphPad Prism (version 7.0 h). Error bars show mean ± S.D.; unpaired, two tailed, T-test revealed a significant difference in fluorescence intensity in forebrain by genotype ($p < 0.01$). n.s.; not significant.

Additional file 8: Figure S8. Primary pathology burden in the M83 transgenic mouse spinal cord relative to M83/G85R-SOD1:YFP mice. M83 only mice (**a**) compared to M83/G85R-SOD1:YFP mice (**b**) after injection with αSyn fibrils to induce αSyn pathology. Sections were stained with the 81A antibody (pSer129 αSyn). Lumbar spinal cord sections are shown. Scale bar; 900 µm.

Additional file 9: Figure S9. Kaplan-Meier survival curves for M83/G85R-SOD1:YFP mice relative to single transgenic M83 controls. All mice were injected intramuscularly with αSyn fibrils to induce pathology. M83 mice expressing the G85R-SOD1:YFP reporter protein that exhibited SOD1 inclusion pathology did not reach an end-stage phenotype significantly faster than M83 transgenic mice. The graphed data originated from 11 bigenic M83/G85R-SOD1:YFP mice (6 female, 5 male) and 15 single transgenic M83 mice (10 male, 5 female) that were littermate controls. Figure generated using GraphPad Prism (version 7.0 h).

Additional file 10: Figure S10. Solubility of αSyn and SOD1 in M83/G85R-SOD1:YFP mice. No changes in soluble versus NP40-insoluble αSyn were observed between M83/G85R-SOD1:YFP versus G85R-SOD1:YFP mice (**a** and **b**). For these immunoblots we used a sequential fractionation protocol that produced a PBS-soluble fraction and an NP40-insoluble fractions (see Methods). Here we controlled sample concentration by resuspending the NP40-insoluble fraction in a volume equivalent to the initial PBS soluble fraction. Equivalent amounts of each fraction were analyzed by SDS-PAGE (30 µL per sample). We used antibodies to GAPDH as a loading control in soluble fractions on the same blot (**a**). Soluble G85R-SOD1:YFP and endogenous mouse SOD1 was detected in both animal groups (**c**), and insoluble G85R-SOD1:YFP was not detected in either group (**d**). αSyn was detected using the 94-3A10 antibody (provided by the laboratory of Benoit Giasson [79]), while mouse/human SOD1 was detected using an in-house generated antibody. $n = 3$ per genotype.

Additional file 11: Table S1. RNAseq expression data for SOD1 in mouse and human tauopathies. Transcriptomic data from studies of the rTg4510 and JNPL3 mouse models, and from studies of humans brain tissues from Alzheimer disease (AD) and progressive supranuclear palsy (PSP) cases available in https://www.synapse.org/#!Synapse:syn2580853/wiki/409840

Additional file 12: Figure S11. G85R-SOD1:YFP expression in spinal cord is 2-fold higher than forebrain in G85R-SOD1:YFP heterozygous mice. Forebrain and spinal cord tissue were extracted and 20 µg of protein was used for immunoblot analysis of SOD1 levels, using an antibody specific for human SOD1 (hSOD1) (**a**). Each lane represents an individual animal (n = 3). Graph represents densitometric quantification of hSOD1 levels normalized to GAPDH (**b**). Statistical analysis was conducted using GraphPad Prism (version 7.0 h) Error bars show mean ± S.D.; unpaired T-test. A.U.; arbitrary units.

Additional file 13: Figure S12. Hypothetical mechanism of differential effects of tauopathy versus synucleinopathy on G85R-SOD1:YFP secondary aggregation in the spinal cord and cortex. In the JNPL3 spinal cord, misfolded tau occupies proteostatic factors (Factor X) that the mutant SOD1 reporter is also dependent upon for folding or degradation. In the cortex of rTg4510 mice, the levels of Factor X could be higher, or other proteostatic factors specific to brain (Factor Y) could be present to prevent the aggregation mutant SOD1. Meanwhile, misfolded αSyn occupies proteostatic factors distinct from those of tau (Factor Z), leaving a sufficient level of Factor X to prevent the aggregation of mutant SOD1.

Abbreviations

AD: Alzheimer's disease; ALS: Amyotrophic lateral sclerosis; CaMKII: Calmodulin kinase II; CHIP: Carboxy-terminal Hsp70-interacting protein; CNS: Central nervous system; FTD: Frontotemporal dementia; G85R-SOD1:YFP: Superoxide dismutase 1 tagged to YFP containing the G85R mutation; GFP: Green fluorescent protein; IACUC: Institutional animal care and use committee; MIF: Macrophage migration inhibitory factor; PD: Parkinson's disease; polyQ: Polyglutamine; TS: Temperature-sensitive; tTA: Tet-transactivator; UPS: Ubiquitin-proteasome system; αSyn: α-synuclein

Acknowledgements

We thank Dr. Qing-Shan Xue and Mr. Matt Collins for help with histological processing of tissues. We thank Doug Smith and the University of Florida Cell and Tissue Analysis Core, supported by an equipment grant from the National Institutes of Health (S10OD020026). We thank Dr. Todd Golde for assistance in accessing RNAseq data on SOD1 expression in mouse models of tauopathy and human tauopathies. We also thank the University of Florida Animal Care Services for help in the care of the animals used in this study.

Funding

This work was supported by a grant from the National Institute of Neurological Disease and Stroke (R21NS083006) to DRB and JL; R01NS089622 to BIG), the National Institute on Aging (P50AG047266 and U01AG046139) and by the SantaFe HealthCare Alzheimer's Disease Research Center.

Authors' contributions

DRB, GX, JL and BIG conceived and coordinated the study; SF and JH assisted in animal maintenance and breeding; BIG provided the M83 mice and αSyn fibrils; MCP and GX performed intramuscular injections of M83 mice, gathered animal tissue and processed it for immunohistochemistry; MCP conducted fluorescent immunohistochemistry and analyzed the data; MCP, GX, and DRB drafted the images for publication; MCP, GX, and DRB wrote the manuscript. All authors read and approved the final manuscript.

Competing interests

The authors declare that they have no competing interests.

Author details

[1]Department of Neuroscience, Center for Translational Research in Neurodegenerative Disease, McKnight Brain Institute, University of Florida, 1275 Center Drive, BMS Building J-491, PO Box, Gainesville, FL 32610-0244, USA. [2]SantaFe Healthcare Alzheimer's Disease Center, Gainesville, FL, USA.

References

1. Carrell RW, Lomas DA. Conformational disease. Lancet. 1997;350:134–8.
2. Dobson CM. Protein misfolding, evolution and disease. Trends Biochem Sci. 1999;24:329–32.
3. Soto C. Unfolding the role of protein misfolding in neurodegenerative diseases. Nat Rev Neurosci. 2003;4:49–60. Available from: http://www.ncbi.nlm.nih.gov/entrez/query.fcgi?cmd=Retrieve&db=PubMed&dopt=Citation&list_uids=12511861.
4. Spillantini MG, Goedert M, Crowther RA, Murrell JR, Farlow MR, Ghetti B. Familial multiple system tauopathy with presenile dementia: a disease with abundant neuronal and glial tau filaments. Proc Natl Acad Sci U S A. [Internet]. 1997;94:4113–8. Available from: http://www.pubmedcentral.nih.gov/articlerender.fcgi?artid=20577&tool=pmcentrez&rendertype=abstract.
5. Bossy-Wetzel E, Schwarzenbacher R, Lipton SA. Molecular pathways to neurodegeneration. Nat Med. 2004;10 Suppl:S2–9.
6. Keller JN, Hanni KB, Markesbery WR. Impaired proteasome function in Alzheimer's disease. J Neurochem. 2000;75:436–9.
7. McKinnon C, Tabrizi SJ. The ubiquitin-proteasome system in neurodegeneration. Antioxid Redox Signal. 2014;21:2302–21. Available from: http://www.ncbi.nlm.nih.gov/pubmed/24437518.
8. Wong E, Cuervo AM. Autophagy gone awry in neurodegenerative diseases. Nat Neurosci. 2010 [cited 2016 May 2];13:805–811. Available from: https://www.ncbi.nlm.nih.gov/pubmed/20581817.
9. Myeku N, Clelland CL, Emrani S, Kukushkin NV, Yu WH, Goldberg AL, et al. Tau-driven 26S proteasome impairment and cognitive dysfunction can be prevented early in disease by activating cAMP-PKA signaling. Nat Med. 2015;6:1–11. Available from: https://www.ncbi.nlm.nih.gov/pmc/articles/PMC4787271/.
10. Emmanouilidou E, Stefanis L, Vekrellis K. Cell-produced α-synuclein oligomers are targeted to, and impair, the 26S proteasome. Neurobiol Aging. 2010;31:953–68. Elsevier Inc., Available from: https://doi.org/10.1016/j.neurobiolaging.2008.07.008.
11. Dyllick-Brenzinger M, D'Souza CA, Dahlmann B, Kloetzel P-M, Tandon A. Reciprocal effects of α-Synuclein overexpression and proteasome inhibition in neuronal cells and tissue. Neurotox Res. 2010;17:215–27. Available from: http://link.springer.com/10.1007/s12640-009-9094-1.
12. Deger JM, Gerson JE, Kayed R. The interrelationship of proteasome impairment and oligomeric intermediates in neurodegeneration. Aging Cell. 2015;14:715–24.
13. Keck S, Nitsch R, Grune T, Ullrich O. Proteasome inhibition by paired helical filament-tau in brains of patients with Alzheimer's disease. J Neurochem. 2003;85:115–22.
14. Han DH, Na H-K, Choi WH, Lee JH, Kim YK, Won C, et al. Direct cellular delivery of human proteasomes to delay tau aggregation. Nat Commun. 2014;5:5633. Nature Publishing Group; Available from: http://www.nature.com/articles/ncomms6633.
15. Tai HC, Serrano-Pozo A, Hashimoto T, Frosch MP, Spires-Jones TL, Hyman BT. The synaptic accumulation of hyperphosphorylated tau oligomers in alzheimer disease is associated with dysfunction of the ubiquitin-proteasome system. Am J Pathol. 2012 [cited 2017 Mar 10];181:1426–1435. Available from: https://ajp.amjpathol.org/article/S0002-9440(12)00514-7/fulltext.
16. Metcalfe MJ, Huang Q, Figueiredo-Pereira ME. Coordination between proteasome impairment and caspase activation leading to TAU pathology: neuroprotection by cAMP. Cell Death Dis. 2012;3:e326. Nature Publishing Group, Available from: http://www.nature.com/articles/cddis201270.
17. Alves-Rodrigues A, Gregori L, Figueiredo-Pereira ME. Ubiquitin, cellular inclusions and their role in neurodegeneration. Trends Neurosci. 1998:516–20.
18. Neumann M, Sampathu DM, Kwong LK, Truax AC, Micsenyi MC, Chou TT, et al. Ubiquitinated TDP-43 in frontotemporal lobar degeneration and amyotrophic lateral sclerosis. Science (80-.). 2006;314:130–3. Available from: http://www.sciencemag.org/cgi/doi/10.1126/science.1134108

19. Shimura H, Schwartz D, Gygi SP, Kosik KS. CHIP-Hsc70 complex Ubiquitinates phosphorylated tau and enhances cell survival. J Biol Chem. 2004;279:4869–76.
20. Sherman MY, Goldberg AL. Cellular defenses against unfolded proteins: a cell biologist thinks about neurodegenerative diseases. Neuron. 2001;29:15–32.
21. Hipp MS, Park SH, Hartl UU. Proteostasis impairment in protein-misfolding and -aggregation diseases. Trends cell biol. 2014;24:506–14. Elsevier Ltd,Available from: https://doi.org/10.1016/j.tcb.2014.05.003.
22. Balch WE, Morimoto RI, Dillin A, Kelly JW. Adapting Proteostasis for disease intervention. Science (80-.). 2008;319:916–9.
23. Powers ET, Balch WE. Diversity in the origins of proteostasis networks-a driver for protein function in evolution. Nat Rev Mol Cell Biol. 2013 [cited 2018 Jan 2]. p. 237–248. Available from: https://www.nature.com/articles/nrm3542.pdf.
24. Haslbeck M, Franzmann T, Weinfurtner D, Buchner J. Some like it hot: the structure and function of small heat-shock proteins. Nat Struct Mol Biol. 2005;12:842–6.
25. Dantuma NP, Bott LC. The ubiquitin-proteasome system in neurodegenerative diseases: precipitating factor, yet part of the solution. Front Mol Neurosci. 2014;7:70. Available from: https://www.frontiersin.org/articles/10.3389/fnmol.2014.00070/full
26. Elsasser S, Finley D. Delivery of ubiquitinated substrates to protein-unfolding machines. Nat Cell Biol. 2005;7:742–9.
27. Kundu M, Thompson CB. Autophagy: basic principles and relevance to disease. Annu Rev Pathol. 2008 [cited 2016 May 2];3:427–455. Available from: https://www.annualreviews.org/doi/10.1146/annurev.pathmechdis.2.010506.091842.
28. Gidalevitz T, Ben-Zvi A, Ho KH, Brignull HR, Morimoto RI. Progressive disruption of cellular protein folding in models of polyglutamine diseases. Science (80-.). 2006 [cited 2016 May 4];311:1471–1474. Available from: http://science.sciencemag.org/content/311/5766/1471.
29. Gidalevitz T, Krupinski T, Garcia S, Morimoto RI. Destabilizing protein polymorphisms in the genetic background direct phenotypic expression of mutant SOD1 toxicity. PLoS Genet. 2009;5
30. Colom-Cadena M, Gelpi E, Charif S, Belbin O, Blesa R, Marti MJ, et al. Confluence of alpha-synuclein, tau, and beta-amyloid pathologies in dementia with Lewy bodies. J Neuropathol Exp Neurol. 2013;72:1203–12.
31. Higashi S, Iseki E, Yamamoto R, Minegishi M, Hino H, Fujisawa K, et al. Concurrence of TDP-43, tau and alpha-synuclein pathology in brains of Alzheimer's disease and dementia with Lewy bodies. Brain Res. 2007 [cited 2016 Jun 16];1184:284–294. Available from: http://www.sciencedirect.com/science/article/pii/S000689930702224X.
32. Spires-Jones TL, Attems J, Thal DR. Interactions of pathological proteins in neurodegenerative diseases. Acta Neuropathol. Springer Berlin Heidelberg. 2017:1–19.
33. Walker L, Kirsty Mcaleese E, Thomas AJ, Johnson M, Martin-ruiz C, et al. Neuropathologically mixed Alzheimer's and Lewy body disease: burden of pathological protein aggregates differs between clinical phenotypes. Acta Neuropathol. 2015 [cited 2017 Jun 27];129:729–748. Available from: https://link.springer.com/content/pdf/10.1007%2Fs00401-015-1406-3.pdf.
34. James BD, Wilson RS, Boyle PA, Trojanowski JQ, Bennett DA, Schneider JA. TDP-43 stage, mixed pathologies, and clinical Alzheimer's-type dementia. Brain. 2016 [cited 2017 Jun 27];139:2983–2993. Available from: https://academic.oup.com/brain/article/139/11/2983/2422129.
35. Clippinger AK, D'Alton S, Lin WL, Gendron TF, Howard J, Borchelt DR, et al. Robust cytoplasmic accumulation of phosphorylated TDP-43 in transgenic models of tauopathy. Acta Neuropathol. 2013;126:39–50.
36. Helferich AM, Ruf WP, Grozdanov V, Freischmidt A, Feiler MS, Zondler L, et al. α-synuclein interacts with SOD1 and promotes its oligomerization. Mol Neurodegener. 2015;10:66. Available from: http://www.molecularneurodegeneration.com/content/10/1/66.
37. Giasson BI, Forman MS, Higuchi M, Golbe LI, Graves CL, Kotzbauer PT, et al. Initiation and synergistic fibrillization of tau and alpha-Synuclein. Science (80-.). 2003;300:636–40. Available from: http://www.sciencemag.org/cgi/doi/10.1126/science.1082324.
38. Guo JL, Covell DJ, Daniels JP, Iba M, Stieber A, Zhang B, et al. Distinct α-Synuclein Strains Differentially Promote Tau Inclusions in Neurons. 2013 [cited 2017 Jun 27]; Available from: https://doi.org/10.1016/j.cell.2013.05.057.

39. Morales R, Moreno-Gonzalez I, Soto C. Cross-seeding of misfolded proteins: implications for etiology and pathogenesis of protein Misfolding diseases. PLoS Pathog. 2013;9:1–4.

40. Guerrero-Muñoz MJ, Castillo-Carranza DL, Krishnamurthy S, Paulucci-Holthauzen AA, Sengupta U, Lasagna-Reeves CA, et al. Amyloid-β oligomers as a template for secondary amyloidosis in Alzheimer's disease. 2014 [cited 2017 Jun 27]; Available from: https://www.sciencedirect.com/science/article/pii/S0969996114002393?via%3Dihub.

41. Vasconcelos B, Stancu IC, Buist A, Bird M, Wang P, Vanoosthuyse A, et al. Heterotypic seeding of tau fibrillization by pre-aggregated Abeta provides potent seeds for prion-like seeding and propagation of tau-pathology in vivo. Acta Neuropathol. Springer Berlin Heidelberg. 2016;131:549–69.

42. Scherzinger E, Sittler A, Schweiger K, Heiser V, Lurz R, Hasenbank R, et al. Self-assembly of polyglutamine-containing huntingtin fragments into amyloid-like fibrils: implications for Huntington's disease pathology. Proc Natl Acad Sci U S A. 1999 [cited 2016 May 6];96:4604–4609. Available from: https://www.ncbi.nlm.nih.gov/pmc/articles/PMC16379/.

43. Ayers JI, Fromholt S, Koch M, DeBosier A, McMahon B, Xu G, et al. Experimental transmissibility of mutant SOD1 motor neuron disease. Acta Neuropathol. 2014;128:791–803.

44. Ayers JI, Fromholt SE, O'Neal VM, Diamond JH, Borchelt DR. Prion-like propagation of mutant SOD1 misfolding and motor neuron disease spread along neuroanatomical pathways. Acta Neuropathol. 2016;131:103–14.

45. Ayers JI, Diamond J, Sari A, Fromholt S, Galaleldeen A, Ostrow LW, et al. Distinct conformers of transmissible misfolded SOD1 distinguish human SOD1-FALS from other forms of familial and sporadic ALS. Acta Neuropathol. Springer Berlin Heidelberg. 2016;132:827–40.

46. Wang J, Farr GW, Zeiss CJ, Rodriguez-Gil DJ, Wilson JH, Furtak K, et al. Progressive aggregation despite chaperone associations of a mutant SOD1-YFP in transgenic mice that develop ALS. Proc Natl Acad Sci U S A. 2009 [cited 2016 May 2];106:1392–1397. Available from: https://www.ncbi.nlm.nih.gov/pmc/articles/PMC2631083/.

47. Lewis J, McGowan E, Rockwood J, Melrose H, Nacharaju P, Van Slegtenhorst M, et al. Neurofibrillary tangles, amyotrophy and progressive motor disturbance in mice expressing mutant (P301L) tau protein. Nat Genet. 2000 [cited 2016 May 2];25:402–405. Available from: http://www.nature.com/articles/ng0800_402.

48. Giasson BI, Duda JE, Quinn SM, Zhang B, Trojanowski JQ, Lee VMY. Neuronal α-synucleinopathy with severe movement disorder in mice expressing A53T human α-synuclein. Neuron. 2002;34:521–33.

49. Ramsden M, Kotilinek L, Forster C, Paulson J, McGowan E, SantaCruz K, et al. Age-dependent neurofibrillary tangle formation, neuron loss, and memory impairment in a mouse model of human tauopathy (P301L). J Neurosci. 2005 [cited 2016 May 2];25:10637–10647. Available from: http://www.jneurosci.org/content/25/46/10637.

50. SantaCruz K, Lewis J, Spires-Jones TL, Paulson J, Kotilinek L, Ingelsson M, et al. Tau suppression in a neurodegenerative mouse model improves memory function. Science (80-). 2005;309:476–81. Available from: http://www.sciencemag.org/cgi/doi/10.1126/science.1113694.

51. Sacino AN, Brooks M, Thomas MA, McKinney AB, Lee S, Regenhardt RW, et al. Intramuscular injection of α-synuclein induces CNS α-synuclein pathology and a rapid-onset motor phenotype in transgenic mice. Proc Natl Acad Sci U S A. 2014 [cited 2016 May 27];111:1–6. Available from: https://www.ncbi.nlm.nih.gov/pmc/articles/PMC4115570/.

52. Wang J, Slunt H, Gonzales V, Fromholt D, Coonfield M, Copeland NG, et al. Copper-binding-site-null SOD1 causes ALS in transgenic mice: aggregates of non-native SOD1 delineate a common feature. Hum Mol Genet. 2003 [cited 2016 May 2];12:2753–2764. Available from: https://academic.oup.com/hmg/article/12/21/2753/558413.

53. Karch CM, Prudencio M, Winkler DD, Hart PJ, Borchelt DR. Role of mutant SOD1 disulfide oxidation and aggregation in the pathogenesis of familial ALS. Proc Natl Acad Sci U S A. 2009;106:7774–9. Available from: https://www.ncbi.nlm.nih.gov/pmc/articles/PMC2675570/.

54. Xu G, Stevens SM, Moore BD, McClung S, Borchelt DR. Cytosolic proteins lose solubility as amyloid deposits in a transgenic mouse model of alzheimer-type amyloidosis. Hum Mol Genet. 2013;22:2765–74.

55. Bruijn LI, Becher MW, Lee MK, Anderson KL, Jenkins NA, Copeland NG, et al. ALS-linked SOD1 mutant G85R mediates damage to astrocytes and promotes rapidly progressive disease with SOD1-containing inclusions. Neuron. 1997;18:327–38.

56. Lewis J, Dickson DW, Lin WL, Chisholm L, Corral A, Jones G, et al. Enhanced neurofibrillary degeneration in transgenic mice expressing mutant tau and

APP. Science. 2001 [cited 2016 Jun 8];293:1487–1491. Available from: http://science.sciencemag.org/content/293/5534/1487.

57. Arai T, Hasegawa M, Akiyama H, Ikeda K, Nonaka T, Mori H, et al. TDP-43 is a component of ubiquitin-positive tau-negative inclusions in frontotemporal lobar degeneration and amyotrophic lateral sclerosis. Biochem Biophys Res Commun. 2006;351:602–11.

58. Israelson A, Ditsworth D, Sun S, Song SW, Liang J, Hruska-Plochan M, et al. Macrophage migration inhibitory factor as a chaperone inhibiting accumulation of misfolded SOD1. Neuron. 2015;86:218–32. Elsevier Inc,Available from: https://doi.org/10.1016/j.neuron.2015.02.034

59. Batulan Z, Shinder GA, Minotti S, He BP, Doroudchi MM, Nalbantoglu J, et al. High threshold for induction of the stress response in motor neurons is associated with failure to activate HSF1. J Neurosci. 2003;23: 5789–98.

60. Kieran D, Kalmar B, Dick JRT, Riddoch-Contreras J, Burnstock G, Greensmith L. Treatment with arimoclomol, a coinducer of heat shock proteins, delays disease progression in ALS mice. Nat Med. 2004;10:402–5.

61. Koch Y, Helferich AM, Steinacker P, Oeckl P, Walther P, Weishaupt JH, et al. Aggregated α-Synuclein increases SOD1 oligomerization in a mouse model of amyotrophic lateral sclerosis. Am J Pathol. 2016 [cited 2017 Jun 27];186: 2152–2161. Available from: http://ajp.amjpathol.org/article/S0002-9440(16)30120-1/pdf.

62. Parakh S, Atkin JD. Protein folding alterations in amyotrophic lateral sclerosis. Brain res. 2016;1648:633–49. Elsevier, Available from: https://doi.org/10.1016/j.brainres.2016.04.010.

63. Nagy M, Fenton WA, Li D, Furtak K, Horwich AL. Extended survival of misfolded G85R SOD1-linked ALS mice by transgenic expression of chaperone Hsp110. Proc Natl Acad Sci. 2016;113:1–5.

64. Sarkar M, Kuret J, Lee G. Two motifs within the tau microtubule-binding domain mediate its association with the hsc70 molecular chaperone. J Neurosci Res. 2008;86:2763–73.

65. Jinwal UK, O'Leary JC, Borysov SI, Jones JR, Li Q, Koren J, et al. Hsc70 rapidly engages tau after microtubule destabilization. J Biol Chem. 2010;285:16798–805.

66. Dou F, Netzer WJ, Tanemura K, Li F, Hartl FU, Takashima A, et al. Chaperones increase association of tau protein with microtubules. Proc Natl Acad Sci U S A. 2003 [cited 2016 Jul 2];100:721–726. Available from: https://www.ncbi.nlm.nih.gov/pmc/articles/PMC141063/.

67. Petrucelli L, Dickson D, Kehoe K, Taylor J, Snyder H, Grover A, et al. CHIP and Hsp70 regulate tau ubiquitination, degradation and aggregation. Hum Mol Genet. 2004;13:703–14.

68. Dickey CA, Kamal A, Lundgren K, Klosak N, Bailey RM, Dunmore J, et al. The high-affinity HSP90-CHIP complex recognizes and selectively degrades phosphorylated tau client proteins. J Clin Invest. 2007;117:648–58.

69. Karagö GE, Duarte AMS, Akoury E, Ippel H, Biernat J, Moran Luengo T, et al. Hsp90-tau complex reveals molecular basis for specificity in chaperone action. Cell. 2014 [cited 2016 Sep 2];156:963–974. Available from: https://doi.org/10.1016/j.cell.2014.01.037.

70. Shimura H, Miura-Shimura Y, Kosik KS. Binding of tau to heat shock protein 27 leads to decreased concentration of Hyperphosphorylated tau and enhanced cell survival. J Biol Chem. 2004 [cited 2017 Jun 28];279:17957–17962. Available from: http://www.jbc.org/content/279/17/17957.full.pdf.

71. Huang C, Cheng H, Hao S, Zhou H, Zhang X, Gao J, et al. Heat Shock Protein 70 Inhibits α-Synuclein Fibril Formation via Interactions with Diverse Intermediates. [cited 2017 Jun 27]; Available from: https://www.sciencedirect.com/science/article/pii/S0022283606011156?via%3Dihub.

72. Auluck PK, Edwin Chan HY, Trojanowski JQ, Lee VM-Y, Bonini NM. Chaperone suppression of α-Synuclein toxicity in a Drosophila model for Parkinson's disease. Science (80-.). 2002;295:865–8. Available from: http://www.sciencemag.org/cgi/doi/10.1126/science.1067389.

73. Luk KC, Mills IP, Trojanowski JQ, Lee VMY. Interactions between Hsp70 and the hydrophobic Core of α-Synuclein inhibit fibril assembly. Biochemistry. 2008;47:12614–25. Available from: https://www.ncbi.nlm.nih.gov/pmc/articles/PMC2648307/.

74. Ebrahimi-Fakhari D, Saidi L-J, Wahlster L. Molecular chaperones and protein folding as therapeutic targets in Parkinson's disease and other synucleinopathies. Acta Neuropathol Commun. 2013:1–79. Available from: http://actaneurocomms.biomedcentral.com/articles/10.1186/2051-5960-1-79.

75. Shin Y, Klucken J, Patterson C, Hyman BT, McLean PJ. The co-chaperone carboxyl terminus of Hsp70-interacting protein (CHIP) mediates α-synuclein degradation decisions between proteasomal and lysosomal pathways. J Biol Chem. 2005;280:23727–34.

76. Bruinsma IB, Bruggink KA, Kinast K, Versleijen AAM, Segers-Nolten IMJ, Subramaniam V, et al. Inhibition of α-synuclein aggregation by small heat shock proteins. Proteins Struct Funct Bioinf. 2011;79:2956–67.

77. Daturpalli S, Waudby CA, Meehan S, Jackson SE. Hsp90 inhibits α-synuclein aggregation by interacting with soluble oligomers. J Mol Biol. 2013;425:4614–28. Elsevier B.V., Available from: https://doi.org/10.1016/j.jmb.2013.08.006.

78. Falsone SF, Kungl AJ, Rek A, Cappai R, Zangger K. The molecular chaperone Hsp90 modulates intermediate steps of amyloid assembly of the Parkinson-related protein α-synuclein. J Biol Chem. 2009 [cited 2017 Jun 27];284:31190–31199. Available from: http://www.jbc.org/content/284/45/31190.full.pdf.

79. Dhillon JKS, Riffe C, Moore BD, Ran Y, Chakrabarty P, Golde TE, et al. A novel panel of α-synuclein antibodies reveal distinctive staining profiles in synucleinopathies. PLoS One. 2017 [cited 2018 Apr 13];12. Available from: https://www.ncbi.nlm.nih.gov/pmc/articles/PMC5599040/.

2

PU.1 regulates Alzheimer's disease-associated genes in primary human microglia

Justin Rustenhoven[1,2†], Amy M. Smith[3†], Leon C. Smyth[1,2], Deidre Jansson[1,2], Emma L. Scotter[1,2], Molly E. V. Swanson[1,4], Miranda Aalderink[1,2], Natacha Coppieters[1,4], Pritika Narayan[2,5], Renee Handley[2,5], Chris Overall[6,7], Thomas I. H. Park[1,2,4], Patrick Schweder[8], Peter Heppner[8], Maurice A. Curtis[1,4], Richard L. M. Faull[1,4] and Mike Dragunow[1,2*] ⓘD

Abstract

Background: Microglia play critical roles in the brain during homeostasis and pathological conditions. Understanding the molecular events underpinning microglial functions and activation states will further enable us to target these cells for the treatment of neurological disorders. The transcription factor PU.1 is critical in the development of myeloid cells and a major regulator of microglial gene expression. In the brain, PU.1 is specifically expressed in microglia and recent evidence from genome-wide association studies suggests that reductions in PU.1 contribute to a delayed onset of Alzheimer's disease (AD), possibly through limiting neuroinflammatory responses.

Methods: To investigate how PU.1 contributes to immune activation in human microglia, microarray analysis was performed on primary human mixed glial cultures subjected to siRNA-mediated knockdown of PU.1. Microarray hits were confirmed by qRT-PCR and immunocytochemistry in both mixed glial cultures and isolated microglia following PU.1 knockdown. To identify attenuators of PU.1 expression in microglia, high throughput drug screening was undertaken using a compound library containing FDA-approved drugs. NanoString and immunohistochemistry was utilised to investigate the expression of PU.1 itself and PU.1-regulated mediators in primary human brain tissue derived from neurologically normal and clinically and pathologically confirmed cases of AD.

Results: Bioinformatic analysis of gene expression upon PU.1 silencing in mixed glial cultures revealed a network of modified AD-associated microglial genes involved in the innate and adaptive immune systems, particularly those involved in antigen presentation and phagocytosis. These gene changes were confirmed using isolated microglial cultures. Utilising high throughput screening of FDA-approved compounds in mixed glial cultures we identified the histone deacetylase inhibitor vorinostat as an effective attenuator of PU.1 expression in human microglia. Further characterisation of vorinostat in isolated microglial cultures revealed gene and protein changes partially recapitulating those seen following siRNA-mediated PU.1 knockdown. Lastly, we demonstrate that several of these PU.1-regulated genes are expressed by microglia in the human AD brain in situ.

Conclusions: Collectively, these results suggest that attenuating PU.1 may be a valid therapeutic approach to limit microglial-mediated inflammatory responses in AD and demonstrate utility of vorinostat for this purpose.

Keywords: Alzheimer's disease, Vorinostat, Phagocytosis, Antigen presentation, Drug screening, Neuroinflammation

* Correspondence: m.dragunow@auckland.ac.nz
†Justin Rustenhoven and Amy M. Smith contributed equally to this work.
[1]Department of Pharmacology and Clinical Pharmacology, The University of Auckland, Private Bag 92019, Auckland 1142, New Zealand
[2]Centre for Brain Research, The University of Auckland, Auckland, New Zealand
Full list of author information is available at the end of the article

Background

Microglia are the resident macrophages in the central nervous system (CNS) and primary mediators of neuro-inflammation. Whilst they are beneficial in pruning unnecessary synapses during development [1] and removing pathogens and cellular debris [2], microglia can also contribute to neurological dysfunction [3]. Elevated microglial-mediated neuroinflammatory responses can perturb neuronal functioning or induce neuronal death [4], and unrestricted phagocytosis of stressed-but-viable cells can lead to inappropriate removal of neurons via phagoptosis [5]. Numerous stimuli can promote microglial inflammatory responses, including microorganism recognition, peripheral inflammation, CNS damage, as well as recognition of misfolded proteins, including amyloid-beta (Aβ) plaques present in Alzheimer's disease (AD) [3, 6].

AD is a progressive neurodegenerative disorder characterized symptomatically by gradual memory impairment and other cognitive deficits [7]. Pathologically, the AD brain displays extensive extracellular deposition of parenchymal Aβ plaques and intracellular neurofibrillary tangles composed of hyperphosphorylated tau [8]. It is well recognized that elevated microglia inflammatory responses precipitated by these misfolded proteins contribute to disease progression [9]. Importantly, microglial inflammatory responses are not unique to AD but are present, and indeed detrimental, in other neurodegenerative disorders (Parkinson's disease [10], Huntington's disease [11], amyotrophic lateral sclerosis [12], and multiple sclerosis [13]), epilepsy, neuropsychiatric disorders (depression [14] and autism [15]), and acute brain injuries (stroke [16] and traumatic brain injuries [17]), making microglia an attractive therapeutic target.

Whilst the exact cause of AD remains elusive, there is a significant genetic component. Approximately 1–6% of all cases are classed as early-onset AD, typically with mutations in amyloid-processing genes (APP, PSEN1 and PSEN2) [18], whilst genome wide-association studies (GWAS) have identified numerous risk variant genes associated with late onset Alzheimer's disease (AD) [19–28]. Interestingly, several of these genes, including TREM2, CD33, ABCA7, HLA-DRB5, and MS4A4, are highly expressed by myeloid cells and are involved in innate and adaptive immune mechanisms [29–31]. These findings have helped shape our understanding of the neuroinflammatory component of this disease. Recently, a genome-wide survival analysis identified a common haplotype, rs1057233[g], in the CELF1 AD risk locus which displayed reduced expression of PU.1 in monocytes and macrophages and delayed age of onset of AD [32]. The transcription factor PU.1 (SPI1) is a master regulator of myeloid cells and controls microglial development and function [33, 34]. In the CNS its expression is limited to microglia and PU.1 knockdown or overexpression in the BV2 rodent microglia cell line identified a hub of differentially expressed genes relating to neuroimmune responses [32]. Additionally, mutant Huntingtin aggregates present in Huntington's disease enhance microglial activation through PU.1 [35], as do hypoxic-ischaemic insults [36], suggesting that PU.1 modulation may be a common feature underlying distinct neurological disorders. Further, overexpression of the CNS-enriched miRNA124 [37] attenuates macrophage inflammatory responses through reduced C/EBPα and PU.1 signalling [38], as well as preventing CNS inflammation and associated epileptogenesis [39]. As such, attenuation of PU.1 may be a valid therapeutic strategy to limit microglia-mediated neuroinflammation in various neurological disorders.

Whilst there is overwhelming evidence implicating microglial gene variants in modifying AD risk [31], exactly how these variants contribute to human disease is uncertain. Current studies concerning PU.1 have been performed solely using in vitro/in vivo rodent models or in vitro human macrophages and whether these findings translate to primary human microglia remains unclear. Human microglia display significant species differences from their more frequently used rodent counterparts [40, 41] and several of the highly differentially expressed genes are risk factors for neurodegenerative diseases, particularly AD [30]. Additionally, RNAseq analysis of isolated microglia and macrophages in mice revealed a distinct gene signature in microglia with differential expression of innate immune system genes [42], whilst macrophages and microglia also differ in their inflammatory profile in acute ischaemia [43]. Additionally, treatment with the histone deacetylase (HDAC) inhibitor valproic acid (VPA) prevented phagocytosis of Aβ$_{1-42}$ by human microglia [66], whilst the reverse was true for the rodent microglial BV2 cell line [44], further necessitating caution when identifying pharmacological agents to modify microglial functions in human disease [40, 45]. Together, such findings suggest caution when extrapolating information obtained from non-human microglia.

Previously, we have demonstrated human microglial expression of PU.1, both in vitro and in situ, and its attenuation was found to prevent microglial phagocytosis of Aβ$_{1-42}$ [33]. Here we sought mechanistic insights into the role of PU.1 in regulating immune functions in primary human microglia. We identified changes in innate and adaptive immune pathways, particularly genes involved in antigen presentation and phagocytosis, and confirmed these changes in isolated microglial cultures. Utilising high throughput screening of 1280 FDA approved compounds in primary human brain mixed glial cultures, we identified the HDAC inhibitor vorinostat as a candidate drug for attenuating PU.1 expression in human microglia and mimicking several of the effects of PU.1 silencing. Finally, we demonstrate that several of these PU.1-regulated genes are expressed and upregulated by microglia in the human

AD brain and suggest that modulating PU.1 expression may be a valid therapeutic target to prevent microglial-mediated neurodegeneration.

Methods

Tissue source

For primary human cell culture and subsequent in vitro studies, human brain tissue was obtained, with informed written patient consent, from various sources of neuro-surgical tissue (Additional file 1: Table S1). For imummuno-histochemical studies, middle temporal gyrus (MTG) from post mortem adult human brain tissue of neurologically normal or clinically and pathologically confirmed cases of AD (Additional file 1: Table S1) was obtained from the Neurological Foundation Douglas Human Brain Bank, processed as described previously [46]. All protocols used in this study were approved by the Northern Regional Ethics Committee (New Zealand) for biopsy tissue and the University of Auckland Human Participants Ethics Committee (New Zealand) for post mortem tissue. All donors underwent a full consent process. All methods were carried out in accordance with the approved guidelines.

Cell isolation and culture

Mixed glial cultures containing astrocytes, pericytes, endothelial cells, and microglia were isolated from human brain tissue as described previously [47] and used at passage two. Isolated pericyte cultures were generated from these initial mixed glial cultures by subsequent passaging in order to dilute out non-proliferating microglia, astrocytes, and endothelial cells as described previously [48]. Isolated microglial cultures were generated as described previously [49]. Cells were harvested using 0.25% trypsin-1 mM EDTA (Gibco, CA, USA) with mixed glial cultures and microglia cultures also utilising gentle detachment with a cell scraper (Falcon, MA, USA) due to strong microglial attachment. Viability was determined by trypan blue exclusion (Gibco). Mixed glial and pericyte cultures were plated at 15,000 cells/cm^2 and isolated microglia were plated at 30,000 cells/cm^2 in Nunc™ microwell plates with Nunclon™ Delta surface (Nunc, Denmark). All cultures were maintained in DMEM/F12 (Gibco), 10% fetal bovine serum (FBS; Moregate, Australia) and 1% penicillin streptomycin glutamine (PSG; Gibco).

siRNA transfection

Cells were transfected with 50 nM PU.1 (*SPI1*) specific siRNA (SASI_Hs02_00315880; Sigma Aldrich, MO, USA) or a non-targeting siRNA sequence (Universal Negative Control #1) using Lipofectamine™ RNAiMAX (Life Technologies, CA, USA). Cells were cultured for a further 7 days to allow for PU.1 knockdown with a full media change performed 48 h post-transfection. This procedure

has previously been shown to generate efficient reduction of PU.1 expression in human brain microglia [33].

Immunocytochemistry and fluorescent microscopy

Cells were fixed for 15 min using 4% paraformaldehyde (Scharlau, Spain) and washed three times in phosphate buffered saline (PBS) with 0.1% Triton™ X-100 (PBS-T; Sigma Aldrich). Cells were incubated with primary antibodies (Additional file 2: Table S2) diluted in goat immuno-buffer (1% goat serum (Gibco), 0.2% triton X-100 and 0.04% thiomersal (Sigma Aldrich) in PBS) at 4 °C overnight, washed three times in PBS-T and incubated with appropriate anti-species fluorescently conjugated secondary antibodies diluted in goat immunobuffer at 4 °C overnight. Cells were washed again in PBS-T and nuclei were counterstained with 20 nM Hoechst 33258 (Sigma Aldrich) for 20 min at room temperature. Images were acquired at 20 x magnification using the ImageXpress® Micro XLS automated fluorescent microscope (Version 5.3.0.1, Molecular Devices, CA, USA). Quantitative analysis of intensity measures and scoring of positively stained cells was performed using the Cell Scoring and Show Region Statistics analysis modules within MetaXpress® software (Molecular Devices). For analysis of microglial morphology by immunocyto-chemistry (ICC), CD45 staining was thresholded and the Integrated Morphometry Analysis tools Elliptical Form Factor (elongation factor; length/breadth) and Shape Factor (roundness factor; $4\pi A/P^2$, P = cell perimeter, A = cell area) were used to determine cell shape.

Cytometric bead array

Conditioned media was collected from cells in 96-well plates, centrifuged for 5 min at 300 x g and the clarified supernatant was stored at − 20 °C. Cytokine concentrations were determined using a multiplexed cytometric bead array (CBA; BD Biosciences, CA, USA) as per the manufacturer's instructions. Data was analysed using FCAP array™ software (version 3.1; BD Biosciences) to convert raw fluorescent values into concentrations using an 11-point standard curve (0–10,000 pg/mL).

High throughput drug screening

High throughput screening to identify compounds which modify PU.1 expression was performed using a Chemical Library (Prestwick Chemical, France) containing 1280 small molecules consisting of mostly FDA approved drugs. Compounds were screened at 10 μM for 48 h in mixed glial cultures before fixing and immunostaining for PU.1 and counterstaining with Hoechst 33258. Cells were imaged using the ImageXpress® Micro XLS automated fluorescent microscope and the percentage of PU.1-positive cells and total Hoechst-positive cells was quantified, allowing alterations in PU.1 expression as well as total cell viability to be assessed. The histone deacetylase (HDAC) inhibitor vorinostat (also known as SAHA) was identified by this screen as an attenuator of PU.1 expression. Validation in two further mixed glial cultures confirmed this effect.

Vorinostat treatment

For subsequent experiments cells were treated with 10 μM vorinostat (Sigma Aldrich) or a vehicle control (0.1% DMSO; Sigma Aldrich) for 24 h.

RNA extraction and cDNA synthesis

For mixed glial and pericyte cultures, RNA was extracted using a TRIzol™(Invitrogen)/chloroform procedure followed by isolation using the RNeasy Mini Kit (Qiagen, Netherlands) as described previously [50]. For isolated microglia samples the RNAqueous™ Micro Total RNA Isolation kit (Ambion, CA, USA) was used to allow for efficient extraction from a small number of cells. For microarray samples, RNA quality was assessed using an Agilent 2100 bioanalyzer (Agilent Technologies, CA, USA) and all samples had RIN values of 10. For all samples, RNA concentration was determined using a Nanodrop (Thermo Fisher). All samples were treated with DNase I (1 μg DNase/1 μg RNA) using the RQ1 RNase-free DNase kit (Promega, WI, USA) and cDNA was prepared using the Superscript® III First-Strand Synthesis kit (Life Technologies).

qRT-PCR

Quantitative real-time PCR (qRT-PCR) was performed using Platinum® SYBR® Green qRT-PCR SuperMix-UDG with Rox (Life Technologies, CA, USA) on a 7900HT Fast Real-Time PCR system (Applied Biosystems, CA, USA). Standard curves were run for all primers and efficiencies were all 100 ± 10% (Additional file 3: Table S3). Relative gene expression analysis was performed using the $2^{-\Delta\Delta Ct}$ method with the housekeeping gene *GAPDH* as described previously [51].

Microarray and bioinformatics analysis

RNA was labelled and hybridised to Affymetrix Genechip® Primeview™ Human Gene Expression Arrays (Santa Clara, CA, USA) according to manufacturer's instructions. Microarray was performed and analysed by New Zealand Genomics Limited (NZGL). Bioinformatics analysis was carried out in the 'R' statistical environment as described previously [50]. Briefly, the ".cel" files from each genechip were quality assessed using the 'AffyQCReport' package and were normalised using the RMA algorithm with background correction. To generate a list of differentially expressed genes, statistical analysis of gene abundance between samples was performed on $\log_2$ transformed data using the LIMMA method. The main queries were identifying differentially expressed genes in PU.1 siRNA samples relative to scrambled siRNA samples in mixed glial cultures and pericyte-only cultures. A list of 180 differentially expressed genes in mixed glial cultures with PU.1 siRNA compared to control siRNA was generated with fold changes > 1.5 and adjusted p-values < 0.001 (Additional file 4: Table S4). Of these 180 genes, 32 were excluded as they also showed fold changes of > 1.5 in pericyte only cultures with PU.1 siRNA relative to scrambled siRNA and were deemed off-target effects. A further 46 genes had multiple genes yielding 102 unique genes recognized using the Database for Annotation, Visualisation and Integrated Discovery (DAVID) gene list conversion. Relationships between the remaining 102 differentially expressed genes were further explored using DAVID (https://david.ncifcrf.gov/) gene ontology tools, including Biological Processes, Cellular components, and Molecular Functions. KEGG pathway analysis was performed in DAVID to determine biological pathway maps which were altered with PU.1 silencing yielding 16 pathways with p-values < 0.001. Further, STRING (https://string-db.org/) was utilised to investigate protein-protein interaction networks of PU.1 regulated genes. PU.1 (*SPI1*) was not in the list of 102 differentially regulated genes but was included in the STRING analysis for interaction purposes. For heatmap generation including unbiased hierarchical clustering the heatmap.2 function was utilised in 'R'.

NanoString

RNA was extracted from fresh frozen human brain tissue taken from the middle frontal gyrus of post-mortem control ($n = 8$) and AD ($n = 8$) cases (Additional file 1: Table S1). Care was taken to dissect only grey matter from the tissue samples (< 30 mg), which were then immediately homogenized in 1 mL TRIzol reagent with 2 mm stainless steel beads (Qiagen) using the Tissuelyser II tissue homogenizer (Qiagen) for 4 min at 25 Hz. Samples were centrifuged at 12,000 x g for 2 min at 4 °C. The supernatant was collected and 200 μL of chloroform added, shaken vigorously for 15 s and incubated for 2–3 min at RT and then centrifuged at 12,000 x g for 15 min at 4 °C. The upper aqueous phase was collected and mixed with an equal volume of 70% ethanol. Subsequent steps were performed using the RNeasy kit (Qiagen) following manufacturer's instructions. DNase I treatment was performed using components from the RNAqueous-Micro kit (Ambion) following manufacturer's instructions. RNA purity and concentrations were determined using Qubit and Bioanalyzer 2100 (Agilent Technologies). Only samples with RIN >5 were used for Nanostring. Samples were shipped on dry ice to the Otago Genomics Facility (Otago, NZ) for further QC and processing on the Nanostring N-Counter using a custom CodeSet that included 5 reference housekeeping genes (*ACTB, PGK1, POL1B, RPLP0,* and *RPL30*) which were used for normalisation. All data passed QC, with no imaging, binding, positive control, or CodeSet content normalisation flags. Background-corrected counts (mean + 1SD) normalised to the geometric mean of both the positive controls (between lane hyb effects) and all nominated reference, housekeeping genes (RNA input effects) for all samples were used for graphs.

Immunohistochemistry and fluorescent microscopy

Imummunohistochemistry (IHC) procedures were performed using free-floating, formalin fixed, 50 μm thick tissue sections, processed as described previously [46]. TSA™ SuperBoost™ kits (ThermoFisher) were used to amplify signal from TREM2 and DAP12 stains as per manufacturer's instructions, while IBA1, HLA-DR,DP,DQ, and CD45 stains were performed using traditional primary-secondary labelling. Heat-induced epitope retrieval was performed in Tris-EDTA (ethylenediamine tetraacetic acid, 1 mM; Tris-HCl, 10 mM, pH 9). Endogenous peroxidase activity was then blocked (1% hydrogen peroxide, 50% methanol), before sections were incubated with primary antibody (72 h, 4 °C) diluted in 1% normal donkey serum (Gibco) in PBS-T. Sections were washed and incubated with fluorescent and biotinylated secondary antibodies raised in donkey (24 h, 4 °C) diluted in 1% normal donkey serum in PBS-T. The following day, sections were washed and incubated with extravidin peroxidase, diluted in 1% normal donkey serum in PBS-T, for 4 h at room temperature. Sections were washed, and tyramide reaction solution (tyramide-488, 1:500; hydrogen peroxide, 0.03% in reaction buffer) added for 15 min at room temperature. The reaction was quenched using stop solution, and Hoechst 33342 nuclear counterstain added (1:10,000, 5 min; Thermo Fisher). Tissue sections were imaged at 20 x magnification using a Nikon Eclipse Ni microscope (Japan). For each section, two 2.00×2.00 mm regions were imaged from grey and white matter across two distant sections were imaged per case ($n = 5$ control, $n = 4$ AD).

Statistical analysis

All cell culture experiments were performed at least three independent times on tissue from three different donors. Statistical analysis was performed using an unpaired Students t test, or a two-way ANOVA with Tukey's *post-hoc* multiple comparison test, as designated in figure legends (Graphpad Prism 7, CA, USA). Statistical analysis of microarray data was performed as previously described [50]. All data is displayed as mean+/– SEM.

Results

Characterisation of culture conditions for microarray analysis

Characterisation of mixed glia isolated from human brain biopsy tissue revealed heterogeneous cultures containing microglia (PU.1), endothelia (PECAM1), astrocytes (GFAP), and pericytes (PDGFRβ; Fig. 1a). In contrast, pericyte cultures displayed PDGFRβ expression whilst lacking PU.1, GFAP, and PECAM1 (Fig. 1a). Transfection of mixed glial cultures with PU.1 siRNA was effective in attenuating microglial PU.1 expression compared to a scrambled siRNA (Fig. 1b), as described previously [33]. As expected, microarray analysis revealed a higher expression of astrocyte (*SLC1A3* and *S100B*), endothelial (*PECAM1* and *VWF*), and microglial (*CD163, CD14, CD86, MRC1, TREM2, LST1, PTPRC, MSR1, AIF1, HLADRA,* and *TYROBP*) genes in scrambled siRNA transfected mixed glial cultures compared to similarly treated pericyte-only cultures (Fig. 1c), reflecting the immunocytochemistry analysis (Fig. 1a). Unbiased hierarchical clustering of the top 250 differentially expressed genes across all samples revealed the similarity of biological replicates obtained from different tissue donors. Further, numerous changes were evident in PU.1 siRNA-transfected samples compared to scrambled siRNA in mixed glial cultures, containing PU.1$^+$ microglia, whilst little change was observed in pericyte-only cultures (Fig. 1d).

Microarray analysis of PU.1 silencing

In order to investigate the effect of PU.1 knockdown in mixed glial cultures by microarray analysis, gene expression in PU.1 siRNA samples was normalised to scrambled siRNA samples in either mixed glial cultures or pericyte-only cultures. The top 180 differentially expressed genes displaying $\log_2$ fold changes > 1.5 and adjusted p-values < 0.001 were selected for further analysis (Additional file 4: Table S4), and the corresponding changes in pericyte-only cultures were determined to identify potential off-target effects of PU.1 siRNA (Fig. 2a). Of the 180 differentially expressed genes, 51 were found to be upregulated in both the pericyte and mixed glial cultures, with 26 uniquely upregulated genes in mixed glial cultures (Fig. 2b). Similarly, 129 downregulated genes were identified, 7 of which were present in both culture conditions revealing 122 uniquely downregulated genes (Fig. 2c). A panel of 17 mostly microglial-specific genes (*LST1, HLA-DRA, SPI1, AIF1, MRC1, CEBPA, TREM2, PTPRC, TYROBP, C3, HLA-DMA, GFAP, CSF1R, BDNF, CEBPB, MMP9,* and *IL6*) displaying large reductions ($\log_2$ FC > – 1.5), moderate reductions ($\log_2$ FC = – 0.5 - -1.5), no change ($\log_2$ FC = – 0.5 – 0.5), small inductions ($\log_2$ FC = 0.5–1.5), and large inductions ($\log_2$ FC > 1.5) in mixed glial cultures were selected (Fig. 2d,e) and validated by qRT-PCR (Fig. 2f) to confirm microarray findings, with gene expression showing good correlation ($R^2 = 0.75$) between methods (Fig. 2g).

Bioinformatic analysis reveals PU.1 as a highly connected hub protein involved in innate and adaptive immunity

To further examine how PU.1 knockdown modified microglial gene expression in mixed glial cultures several

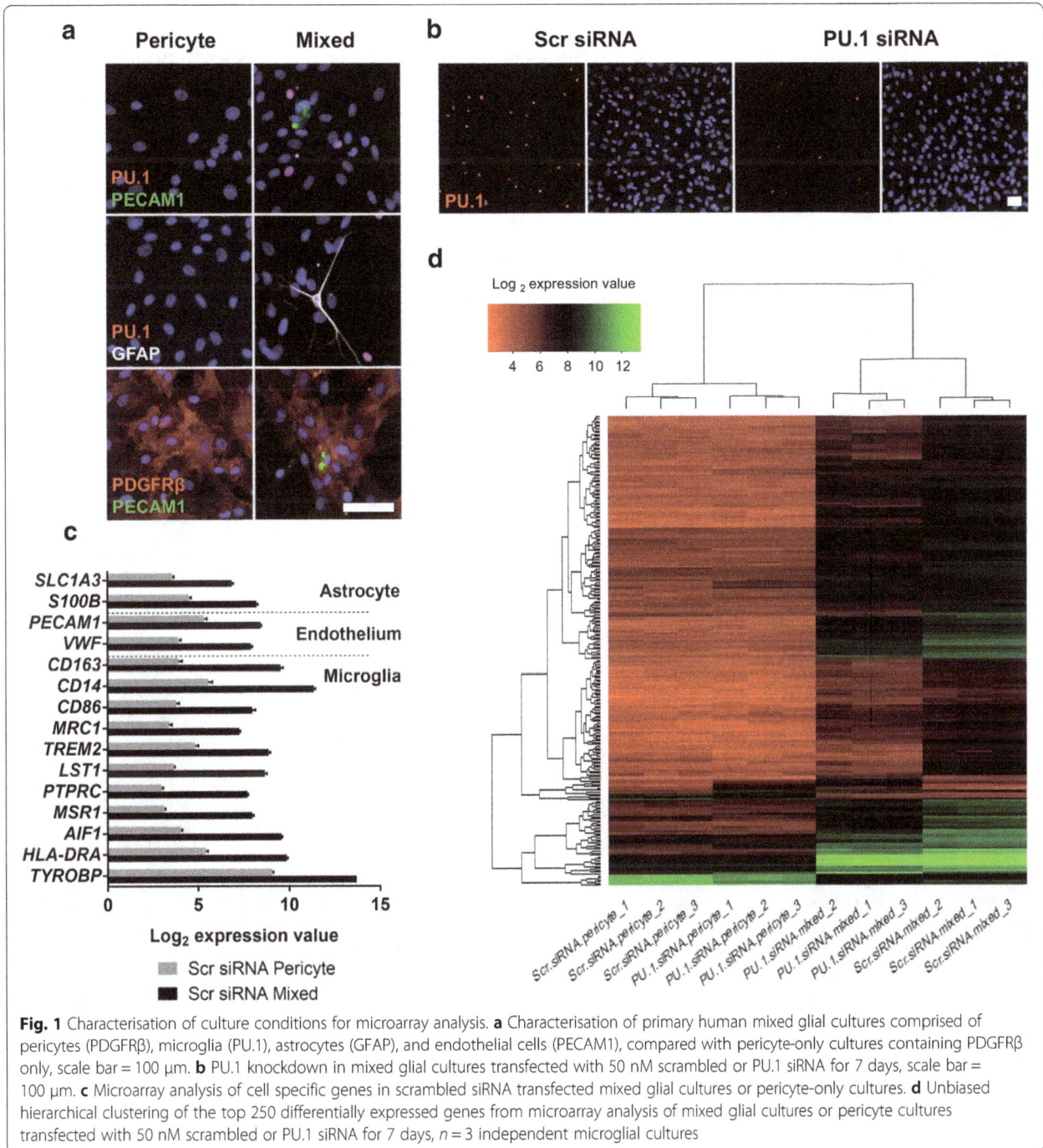

Fig. 1 Characterisation of culture conditions for microarray analysis. **a** Characterisation of primary human mixed glial cultures comprised of pericytes (PDGFRβ), microglia (PU.1), astrocytes (GFAP), and endothelial cells (PECAM1), compared with pericyte-only cultures containing PDGFRβ only, scale bar = 100 μm. **b** PU.1 knockdown in mixed glial cultures transfected with 50 nM scrambled or PU.1 siRNA for 7 days, scale bar = 100 μm. **c** Microarray analysis of cell specific genes in scrambled siRNA transfected mixed glial cultures or pericyte-only cultures. **d** Unbiased hierarchical clustering of the top 250 differentially expressed genes from microarray analysis of mixed glial cultures or pericyte cultures transfected with 50 nM scrambled or PU.1 siRNA for 7 days, n = 3 independent microglial cultures

bioinformatic approaches were employed. A STRING protein-protein interaction network of the top 102 differentially expressed genes specific to mixed glial cultures, with inclusion of PU.1 (SPI1), revealed PU.1 as a highly connected hub protein (Fig. 3a). Through gene ontology analysis of differentially regulated genes, PU.1 silencing was found to modify several innate and adaptive biological processes including "immune response", "antigen processing and presentation", and "T cell costimulation" (Fig. 3b). Analysis of the cellular components revealed that the majority of modified genes localised to the extracellular region, MHCII protein complexes, and various endocytic vesicle structures (Fig. 3c). Collectively, these revealed changes in molecular functions, including "actin filament binding" and "MHC class II receptor activity" (Fig. 3c) which are implicated in phagocytosis and antigen presentation respectively

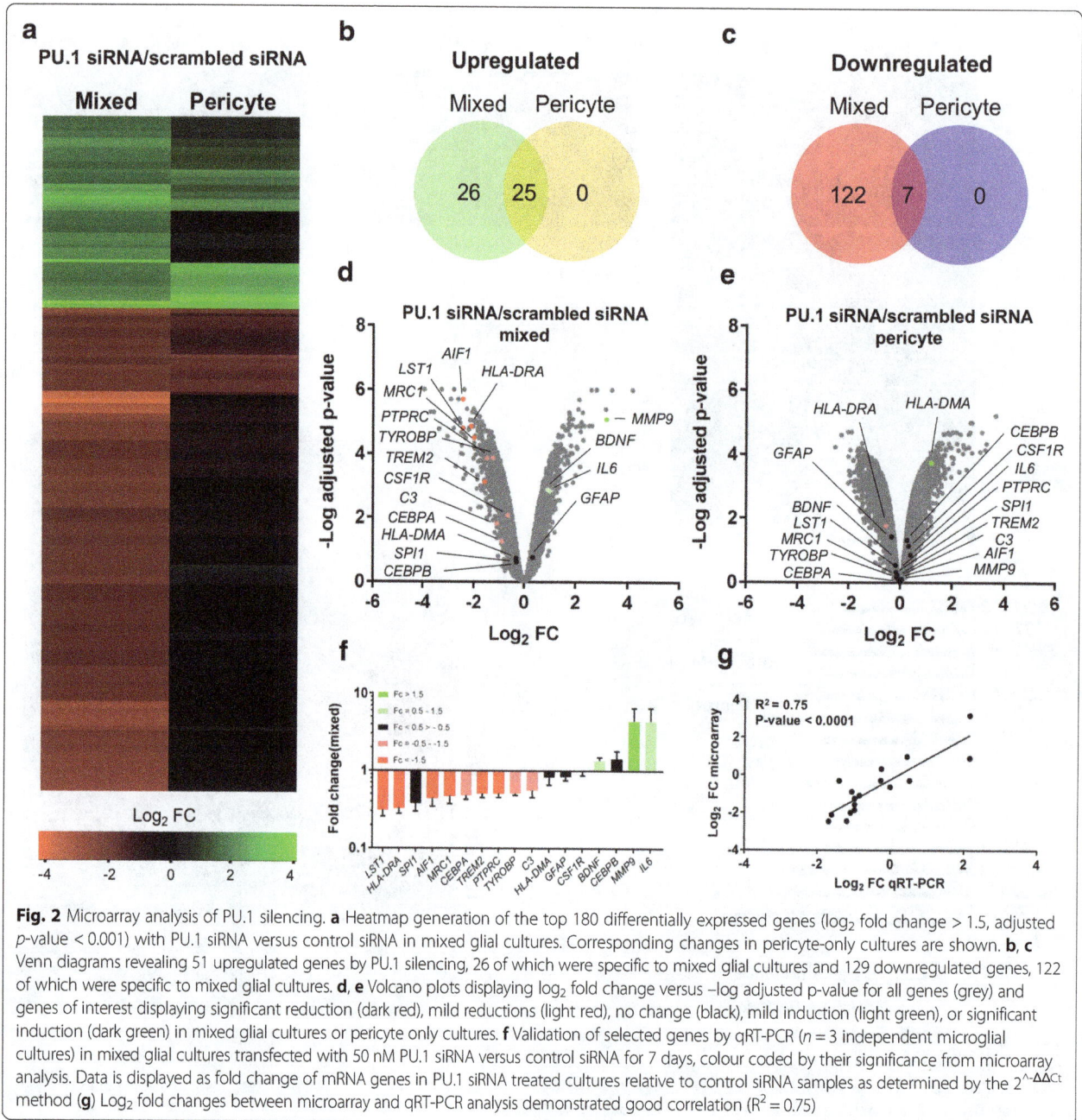

Fig. 2 Microarray analysis of PU.1 silencing. **a** Heatmap generation of the top 180 differentially expressed genes (log$_2$ fold change > 1.5, adjusted p-value < 0.001) with PU.1 siRNA versus control siRNA in mixed glial cultures. Corresponding changes in pericyte-only cultures are shown. **b, c** Venn diagrams revealing 51 upregulated genes by PU.1 silencing, 26 of which were specific to mixed glial cultures and 129 downregulated genes, 122 of which were specific to mixed glial cultures. **d, e** Volcano plots displaying log$_2$ fold change versus –log adjusted p-value for all genes (grey) and genes of interest displaying significant reduction (dark red), mild reductions (light red), no change (black), mild induction (light green), or significant induction (dark green) in mixed glial cultures or pericyte only cultures. **f** Validation of selected genes by qRT-PCR ($n = 3$ independent microglial cultures) in mixed glial cultures transfected with 50 nM PU.1 siRNA versus control siRNA for 7 days, colour coded by their significance from microarray analysis. Data is displayed as fold change of mRNA genes in PU.1 siRNA treated cultures relative to control siRNA samples as determined by the $2^{\wedge-\Delta\Delta Ct}$ method (**g**) Log$_2$ fold changes between microarray and qRT-PCR analysis demonstrated good correlation (R^2 = 0.75)

(Fig. 3d). Lastly, KEGG analysis of differentially expressed genes identified 16 biological pathways, including "phagosome" (Additional file 5: Figure S1) and "antigen processing and presentation" (Additional file 5: Figure S1) containing the largely overlapping genes lists (*CLEC7A, FCGR3A, CTSS, CYBB, HLA-DMB, HLA-DPA1, HLA-DQA1, HLA-DQB1, HLA-DR,* and *MRC1*) and (*CD74, CTSS, HLA-DMB, HLA-DPA1, HLA-DQA1, HLA-DQB1,* and *HLA-DRA*) respectively. Additional bioinformatic analysis using GSEA displayed largely similar pathways modified by PU.1 expression (Additional file 6: Table S5).

Confirmation of microarray analysis in isolated human brain microglia

In order to ensure the aforementioned changes in mixed glial cultures were a result of microglial changes with PU.1 silencing and not effects mediated by other cell types, or changes resulting from a gross loss of microglia, further studies were performed using isolated human microglial cultures. Characterisation of isolated microglia with PU.1 knockdown revealed no change in overall cell number (Fig. 4a) or microglial purity (Fig. 4b). Contaminating cells in microglial cultures were identified

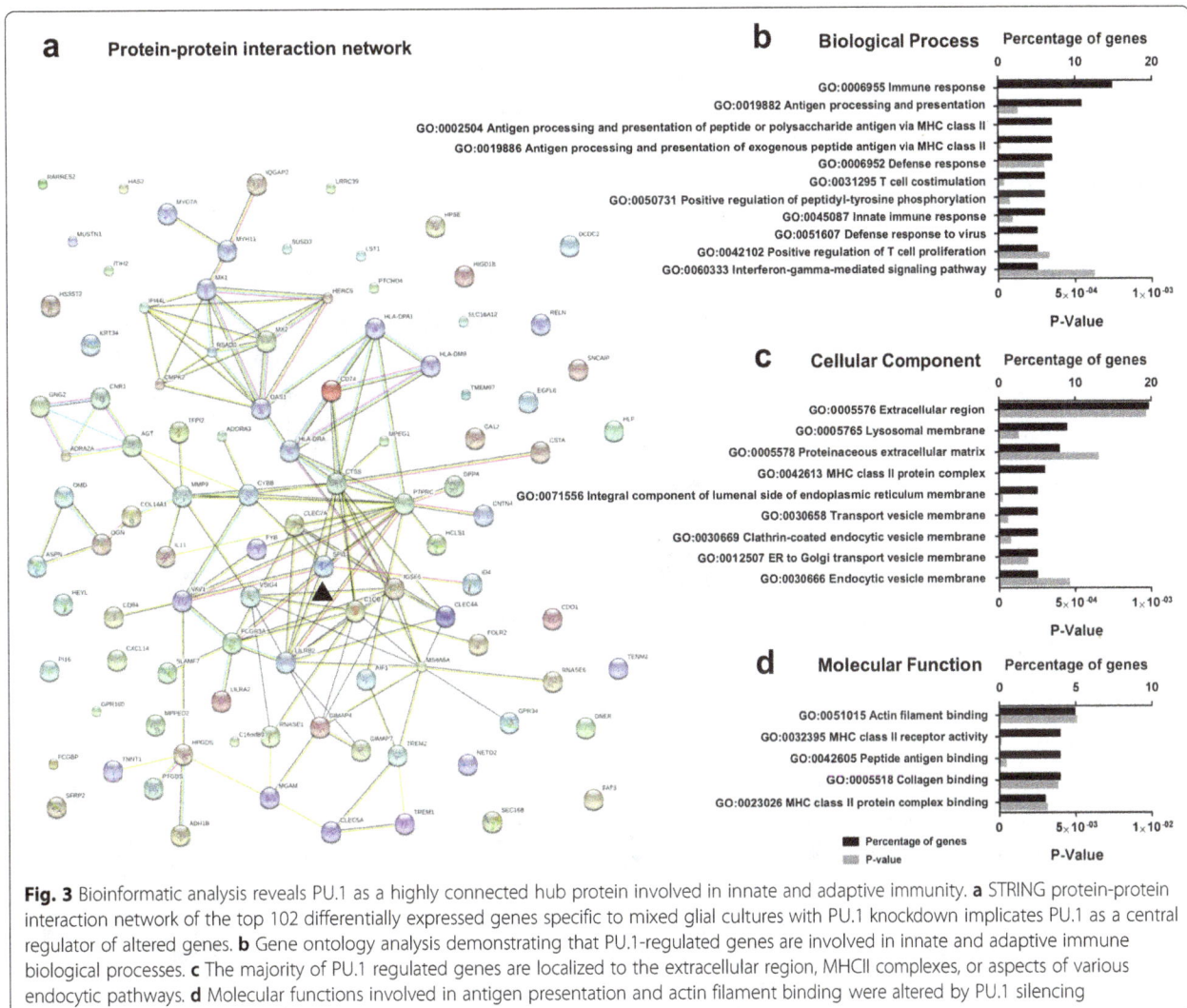

Fig. 3 Bioinformatic analysis reveals PU.1 as a highly connected hub protein involved in innate and adaptive immunity. **a** STRING protein-protein interaction network of the top 102 differentially expressed genes specific to mixed glial cultures with PU.1 knockdown implicates PU.1 as a central regulator of altered genes. **b** Gene ontology analysis demonstrating that PU.1-regulated genes are involved in innate and adaptive immune biological processes. **c** The majority of PU.1 regulated genes are localized to the extracellular region, MHCII complexes, or aspects of various endocytic pathways. **d** Molecular functions involved in antigen presentation and actin filament binding were altered by PU.1 silencing

to be pericytes as described previously [49]. PU.1 siRNA produced a ~ 60% reduction in PU.1 protein expression after 7 days of transfection (Fig. 4c, g). Consistent with gene changes, reductions in DAP12 and HLA-DR, DP, DQ were observed, however there was no change in CD45 (Fig. 4d, g). Analysis of microglial morphology revealed a non-significant increase in rounding (Fig. 4e) and significantly decreased elongation (Fig. 4f). Gene expression, measured by qRT-PCR, reflected changes observed in mixed glial cultures (Fig. 4h, i). Interestingly, overall, inflammatory cytokines and chemokines were largely unaltered in glial cultures with PU.1 knockdown. However, given that gene changes often do not correlate with protein changes, we sought to examine whether PU.1 silencing altered microglial inflammatory cell secretions under both basal and LPS-stimulated conditions. No change was observed in the production of IL-1β (Fig. 4j), TNFα (Fig. 4k), IL-6 (Fig. 4l), or MCP-1 (Fig. 4m), whilst a reduction was observed in IL-8 (Fig. 4n), confirming the lack of effect of PU.1 knockdown on cytokine and chemokine gene expression.

PU.1-regulated proteins demonstrate microglial expression in the human AD brain

PU.1 silencing revealed changes in several genes expressed by microglia in vitro. To investigate the relevance of these microglial genes in vivo, RNA was isolated from neurologically normal and pathologically and clinically confirmed AD human brain middle frontal gyrus (MFG) tissue and the expression of several microglial genes was determined by NanoString analysis. An increase in *SPI1* (Fig. 5a), *TYROBP* (Fig. 5b), *HLA-DRA* (Fig. 5c), *TREM2* (Fig. 5d), *PTPRC* (Fig. 5e), and *AIF1* (Fig. 5f) was observed in AD tissue compared to neurologically normal controls, however, this may reflect an alteration in cell populations in the AD brain, including microglial proliferation or neuronal loss, as opposed to changes in individual microglia. Utilising IHC staining, colocalisation of DAP12 (Fig. 5g), HLA-DR, DP,

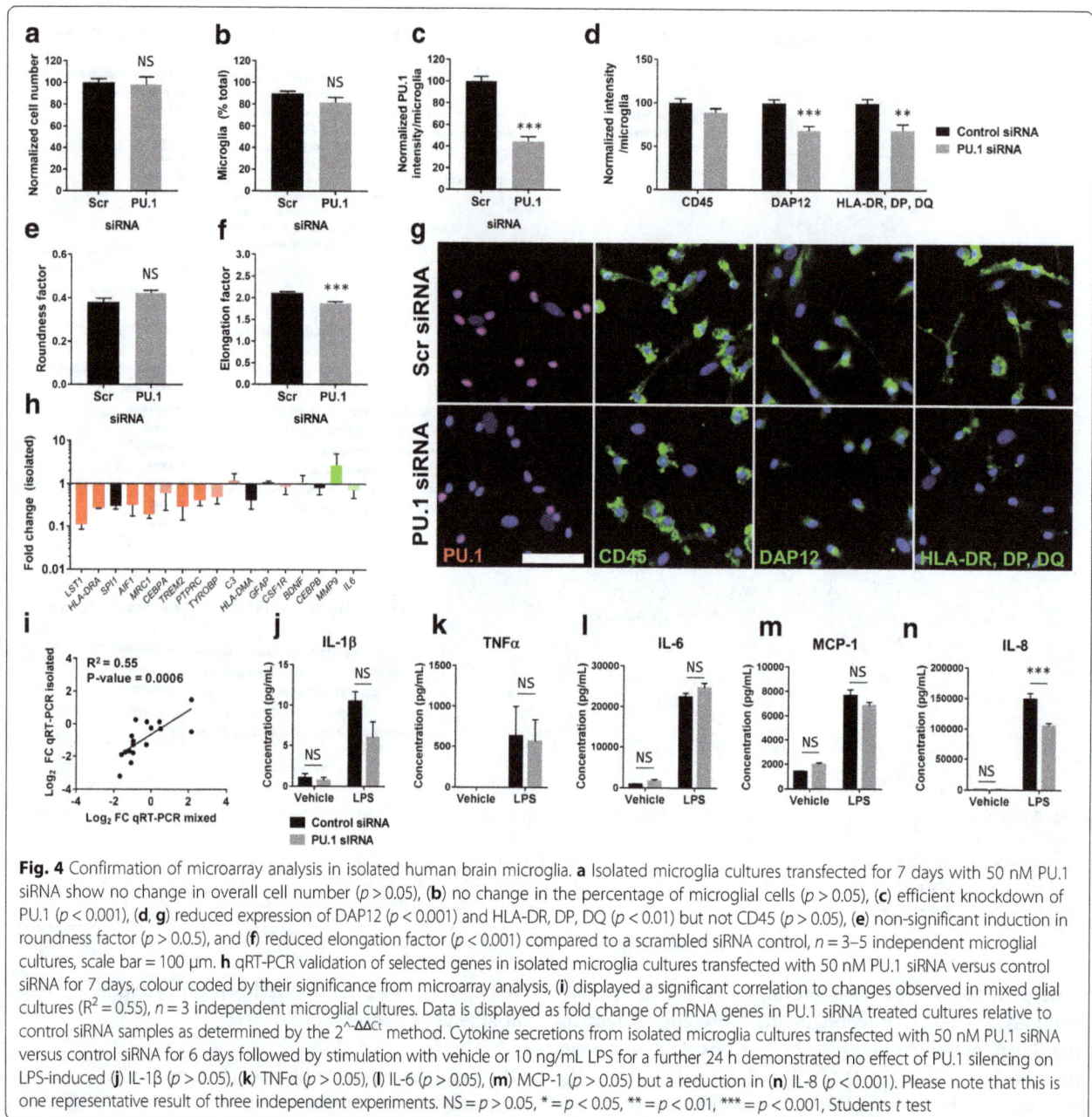

Fig. 4 Confirmation of microarray analysis in isolated human brain microglia. **a** Isolated microglia cultures transfected for 7 days with 50 nM PU.1 siRNA show no change in overall cell number ($p > 0.05$), (**b**) no change in the percentage of microglial cells ($p > 0.05$), (**c**) efficient knockdown of PU.1 ($p < 0.001$), (**d, g**) reduced expression of DAP12 ($p < 0.001$) and HLA-DR, DP, DQ ($p < 0.01$) but not CD45 ($p > 0.05$), (**e**) non-significant induction in roundness factor ($p > 0.05$), and (**f**) reduced elongation factor ($p < 0.001$) compared to a scrambled siRNA control, $n = 3–5$ independent microglial cultures, scale bar = 100 μm. **h** qRT-PCR validation of selected genes in isolated microglia cultures transfected with 50 nM PU.1 siRNA versus control siRNA for 7 days, colour coded by their significance from microarray analysis, (**i**) displayed a significant correlation to changes observed in mixed glial cultures ($R^2 = 0.55$), $n = 3$ independent microglial cultures. Data is displayed as fold change of mRNA genes in PU.1 siRNA treated cultures relative to control siRNA samples as determined by the $2^{-\Delta\Delta Ct}$ method. Cytokine secretions from isolated microglia cultures transfected with 50 nM PU.1 siRNA versus control siRNA for 6 days followed by stimulation with vehicle or 10 ng/mL LPS for a further 24 h demonstrated no effect of PU.1 silencing on LPS-induced (**j**) IL-1β ($p > 0.05$), (**k**) TNFα ($p > 0.05$), (**l**) IL-6 ($p > 0.05$), (**m**) MCP-1 ($p > 0.05$) but a reduction in (**n**) IL-8 ($p < 0.001$). Please note that this is one representative result of three independent experiments. NS = $p > 0.05$, * = $p < 0.05$, ** = $p < 0.01$, *** = $p < 0.001$, Students t test

DQ (Fig. 5h), TREM2 (Fig. 5i), and CD45 (Fig. 5j) was observed in IBA1+ microglia in both control and AD brains, demonstrating that PU.1-regulated genes are expressed by human microglia in situ.

High throughput drug screening identified vorinostat as an effective inhibitor of PU.1 that partially mimics the effects of PU.1 silencing

Having identified that PU.1 silencing modified microglial gene expression involved in antigen presentation/processing and phagocytic functions, we sought to identify potential pharmacological compounds to modify PU.1 expression. Utilising high throughput screening of 1280

compounds (at 10 μM) approved by major regulatory agencies in mixed glial cultures, the HDAC inhibitor vorinostat was found to be highly effective at reducing PU.1 expression (Fig. 6a). Follow up screens in two independent cases confirmed a dramatic reduction in the number of cells displaying PU.1 expression levels compared to vehicle controls (Fig. 6b), whilst a moderate reduction in overall cell number was also observed (Fig. 6c). Further ICC analysis demonstrated that this change was not simply a result of overt microglial loss, as CD45+ microglia largely devoid of nuclear PU.1 were observed (Fig. 6d). Further confirmation of this effect was performed in isolated microglia cultures with a 24 h

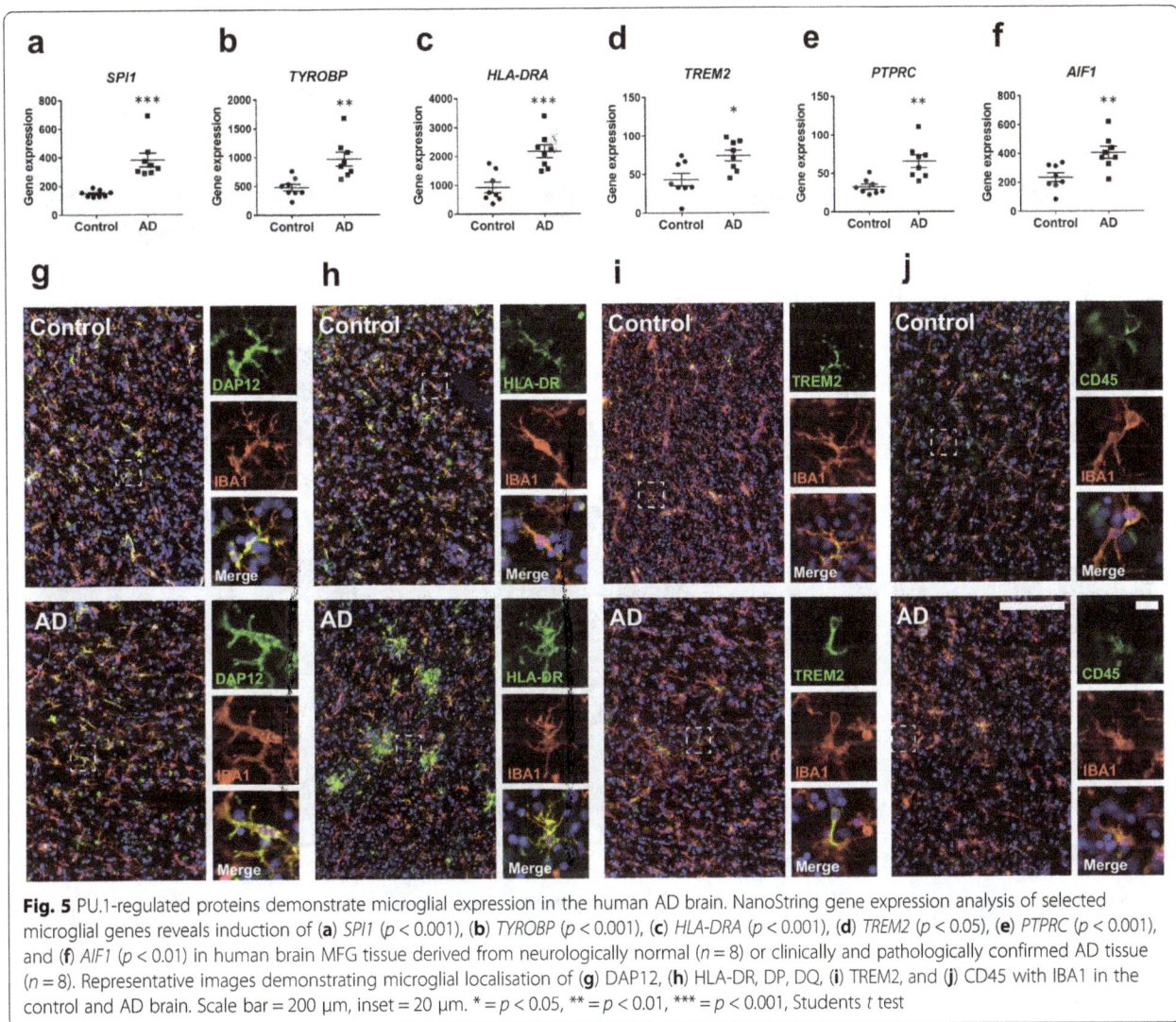

Fig. 5 PU.1-regulated proteins demonstrate microglial expression in the human AD brain. NanoString gene expression analysis of selected microglial genes reveals induction of (**a**) SPI1 ($p < 0.001$), (**b**) TYROBP ($p < 0.001$), (**c**) HLA-DRA ($p < 0.001$), (**d**) TREM2 ($p < 0.05$), (**e**) PTPRC ($p < 0.001$), and (**f**) AIF1 ($p < 0.01$) in human brain MFG tissue derived from neurologically normal ($n = 8$) or clinically and pathologically confirmed AD tissue ($n = 8$). Representative images demonstrating microglial localisation of (**g**) DAP12, (**h**) HLA-DR, DP, DQ, (**i**) TREM2, and (**j**) CD45 with IBA1 in the control and AD brain. Scale bar = 200 µm, inset = 20 µm. * = $p < 0.05$, ** = $p < 0.01$, *** = $p < 0.001$, Students t test

treatment with 10 µM vorinostat which revealed a ~ 20% reduction in total cell number (Fig. 6e) but no alteration in the microglial purity (Fig. 6f). Strong reduction in PU.1 expression by ~ 70% was detected following vorinostat treatment (Fig. 6g, k) and a reduction in DAP12, but not CD45 or HLA-DR, DP, DQ was observed (Fig. 6h, k), partially recapitulating the effects of direct PU.1 silencing with siRNA. No changes in microglial morphology, either through altered elongation (Fig. 6i) or rounding was observed (Fig. 6j). Gene expression analysis by qRT-PCR revealed a moderate correlation with genes altered by siRNA-mediated PU.1 knockdown (Fig. 6l, m).

Discussion

Microarray and bioinformatic analysis of PU.1 silencing in primary human mixed glial cultures revealed a network of PU.1-regulated genes involved in innate and adaptive immune functions, particularly phagocytic and antigen presentation pathways. These changes were confirmed in isolated cultures of primary human microglia obtained from various neurosurgical samples. Utilising high throughput drug screening of 1280 FDA-approved compounds, the HDAC inhibitor vorinostat was found to attenuate PU.1 expression and mimic several of the changes seen with PU.1 siRNA-mediated silencing. Utilising NanoString analysis of human brain tissue from neurologically normal and pathologically confirmed cases of AD, an induction in SPI1 and several PU.1-regulated genes, including TYROBP, HLA-DRA, TREM2, PTPRC, and IBA1 was observed. IHC analysis revealed that these markers were all expressed by microglia in neurologically normal and AD brain tissue. Taken together, these data suggest that targeting PU.1 could be beneficial in limiting microglia-mediated immune functions in AD (Fig. 7).

PU.1 is a master regulator of myeloid development and microglial gene expression [33, 34]. Recent evidence suggests that PU.1 also modulates inflammatory responses in rodent BV2 microglia [32] and its attenuation through

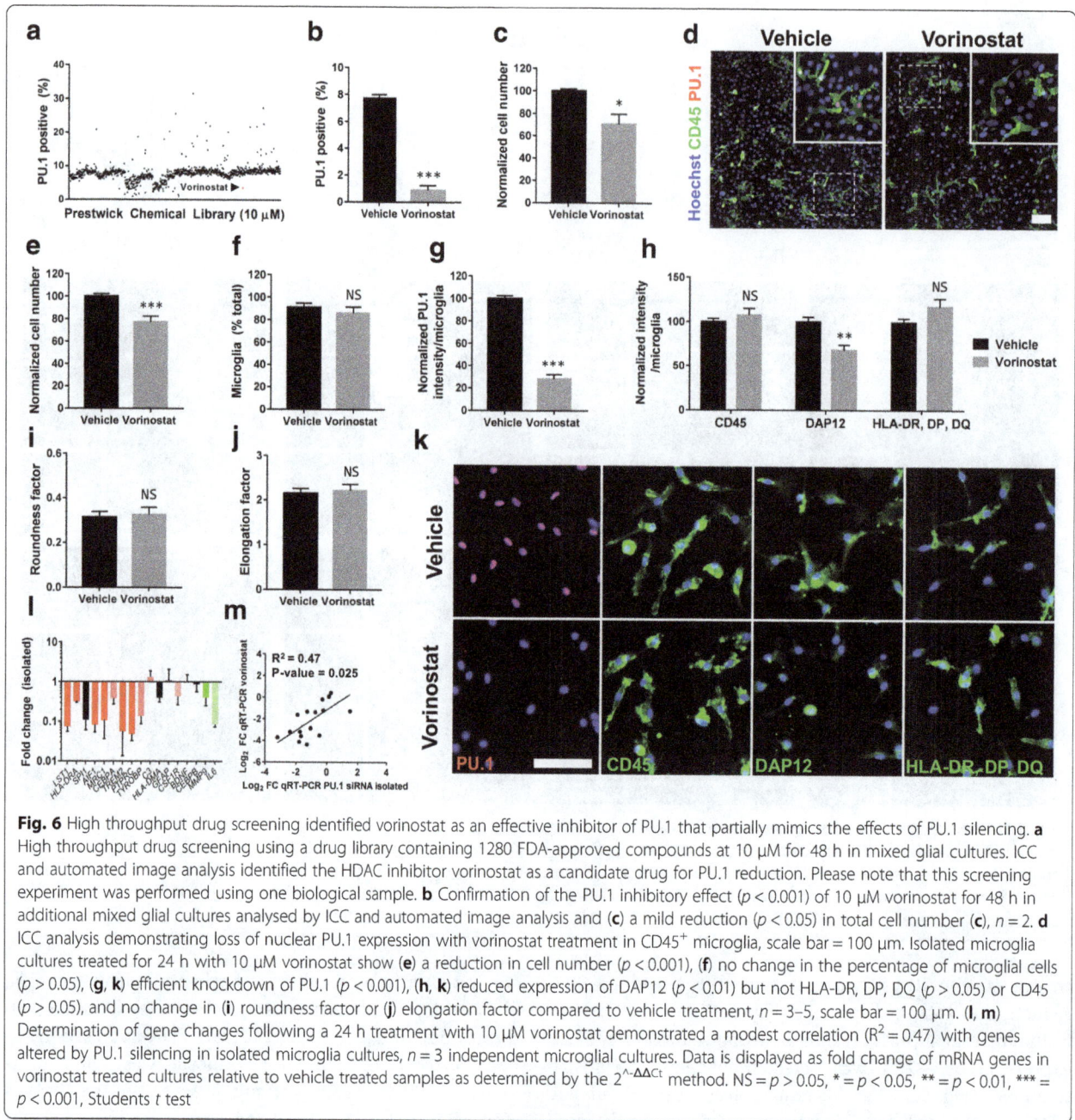

Fig. 6 High throughput drug screening identified vorinostat as an effective inhibitor of PU.1 that partially mimics the effects of PU.1 silencing. **a** High throughput drug screening using a drug library containing 1280 FDA-approved compounds at 10 μM for 48 h in mixed glial cultures. ICC and automated image analysis identified the HDAC inhibitor vorinostat as a candidate drug for PU.1 reduction. Please note that this screening experiment was performed using one biological sample. **b** Confirmation of the PU.1 inhibitory effect ($p < 0.001$) of 10 μM vorinostat for 48 h in additional mixed glial cultures analysed by ICC and automated image analysis and (**c**) a mild reduction ($p < 0.05$) in total cell number (**c**), $n = 2$. **d** ICC analysis demonstrating loss of nuclear PU.1 expression with vorinostat treatment in CD45$^+$ microglia, scale bar = 100 μm. Isolated microglia cultures treated for 24 h with 10 μM vorinostat show (**e**) a reduction in cell number ($p < 0.001$), (**f**) no change in the percentage of microglial cells ($p > 0.05$), (**g, k**) efficient knockdown of PU.1 ($p < 0.001$), (**h, k**) reduced expression of DAP12 ($p < 0.01$) but not HLA-DR, DP, DQ ($p > 0.05$) or CD45 ($p > 0.05$), and no change in (**i**) roundness factor or (**j**) elongation factor compared to vehicle treatment, $n = 3–5$, scale bar = 100 μm. (**l, m**) Determination of gene changes following a 24 h treatment with 10 μM vorinostat demonstrated a modest correlation ($R^2 = 0.47$) with genes altered by PU.1 silencing in isolated microglia cultures, $n = 3$ independent microglial cultures. Data is displayed as fold change of mRNA genes in vorinostat treated cultures relative to vehicle treated samples as determined by the $2^{\wedge-\Delta\Delta Ct}$ method. NS = $p > 0.05$, * = $p < 0.05$, ** = $p < 0.01$, *** = $p < 0.001$, Students t test

miRNA124-mediated silencing prevents neuroinflammatory responses in macrophages through reduced MHC-II, TNFα, and iNOS expression [38]. GWAS has identified a common variant in the *CELF1* locus which correlates with reduced PU.1 expression and elevated age of onset for AD, potentially through limiting immune functions [32]. Collectively, these data suggest that mechanisms to reduce PU.1 expression could prove beneficial in limiting microglial-mediated pro-inflammatory contributions in AD. Through ChIP-Seq analysis, several potential target genes for PU.1 have been identified in rodent microglia BV2 cells, including *Csf1r*, *Aif1*, *Trem2*, and *Tyrobp* [52].

Additionally, *Aif1*, *Csf1r*, and *Tyrobp* were found to be attenuated with shRNA-mediated PU.1 knockdown in BV2 cells, implicating these as important genes under PU.1 regulatory control [32]. Importantly, the aforementioned studies were performed in either macrophages or rodent microglia, both of which display unique gene signatures, particularly with respect to several disease-related genes [30, 40, 42]. It is reassuring to confirm several of these changes in human microglia, particularly phagocytosis-related genes including *AIF1*, *TYROBP*, and *TREM2*, in addition to previously unidentified genes. KEGG pathway analysis of differentially regulated genes identified several other genes

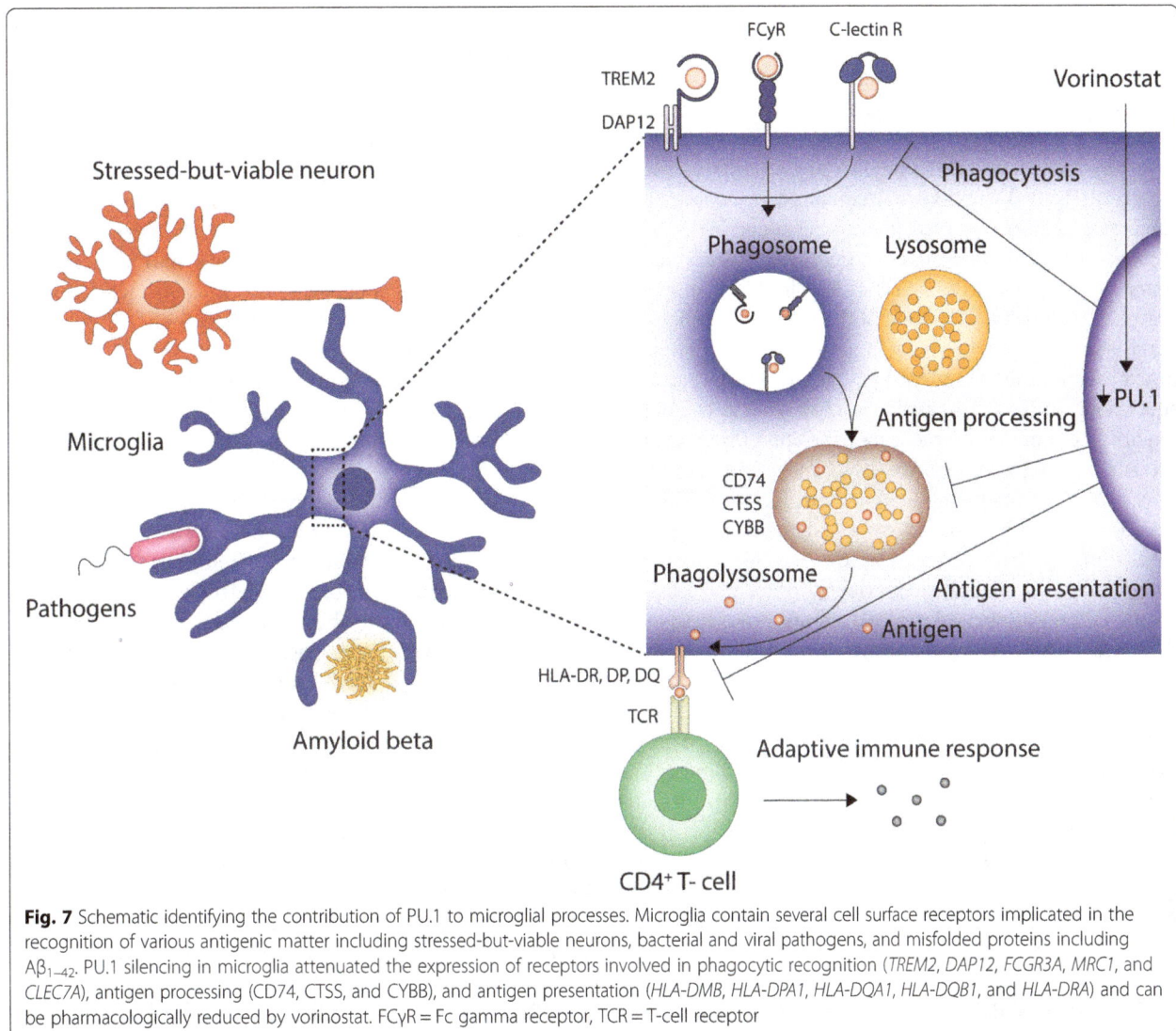

Fig. 7 Schematic identifying the contribution of PU.1 to microglial processes. Microglia contain several cell surface receptors implicated in the recognition of various antigenic matter including stressed-but-viable neurons, bacterial and viral pathogens, and misfolded proteins including $A\beta_{1-42}$. PU.1 silencing in microglia attenuated the expression of receptors involved in phagocytic recognition (*TREM2, DAP12, FCGR3A, MRC1,* and *CLEC7A*), antigen processing (*CD74, CTSS,* and *CYBB*), and antigen presentation (*HLA-DMB, HLA-DPA1, HLA-DQA1, HLA-DQB1,* and *HLA-DRA*) and can be pharmacologically reduced by vorinostat. FCγR = Fc gamma receptor, TCR = T-cell receptor

involved in the phagocytic pathway, including an IgG receptor (*FCGGR3A*), C-lectin receptors (*CLEC7A, MRC1*), as well as degradation enzymes of the phagolysosome (*CTSS*) and NADPH oxidase complex (*CYBB*). Altered expression of several genes involved in the antigen processing (*CD74, CTSS*) and presentation pathway (*HLA-DMB, HLA-DPA1, HLA-DQA1, HLA-DQB1,* and *HLA-DRA*), a common occurrence following phagocytosis, were also observed. Further, it is critical to ensure that gene changes correspond with altered protein expression. Whilst this was observed with DAP12 and HLA-DR, DP, DQ following PU.1 silencing, CD45 displayed no change, highlighting the importance of confirming these changes when predicting biological functions from microarray or RNA-seq datasets.

Whether a reduction in phagocytosis is likely to be beneficial in AD remains controversial. Removal of parenchymal Aβ plaques has historically been considered to be advantageous through limiting microglial-mediated inflammation, however, whilst recent Aβ immunisation trials were effective in reducing plaque burden, they did not prevent progressive neurodegeneration [53]. Such studies suggest that removal of parenchymal Aβ plaques is not an effective strategy in AD. In contrast, uncontrolled phagocytosis can contribute to inappropriate neuronal removal through phagoptosis, and the TREM2/DAP12 complex has been implicated in this process [54, 55]. Further, inhibition of phagocytosis is sufficient to prevent removal of stressed-but-viable neurons expressing "eat me" signatures, particularly phosphatidylserine, with sub-toxic inflammatory exposures [4, 5, 56–59]. In the AD brain, attenuating phagocytosis/phagoptosis of neuronal cells (or perhaps attenuating synaptic pruning), through PU.1 silencing could prove beneficial in attenuating microglia-mediated neurodegeneration.

Whilst a role for PU.1 in phagocytosis has been previously implicated [33], the contribution of this transcription factor in antigen presentation has been less studied. By virtue of the BBB, the CNS was historically considered an immune privileged site; however, overwhelming evidence now suggests immune surveillance of circumventricular organs, a meningeal lymphatic system, and some degree of parenchymal leucocyte infiltration [60]. As a likely consequence of BBB disruption [61] enhanced extravasation of leucocytes is also observed in the AD brain [62]. In the absence of typical dendritic cells, microglia function as the primary antigen presenting cells (APC) in the brain parenchyma. Whilst the exact extent of their APC capabilities remains somewhat controversial, microglia can be stimulated to express appropriate MHCII (HLA-DR, DP, DQ human equivalent) antigen presentation complexes and contain all required co-stimulatory molecules for appropriate antigen presentation, including CD40, CD80 and CD86, and adhesion molecules including LFA-1 and ICAM-1 [63–65]. Additionally, whilst isolated naïve microglia can activate T-cells, in the brain parenchyma they are likely to be involved in re-stimulation of previously primed T-cells following extravasation, and indeed they are more efficient at this process [65]. Antigen presentation to infiltrated CD4$^+$ T-cells resulting in activation or re-priming of CD4$^+$ T-cells to a Th1 phenotype could exacerbate inflammatory responses and its attenuation is likely beneficial [62]. Furthermore, it has been suggested that MHCII molecules themselves can function as signal transduction cascades and this MHCII-TCR interaction with T-cells, or indeed other mediators, can promote a pro-inflammatory microglial phenotype [63]. In such instances, preventing the APC properties of microglia may prove advantageous.

We have previously shown that chronic stimulation with the HDAC inhibitor valproic acid (VPA) attenuated human microglial PU.1 expression and AB$_{1-42}$ phagocytosis [66]. Furthermore, its ability to promote neurogenesis and neuroprotection suggested it could prove beneficial in AD patients [67]. However, a randomised control trial utilising VPA was found to accelerate brain atrophy in AD patients with potentially greater cognitive decline [68]. This may be a result of hyper acetylation in the human AD brain [69] which would be further increased by VPA-mediated inhibition of histone deacetylation. Utilising high throughput drug screening of 1280 FDA approved compounds we identified vorinostat, a more potent HDAC inhibitor, to attenuate PU.1 after a single acute exposure at 10 μM. HDAC1 was recently found to activate PU.1 expression by regulating TAF9 deacetylation and IID transcription factor assembly, suggesting that HDAC1 inhibition is an attractive common pathway to modify PU.1 levels [70]. Further, the vorinostat-induced attenuation of DAP12 reflected effects seen in PU.1-knockdown experiments, suggesting that changes may be PU.1-regulated. Whilst vorinostat-altered genes correlated somewhat to PU.1 siRNA in isolated cultures, this was not true for all

proteins, including HLA-DR, DP, DQ. Currently, a phase I clinical trial is underway to assess the tolerability of vorinostat in AD patients [71] and whilst modifications in microglial-mediated immune functions are not the primary endpoint of such trials, if found to be tolerable this anti-inflammatory contribution could be beneficial in limiting microglial-mediated neurodegeneration through a PU.1-mediated mechanism. Importantly, vorinostat also displays BBB permeability in both the normal brain and during neurodegenerative disease [72, 73], suggesting appropriate distribution of this drug to the CNS to target microglial-mediated immunity.

Importantly, vorinostat displays broad inhibition of class I and II HDACs enzymes, resulting in widespread gene alterations [74]. As such, vorinostat also displays several PU.1-independent effects, including cell cycle arrest and pro-apoptotic functions [74]. Whilst a reduction in overall cell number was observed, the percentage of microglia remained consistent, suggesting subtle cell type-independent toxicity of 10 μM vorinostat after 24 h. Importantly, the ability to attenuate PU.1 exceeded the toxicity of vorinostat, suggesting that additional titration of vorinostat concentrations could eliminate this toxicity. Further, genetic deletion of PU.1 is embryonically lethal, likely due to aberrant myeloid cell production/differentiation [75], whilst conditional deletion during adulthood [76], as well as significant loss in PU.1 expression in rodents carrying hypomorphic *spi1* alleles [77] precipitated the development of acute myeloid leukemia. As such, any considerations when targeting PU.1 expression should seek simply to attenuate its expression in microglia, as observed with vorinostat treatment, rather than obtain complete removal.

Whilst experiments utilising mixed glial cultures, including microarray analysis, were all performed using cells derived from adult human brain epilepsy tissue, subsequent studies were performed using additional sources of neurosurgical tissue, including various tumour resections and paediatric specimens. This difference, including alterations in age, gender, and disease status could contribute to the partial correlation between isolated and mixed glial cultures gene expression with PU.1 silencing. Such changes could also be explained by alterations in non-microglial cells, including astrocytes and endothelial cells which were present in mixed glial cultures and may respond to changes in microglia functions following PU.1 knockdown. Additionally, microglial gene expression profiles change rapidly after removal from the brain microenvironment and subsequent in vitro culture [30]. Whilst this is an inevitable caveat of in vitro human studies, combining primary human samples and in vivo animal models of PU.1 silencing will be beneficial to fully elucidate the role of PU.1 in microglial-mediated immune functions during neurodegeneration. The finding that attenuating

PU.1 expression revealed similar changes independent of the tissue source, and largely the microglial source, is useful in demonstrating the robustness of PU.1 silencing in microglial-modified immune changes.

To investigate whether the aforementioned genes represented valid microglial targets in the human brain, the expression of *SPI1* and several PU.1-regulated genes, *AIF1*, *HLA-DRA*, *TREM2*, *TYROBP*, and *PTPRC*, was determined in post mortem neurologically normal and pathologically confirmed AD MFG tissue. All investigated microglial genes demonstrated elevated expression in the AD brain compared to neurologically normal controls, although this could also be a result of altered cell populations in the AD brain. Furthermore, using IHC we show that all tested markers demonstrated exclusively microglial localisation in both the neurologically normal and AD-brain, suggesting that mechanisms to modulate their expression could prove beneficial in limiting microglial phagocytosis and antigen presentation.

Aside from its role in AD risk, PU.1 has been associated with other neurological disorders including Huntington's disease [35], and hypoxia-ischaemic injury [36]. Microarray analysis in mixed glial cultures revealed that several genes altered by PU.1 silencing were also risk variants [30] for other neurological diseases with a microglial-mediated inflammatory component, including Parkinson's disease (*HLA-DRA*, *HLA-DRB5*, *GPNMB*, and *LRRK2*) and multiple sclerosis (*HLA-DRB1*, *HLA-DRA*, and *CXCR4*) (Additional file 7: Figure S2). Whilst these data should be confirmed by functional protein changes, these findings reinforce the dogma of microglial involvement in numerous neurological disorders and highlight the importance of PU.1 in homeostasis and neurodegeneration.

Conclusion

Preventing microglial-mediated inflammatory responses is likely to prove favourable in limiting neurodegeneration in a diverse range of neurological disorders, including AD. PU.1 silencing was found to attenuate several genes expressed by microglia in the human brain involved in phagocytic and antigen presentation pathways. High throughput drug screening identified vorinostat as an effective attenuator of microglial PU.1 and this partially recapitulated the effects of siRNA-mediated PU.1 silencing and could prove beneficial in limiting microglial immune contributions to AD pathogenesis.

Additional files

Additional file 1: Table S1. List of cases. List of cases used for all studies.

Additional file 2: Table S2. List of antibodies and reagents for ICC and IHC

Additional file 3: Table S3. List of primers used for qRT-PCR

Additional file 4: Table S4. List of the top 180 differentially expressed genes from microarray analysis

Additional file 5: Figure S1. KEGG pathway analysis of PU.1 regulated genes. The top 102 uniquely modified genes regulated by PU.1-silencing in mixed glial cultures were subjected to KEGG pathway analysis using DAVID bioinformatics software. Pathways including (a) "Phagosome" and (b) "Antigen Presentation and Processing" were amongst the most changed (c) and reflected the modified genes by Gene Ontology analysis

Additional file 6: Table S5. GSEA of PU.1 regulated genes. In attempt to identify additional pathways modified by PU.1 silencing in primary human microglia, functionally enriched GO and KEGG gene sets were identified using Gene Set Enrichment Analysis (GSEA) [78, 79] as implemented in WebGestalt [80–82]. The identified pathways (Biological Processes, Molecular Functions, Cellular components, and KEGG analysis) were largely similar to those observed by Fisher's overrepresentation analysis (Fig. 3b-d), suggesting the significance of PU.1 in the regulation of these functions.

Additional file 7: Figure S2. PU.1-regulated genes involved in Alzheimer's disease, Parkinson's disease and multiple sclerosis risk. A list of risk variants associated with (a) Alzheimer's disease, (b) Parkinson's disease, and (c) multiple sclerosis was obtained from [30]. The Log_2 fold change of these risk variants in PU.1 siRNA versus control siRNA in mixed and pericyte only cultures is displayed.

Abbreviations

AD: Alzheimer's disease; APC: Antigen presenting cell; Aβ: Amyloid beta; CBA: Cytometric bead array; CNS: Central nervous system; GWAS: Genome wide association studies; HDAC: Histone deacetylase; ICC: Immunocytochemistry; IHC: Immunohistochemistry; MFG: Middle frontal gyrus; MTG: Middle temporal gyrus; qRT-PCR: Quantitative real-time PCR; VPA: Valproic acid

Acknowledgements

We would like to thank the donors for their generous gift of brain tissue for research. We also thank staff at Auckland Hospital and Marika Eszes (research technician at the Neurological Foundation of New Zealand Douglas Human Brain Bank).

Funding

This work was supported by a Programme Grant from the Health Research Council of New Zealand, the Sir Thomas and Lady Duncan Trust, the Coker Charitable Trust and the Hugh Green Foundation.

Authors' contributions

Conceived the experiments: JR, AMS, MD. Performed experiments and analysed data: JR, AMS, LCS, DJ, ELS, MEVS, MA, NC, PN, RH. Contributed materials and expertise: TIHP, PS, PH, MAC, RLMF, MD. Wrote the manuscript: JR. All authors approved the final manuscript.

Competing interests

The authors declare that they have no competing interests.

Author details

[1]Department of Pharmacology and Clinical Pharmacology, The University of Auckland, Private Bag 92019, Auckland 1142, New Zealand. [2]Centre for Brain Research, The University of Auckland, Auckland, New Zealand. [3]Division of Brain Sciences, Department of Medicine, Imperial College London, London, UK. [4]Department of Anatomy and Medical Imaging, The University of Auckland, Auckland, New Zealand. [5]School of Biological Sciences, The University of Auckland, Auckland, New Zealand. [6]Center for Brain Immunology and Glia, University of Virginia, Charlottesville, Virginia, USA. [7]Departmemt of Neuroscience, University of Virginia, Charlottesville, Virginia, USA. [8]Auckland City Hospital, Auckland, New Zealand.

References

1. Paolicelli RC, et al. Synaptic pruning by microglia is necessary for normal brain development. Science. 2011;333(6048):1456–8.
2. Fu R, et al. Phagocytosis of microglia in the central nervous system diseases. Mol Neurobiol. 2014;49(3):1422–34.
3. Perry VH, Nicoll JA, Holmes C. Microglia in neurodegenerative disease. Nat Rev Neurol. 2010;6(4):193–201.
4. Brown GC, Vilalta A. How microglia kill neurons. Brain Res. 2015;1628(Pt B):288–97.
5. Brown GC, Neher JJ. Microglial phagocytosis of live neurons. Nat Rev Neurosci. 2014;15(4):209–16.
6. Perry VH. Contribution of systemic inflammation to chronic neurodegeneration. Acta Neuropathol. 2010;120(3):277–86.
7. McKhann G, et al. Clinical diagnosis of Alzheimer's disease report of the NINCDS-ADRDA Work Group* under the auspices of Department of Health and Human Services Task Force on Alzheimer's Disease. Neurology. 1984; 34(7):939–44.
8. Braak H, Braak E. Neuropathological stageing of Alzheimer-related changes. Acta Neuropathol. 1991;82(4):239–59.
9. Mandrekar-Colucci S, Landreth GE. Microglia and inflammation in Alzheimer's disease. CNS Neurol Disord Drug Targets. 2010;9(2):156–67.
10. Qian L, Flood PM. Microglial cells and Parkinson's disease. Immunol Res. 2008;41(3):155.
11. Crotti A, Glass CK. The choreography of neuroinflammation in Huntington's disease. Trends Immunol. 2015;36(6):364–73.
12. Henkel JS, et al. Microglia in ALS: the good, the bad, and the resting. J Neuroimmune Pharmacol. 2009;4(4):389–98.
13. Jack C, et al. Microglia and multiple sclerosis. J Neurosci Res. 2005;81(3):363–73.
14. Yirmiya R, Rimmerman N, Reshef R. Depression as a microglial disease. Trens Neurosci. 2015;38(10):637–58.
15. Rodriguez JI, Kern JK. Evidence of microglial activation in autism and its possible role in brain underconnectivity. Neuron Glia Biol. 2011;7(2–4):205–13.
16. Patel AR, et al. Microglia and ischemic stroke: a double-edged sword. Int J Physiol Pathophysiol Pharmacol. 2013;5(2):73.
17. Karve IP, Taylor JM, Crack PJ. The contribution of astrocytes and microglia to traumatic brain injury. Br J Pharmacol. 2016;173(4):692–702.
18. Bekris LM, et al. Genetics of Alzheimer disease. J Geriatr Psychiatry Neurol. 2010;23(4):213–27.
19. Corder E, et al. Gene dose of apolipoprotein E type 4 allele and the risk of Alzheimer's disease in late onset families. Science. 1993;261(5123):921–3.
20. Genin E, et al. APOE and Alzheimer disease: a major gene with semi-dominant inheritance. Mol Psychiatry. 2011;16(9):903.
21. Lambert J, et al. European Alzheimer's disease initiative investigators. Genome-wide association study identifies variants at CLU and CR1 associated with Alzheimer's disease. Nat Genet. 2009;41(10):1094–9.
22. Harold D, et al. Genome-wide association study identifies variants at CLU and PICALM associated with Alzheimer's disease. Nat Genet. 2009;41(10):1088–93.
23. Seshadri S, et al. Genome-wide analysis of genetic loci associated with Alzheimer disease. Jama. 2010;303(18):1832–40.
24. Hollingworth P, et al. Common variants at ABCA7, MS4A6A/MS4A4E, EPHA1, CD33 and CD2AP are associated with Alzheimer's disease. Nat Genet. 2011;43(5):429–35.
25. Naj AC, et al. Common variants at MS4A4/MS4A6E, CD2AP, CD33 and EPHA1 are associated with late-onset Alzheimer's disease. Nat Genet. 2011;43(5):436–41.
26. Guerreiro R, et al. TREM2 variants in Alzheimer's disease. NEJM. 2013;368(2):117–27.
27. Jonsson T, et al. Variant of TREM2 associated with the risk of Alzheimer's disease. NEJM. 2013;368(2):107–16.
28. Sims R, et al. Rare coding variants in PLCG2, ABI3, and TREM2 implicate microglial-mediated innate immunity in Alzheimer's disease. Nat Genet. 2017;49(9):1373–84.
29. Lambert J-C, et al. Meta-analysis of 74,046 individuals identifies 11 new susceptibility loci for Alzheimer's disease. Nat Genet. 2013;45(12):1452–8.
30. Gosselin D, et al. An environment-dependent transcriptional network specifies human microglia identity. Science. 2017;356:eaal3222.
31. Efthymiou AG, Goate AM. Late onset Alzheimer's disease genetics implicates microglial pathways in disease risk. Mol Neurodegen. 2017;12(1):43.
32. Huang K, et al. A common haplotype lowers PU. 1 expression in myeloid cells and delays onset of Alzheimer's disease. Nat Neurosci. 2017;20(8):1052–61.
33. Smith AM, et al. The transcription factor PU.1 is critical for viability and function of human brain microglia. Glia. 2013;61(6):929–42.
34. Kierdorf K, et al. Microglia emerge from erythromyeloid precursors via Pu.1- and Irf8-dependent pathways. Nat Neurosci. 2013;16(3):273–80.
35. Crotti A, et al. Mutant huntingtin promotes autonomous microglia activation via myeloid lineage-determining factors. Nat Neurosci. 2014;17(4):513–21.
36. Walton MR, et al. PU.1 expression in microglia. J Neuroimmunol. 2000; 104(2):109–15.
37. Sun Y, et al. An updated role of microRNA-124 in central nervous system disorders: a review. Front Cell Neurosci. 2015;9:193.
38. Ponomarev ED, et al. MicroRNA-124 promotes microglia quiescence and suppresses EAE by deactivating macrophages via the C/EBP-alpha-PU.1 pathway. Nat Med. 2011;17(1):64–70.
39. Brennan GP, et al. Dual and opposing roles of microRNA-124 in epilepsy are mediated through inflammatory and NRSF-dependent gene networks. Cell Rep. 2016;14(10):2402–12.
40. Smith AM, Dragunow M. The human side of microglia. Trends Neurosci. 2014;37(3):125–35.
41. Gross TJ, et al. Epigenetic silencing of the human NOS2 gene: rethinking the role of nitric oxide in human macrophage inflammatory responses. J Immunol. 2014;192(5):2326–38.
42. Hickman SE, et al. The microglial sensome revealed by direct RNA sequencing. Nat Neurosci. 2013;16(12):1896–905.
43. Zarruk JG, Greenhalgh AD, David S. Microglia and macrophages differ in their inflammatory profile after permanent brain ischemia. Exp Neurol. 2018; 301:120–32.
44. Smith AM, Gibbons HM, Dragunow M. Valproic acid enhances microglial phagocytosis of amyloid-beta(1-42). Neuroscience. 2010;169(1):505–15.
45. Dragunow M. The adult human brain in preclinical drug development. Nat Rev Drug Discov. 2008;7(8):659.
46. Waldvogel HJ, et al. Immunohistochemical staining of post-mortem adult human brain sections. Nat Protoc. 2006;1(6):2719–32.
47. Gibbons HM, et al. Cellular composition of human glial cultures from adult biopsy brain tissue. J Neurosci Methods. 2007;166(1):89–98.
48. Rustenhoven J, et al. An anti-inflammatory role for C/EBPdelta in human brain pericytes. Sci Rep. 2015;5:12132.
49. Rustenhoven J, et al. Isolation of highly enriched primary human microglia for functional studies. Sci Rep. 2016;6:19371.
50. Jansson D, et al. A role for human brain pericytes in neuroinflammation. J Neuroinflammation. 2014;11(1):104.
51. Rustenhoven J, et al. TGF-beta1 regulates human brain pericyte inflammatory processes involved in neurovasculature function. J Neuroinflammation. 2016;13(1):1–15.
52. Satoh J, et al. A Comprehensive Profile of ChIP-Seq-Based PU. 1/Spi1 Target Genes in Microglia. Gene Regul Syst Biol. 2014;8:127.
53. Holmes C, et al. Long-term effects of Aβ 42 immunisation in Alzheimer's disease: follow-up of a randomised, placebo-controlled phase I trial. Lancet. 2008;372(9634):216–23.
54. Takahashi K, Rochford CD, Neumann H. Clearance of apoptotic neurons without inflammation by microglial triggering receptor expressed on myeloid cells-2. J Exp Med. 2005;201(4):647–57.
55. Hsieh CL, et al. A role for TREM2 ligands in the phagocytosis of apoptotic neuronal cells by microglia. J Neurochem. 2009;109(4):1144–56.

56. Fricker M, Oliva-Martin MJ, Brown GC. Primary phagocytosis of viable neurons by microglia activated with LPS or Abeta is dependent on calreticulin/LRP phagocytic signalling. J Neuroinflammation. 2012;9:196.

57. Neher JJ, Neniskyte U, Brown GC. Primary phagocytosis of neurons by inflamed microglia: potential roles in neurodegeneration. Front Pharmacol. 2012;3

58. Neher JJ, et al. Inhibition of microglial phagocytosis is sufficient to prevent inflammatory neuronal death. J Immunol. 2011;186(8):4973–83.

59. Brown GC, Neher JJ. Inflammatory neurodegeneration and mechanisms of microglial killing of neurons. Mol Neurbiol. 2010;41(2–3):242–7.

60. Galea I, Bechmann I, Perry VH. What is immune privilege (not)? Trends Immunol. 2007;28(1):12–8.

61. Sagare AP, et al. Pericyte loss influences Alzheimer-like neurodegeneration in mice. Nat Commun. 2013;4:2932.

62. Town T, et al. T-cells in Alzheimer's disease. NeuroMolecular Med. 2005;7(3):255–64.

63. Benveniste EN, Nguyen VT, O'Keefe GM. Immunological aspects of microglia: relevance to Alzheimer's disease. Neurochem Int. 2001;39(5):381–91.

64. Kreutzberg GW. Microglia: a sensor for pathological events in the CNS. Trends Neurosci. 1996;19(8):312–8.

65. Aloisi F, Ria F, Adorini L. Regulation of T-cell responses by CNS antigen-presenting cells: different roles for microglia and astrocytes. Immunol Today. 2000;21(3):141–7.

66. Gibbons HM, et al. Valproic acid induces microglial dysfunction, not apoptosis, in human glial cultures. Neurobiol Dis. 2011;41(1):96–103.

67. Zhang X-Z, Li X-J, Zhang H-Y. Valproic acid as a promising agent to combat Alzheimer's disease. Brain Red Bull. 2010;81(1):3–6.

68. Fleisher A, et al. Chronic divalproex sodium use and brain atrophy in Alzheimer disease. Neurology. 2011;77(13):1263–71.

69. Narayan PJ, et al. Increased acetyl and total histone levels in post-mortem Alzheimer's disease brain. Neurobiol Dis. 2015;74:281–94.

70. Jian W, et al. Histone deacetylase 1 activates PU. 1 gene transcription through regulating TAF9 deacetylation and geneion factor IID assembly. FASEB J. 2017; https://doi.org/10.1096/fj.201700022R.

71. VostatAD01, Clinical Trial to Determine Tolerable Dosis of Vorinostat in Patients With Mild Alzheimer Disease (VostatAD01). 2017, https://ClinicalTrials.gov/show/NCT03056495.

72. Hockly E, et al. Suberoylanilide hydroxamic acid, a histone deacetylase inhibitor, ameliorates motor deficits in a mouse model of Huntington's disease. PNAS. 2003;100(4):2041–6.

73. Palmieri D, et al. Vorinostat inhibits brain metastatic colonization in a model of triple-negative breast cancer and induces DNA double-strand breaks. Clin Cancer Res. 2009;15(19):6148–57.

74. Bubna AK. Vorinostat—An Overview. Indian J Dermatol. 2015;60(4):419.

75. Lloberas J, Soler C, Celada A. The key role of PU. 1/SPI-1 in B cells, myeloid cells and macrophages. Immunol Today. 1999;20(4):184–9.

76. Metcalf D, et al. Inactivation of PU. 1 in adult mice leads to the development of myeloid leukemia. PNAS. 2006;103(5):1486–91.

77. Rosenbauer F, et al. Acute myeloid leukemia induced by graded reduction of a lineage-specific geneion factor, PU. 1. Nat Genet. 2004;36(6):624.

78. Mootha VK, et al. PGC-1α-responsive genes involved in oxidative phosphorylation are coordinately downregulated in human diabetes. Nat Genet. 2003;34(3):267.

79. Subramanian A, et al. Gene set enrichment analysis: a knowledge-based approach for interpreting genome-wide expression profiles. PNAS. 2005;102(43):15545–50.

80. Zhang B, Kirov SA, Snoddy JR. WebGestalt: an integrated system for exploring gene sets in various biological contexts. Nucleic Acids Res. 2005;33(Web Server issue):W741–8.

81. Wang J, Duncan D, Shi Z, Zhang B. WEB-based GEne SeT AnaLysis Toolkit (WebGestalt): update 2013. Nucleic Acids Res. 2013;41(Web Server issue): W77–83.

82. Wang J, Vasaikar S, Shi Z, Greer M, Zhang B. WebGestalt 2017: a more comprehensive, powerful, flexible and interactive gene set enrichment analysis toolkit. Nucleic Acids Res. 2017;45(W1):W130–7.

3

Large-scale transcriptomic analysis reveals that pridopidine reverses aberrant gene expression and activates neuroprotective pathways in the YAC128 HD mouse

Rebecca Kusko[1†], Jennifer Dreymann[2†], Jermaine Ross[1], Yoonjeong Cha[1], Renan Escalante-Chong[1], Marta Garcia-Miralles[3], Liang Juin Tan[3], Michael E. Burczynski[2], Ben Zeskind[1], Daphna Laifenfeld[2], Mahmoud Pouladi[3,5], Michal Geva[2], Iris Grossman[2] and Michael R. Hayden[2,3,4,5*]

Abstract

Background: Huntington Disease (HD) is an incurable autosomal dominant neurodegenerative disorder driven by an expansion repeat giving rise to the mutant huntingtin protein (mHtt), which is known to disrupt a multitude of transcriptional pathways. Pridopidine, a small molecule in development for treatment of HD, has been shown to improve motor symptoms in HD patients. In HD animal models, pridopidine exerts neuroprotective effects and improves behavioral and motor functions. Pridopidine binds primarily to the sigma-1 receptor, (IC50 ~ 100 nM), which mediates its neuroprotective properties, such as rescue of spine density and aberrant calcium signaling in HD neuronal cultures. Pridopidine enhances brain-derived neurotrophic factor (BDNF) secretion, which is blocked by putative sigma-1 receptor antagonist NE-100, and was shown to upregulate transcription of genes in the BDNF, glucocorticoid receptor (GR), and dopamine D1 receptor (D1R) pathways in the rat striatum. The impact of different doses of pridopidine on gene expression and transcript splicing in HD across relevant brain regions was explored, utilizing the YAC128 HD mouse model, which carries the entire human mHtt gene containing 128 CAG repeats.

Methods: RNAseq was analyzed from striatum, cortex, and hippocampus of wild-type and YAC128 mice treated with vehicle, 10 mg/kg or 30 mg/kg pridopidine from the presymptomatic stage (1.5 months of age) until 11. 5 months of age in which mice exhibit progressive disease phenotypes.

Results: The most pronounced transcriptional effect of pridopidine at both doses was observed in the striatum with minimal effects in other regions. In addition, for the first time pridopidine was found to have a dose-dependent impact on alternative exon and junction usage, a regulatory mechanism known to be impaired in HD. In the striatum of YAC128 HD mice, pridopidine treatment initiation prior to symptomatic manifestation rescues the impaired expression of the BDNF, GR, D1R and cAMP pathways.

(Continued on next page)

* Correspondence: Michael.Hayden@teva.co.il; mrh@cmmt.ubc.ca
†Rebecca Kusko and Jennifer Dreymann contributed equally to this study.
[2]Research and Development, Teva Pharmaceutical Industries Ltd, Netanya, Israel
[3]Translational Laboratory in Genetic Medicine, Agency for Science, Technology and Research, Singapore (A*STAR), Singapore 138648, Singapore
Full list of author information is available at the end of the article

(Continued from previous page)

Conclusions: Pridopidine has broad effects on restoring transcriptomic disturbances in the striatum, particularly involving synaptic transmission and activating neuroprotective pathways that are disturbed in HD. Benefits of treatment initiation at early disease stages track with trends observed in the clinic.

Keywords: Huntington disease, Movement disorders, Neurodegeneration

Background

Huntington Disease (HD) is a progressive and neurological disorder caused by an autosomal dominant CAG trinucleotide expansion in the *Htt* gene [1], characterized by psychiatric, cognitive and motor disturbances, manifesting usually between 40 and 50 years of age and worsening until death [2]. Htt plays a role in facilitating axonal transport of brain-derived neurotrophic factor (BDNF) in the corticostriatal pathway of the motor circuit in wild-type animals (Fig. 1a and b) [3]. Consistently, in animal models of HD, mHtt disrupts several neuronal functions including corticostriatal communication [4] and cortical release of BDNF [5] (Fig. 1c). Breakdown of corticostriatal transmission reduces synaptic activity of striatal neurons [6] and influences downstream signal transduction within the striatum. In addition to the deficiencies in BDNF-TrkB signaling previously reported in mouse models of HD [7, 8], cyclic AMP (cAMP) signaling is disrupted in the striatum of presymptomatic R6/2 HD mice [9].

Pridopidine, a small molecule in development for the treatment of HD, improved motor function in HD patients in two large, double-blind, placebo-controlled studies (HART and MermaiHD) as exhibited by UHDRS–Total Motor Score (TMS), but did not meet primary endpoint of changes from baseline to week 12 in Modified Motor Score [10, 11]. Pridopidine is a high affinity sigma-1 receptor [12] ligand and exerts low-binding affinity towards additional CNS receptors, such as Dopamine D2, Adrenergic a2C, Serotonin 5HT-1A and Histamine H3 [13, 14]. Further, an in-vivo PET imaging study in rats confirmed that pridopidine occupies the sigma-1 receptor at low doses (3 and 15 mg/kg), and the D2R only at higher doses (60 mg/kg). Pridopidine normalizes endoplasmic reticulum (ER) calcium levels in YAC128 corticostriatal co-cultures [15], mediated by the sigma-1 receptor (Fig. 1d). The sigma-1 receptor also mediates pridopidine-induced BDNF in rat neuroblastoma cells [15]. In the striatum of R6/2 HD mice [16, 17], pridopidine treatment increases BDNF protein levels in the striatum (Fig. 1d). Finally, a gene expression analysis in WT rat striatum demonstrates pridopidine induces differential expression (DE) of genes enriched for the BDNF, D1R, and glucocorticoid receptor pathways, presumably mediated via sigma-1 receptor activation.

The effect of different doses of chronic pridopidine treatment, initiated at pre-symptomatic stages, on gene expression and transcript splicing in the context of HD was evaluated using single nucleotide resolution RNA sequencing in YAC128 mice, examining specificity of effects across brain regions.

Methods

Animals

YAC128 HD mice [18] (referred to herein as YAC128), maintained on the FVB/N strain were used. Mice were bred and housed according to Garcia-Miralles 2017 [19]. All mouse experiments were performed with the approval of and in accordance with the Institutional Animal Care and Use Committee at the Biomedical Sciences Institute at the Agency for Science, Technology and Research. Pridopidine synthesized by Teva Pharmaceutical Industries was dissolved in sterile water for oral administration. Pridopidine or vehicle was given every day by an oral gavage for 5 days/week for 10 months starting at a presymptomatic stage (1.5 months of age). Mice were split into three treatment groups: vehicle (sterile water), 10 mg/kg of pridopidine ("low dose"), or 30 mg/kg of pridopidine ("high dose").

A second group of WT mice (C57Bl6) were bred and housed at the Department of Experimental Medical Science of Lund University (Sweden), and treated with pridopidine 30 mg/kg for 10 days.

Sample preparation and RNA extraction

Mice were anaesthetised and perfused with ice-cold phosphate-buffered saline followed by ice-cold 4% paraformaldehyde in phosphate-buffered saline as described in Garcia-Miralles 2017 [19]. Brains were removed from YAC128 and WT, striatum, hippocampus, and cortex were frozen on dry ice, mounted with Tissue-TEK O.C.T. compound (Sakura, Torrance, CA, USA), and sliced coronally into 25-µm sections on a cryostat (Microm HM 525, Thermo Fisher Scientific, Waltham, Massachusetts, USA). The sections were collected and kept in RNAlater solution (Ambion, AM7021) overnight at 4 °C and then stored at − 80 °C until use. Total RNA was isolated by EA Genomics from tissue biopsies from mouse brain regions using the miRNeasy mini kit (Qiagen). RNA was also extracted from blood samples of the same mice using RNeasy Protect Animal Blood Kit EA. RNA integrity was assessed using an Agilent Bioanaylzer and only RNA samples with RIN scores

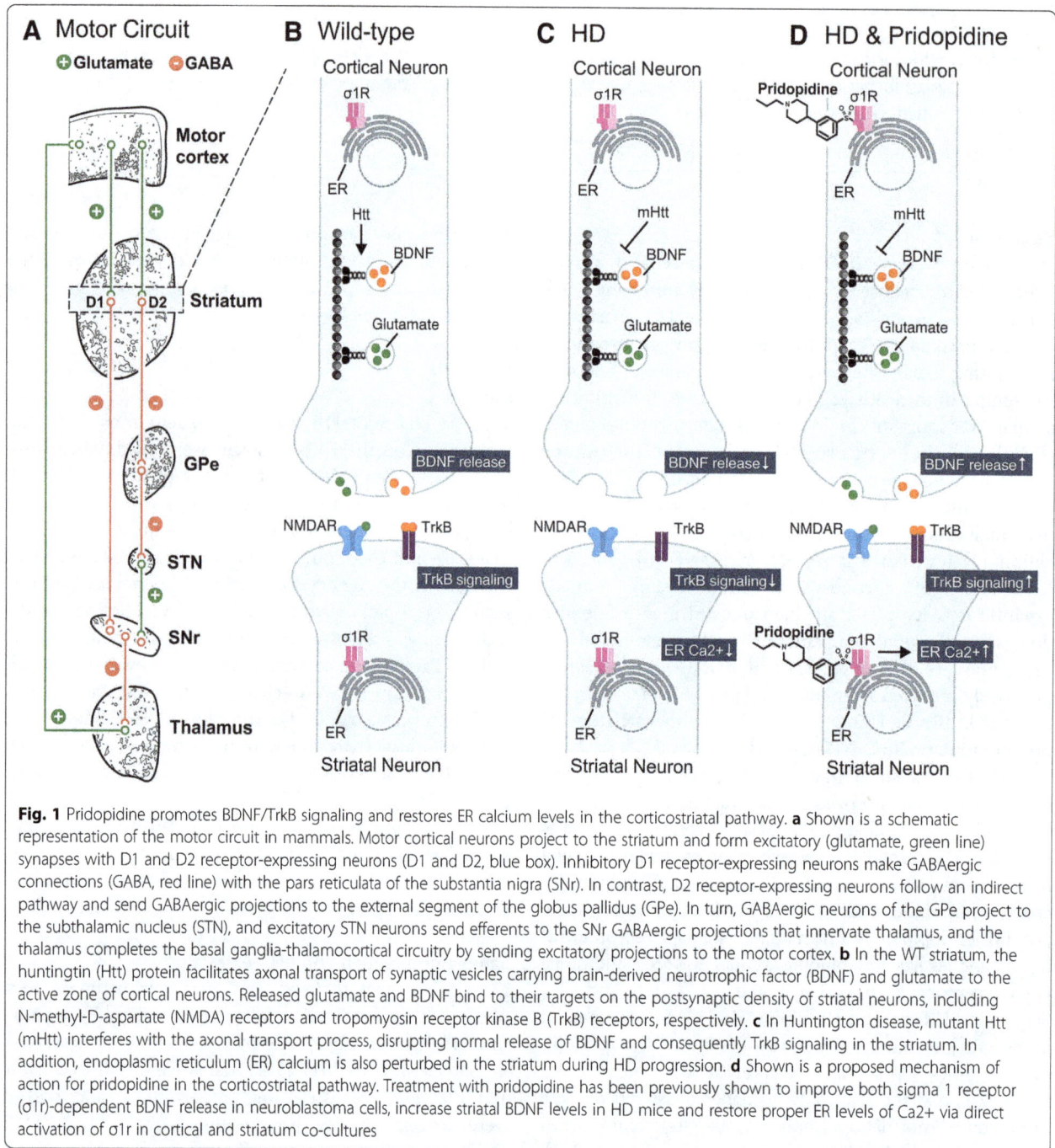

Fig. 1 Pridopidine promotes BDNF/TrkB signaling and restores ER calcium levels in the corticostriatal pathway. **a** Shown is a schematic representation of the motor circuit in mammals. Motor cortical neurons project to the striatum and form excitatory (glutamate, green line) synapses with D1 and D2 receptor-expressing neurons (D1 and D2, blue box). Inhibitory D1 receptor-expressing neurons make GABAergic connections (GABA, red line) with the pars reticulata of the substantia nigra (SNr). In contrast, D2 receptor-expressing neurons follow an indirect pathway and send GABAergic projections to the external segment of the globus pallidus (GPe). In turn, GABAergic neurons of the GPe project to the subthalamic nucleus (STN), and excitatory STN neurons send efferents to the SNr GABAergic projections that innervate thalamus, and the thalamus completes the basal ganglia-thalamocortical circuitry by sending excitatory projections to the motor cortex. **b** In the WT striatum, the huntingtin (Htt) protein facilitates axonal transport of synaptic vesicles carrying brain-derived neurotrophic factor (BDNF) and glutamate to the active zone of cortical neurons. Released glutamate and BDNF bind to their targets on the postsynaptic density of striatal neurons, including N-methyl-D-aspartate (NMDA) receptors and tropomyosin receptor kinase B (TrkB) receptors, respectively. **c** In Huntington disease, mutant Htt (mHtt) interferes with the axonal transport process, disrupting normal release of BDNF and consequently TrkB signaling in the striatum. In addition, endoplasmic reticulum (ER) calcium is also perturbed in the striatum during HD progression. **d** Shown is a proposed mechanism of action for pridopidine in the corticostriatal pathway. Treatment with pridopidine has been previously shown to improve both sigma 1 receptor (σ1r)-dependent BDNF release in neuroblastoma cells, increase striatal BDNF levels in HD mice and restore proper ER levels of Ca2+ via direct activation of σ1r in cortical and striatum co-cultures

>8 were used. RNA samples were quantified by NanoDrop for RNAseq.

RNA sequencing and mapping

EA Genomics performed the RNA sequencing on both mouse studies: 1. Striatum, hippocampus, and cortex of chronic pridopidine or vehicle treated YAC128 or WT mouse and 2. Blood from acute pridopidine treated WT mice. Sequencing was performed using the Illumina TruSeq Stranded mRNA Kit with HiSeq 2x50nt paired end sequencing. Star v.2.5.0a was used to align FASTQ files [20], using the GRCm38 primary assembly annotation and standard options. PCA plots of the samples were used to select outliers and to adjust for possible covariates. Transcripts that had less than 10 reads on average were filtered out. CalcNormFactors from the edgeR R package [21] was used to normalize the counts via the TMM method.

RNAseq analysis

Following the lead of MAQC [22], the limma v3.28.21 [23] R-package was used to transform and model the gene-level quantification data. Limma::voom was used to transform the count data to log2-counts per million and calculate the mean-variance relationship. Limma::lmFit was used to fit a linear model for each gene based on the experimental design matrix. Limma::eBayes was used to calculate the empirical Bayes moderated t-statistic for contrast significance. Multiple hypothesis adjusted p-values were calculated using limma::topTable, which implemented the Benjamini-Hochberg procedure to control FDR. In order to decrease the chance of finding a differential expression signature by chance, we utilized pvalue correction to adjust for the number of hypothesis (genes) we were testing Differential expression contrasts were independently calculated for all three tissues between: **A.** untreated YAC128 and untreated WT samples, **B.** 30 mg/kg pridopidine YAC128 and untreated YAC128 samples, **C.** 10 mg/kg pridopidine YAC128 and untreated YAC128 samples, **D.** 30 mg/kg pridopidine WT and untreated WT samples. In order to compare the magnitude of, and concordance between brain transcriptional signatures and peripheral blood profiles, indicative of the potential to develop biomarkers of disease and response to therapy, we examined samples obtained from a 10-day treatment study, contrasting 30 mg/kg pridopidine WT and untreated WT blood (**E.**).

To test whether the treatment gene expression signature is enriched for relevant pathways, Gene Set Enrichment Analysis (GSEA) [24] was used. All genes tested for differential expression were ranked by limma generated t-statistic for a given contrast. This was input as the "ranked list" in GSEA pre-ranked analysis. Moreover, gene sets were made from lists of differentially expressed genes from literature [25–27] in order to assess whether genes regulated by pridopidine enriched for genes downstream of Dopamine 1 Receptor, BDNF, and Glucocorticoid Receptor. In order to further filter before pathway analysis, we employ a strict version of what is recommended by MAQC, combining a fold change cutoff with an adjusted pvalue cutoff [28]. Hypothesis free broad pathway and transcription factor enrichment was done using Enrichr [29], selecting striatal differential expressed genes combining a fold change with a p-value cutoff according to MAQC guidance [28] (absolute linear fold change > 1.25 and adjusted p-value < 0.05). For all differential expression, splicing, pathway, and transcription factor analyses we consider "significant" to mean Adj. pval < 0.05 unless otherwise stated.

A signature of genes modulated in HD patient tissue was assembled through a meta-analysis of LIMMA results from two publicly available gene expression datasets from caudate nucleus of 48 total HD patients and 42 controls (GSE26927 and GSE3790). A signature of genes modulated in YAC128 striatum was assembled using LIMMA results from 9 YAC128 mice and 6 WT mice, aged 11.5 months. The HD and YAC128 disease signatures were queried against our expression signatures for pridopidine in striatum of YAC128 mice treated for 10 months at 10 or 30 mg/kg daily using cosine similarity of the moderated t-statistic to assess gene expression reversal.

Exon and splice junction analysis

Star aligned reads were processed using Quality of RNA-Seq Toolset (QoRTS) with the parameter –stranded. A flat annotation file for GRCm38.p4 was generated using QoRTs and used for subsequent analysis. Differential usage of exon and splice junction (DUEJ) analysis was performed using the JunctionSeq Bioconductor package. JunctionSeq uses a multivariate generalized linear model using a negative binomial distribution to detect exons and splice junctions whose expression changes between conditions relative to the expression of their respective genes. To determine differential usage of exons and splice junctions an adjusted p-value cutoff of 0.05 was used.

Results

Pridopidine induces striatal gene expression changes in YAC128 HD mice

In a previous study, behavioral and motor effects of pridopidine were evaluated longitudinally, demonstrating improvements in motor coordination, reduced anxiety and depressive like phenotypes, concordant with reversal of specific striatal transcriptional deficits [19]. Here, to characterize the underlying mechanisms, the effect of pridopidine on the YAC128 HD model, gene expression was assessed through the comparison of transcriptomic profiles in YAC128 mice treated with pridopidine (10 or 30 kg/mg, p.o.) or vehicle (5 days/week) and WT mice treated with 30 mg/kg of pridopidine or vehicle (5 days/week). In parallel with the previously described behavioral study [19], animals were treated starting at 1.5 months of postnatal life (presymptomatic) and sacrificed at 11.5 months of age (robust HD phenotype). Gene expression from the striatum, hippocampus, and cortex was evaluated using large RNAseq.

To further identify disease-specific gene expression patterns, vehicle-treated YAC128 mice were compared to vehicle-treated wild-type (WT) mice, demonstrating gene expression changes largely restricted to the striatum. We identified 1346 differentially expressed genes (DEGs) in the striatum (Adj. p-val < 0.05, Table 1) compared to 340 DEGs in the hippocampus and 7 DEGs in the cortex (Adj. p-val < 0.05, Table 1). Fold change and pvalue ranges are in Additional file 1: Table S1.

Table 1 Summary of genes with differential expression or alternative junction/exon usage

Number of Differentially Expressed Genes

Contrast	Striatum	Hippocampus	Cortex
YAC128 Veh-WT Veh	1346	340	7
YAC128 10 mg/kg-YAC128 Veh	73	0	0
YAC128 30 mg/kg-YAC128 Veh	221	0	0
WT 30 mg/kg-WT Veh	17	0	0
Number of Genes with Alternative Junction/Exon usage			
YAC128 Veh-WT Veh	39	14	4
YAC128 10 mg/kg-YAC128 Veh	1	0	0
YAC128 30 mg/kg-YAC128 Veh	565	1	4
WT 30 mg/kg-WT Veh	0	4	2

An Adj. p-val cutoff of 0.05 was used as pre-requisite criterion to identify differentially expressed genes (top) and alternative exon/junction usage cases (bottom) for each contrast and each tissue

To test if disease progression and/or pridopidine induced gene expression signatures can also be observed outside of the brain, and thus potentially produce biomarkers useful for therapeutic development and monitoring, transcriptomic signals were examined in blood from WT mice treated with pridopidine for 10 days. Only one gene was found to be significantly differentially expressed between 30 mg and vehicle treated mice (IL7R adj pval = 0.03, linear FC 2.11).

In the YAC128 HD model, a dose-dependent effect of pridopidine (vs vehicle) was observed in striatum (Adj. p-val < 0.05, Table 1): 10 mg/kg of pridopidine treatment induced significant differential expression of 73 genes, with 30 mg/kg pridopidine inducing roughly three times as many genes as the 10 mg dose (221 striatal DEGs, Adj. *p*-val < 0.05, Table 1, 55 genes overlap the two lists). No detectable differences in gene expression were observed in the YAC128 hippocampus or cortex after pridopidine treatment (Adj. *p*-val < 0.05, Table 1), suggesting that a robust pridopidine signature is brain compartment specific and not an off target effect. In WT mice, treatment with 30 mg/kg of pridopidine resulted in striatal differential expression of only 17 genes (Adj. *p*-val < 0.05, Table 1). Among these genes, four were also

described in a recent microarray study that identified 16 DEGs in the striatum of wild-type rats after treatment with pridopidine (60 mg/kg) [30]. The four overlapping genes are *Junb*, *Egr2*, *Nr4a1*, and *Per1*. With the exception of *Junb*, these genes are also downregulated in the YAC128 mouse model of HD. Taken together, the data demonstrate that the effect of pridopidine on gene expression is more pronounced in a disease model than in WT animals, and is primarily limited to the striatum.

Pridopidine reverses YAC128 HD mouse model and human HD disease gene expression signatures

We next quantified the extent to which the genes with expression modulated by 10 and 30 mg/kg of pridopidine reverse: 1) genes with expression modulated in HD patient tissue relative to healthy controls (from GSE26927 and GSE3790, described in methods), and 2) genes with expression modulated in YAC128 striatum compared to WT controls. In agreement with Garcia-Miralles 2017 [19], we observed that treatment with 10 and 30 mg/kg of pridopidine significantly reversed the YAC128 disease signature (Fig. 2, Table 2). Moreover, in this study, we additionally observe reversal of our HD patient signature (derived from GSE26927 and GSE3790). The results demonstrate the effectiveness of pridopidine to reverse genes modulated in human HD and the YAC128 mouse model of HD.

BDNF, GR, and D1R pathways are downregulated in HD [5, 9, 31], while pridopidine upregulates these pathways in WT rat striatum [30]. We investigated whether pridopidine upregulation of these pathways is recapitulated in WT and/or YAC128 mice. We performed Gene Set Enrichment Analysis (GSEA) using manually-curated BDNF, GR, and D1R gene sets. In YAC128 mice, we observed the expected reduction of the BDNF pathway via negative GSEA enrichment in the cortex and striatum, along with downregulation of the D1R pathway in the cortex (Adj. *p*-val < 0.05, Fig. 3). Consistent with previous reports, GSEA pathway analysis revealed positive enrichment of BDNF, GR, and D1R pathway genes in WT mouse striatum after 30 mg/kg pridopidine treatment (Adj. *p*-val < 0.05, Fig. 3). Enrichment analysis also confirmed upregulation of the BDNF pathways in the

Table 2 Pridopidine treatment signal significantly reverses YAC128 HD signal. Numbers shown are adjusted *p*-values from Gene Set Enrichment Analysis

Dose	Direction	Striatum	Hippocampus	Cortex
10 mg/kg	Up in YAC128, Down with pridopidine	3.58E-04	3.78E-04	2.40E-04
	Down in YAC128, Up with pridopidine	3.64E-04	4.99E-02	2.40E-04
30 mg/kg	Up in YAC128, Down with pridopidine	3.15E-04	3.46E-04	2.35E-04
	Down in YAC128, Up with pridopidine	3.37E-04	3.53E-03	2.35E-04

Reversal was significant for all doses of pridopidine across the striatum, hippocampus, and cortex of YAC128 mice

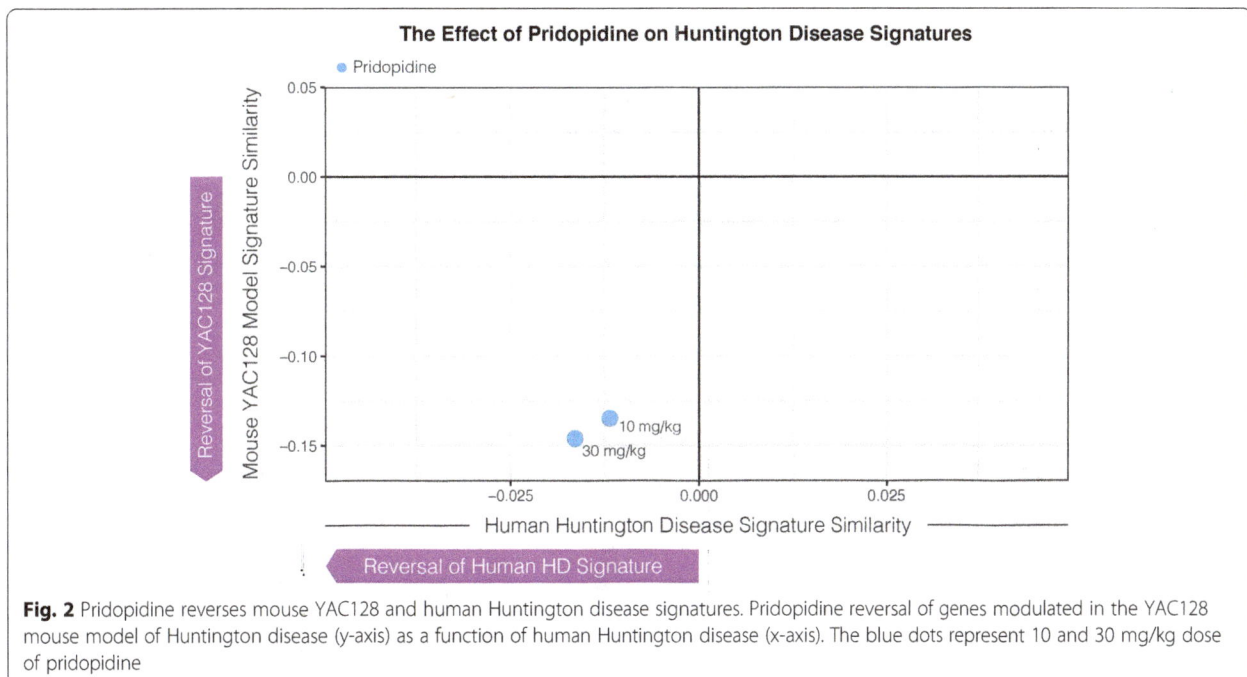

Fig. 2 Pridopidine reverses mouse YAC128 and human Huntington disease signatures. Pridopidine reversal of genes modulated in the YAC128 mouse model of Huntington disease (y-axis) as a function of human Huntington disease (x-axis). The blue dots represent 10 and 30 mg/kg dose of pridopidine

striatum, hippocampus, and cortex of YAC128 animals after treatment with either the 10 or 30 mg/kg dose of pridopidine (Adj. p-val < 0.05, Fig. 3). In addition, D1R and GR pathways were positively enriched across all three tissues after either 10 or 30 mg/kg treatment of pridopidine, with two exceptions: no significant enrichments were observed 1) for the GR pathway in the cortex after 10 mg/kg treatment; and 2) for the D1R pathway in the hippocampus after 30 mg/kg treatment.

Database-driven enrichment analysis reveals that pridopidine enhances relevant biological pathways altered in the YAC128 HD striatum

While GSEA provides a robust approach for pathway analysis, the method is limited to the manual curation of gene sets. To expand systematically our search for biological processes modulated by pridopidine, we next employed the enrichment tool Enrichr, which utilizes several comprehensive datasets including the Gene Ontology (GO) database. Our analysis focused on DEGs identified in the striatum, where the effect of pridopidine was most pronounced. Enrichment analysis was performed to identify pathways that are downregulated in vehicle-treated YAC128 and upregulated in pridopidine-treated YAC128 mice. Top 10 (of 63) downregulated pathways in the YAC128-vehicle mice (Adj. p-val < 0.05, Additional file 2: Table S2), include impaired synaptic transmission processes, MAP kinase activity, cAMP metabolism, and adenylate cyclase signaling, as well as response to amphetamine and cocaine (Adj. p-val < 0.05, Fig. 4).

Pridopidine treatment upregulated cAMP and kinase activity pathways impaired in the YAC128 striatum. Enrichment analysis revealed upregulation of enhanced biological pathways in the YAC128 striatum, with the cAMP response biological process showing a robust, statistically significant signal, ranking 1st after treatment with either the 10 or 30 mg/kg dose of pridopidine (Adj. p-val = 2.49E-09 and 2.53E-09 respectively, Fig. 4). For both doses of pridopidine, other highly ranked biological processes include negative regulation of kinase and phosphorylation (Adj. p-val < 0.05, Fig. 4 and Additional file 2: Table S2). In the YAC128 striatum, there were no significant GO enrichments using DEGs 1) upregulated after vehicle treatment, or 2) downregulated after pridopidine treatment. In wild-type mice, pridopidine induced enrichment of cAMP and p38-MAPK regulation pathways (Adj. p-val < 0.05, Fig. 4, Additional file 2: Table S2).

To identify enriched transcriptional factors (TFs) constituting upstream regulatory mechanisms, ENCODE and ChIP Enrichment Analysis (ChEA) databases were queried via Enrichr using DEGs that were: 1) downregulated in the YAC128 versus WT striatum, or 2) upregulated in the pridopidine treatment group. TF analysis of genes downregulated in YAC128 striatum revealed enrichment for gene targets of the transcription factor SUZ12 (Adj. p-val < 0.05, Additional file 3: Table S3). These enrichments are consistent with previous studies showing that SUZ12 is perturbed due to epigenetic dysregulation in HD [32].

TF analysis of DEGs upregulated in the pridopidine treatment group revealed CREB1 transcription factor as a highly significantly enriched gene set (10 and 30 mg/

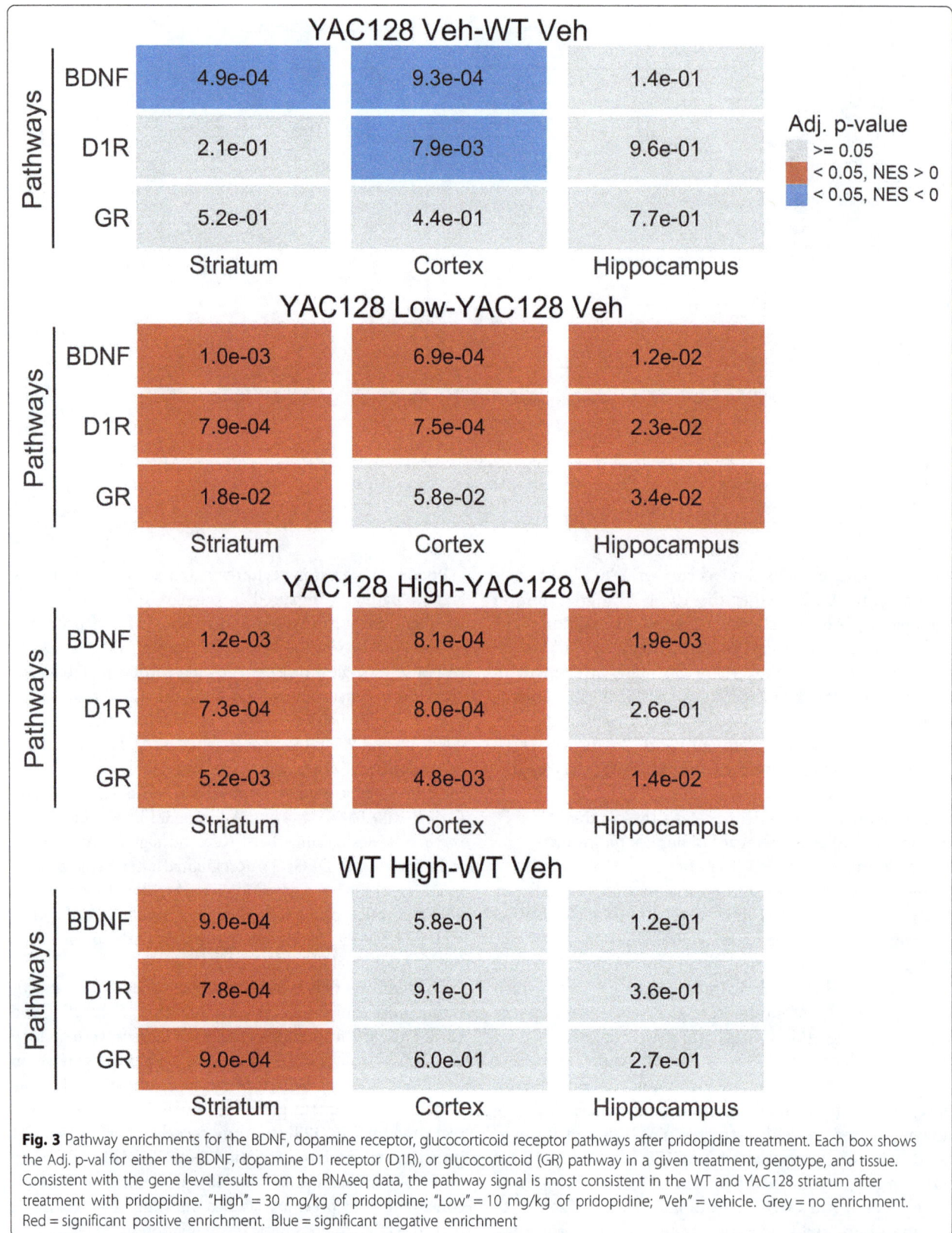

YAC128 Veh-WT Veh

	Striatum	Cortex	Hippocampus
BDNF	4.9e-04	9.3e-04	1.4e-01
D1R	2.1e-01	7.9e-03	9.6e-01
GR	5.2e-01	4.4e-01	7.7e-01

Pathways

Adj. p-value
- >= 0.05
- < 0.05, NES > 0
- < 0.05, NES < 0

YAC128 Low-YAC128 Veh

	Striatum	Cortex	Hippocampus
BDNF	1.0e-03	6.9e-04	1.2e-02
D1R	7.9e-04	7.5e-04	2.3e-02
GR	1.8e-02	5.8e-02	3.4e-02

Pathways

YAC128 High-YAC128 Veh

	Striatum	Cortex	Hippocampus
BDNF	1.2e-03	8.1e-04	1.9e-03
D1R	7.3e-04	8.0e-04	2.6e-01
GR	5.2e-03	4.8e-03	1.4e-02

Pathways

WT High-WT Veh

	Striatum	Cortex	Hippocampus
BDNF	9.0e-04	5.8e-01	1.2e-01
D1R	7.8e-04	9.1e-01	3.6e-01
GR	9.0e-04	6.0e-01	2.7e-01

Pathways

Fig. 3 Pathway enrichments for the BDNF, dopamine receptor, glucocorticoid receptor pathways after pridopidine treatment. Each box shows the Adj. p-val for either the BDNF, dopamine D1 receptor (D1R), or glucocorticoid (GR) pathway in a given treatment, genotype, and tissue. Consistent with the gene level results from the RNAseq data, the pathway signal is most consistent in the WT and YAC128 striatum after treatment with pridopidine. "High" = 30 mg/kg of pridopidine; "Low" = 10 mg/kg of pridopidine; "Veh" = vehicle. Grey = no enrichment. Red = significant positive enrichment. Blue = significant negative enrichment

Large-scale transcriptomic analysis reveals that pridopidine reverses aberrant gene expression and activates...

39

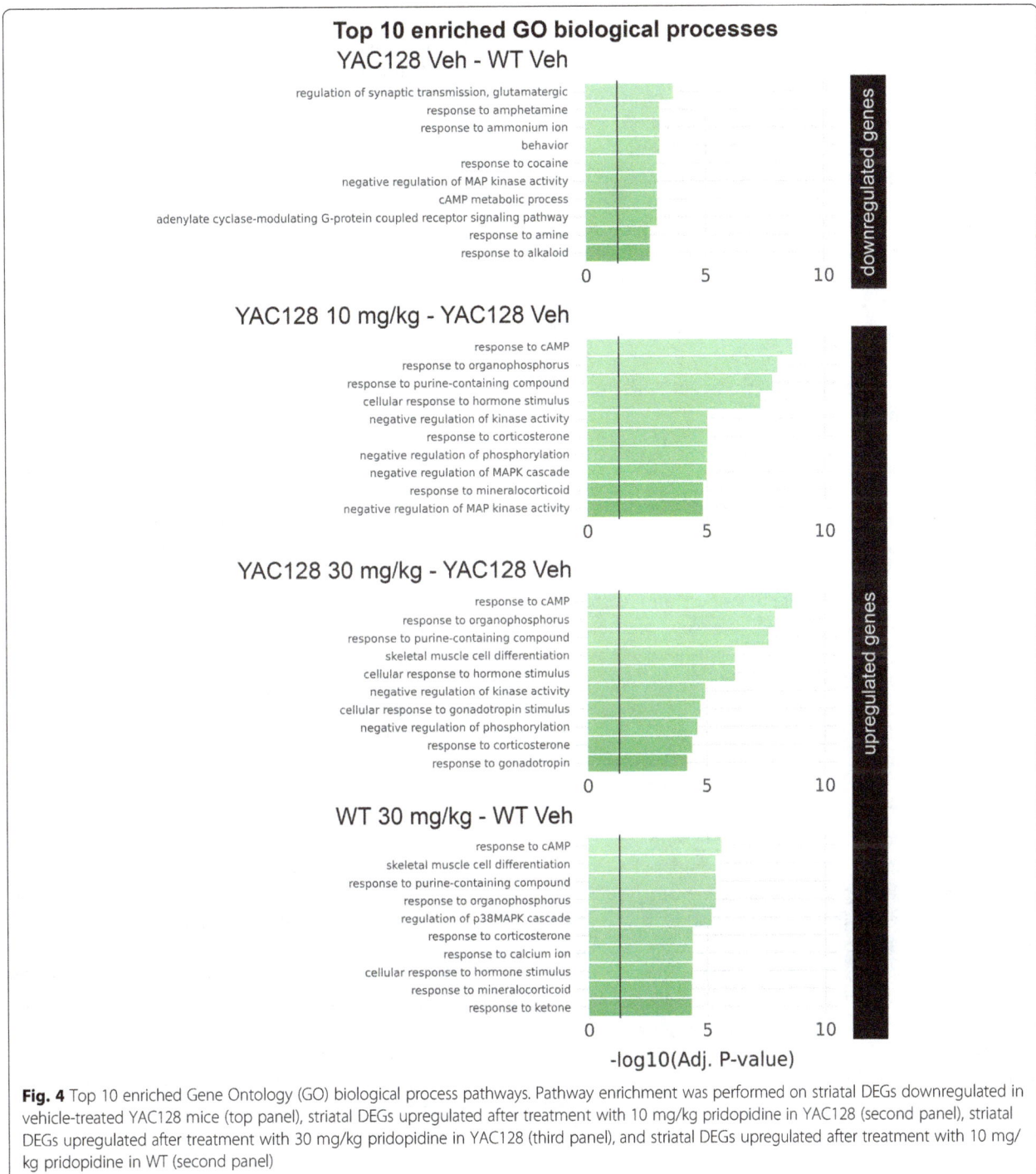

Fig. 4 Top 10 enriched Gene Ontology (GO) biological process pathways. Pathway enrichment was performed on striatal DEGs downregulated in vehicle-treated YAC128 mice (top panel), striatal DEGs upregulated after treatment with 10 mg/kg pridopidine in YAC128 (second panel), striatal DEGs upregulated after treatment with 30 mg/kg pridopidine in YAC128 (third panel), and striatal DEGs upregulated after treatment with 10 mg/kg pridopidine in WT (second panel)

kg) in the YAC128 striatum (Adj. p-val < 0.05, Additional file 3: Table S3). This is consistent with both disrupted CREB activity in HD [33] and the identification of up-regulation of cAMP-response genes after pridopidine treatment (Adj. p-val < 0.05, see Additional file 2: Table S2). CREB1 gene set was also enriched after 30 mg/kg pridopidine treatment in WT striatum (Adj. *p*-val < 0.05, Additional file 3: Table S3). Taken together, these

observations suggest that pridopidine treatment may induce gene expression regulated via the CREB transcriptional pathway, known to be disrupted in HD.

Pridopidine reverses compromised cAMP response gene activity in the YAC128 HD striatum

In YAC128 striatum, pridopidine enrichment of cAMP response is composed of 8 upregulated genes (*Dusp1,*

Egr1, Egr2, Egr4, Fos, Fosb, Fosl2, and *Junb*) after treatment with 10 mg/kg of pridopidine, and 9 upregulated genes (*Dusp1, Egr1, Egr2, Egr3, Egr4, Fos, Fosb, Fosl2,* and *Junb*) after treatment with 30 mg/kg of pridopidine (Adj. p-val < 0.05, Figs. 5 and 6). In addition, we also identified another cAMP-regulated gene, *Rgs2* [34], upregulated after pridopidine treatment (Fig. 6). Five of these genes (*Dusp1, Egr1, Egr2, Fosl2, and Rgs2*) are downregulated in the striatum of vehicle-treated YAC128 mice (Adj. p-val < 0.05, Fig. 5, Additional file 4: Table S4). qPCR confirmed pridopidine reversed the expression of *Dusp1,* and *Egr2,* and *Fosl2* (Adj. p-val < 0.05, Fig. 5 and Additional file 4: Table S4).

Pridopidine modulates exon and transcript junction in the striatum of HD mice

Alternative splicing represents a key transcriptomic regulatory mechanism required for many basic cellular functions. Recent evidence suggests alternative splicing may be perturbed in HD. To determine if alternative splicing also occurs in YAC128 mice, we performed differential usage of exon and splice junction (DUEJ) analysis in the striatum, hippocampus, and cortex. In YAC128 mice compared to WT controls, we observed 39, 14, and 4 DUEJs in striatal, hippocampal, and cortical genes, respectively (all Adj. p-val < 0.05, Table 1). In concordance with gene level differential expression, the majority of DUEJ occurred in the striatum.

We then examined whether treatment with pridopidine compared to vehicle induces DUEJ in the brains of WT and YAC128 mice. In the YAC128 striatum, pridopidine induced dose-dependent DUEJ, with 565 genes significant in the 30 mg/kg group compared to only a single gene in 10 mg/kg pridopidine-group (both Adj. p-val < 0.05, Table 1). In WT mice, treatment with pridopidine did not lead to any DUEJ differences in striatum (all Adj. p-val < 0.05, Table 1). Eleven genes (*Kifap3, Zwint, Cltc, Rtn1, Acin1, Ano3, Dclk1, Ppp3ca, Atp2b2, Arpp19,* and *Arpp21*) demonstrated significant DUEJ and reversal after 30 mg/kg pridopidine treatment in the YAC128 striatum (Adj. *p*-val < 0.05). Pridopidine induced minimal to no DUEJ changes in hippocampus and cortex (Table 1). These results are consistent with the dose-dependent effect of pridopidine on gene expression restricted to the YAC128 striatum.

Pathway analysis on the 565 genes demonstrating DUEJ after 30 mg/kg pridopidine treatment in YAC128 mice showed enrichments for pathways previously described to be involved in pridopidine's mechanism of action such as calcium regulation (adj.pval = 3.6E-06), and Synaptic Vesicle (3.4E-06). Additional pathways of interest previously reported as part of pridopidine's mechanism of action include: BDNF signaling and G protein signaling, (Adj. *p*-val < 0.05, Fig. 7a, b and

Additional file 5: Table S5). Taken together, these results demonstrate that the 30 mg/kg of pridopidine induces exon and junction level changes in pathways that are relevant to HD pathology.

Discussion

It has recently been demonstrated that 30 mg/kg of pridopidine rescues motor behavioral deficits in YAC128 mouse model of HD [19]. To identify potential mechanisms by which pridopidine confers motor benefits, this study focuses on pridopidine induced changes in transcription across multiple brain regions and dose regimens. To characterize the functional relevance of transcriptomic changes, RNAseq data was analyzed for expression signaling, as well as splice variant modifications in pre-specified pathways, as well as across the genome unbiasedly. Testing was performed on WT and YAC128 striatum, cortex, and hippocampus after treatment with vehicle, 10 or 30 mg/kg pridopidine from a presymptomatic stage through disease progression. Both doses of pridopidine had a significant effect on gene and transcript levels in the striatum, with modest to unobserved effects in the cortex and hippocampus. However, the transcriptional effect of pridopidine in YAC128 striatum is dose-dependent. The two doses tested herein suggest linearity of the effect, which future studies employing additional doses will serve to shed further light on. While this study cannot directly query whether pridopidine's behavioral benefits are transcriptionally mediated, the fact that pridopidine's main transcriptomic effect is detected in the striatum supports this hypothesis. Moreover, the dose dependent functional expression signals induced by pridopidine track well with the dose-dependent behavioral benefits induced it induces at parallel experimental conditions (Garcia-Miralles et al., 2017). Lastly, genes with perturbed expression in YAC128 pathology are oppositely modulated by pridopidine in the striatum, far more so than expected by chance.

The transcriptional footprint of pridopidine demonstrates a reversal of the disease-specific gene expression and alternative splicing. The disease mechanisms reversed by pridopidine include critical neuroprotective pathways such as BDNF, D1R and glucocorticoid pathways previously reported. qPCR confirmed differential expression of many genes in these pathways. In addition, pridopidine induced gene expression triggered by cAMP transduction, also supported by modulation of downstream transcription factors (e.g. CREB1). Together, these findings provide robust data to demonstrate pridopidine restores mechanisms impaired in HD, specifically in the striatum.

Previous studies reported rescue of several aspects of HD, including phenotype and behavior, in the YAC128 mouse

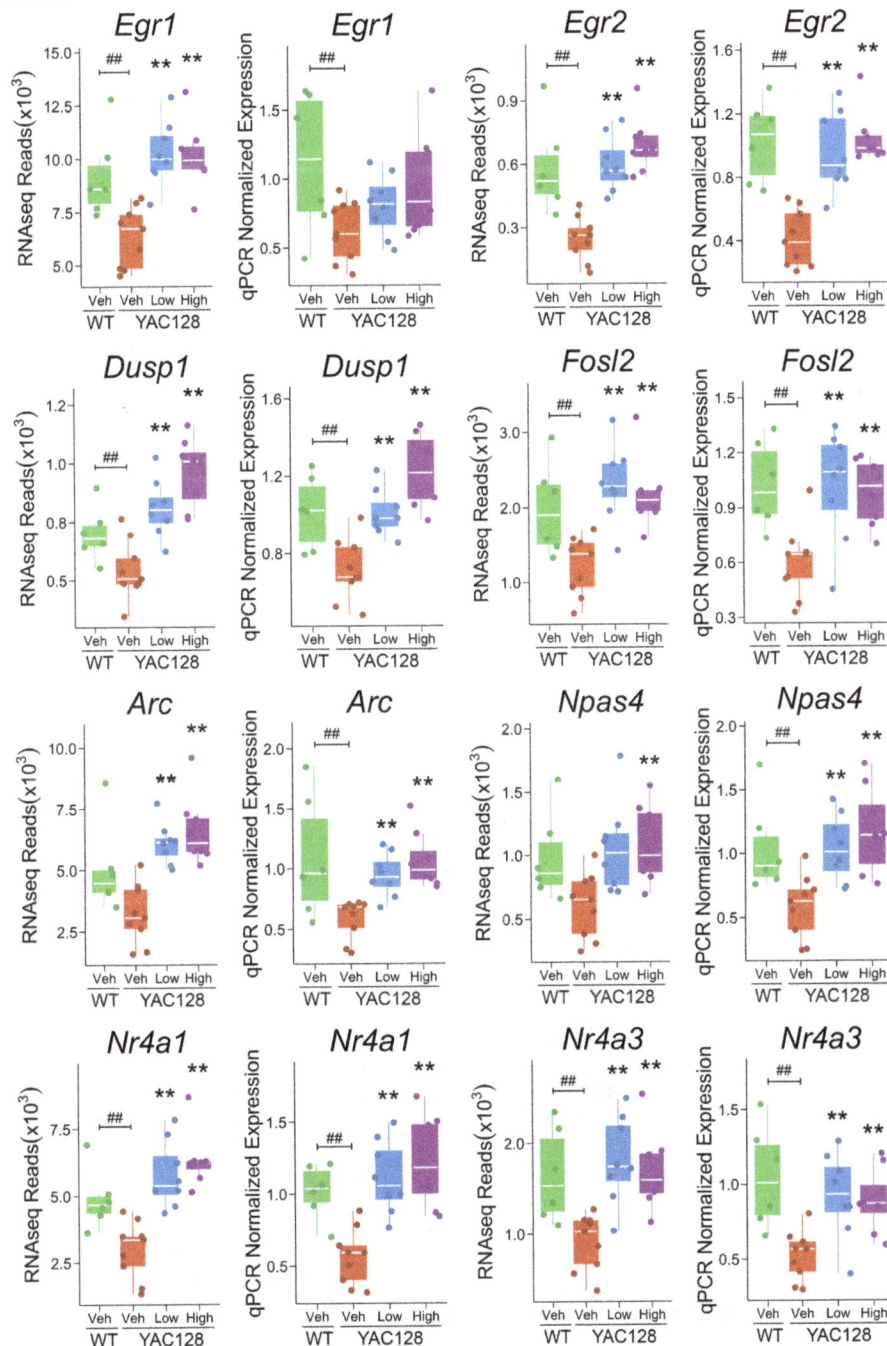

Fig. 5 qPCR validation of differential expression of striatal genes in YAC128 mice. Shown are RNAseq and qPCR results for genes differentially expressed in the striatum of YAC128 mice after pridopidine treatment. "**" and "##" represent significant (Adj. p-val < 0.05) differential expression in YAC128 Veh-WT Veh and YAC128 Low/High-YAC128 Veh contrasts, respectively. "High" = 30 mg/kg of pridopidine; "Low" = 10 mg/kg of pridopidine; "Veh" = vehicle

through BDNF overexpression [35]. Dexamethasone, a glucocorticoid that activates the GR pathway, also dampens disease progression in a HD animal model [36]. Both 10 and 30 mg/kg pridopidine treatment in YAC128 mice significantly induced the BDNF, GR and D1R pathways in the striatum, hippocampus, and cortex, consistent with prior reports in WT rat [30]. As pridopidine does not directly bind GR (internal data, not shown), it suggests that the upregulation of the GR pathway may be indirect. Pridopidine increases dopamine efflux in the striatum [37], which may explain the observed upregulation of expression for D1R pathway genes after pridopidine treatment.

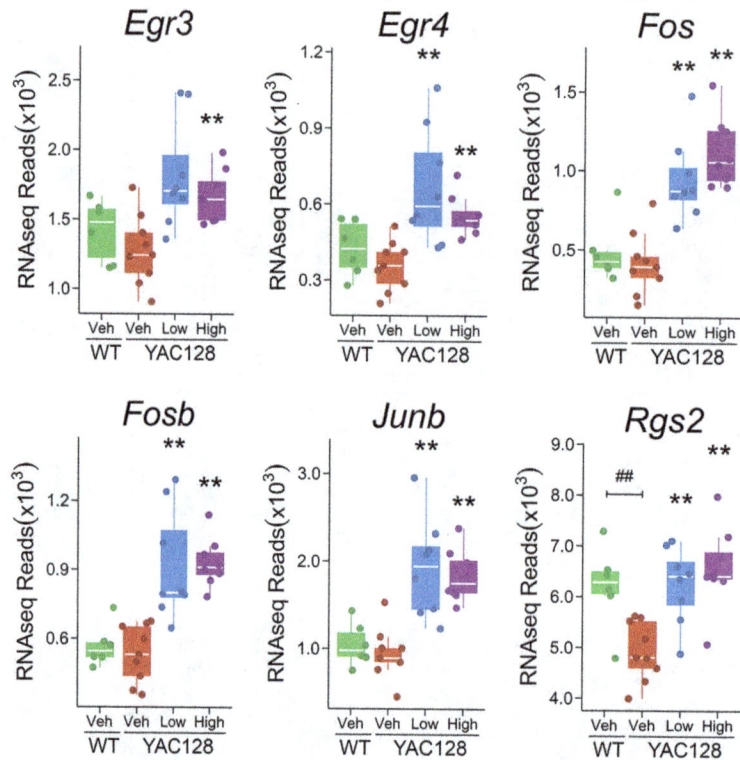

Fig. 6 RNAseq differential expression analysis of cAMP-related genes in the YAC128 striatum. Shown are RNAseq results for differentially expressed genes in the YAC128 striatum after pridopidine treatment. "**" and "##" represent significant (Adj. p-val < 0.05) differential expression in YAC128 Veh-WT Veh and YAC128 Low/High-YAC128 Veh contrasts, respectively. "High" = 30 mg/kg of pridopidine; "Low" = 10 mg/kg of pridopidine; "Veh" = vehicle

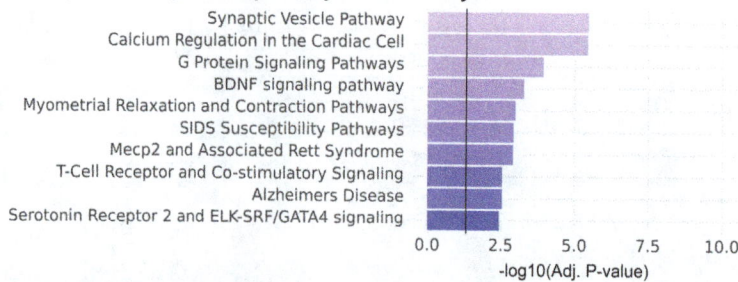
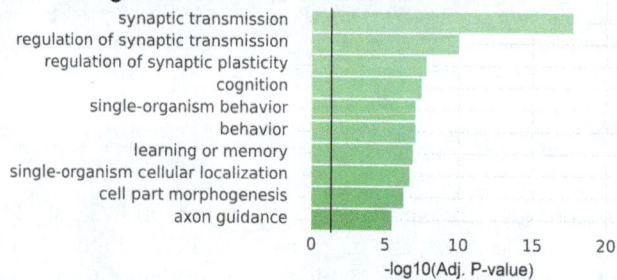

Fig. 7 Pathway and differential exon/splice junction analysis in the YAC128 striatum after pridopidine treatment. Pathway analysis was performed on genes that demonstrated pridopidine induced alternative exon/junction usage at a high dose (30 mg/kg). **a** Top 10 significant (Adj. p-val < 0.05) pathways from the WikiPathway database. **b** Top 10 significant (Adj. p-val < 0.05) pathways from the Gene Ontology (GO) pathway database

In the WT striatum, dopamine is a central regulator of cAMP activity in both D1 and D2 receptor-expressing neurons, namely, medium spiny neurons, where D1Rs and D2Rs have opposing effects on cAMP levels [38]. Previous studies of HD postmortem brain tissue and animal models have shown that cAMP signaling becomes deregulated in the striatum of humans and animal HD models [9, 39, 40]. Restoration of cAMP levels reduced mHtt aggregates in the striatum of R6/2 HD mice [40], underscoring the importance of rescuing striatal cAMP signaling. In the YAC128 striatum, we observed downregulation of cAMP pathway genes, which are upregulated after treatment with pridopidine (Figs. 5, 6, and 8).

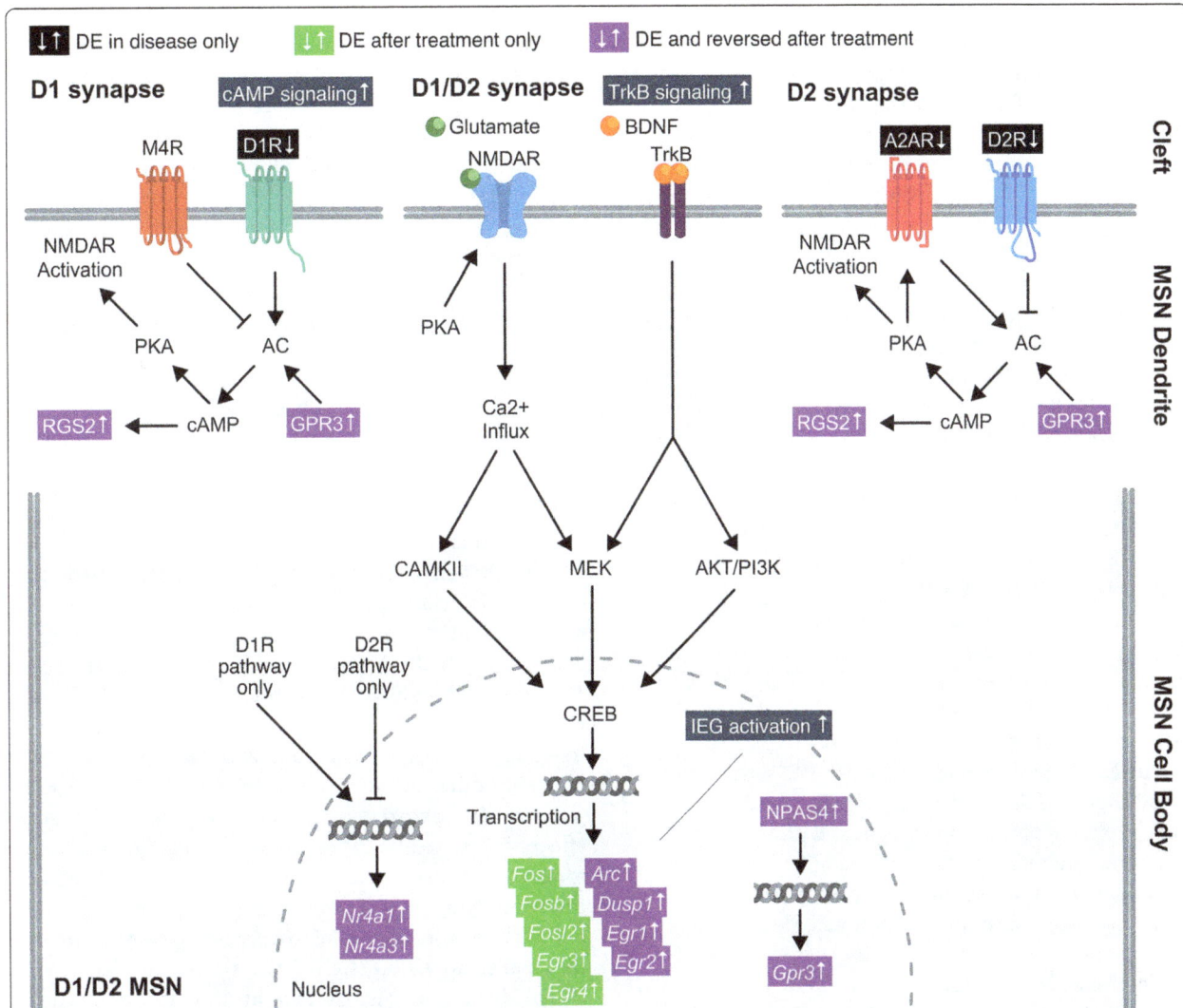

Fig. 8 Pridopidine enhances cAMP/PKA and TrkB pathway genes in the YAC128 striatum. Shown is a model of gene regulation after treatment with pridopidine in the YAC128 striatum. Dopamine transmission directs the activation of dopamine D1 and D2 receptors (D1R and D2R, respectively) in medium spiny neurons (MSNs) of the striatum. On the WT postsynaptic density of a D1 synapse, D1Rs activate adenylyl cyclase (AC) in MSNs, whereas muscarinic acetylcholine receptor M4 (M4R) inhibits AC activity. In contrast, D2Rs negatively regulate AC in MSNs, while A2ARs are AC agonists. GPR3 activates AC in both D1R and D2R-expressing MSNs, where RGS2 is a target of cAMP signaling. Activation of AC is upstream of cAMP and PKA, which augments NMDAR activity. Dopamine D1 and D2 receptor genes (*Drd1* and *Drd2*) and A2AR gene (*Adora2a*) are differentially expressed (DE) and downregulated in the YAC128 striatum, but unchanged after pridopidine treatment (black highlighting). Both *Rgs2* and *Gpr3* are downregulated in YAC128 striatum (Adj. p-val < 0.05) and upregulated after treatment of pridopidine. NMDARs and TrkB receptors are expressed in both D1R and D2R-expression MSNs. NMDAR and TrkB receptors both indirectly activate the transcription factor (TF) CREB in the nucleus via downstream pathways. In turn, CREB activates gene expression of several targets. Genes *Arc*, *Dusp1*, *Egr1* and *Egr2* are downregulated in the YAC128 striatum, but upregulated after pridopidine treatment (Adj. p-val < 0.05). *Fos*, *Fosb*, *Fosl2*, *Egr3*, and *Egr4* are unperturbed in the striatum of YAC128 mice, but expression of these genes is restored after treatment with pridopidine (Adj. *p*-val < 0.05). Dopamine pathway genes *Nr4a1* and *Nr4a3* and TF gene *Npas4* are downregulated in YAC128 and upregulated after pridopidine treatment (Adj. *p*-val < 0.05). NPAS4 regulates *Gpr3* gene expression

In agreement with Garcia-Miralles et al. [19], we noted reversal of compromised expression of dopamine receptor genes (*Drd1* and *Drd2*) after pridopidine treatment in the YAC128 striatum. However, reversal of *Drd1* and *Drd2* expression was only nominally significant after treatment with either the 10 or 30 mg/kg dose of pridopidine [19]. Therefore, pridopidine could partly restore dopamine-cAMP signaling via compensatory mechanisms. One possibility is that pridopidine induces post-translational regulation of the D1R protein. PSD-95 has been shown to increase D1R surface level expression [41], regulate D1R internalization, and D1R-cAMP signaling [42, 43]. In the striatum, wild-type HTT binds to postsynaptic density protein 95 and promotes its clustering (PSD-95) [42, 44], whereas mHTT lacks binding affinity to PSD-95 [44]. In agreement with increased D1R activity, compromised expression of D1R-regulated genes *Nr4a1* and *Nr4a3* is rescued after treatment with either 10 or 30 mg/kg pridopidine in the YAC128 striatum (Adj. p-val < 0.05, Fig. 5).

In addition to dopamine signaling, other signal transduction pathways regulate cAMP response targets, which may also explain the putative effect of pridopidine on cAMP signaling. For example, we identified two additional cAMP-related DEGs (*Npas4* and *Gpr3*) upregulated after treatment with pridopidine in the YAC128 striatum (Additional file 6: Figure S1). Activity-dependent NPAS4 has been shown to upregulate both *BDNF* and *Gpr3* expression in cultured excitatory and inhibitory neurons, respectively [45]. GPR3 is a constitutive activator of cAMP signaling via adenylyl cyclase (AC) [46, 47]. Interestingly, *Npas4* gene expression is compromised in the YAC128 striatum, but rescued after pridopidine treatment with either dose (10 or 30 mg/kg, Adj. p-val < 0.05, Fig. 5). In addition, *Gpr3* gene expression is downregulated in the YAC128 striatum, whereas striatal expression of *Gpr3* is upregulated after either 10 or 30 mg/kg pridopidine treatment in YAC128 mice (Additional file 5: Figure S5, Adj. p-val < 0.05). Taken together, this suggests that pridopidine could partly rescue dysregulated cAMP signaling by modulating *Npas4* and *Gpr3* gene expression. In addition to the GPR3-cAMP pathway, BDNF-TrkB signaling has also been shown to activate cAMP response element binding (CREB) protein activity and thus facilitate gene expression in cultured striatal neurons [26]. In other words, pridopidine may induce transcription by binding to S1R, which leads to enhanced BDNF activity, in turn activating gene and splice-variant expression. This alternative mechanism is also supported by the fact that pridopidine induces BDNF release in neuroblastoma cells [30].

Recently, it was demonstrated that treatment with 30 mg/kg of pridopidine rescues motor deficiencies in YAC128 mice, whereas no effect was detected in YAC128 animals treated with 10 mg/kg of pridopidine [19]. In agreement with this observation, we report a broader effect of 30 mg/kg pridopidine on gene expression in the YAC128 striatum compared to the 10 mg/kg dose, but also report that either dose reverses disease associated gene expression. The effect of 30 mg/kg pridopidine on motor function diminishes during the progression of the disease [19], and the lowest locomotor performance is observed between 10 and 12 months of age when mice are very ill. Given that RNA samples for this study were collected during the decline of motor activity in 30 mg/kg pridopidine-treated YAC128 mice, it is difficult to correlate improvement in motor deficit and pridopidine-induced gene expression in the striatum of YAC128 animals. Moreover, our study showed that pridopidine induces a robust gene expression signal when treatment begins early in disease course. This may suggest that in humans, pridopidine may be more effective if started in early disease stages. For both of these reasons, a longitudinal study with earlier time points would better illuminate the link between gene expression and motor behavior after treatment with pridopidine in YAC128 mice.

Conclusions

In conclusion, pridopidine reverses HD associated changes in transcription at the pathway, gene and splice-variant level. Pathways with transcriptomic aberrations in the YAC128 mouse that are restored to WT levels by pridopidine treatment include BDNF, D1R, GR, cAMP, and calcium signaling. These pathways together are known to interact, and likely positively feed into each other downstream of pridopidine treatment, to relieve HD associated motor symptoms. Beneficial effects when treatment is initiated early, before symptoms are manifest, tracks with trends observed in clinical trials. Studying the effect of pridopidine at multiple time points over the course of treatment against transcriptomic aberrations in YAC128 will reveal additional regulatory dynamics. The results in this study, all taken together, support exploring pridopidine's role as a therapeutic for neuroprotection in HD and similar neurological movement disorders.

Additional files

Additional file 1: Table S1. Adjusted p-val range and fold change range for differential expression and DUEJ genes meeting adj p-val < 0.05 cutoff.

Additional file 2: Table S2. Gene Ontology pathway analysis of genes differentially expressed in the mouse striatum.

Additional file 3: Table S3. Transcription factor enrichment analysis of genes differentially expressed in the mouse striatum.

Additional file 4: Table S4. qPCR validation of striatal gene expression identified in RNAseq and pathway analysis.

Additional file 5: Table S5. Pathway analysis of alternatively spliced genes identified after high dose treatment with pridopidine.

Additional file 6: Figure S1. Pridopidine reverses downregulation of *G Protein-Coupled Receptor 3* (*Gpr3*) gene expression in the striatum of YAC128 mice. Shown are RNAseq results for Gpr3 in the YAC128 striatum after pridopidine treatment. "**" and "##" represent significant (Adj. p-val < 0.05) differential expression in YAC128 Veh-WT Veh and YAC128 Low/ High-YAC128 Veh contrasts, respectively. "High" = 30 mg/kg of pridopidine; "Low" = 10 mg/kg of pridopidine; "Veh" = vehicle.

Abbreviations

AC: Adenylyl cyclase; BDNF: Brain-derived neurotrophic factor; cAMP: Cyclic AMP; ChEA: ChIP Enrichment Analysis; CREB: cAMP response element binding; D1R: Dopamine D1 receptor; DE: Differential expression; DUEJ: Differential usage of exon and splice junction; ER: Endoplasmic reticulum; GO: Gene ontology; GPe: External segment of the globus pallidus; Gpr3: G protein-coupled receptor 3; GR: Glucocorticoid receptor; GSEA: Gene set enrichment analysis; HD: Huntington disease; Htt: Huntingtin; M4R: Muscarinic acetylcholine receptor M4; MAQC: MicroArray quality control; mHtt: Mutant Htt; MSNs: Medium spiny neurons; NMDA: N-methyl-D-aspartate; QoRTs: Quality of RNA-Seq toolset; SNr: Pars reticulata of the substantia nigra; STN: Subthalamic nucleus; TF: Transcriptional factors; TMS: Total Motor Score; TrkB: Tropomyosin receptor kinase B; WT: Wild-type; σ1r: Sigma-1 receptor

Funding

Teva Pharmaceuticals provided funding for the study.

Authors' contributions

All authors discussed the results and contributed to the manuscript. RK, JD, MG, MP, DL, MGM, LJT, MEB, and MRH designed the study and participated in its design and coordination. RK, JR, YC, and REC processed and analyzed gene expression data. RK, JD, JR, MG, DL, IG, MEB, MP, BZ, and MRH drafted and revised the manuscript. All authors read and approved the final manuscript.

Authors' information

Information for all the co-authors is listed in the title page.

Ethics approval

All mouse experiments were performed with the approval of and in accordance with the Institutional Animal Care and Use Committee at the Biomedical Sciences Institute at the Agency for Science, Technology and Research.

Competing interests

RK, JR, YC, REC, BZ are employees of Immuneering Corporation. JD, MEB, DL, MG, IG, and MRH are employees of Teva Pharmaceutical. Teva Pharmaceuticals played no role in the treatment or testing of animals, or the collection, or analysis of the results.

Author details

[1]Immuneering Corporation, Cambridge, MA 02142, USA. [2]Research and Development, Teva Pharmaceutical Industries Ltd, Netanya, Israel. [3]Translational Laboratory in Genetic Medicine, Agency for Science, Technology and Research, Singapore (A*STAR), Singapore 138648, Singapore. [4]Centre for Molecular Medicine and Therapeutics, Child and Family Research Institute, University of British Columbia, Vancouver, BC V5Z 4H4, Canada.

[5]Department of Medicine, Yong Loo Lin School of Medicine, National University of Singapore, Singapore 117597, Singapore.

References

1. Macdonald M. A novel gene containing a trinucleotide repeat that is expanded and unstable on Huntington's disease chromosomes. Cell. 1993; 72:971–83.
2. Foroud T, Gray J, Ivashina J, Conneally PM. Differences in duration of Huntington's disease based on age at onset. J Neurol Neurosurg Psychiatry. 1999;66:52–6.
3. Colin E, Zala D, Liot G, Rangone H, Borrell-Pagès M, Li X-J, et al. Huntingtin phosphorylation acts as a molecular switch for anterograde/retrograde transport in neurons. EMBO J. 2008;27:2124–34.
4. Miller BR, Bezprozvanny I. Corticostriatal circuit dysfunction in Huntington's disease: intersection of glutamate, dopamine and calcium. Future Neurol. 2010;5:735–56.
5. Gauthier LR, Charrin BC, Borrell-Pagès M, Dompierre JP, Rangone H, Cordelières FP, et al. Huntingtin controls neurotrophic support and survival of neurons by enhancing BDNF vesicular transport along microtubules. Cell. 2004;118:127–38.
6. André VM, Fisher YE, Levine MS. Altered balance of activity in the striatal direct and indirect pathways in mouse models of Huntington's disease. Front Syst Neurosci. 2011;5:46.
7. Plotkin JL, Day M, Peterson JD, Xie Z, Kress GJ, Rafalovich I, et al. Impaired TrkB receptor signaling underlies corticostriatal dysfunction in Huntington's disease. Neuron. 2014;83:178–88.
8. Nguyen KQ, Rymar VV, Sadikot AF. Impaired TrkB signaling underlies reduced BDNF-mediated trophic support of striatal neurons in the R6/2 mouse model of Huntington's disease. Front Cell Neurosci. 2016;10:37.
9. Bibb JA, Yan Z, Svenningsson P, Snyder GL, Pieribone VA, Horiuchi A, et al. Severe deficiencies in dopamine signaling in presymptomatic Huntington's disease mice. Proc Natl Acad Sci U S A. 2000;97:6809–14.
10. de Yebenes JG, Landwehrmeyer B, Squitieri F, Reilmann R, Rosser A, Barker RA, et al. Pridopidine for the treatment of motor function in patients with Huntington's disease (MermaiHD): a phase 3, randomised, double-blind, placebo-controlled trial. Lancet Neurol. 2011;10:1049–57.
11. The Huntington Study Group HART Investigators. A randomized, double-blind, placebo-controlled trial of pridopidine in Huntington's disease. Mov Disord. 2013;28:1407–15.
12. Sahlholm K, Sijbesma JWA, Maas B, Kwizera C, Marcellino D, Ramakrishnan NK, et al. Pridopidine selectively occupies sigma-1 rather than dopamine D2 receptors at behaviorally active doses. Psychopharmacology. 2015;232:3443–53.
13. Ponten H, Kullingsjö J, Sonesson C, Waters S, Waters N, Tedroff J. The dopaminergic stabilizer pridopidine decreases expression of L-DOPA-induced locomotor sensitisation in the rat unilateral 6-OHDA model. Eur J Pharmacol. 2013;698:278–85.
14. Dyhring T, Nielsen EØ, Sonesson C, Pettersson F, Karlsson J, Svensson P, et al. The dopaminergic stabilizers pridopidine (ACR16) and (−)-OSU6162 display dopamine D2 receptor antagonism and fast receptor dissociation properties. Eur J Pharmacol. 2010;628:19–26.
15. Ryskamp D, Wu J, Geva M, Kusko R, Grossman I, Hayden M, et al. The sigma-1 receptor mediates the beneficial effects of pridopidine in a mouse model of Huntington disease. Neurobiol Dis. 2017;97:46–59.
16. Squitieri F, Di Pardo A, Favellato M, Amico E, Maglione V, Frati L. Pridopidine, a dopamine stabilizer, improves motor performance and shows neuroprotective effects in Huntington disease R6/2 mouse model. J Cell Mol Med. 2015;19(11):2540–548.
17. Altar CA, Cai N, Bliven T, Juhasz M, Conner JM, Acheson AL, et al. Anterograde transport of brain-derived neurotrophic factor and its role in the brain. Nature. 1997;389:856–60.
18. Slow EJ, van Raamsdonk J, Rogers D, Coleman SH, Graham RK, Deng Y, et al. Selective striatal neuronal loss in a YAC128 mouse model of Huntington disease. Hum Mol Genet. 2003;12:1555–67.
19. Garcia-Miralles M, Geva M, Tan JY, et al. Early pridopidine treatment improves behavioral and transcriptional deficits in YAC128 Huntington disease mice. JCI Insight. 2017;2(23):e95665. https://doi.org/10.1172/jci.insight.95665.
20. Dobin A, Davis CA, Schlesinger F, Drenkow J, Zaleski S, Jha S, et al. STAR: ultrafast universal RNA-seq aligner. Bioinformatics. 2013;29:15–21.

21. Robinson MD, McCarthy DJ, Smyth GK. edgeR: a Bioconductor package for differential expression analysis of digital gene expression data. Bioinformatics. 2010;26:139–40.

22. Su Z, Łabaj PP, Li S, Thierry-Mieg J, Thierry-Mieg D, et al. Seqc/Maqc-Iii Consortium. A comprehensive assessment of RNA-seq accuracy, reproducibility and information content by the sequencing quality control consortium. Nat Biotechnol 2014;32:903–914.

23. Ritchie ME, Phipson B, Wu D, Hu Y, Law CW, Shi W, et al. Limma powers differential expression analyses for RNA-sequencing and microarray studies. Nucleic Acids Res. 2015;43:e47.

24. Subramanian A, Tamayo P, Mootha VK, Mukherjee S, Ebert BL, Gillette MA, et al. Gene set enrichment analysis: a knowledge-based approach for interpreting genome-wide expression profiles. Proc Natl Acad Sci. 2005;102: 15545–50.

25. Sato H, Horikawa Y, Iizuka K, Sakurai N, Tanaka T, Shihara N, et al. Large-scale analysis of glucocorticoid target genes in rat hypothalamus. J Neurochem. 2008;106:805–14.

26. Gokce O, Runne H, Kuhn A, Luthi-Carter R. Short-term striatal gene expression responses to brain-derived neurotrophic factor are dependent on MEK and ERK activation. PLoS One. 2009;4:e5292.

27. Cadet JL, Jayanthi S, McCoy MT, Beauvais G, Cai NS. Dopamine D1 receptors, regulation of gene expression in the brain, and neurodegeneration. CNS Neurol Disord Drug Targets. 2010;9:526–38.

28. Maqc Consortium SL, Shi L, Reid LH, Jones WD, Shippy R, et al. The MicroArray quality control (MAQC) project shows inter- and intraplatform reproducibility of gene expression measurements. Nat Biotechnol. 2006;24:1151–61.

29. Chen EY, Tan CM, Kou Y, Duan Q, Wang Z, Meirelles GV, et al. Enrichr: interactive and collaborative HTML5 gene list enrichment analysis tool. BMC Bioinformatics. 2013;14:1–14.

30. Geva M, Kusko R, Soares H, Fowler KD, Birnberg T, Barash S, et al. Pridopidine activates neuroprotective pathways impaired in Huntington disease. Hum Mol Genet. 2016;25(18):3975–987.

31. Aziz NA, Pijl H, Frölich M, van der Graaf AWM, Roelfsema F, Roos RAC. Increased hypothalamic-pituitary-adrenal axis activity in Huntington's disease. J Clin Endocrinol Metab. 2009;94:1223–8.

32. Dong X, Tsuji J, Labadorf A, Roussos P, Chen J-F, Myers RH, et al. The role of H3K4me3 in transcriptional regulation is altered in Huntington's disease. PLoS One. 2015;10:e0144398.

33. Choi Y-S, Lee B, Cho H-Y, Reyes IB, Pu X-A, Saido TC, et al. CREB is a key regulator of striatal vulnerability in chemical and genetic models of Huntington's disease. Neurobiol Dis. 2009;36:259–68.

34. Taymans J-M, Leysen JE, Langlois X. Striatal gene expression of RGS2 and RGS4 is specifically mediated by dopamine D1 and D2 receptors: clues for RGS2 and RGS4 functions. J Neurochem. 2003;84:1118–27.

35. Xie Y, Hayden MR, Xu B. BDNF overexpression in the forebrain rescues Huntington's disease phenotypes in YAC128 mice. J Neurosci. 2010;30:14708–18.

36. Maheshwari M, Bhutani S, Das A, Mukherjee R, Sharma A, Kino Y, et al. Dexamethasone induces heat shock response and slows down disease progression in mouse and fly models of Huntington's disease. Hum Mol Genet. 2014;23:2737–51.

37. Ponten H, Kullingsjö J, Lagerkvist S, Martin P, Pettersson F, Sonesson C, et al. In vivo pharmacology of the dopaminergic stabilizer pridopidine. Eur J Pharmacol. 2010;644:88–95.

38. Nagai T, Yoshimoto J, Kannon T, Kuroda K, Kaibuchi K. Phosphorylation signals in striatal medium spiny neurons. Trends Pharmacol Sci. 2016;37:858–71.

39. Gines S, Seong IS, Fossale E, Ivanova E, Trettel F, Gusella JF, et al. Specific progressive cAMP reduction implicates energy deficit in presymptomatic Huntington's disease knock-in mice. Hum Mol Genet. 2003;12:497–508.

40. Lin J-T, Chang W-C, Chen H-M, Lai H-L, Chen C-Y, Tao M-H, et al. Regulation of feedback between protein kinase a and the proteasome system worsens Huntington's disease. Mol Cell Biol. 2013;33:1073–84.

41. Porras G, Berthet A, Dehay B, Li Q, Ladepeche L, Normand E, et al. PSD-95 expression controls l-DOPA dyskinesia through dopamine D1 receptor trafficking. J Clin Invest. 2012;122:3977–89.

42. Parsons MP, Kang R, Buren C, Dau A, Southwell AL, Doty CN, et al. Bidirectional control of postsynaptic density-95 (PSD-95) clustering by huntingtin. J Biol Chem. 2014;289:3518–28.

43. Zhang J, Vinuela A, Neely MH, Hallett PJ, Grant SGN, Miller GM, et al. Inhibition of the dopamine D1 receptor signaling by PSD-95. J Biol Chem. 2007;282:15778–89.

44. Sun Y, Savanenin A, Reddy PH, Liu YF. Polyglutamine-expanded huntingtin promotes sensitization of N-methyl-D-aspartate receptors via post-synaptic density 95. J Biol Chem. 2001;276:24713–8.

45. Spiegel I, Mardinly A, Gabel H, Bazinet J, Couch C, Tzeng C, et al. Npas4 regulates excitatory-inhibitory balance within neural circuits through cell type-specific gene programs. Cell. 2014;157:1216–29.

46. Eggerickx D, Denef JF, Labbe O, Hayashi Y, Refetoff S, Vassart G, et al. Molecular cloning of an orphan G-protein-coupled receptor that constitutively activates adenylate cyclase. Biochem J. 1995;309(Pt 3):837–43.

47. Valverde O, Célérier E, Baranyi M, Vanderhaeghen P, Maldonado R, Sperlagh B, et al. GPR3 receptor, a novel actor in the emotional-like responses. PLoS One. 2009;4:e4704.

4

Protective paraspeckle hyper-assembly downstream of TDP-43 loss of function in amyotrophic lateral sclerosis

Tatyana A. Shelkovnikova[1][*] ⓘ, Michail S. Kukharsky[1,2], Haiyan An[1], Pasquale Dimasi[1], Svetlana Alexeeva[1], Osman Shabir[3], Paul R. Heath[3] and Vladimir L. Buchman[1,2]

Abstract

Background: Paraspeckles are subnuclear bodies assembled on a long non-coding RNA (lncRNA) NEAT1. Their enhanced formation in spinal neurons of sporadic amyotrophic lateral sclerosis (ALS) patients has been reported but underlying mechanisms are unknown. The majority of ALS cases are characterized by TDP-43 proteinopathy. In current study we aimed to establish whether and how TDP-43 pathology may augment paraspeckle assembly.

Methods: Paraspeckle formation in human samples was analysed by RNA-FISH and laser capture microdissection followed by qRT-PCR. Mechanistic studies were performed in stable cell lines, mouse primary neurons and human embryonic stem cell-derived neurons. Loss and gain of function for TDP-43 and other microRNA pathway factors were modelled by siRNA-mediated knockdown and protein overexpression.

Results: We show that de novo paraspeckle assembly in spinal neurons and glial cells is a hallmark of both sporadic and familial ALS with TDP-43 pathology. Mechanistically, loss of TDP-43 but not its cytoplasmic accumulation or aggregation augments paraspeckle assembly in cultured cells. TDP-43 is a component of the microRNA machinery, and recently, paraspeckles have been shown to regulate pri-miRNA processing. Consistently, downregulation of core protein components of the miRNA pathway also promotes paraspeckle assembly. In addition, depletion of these proteins or TDP-43 results in accumulation of endogenous dsRNA and activation of type I interferon response which also stimulates paraspeckle formation. We demonstrate that human or mouse neurons in vitro lack paraspeckles, but a synthetic dsRNA is able to trigger their de novo formation. Finally, paraspeckles are protective in cells with compromised microRNA/dsRNA metabolism, and their assembly can be promoted by a small-molecule microRNA enhancer.

Conclusions: Our study establishes possible mechanisms behind paraspeckle hyper-assembly in ALS and suggests their utility as therapeutic targets in ALS and other diseases with abnormal metabolism of microRNA and dsRNA.

Keywords: ALS, TDP-43, Paraspeckle, NEAT1

Background

Amyotrophic lateral sclerosis (ALS), the most common form of motor neuron disease, is a severe adult-onset neuromuscular disease affecting motor neurons in the spinal cord, brainstem and motor cortex. Up to 90% of ALS cases are sporadic (sALS), the rest 10% bear a strong genetic component (familial ALS, fALS), and

* Correspondence: shelkovnikovat@cardiff.ac.uk
[1]School of Biosciences, Cardiff University, Museum Avenue, Cardiff CF10 3AX, UK
Full list of author information is available at the end of the article

currently mutations in more than 20 genes are known to cause fALS [1]. The complexity of the disease hinders development of ALS therapeutics, and those two drugs that have been approved for the treatment of ALS so far, riluzole and edaravone, have very limited efficacy.

A multifunctional RNA-binding protein TDP-43 encoded by *TARDBP* gene is believed to be the main culprit in ALS: TDP-43 pathology is typical for ~ 95% of sALS cases and for fALS cases caused by *C9ORF72* gene mutation [2]; in addition, dozens of mutations in *TARDBP* have been identified in fALS and sALS patients

[3, 4]. Hallmarks of all these ALS cases include protein clearance from the nucleus, its cytoplasmic accumulation and aggregation [5, 6]. Therefore, both loss and gain of TDP-43 function are implicated in ALS however the relative contribution of these two mechanisms is still debated.

The paraspeckle is a prototypical nuclear body localized on the border of splicing speckles [7]. A long non-coding RNA (lncRNA) NEAT1 serves as a scaffold for paraspeckles, spatially organizing a variety of proteins by direct binding or piggy-back mechanism [8–11]. The NEAT1 locus produces two transcripts, NEAT1_1 and NEAT1_2. The longer NEAT1 isoform, NEAT1_2, is essential for paraspeckle assembly [10, 12]. Functions of paraspeckles described so far include nuclear retention of specific RNAs, including inverted Alu repeat-containing transcripts; regulation of gene expression by sequestration of transcription factors; and modulation of miRNA biogenesis [13–16].

There is an established association of paraspeckles and their components with a variety of pathological states and conditions, from cancer to neurodegeneration. Paraspeckles protect cancer cells against DNA damage and replication stress, regulate hormone receptor signaling and hypoxia-associated pathways thereby increasing their survival [17–19]. Paraspeckles become enlarged in cells primed by viral or synthetic double-stranded (ds) RNAs and play an important role in antiviral response [14]. An unusually tight association of paraspeckle components with neurodegenerative conditions, and ALS in particular, has recently emerged. Firstly, enhanced paraspeckle formation has been reported in spinal motor neurons of sALS patients [20]. This finding was surprising because levels of the longer NEAT1 isoform, NEAT1_2, essential for paraspeckle formation, are very low in the adult nervous system [21]. Secondly, at least seven paraspeckle proteins, including TDP-43 and FUS, are genetically linked to ALS and a related condition, frontotemporal lobar degeneration (FTLD) [22–25]. FUS, a protein structurally and functionally similar to TDP-43, is required to build paraspeckles [8, 23]. TDP-43 association with paraspeckles has also been reported [8]. TDP-43 directly binds NEAT1, and this interaction is increased in the brain of FTLD patients [26, 27]. Overall, currently available data support the role of paraspeckles in molecular pathology of ALS, however the underlying mechanisms of their enhanced formation in spinal neurons are not understood.

In current study we show that loss of TDP-43 is sufficient to stimulate paraspeckle formation – a phenomenon likely linked to the function of TDP-43 in microRNA (miRNA) processing and as an RNA chaperone. Furthermore, we provide evidence that paraspeckles are protective in cells with impaired function of the miRNA machinery and those with activated dsRNA response. Finally, we show that enoxacin, an enhancer of the miRNA pathway, promotes paraspeckle formation.

Methods

Stable cell line maintenance, transfection and treatments

SH-SY5Y neuroblastoma cells and MCF7 cells were maintained in 1:1 mixture of Dulbecco's Modified Eagle's Medium and F12 medium supplemented with 10% fetal bovine serum (FBS), penicillin-streptomycin and glutamine (all Gibco, Invitrogen). For differentiation into neuron-like cells, SH-SY5Y cells were grown on poly-L-lysine (Sigma) coated coverslips in advanced DMEM/F12 (ADF)/Neurobasal A mixture supplemented with 10 µM all-trans retinoic acid (Sigma), B27 (Life Technologies) and BDNF (Miltenyi, 10 ng/ml) for 6 days. The following gene-specific siRNAs were used: ADAR1; Dicer; Drosha; FUS; Ago2; IFNB1 (all Life Technologies, Silencer®); TARDBP (Silencer Select®, s23829 and EHU109221, Mission® esiRNA, Sigma); NEAT1 (Silencer Select®, n272456). Scrambled negative control was AllStars from Qiagen. Plasmids for expression of TDP-43 dNLS and TDP-43 C-termical fragment are described elsewhere [28]. Cells were transfected with siRNA (400 ng/well), plasmid DNA (200 ng/well) or poly(I:C) (Sigma, 250 ng/well) using Lipofectamine2000 (Life Technologies) in 24-well plates. TDP-43 specific shRNA plasmid was from Sigma (MISSION® SHCLNG-NM_007375). To delete the NLS of endogenous TDP-43, Feng Zhang lab's Target Finder (http://crispr.mit.edu/) was used to identify guide RNA target sequences flanking the genomic region of TARDBP gene encoding NLS. Respective forward and reverse oligonucleotides for two pairs of guides were annealed and cloned into pX330-U6-Chimeric_BB-CBh-hSpCas9 (pX330) vector provided by Feng Zhang (Addgene deposited plasmid) as described [29]. MCF7 cells were transfected with plasmids encoding upstream and downstream guide RNAs (500 ng/well) using Lipofectamine2000 and analysed after 72 h. Guide RNA sequences: T1: 5'-TTATTTAGATAACAAAAGAAAAA-3', T2: 5'-AACATCCGATTTAATAGTGT-3', T3: 5'-GGAATTCTGCATGCCCCAGATGC-3', T4: 5'-ACATCCGATTTAATAGTGTT-3'. Cellular treatments were as follows: 1×10^4 IU interferon beta-1a (IFNbeta), 0.5 µg/ml LPS, 100 µg/ml zymosan, 50 µM suramin, 500 nM TSA, 2 mM sodium butyrate, 10 and 50 µM enoxacin, 10 µM riluzole, 10 µM edaravone (all Sigma). Human ES cell derived neurons were transfected with 15 µg/well of poly(I:C) using FuGENE®HD (Promega). Enoxacin, edaravone and riluzole toxicity was assessed using resazurin-based CellTiter-Blue Cell Viability Assay (Promega).

Primary culture of mouse neurons

Primary cultures of mouse hippocampal neurons were prepared from P0 CD1 mice as described [28] and maintained for 5–14 days.

Differentiation of human ES cells into motor neuron enriched cultures

Cultures of human neural precursor cells (NPCs) and motor neurons differentiated from H9 hES cell line were prepared as described previously [30]. Briefly, hES cells were maintained in mTESR2 media (Stemcell Technologies) on Matrigel® (Corning) coated dishes. Confluent hES H9 cultures were switched to differentiation medium composed of ADF supplemented with SB431542 (10 μM, Abcam). Purmorphamine (1 μM, Cayman Chemicals) and retinoic acid (0.1 μM, Sigma) were added on Day 4. On Day 8, cells were split in 1:2 ratio and on Day 16, NPCs were dissociated using Accutase®, plated onto Matrigel® coated dishes and cultured in ADF with GlutaMAX, penicillin-streptomycin, B27 (12587–010) and N2 supplements (all Life Technologies) and BDNF (Miltenyi, 10 ng/ml). On Day 23, Accutase® was used to re-plate neurons on dishes/coverslips at desired density. Neurons were cultured in 50:50 mixture of ADF/Neurobasal A with the above supplements until Day 40.

Immunocytochemistry and RNA-FISH on cultured cells

Cells were fixed on coverslips with 4% paraformaldehyde on ice for 15 min and permeabilized in cold methanol (or 70% ethanol in case of RNA-FISH). Coverslips were incubated with primary antibodies diluted in blocking solution (5% goat serum in 0.1% Triton X-100/PBS) for 1 h at RT or at 4 °C overnight. Secondary Alexa488- or Alexa546-conjugated antibody was added for 1 h at RT. For RNA-FISH, commercially available NEAT1 and MALAT1 probes (Stellaris® FISH Probes against human NEAT1, middle segment or 5′ segment, or human MALAT1, all Biosearch Technologies) were used as per standard protocol. Fluorescent images were taken using BX61 microscope equipped with F-View II camera and processed using CellF software (all Olympus). Paraspeckle quantification (number of individual paraspeckles per DAPI-visualised nucleus) was performed manually, by the same person for all conditions, blinded to the experimental condition. Clusters of paraspeckles were counted as a single paraspeckle. For quantification of cleaved caspase 3 positive cells, 'Analyze particles' tool of Image J software was used (8–10 fields were analysed per condition).

RNA analysis

Total cellular RNA was extracted using GenElute total RNA kit (Sigma) and possible DNA contamination was removed using RNase free DNase kit (Qiagen). First-strand cDNA synthesis were performed using random primers and Superscript IV (Invitrogen). For analysis of miRNA levels, RNA was extracted with QIAzol (Qiagen) followed by reverse transcription with Qiagen miScript II RT Kit. Real-time qPCR was conducted using SYBR green master mix as described [28]. For miRNA quantification, forward miRNA-specific primers were used in combination with the universal reverse primer (unimiR). All primer sequences are given in Table 1.

RNA immunoprecipitation (RIP) and PCR analysis

MCF7 cells were transfected with equal amounts of plasmids to express GFP-tagged FUS or NONO together with TARDBP siRNA or scrambled control siRNA. After 48 h, cells were scraped in RIP buffer prepared using RNase-free water (1xPBS with 1% Triton-X100 and protease inhibitors cocktail). Cells were left on ice for 10 min with periodic vortexing, and the lysate was centrifuged at 13,000 rpm for 10 min. GFP-Trap® beads (Chromotek) were washed in RIP buffer 4 times and added directly to cleared cell lysates with subsequent rotation at + 4 °C for 3 h. Beads were washed 4 times in RIP buffer and RNA was eluted by resuspension in TRI-reagent (Sigma). RNA was purified according to manufacturer's protocol, and equal amounts of RNA were used for cDNA synthesis as described above.

Protein analysis

Total cell lysates were prepared for Western blot by lysing cells in wells in 2× Laemmli (loading) buffer followed by denaturation at 100 °C for 5 min. Proteins were resolved by SDS-PAGE and transferred to PVDF membrane (Amersham) by semi-dry transfer. The membrane was blocked in 4% non-fat milk in TBST and incubated in primary antibodies prepared in milk or 5% BSA overnight. Secondary HRP-conjugated antibodies were from Amersham. For detection of proteins, WesternBright Sirius ECL reagent (Advansta) was used. β-actin was used for normalisation.

Primary antibodies

The following commercial primary antibodies were used: TDP-43 (rabbit polyclonal, 10782–2-AP, Proteintech and mouse monoclonal, MAB7778-SP, R&D Biosystems); FUS (rabbit polyclonal, Proteintech, 11570–1-AP); p54nrb/NONO (rabbit polyclonal C-terminal, Sigma); PSF/SFPQ (rabbit monoclonal, ab177149, Abcam); Tuj (β-Tubulin III, mouse monoclonal, Sigma); dsRNA (mouse monoclonal, J2, Kerafast); cleaved caspase 3 (rabbit polyclonal, 9661, Cell Signaling); NF-κB p65 (rabbit monoclonal, D14E12, Cell Signaling); IFIT3 (rabbit polyclonal, Bethyl); p-eIF2α (rabbit monoclonal, ab32157, Abcam); p-PKR (rabbit polyclonal, Thr451, ThermoFisher); PKR (mouse monoclonal, MAB1980-SP, R&D Systems); eIF2α (rabbit monoclonal, D7D3, Cell

Table 1 Primers used in the study

Target	Forward	Reverse
GAPDH	5'-TCGCCAGCCGAGCCA-3'	5'-GAGTTAAAAGCAGCCCTGGTG – 3'
NEAT1 total	5'-CTCACAGGCAGGGGAAATGT-3'	5'-AACACCCACACCCCAAACAA-3'
NEAT1_2	5'-AGAGGCTCAGAGAGGACTGTAACCTG-3'	5'-TGTGTGTGTAAAAGAGAGAAGTTGTGG-3'
TDP-43	5'-TCAGGGCCTTTGCCTTTGTT-3'	5'-TGCTTAGGTTCGGCATTGGAT-3'
IL8	5'-ACACTGCGCCAACACAGAAA-3'	5'-CCTCTGCACCCAGTTTTCCT-3'
ADARB2	ATATTCGTGCGGTTAAAAGAAGGTG	ATCTCGTAGGGAGAGTGGAGTCTTG
Alu RNA	5'-GAGGCTGAGGCAGGAGAATCG-3'	5'-GTCGCCCAGGCTGGAGTG-3'
DICER	5'-TTAACCTTTTGGTGTTTGATGAGTGT-3'	5'-GCGAGGACATGATGGACAATT-3'
DROSHA	5'-CGGCCCGAGAGCCTTTTAT-3'	5'-TGCACACGTCTAACTCTTCCA-3'
ADAR1	5'-TTGTCAACCACCCCAAGGT-3'	5'-CCATCAGCCAGACACCAGTT-3'
AGO2	5'-CACCATGTACTCGGGAGCC-3'	5'-TCCCAAAGTCGGGTCTAGGT-3'
FUS	5'-GCGGGGCTGCTCAGT-3'	5'-TTGGGTTGCTTGTTGGGTAT-3'
CHOP	5'-TTAAAGATGAGCGGGTGGC-3'	5'-GCTTTCAGGTGTGGTGATGTA-3'
CXCL10	5'-TGCCATTCTGATTTGCTGCC-3'	5'-ATGCTGATGCAGGTACAGCG-3'
IFNB1	5'-ACGCCGCATTGACCATCTAT-3'	5'-AGCCAGGAGGTTCTCAACAA-3'
IFNA1	5'-TCTGCTATGACCATGACACGAT-3'	5'-CAGCATGGTCCTCTGTAAGGG-3'
IFNA2	5'-AGGAGGAAGGAATAACATCTGGTC-3'	5'-GCAGGGGTGAGAGTCTTTGAA-3'
MALAT1	5'-GGATCCTAGACCAGCATGCC-3'	5'- AAAGGTTACCATAAGTAAGTTCCAGAAAA-3'
IFIH1	5'-GCATGGAGGAGGAACTGTTGA-3'	5'-GCATGGAGGAGGAACTGTTGA-3'
CYCS	5'-TCGTTGTGCCAGCGACTAAA-3'	5'-GCTTGCCTCCCTTTTCAACG-3'
STAT1	5'-CTGTGCGTAGCTGCTCCTTT-3'	5'-GGTGAACCTGCTCCAGGAAT-3'
MYD88	5'-TGACCCCCTGGGGCAT-3'	5'-AGTTGCCGGATCATCTCCTG-3'
Pri-miR-17–92	5'-CAGTAAAGGTAAGGAGAGCTC AATCTG-3'	5'-CATACAACCACTAAGCTAAAGAAT AATCTGA-3'
Pri-miR-15a	5'-CCTTGGAGTAAAGTAGCAGCAC-3'	5'-CCTTGTATTTTTGAGGCAGCAC-3'
miR-18a	5'-CATCATCGGTAAGGTGCATC-3'	5'-GAATCGAGCACCAGTTACGC-3' (unimiR)
miR-92a	5'-GAGTCTATTGCACTTGTCCC-3'	unimiR
miR-106a	5'-AAAAGTGCTTACAGTGCAGGTAG-3'	unimiR

Signaling); β-actin (mouse monoclonal, A5441, Sigma). Antibodies were used at 1:500–1:1000 dilution for all applications.

Analysis of human tissue samples

Human spinal cord paraffin sections from a panel of clinically and histopathologically characterised ALS cases and neurologically healthy individuals were obtained from the Sheffield Brain Tissue Bank and MRC London Neurodegenerative Diseases Brain Bank (Institute of Psychiatry, King's College London). Consent was obtained from all subjects for autopsy, histopathological assessment and research were performed in accordance with local and national Ethics Committee approved donation. Human spinal cord sections were 7 μm thick. For conventional RNA-FISH, slides were boiled in citrate buffer for 10 min, washed in 2xSSC prepared with DEPC-treated water and incubated with NEAT1 probe (Stellaris® FISH Probes against human NEAT1 5′ segment, Biosearch Technologies) diluted in hybridisation buffer (10% formamide/2xSSC, 5 μl probe in 200 μl buffer per slide under a 24 × 60 mm coverslip) in a humidified chamber at 37 °C overnight. Nuclei were co-stained with DAPI. Paraspeckles were analysed using BX61 microscope/F-View II camera (Olympus) at 100× magnification. For RNAscope® ISH analysis, Hs-NEAT1-long (411541) probe (Advanced Cell Diagnostics) was used according to manufacturer's instructions. For qRT-PCR analysis, total RNA was extracted from thick frozen spinal cord sections and cDNA prepared using Ready-To-Go You-Prime First-Strand Beads (GE Healthcare). For laser capture microdissection (LCM), frozen spinal cord sections (total of 5 sections per patient/case) were cut into 5–10 μm thin sections using a cryostat, mounted on glass slides and fixed in cold acetone for 3 min. Sections were stained using toluidine blue, dehydrated in ascending alcohol series for 30 s and placed in xylene for 1 min. The PixCell® II Microdissection system (Applied Biosystems) was used for LCM. Motor neurons from the anterior grey horn were laser captured (300–500 or 30–80 per patient for healthy controls and ALS cases respectively), with the Macro-LCM cap films peeled and placed in test tubes with 50 μl extraction buffer (Pico Pure® RNA Isolation Kit; Thermo Fisher Scientific) on ice. The extracted films were incubated at 42 °C with the extraction buffer for 30 min and frozen at -80 °C until RNA extraction. Total RNA purification was performed using the above kit as per manufacturer's instructions. RNA samples were analysed using the Agilent RNA 6000 Pico Kit (Agilent Technologies®) and used for qRT-PCR.

Statististical analysis

GraphPad Prism software was used for statistical analysis. Statistical test used in each case is indicated in the figure legend. N indicates the number of biological replicates. On all graphs, error bars represent SEM.

Results
Presence of paraspeckles in the spinal cord neurons is a hallmark of sALS and fALS

Augmented paraspeckle assembly has been previously reported in sALS spinal cord neurons as compared to non-ALS controls [20]. We sought to verify this result in a separate cohort of sALS cases as well as to extend this analysis to fALS. In total, 7 sALS cases, 2 cases with *TARDBP* mutations and 4 cases with *C9ORF72* mutations alongside with 6 healthy controls were examined by RNA-FISH with NEAT1 probe. No neurons with paraspeckles were detected in the spinal cord of healthy individuals (97 neurons analysed), however such neurons were present in up to 40% of neurons in all ALS cases examined (Fig. 1a and b). We also confirmed the presence of paraspeckles in ALS motor neurons using RNA-scope® ISH (Fig. 1c). Consistently, qRT-PCR analysis of spinal cord tissue from four healthy controls and four ALS patients demonstrated elevated NEAT1 levels in the latter group (Fig. 1d). We further performed laser capture microdissection (LCM) of spinal neurons in the ventral horn and analysed NEAT1_2 levels by qRT-PCR (*n* = 3 for controls and *n* = 6 for ALS patients, including three sALS and three ALS-C9 cases). NEAT1_2 levels were indeed significantly upregulated in LCM neurons of ALS patients (Fig. 1e). Finally, using RNAscope® ISH, we also analysed the presence of paraspeckles in non-neuronal cells. Wide-spread paraspeckle assembly in glial cells in ALS spinal cord was observed (n = 6 for controls and *n* = 4 for ALS patients, including two sALS, one ALS-TDP and one ALS-C9 case) (Fig. 1f).

Thus, de novo paraspeckle formation is typical for spinal motor neurons and glial cells of individuals affected by ALS with primary or secondary TDP-43 pathology.

Loss of TDP-43 but not its cytoplasmic accumulation or aggregation results in paraspeckle hyper-assembly

We next sought to determine possible mechanisms underlying paraspeckle hyper-assembly in ALS. TDP-43 pathology in the spinal cord is very common in ALS, being present in almost all sALS cases, fALS cases caused by mutations in *TARDBP* gene itself as well as those caused by *C9ORF72* gene repeat expansions [2–4, 31]. TDP-43 has been identified as a paraspeckle protein [20], thus we tested the possibility that TDP-43 dysfunction affects paraspeckle assembly.

Hallmarks of TDP-43 proteinopathy are clearance of the protein from the nucleus and its accumulation and aggregation in the cytoplasm [5, 6]. We first modelled loss of TDP-43 function in two stable cell lines. By using specific siRNA, ~ 90 and 50% TDP-43 knockdown was achieved in MCF7 and neuroblastoma SH-SY5Y cells, respectively (Fig. 2a; Additional file 1: Fig. S1a). TDP-43 depletion led to a significant increase of the number of paraspeckles per nucleus (Fig. 2b and c; Additional file 1: Fig. S1b). Consistently, the paraspeckle-specific NEAT1 isoform, NEAT1_2, was upregulated in cells transfected with TDP-43 siRNA (Fig. 2a; Additional file 1: Fig. S1a). Similar results were obtained using an independent TDP-43 siRNA pool and an shRNA targeting TDP-43 (Additional file 1: Fig. S1c and d). In contrast, we did not observe changes in the levels or distribution of another abundant lncRNA, MALAT1, a component of splicing speckles (Fig. 2a; Additional file 1: Fig. S1e). Levels of core paraspeckle proteins SFPQ, NONO and FUS were also unaffected by TDP-43 knockdown (Additional file 1: Fig. S1f). We next examined whether TDP-43 knockdown would result in enhanced association of core paraspeckle proteins with NEAT1_2. Plasmids to overexpress GFP-tagged FUS or NONO proteins were co-transfected with scrambled or TDP-43 siRNA followed by RNA immunoprecipitation with GFP-Trap beads. Indeed, by PCR, both FUS and NONO demonstrated increased association with NEAT1_2 in TDP-43 depleted cells (Fig. 2d). To verify that paraspeckles formed in TDP-43 depleted cells are functional, we measured the expression of established paraspeckle-dependent genes, *IL8* and *ADARB2*, known to be positively and negatively regulated by paraspeckles, respectively [13, 14]. Indeed, IL8 mRNA was upregulated and ADARB2 mRNA decreased upon TDP-43 knockdown (Fig. 2e).

Since nuclear clearance of TDP-43 in ALS is coupled to its cytoplasmic accumulation and aggregation, we next evaluated the effect of cytoplasmic TDP-43 on paraspeckles. TDP-43 lacking nuclear localization signal

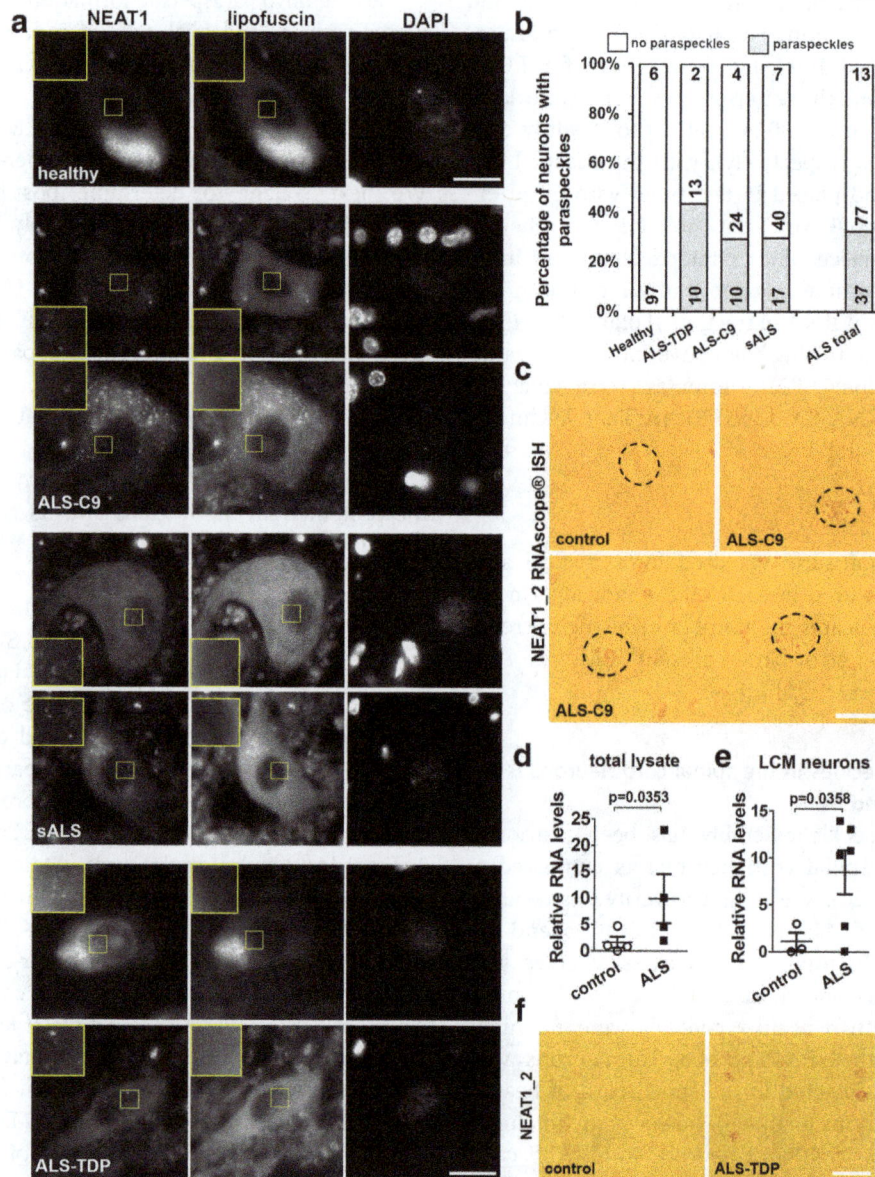

Fig. 1 Paraspeckles are formed in the spinal cord of sALS and fALS patients but not healthy controls. **a** and **b** Examples of spinal motor neurons with paraspeckles (**a**) and their quantification (**b**) in ALS patients with different disease aetiology. Paraspeckles were visualised in the spinal cord sections of a cohort of fALS and sALS patients as well as neurologically normal control individuals using RNA-FISH with a fluorescent (Quasar 570) probe mapping to the 5′ portion of NEAT1. Images were also taken in the FITC channel to distinguish between specific NEAT1 signal and green autofluorescence from lipofuscin (**a**). The fraction of neurons with identifiable paraspeckles in the spinal anterior horn of aetiologically different ALS cases and control individuals was quantified and plotted separately for fALS with *TARDBP* mutations (ALS-TDP), fALS with *C9ORF72* repeat expansion (ALS-C9) and sALS cases (**b**). The top figure within each bar corresponds to the number of cases analysed and the figures below - to the number of individual neurons negative or positive for the presence of paraspeckles. Scale bars, 10 μm. **c** Examples of paraspeckle-containing neurons in the ALS spinal cord visualised with RNAscope® NEAT1_2 specific probe. In the bottom panel, a paraspeckle-positive (right) and a paraspeckle-negative (left) neurons, found adjacent to each other, are shown. Nuclei are circled. Scale bar, 10 μm. **d** NEAT1 levels in the total RNA samples extracted from transversely cut spinal cord blocks of ALS patients and healthy controls analysed by qRT-PCR (*n* = 4 for control and ALS patients, including two sALS and two ALS-C9 cases, Mann-Whitney *U*-test). **e** NEAT1_2 levels in neurons microdissected from the spinal anterior horn of ALS patients and healthy controls analysed by qRT-PCR (*n* = 3 for control and *n* = 6 for ALS cases, including three sALS and three ALS-C9 cases, Mann-Whitney *U*-test). **f** Paraspeckles in glial cells in the ALS spinal cord visualised with RNAscope® ISH using NEAT1_2 specific probe. Representative images of the spinal cord for a control individual and an ALS patient are shown. Scale bar, 20 μm

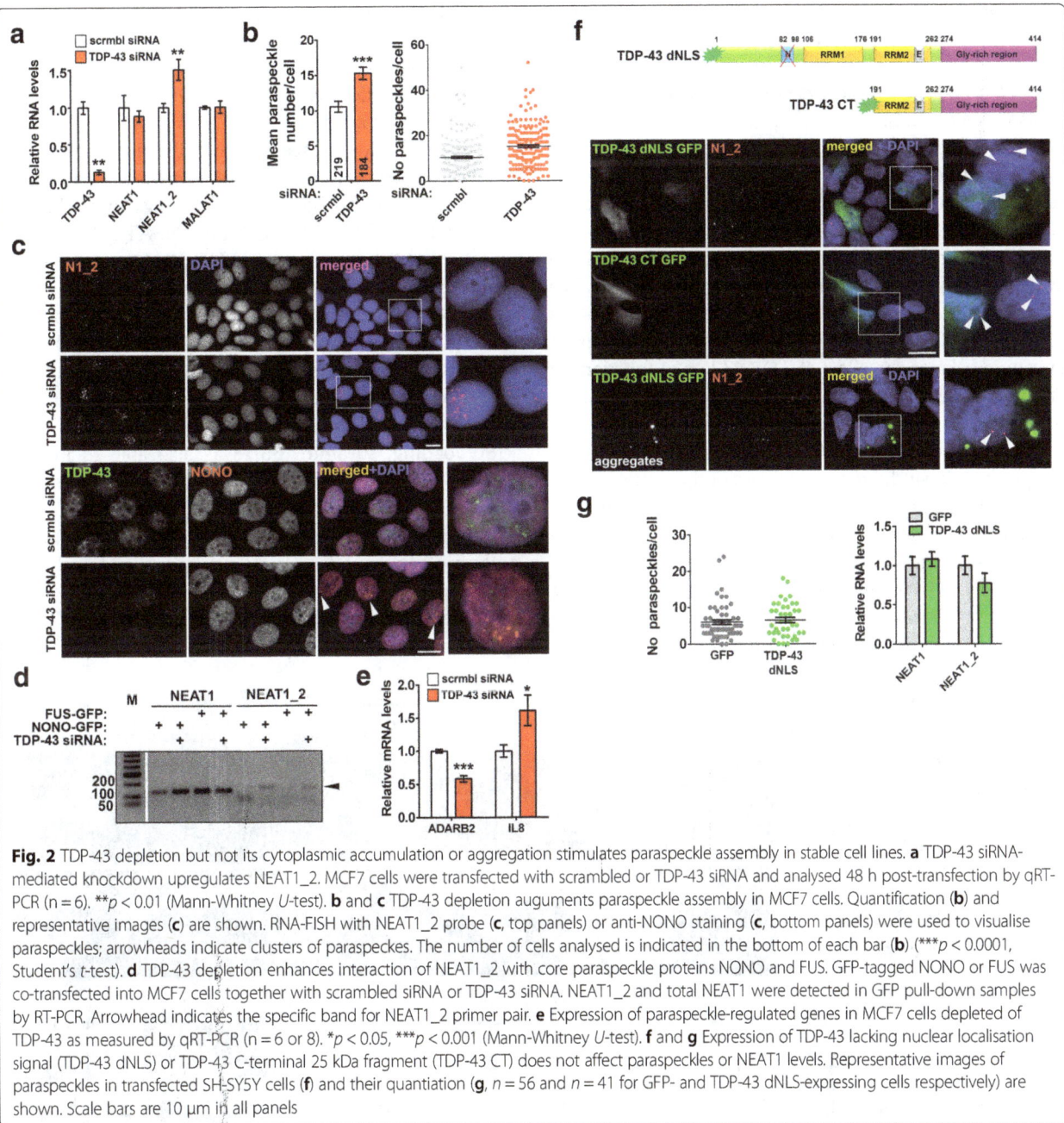

Fig. 2 TDP-43 depletion but not its cytoplasmic accumulation or aggregation stimulates paraspeckle assembly in stable cell lines. **a** TDP-43 siRNA-mediated knockdown upregulates NEAT1_2. MCF7 cells were transfected with scrambled or TDP-43 siRNA and analysed 48 h post-transfection by qRT-PCR (n = 6). **$p < 0.01$ (Mann-Whitney U-test). **b** and **c** TDP-43 depletion auguments paraspeckle assembly in MCF7 cells. Quantification (**b**) and representative images (**c**) are shown. RNA-FISH with NEAT1_2 probe (**c**, top panels) or anti-NONO staining (**c**, bottom panels) were used to visualise paraspeckles; arrowheads indicate clusters of paraspeckes. The number of cells analysed is indicated in the bottom of each bar (**b**) (***$p < 0.0001$, Student's t-test). **d** TDP-43 depletion enhances interaction of NEAT1_2 with core paraspeckle proteins NONO and FUS. GFP-tagged NONO or FUS was co-transfected into MCF7 cells together with scrambled siRNA or TDP-43 siRNA. NEAT1_2 and total NEAT1 were detected in GFP pull-down samples by RT-PCR. Arrowhead indicates the specific band for NEAT1_2 primer pair. **e** Expression of paraspeckle-regulated genes in MCF7 cells depleted of TDP-43 as measured by qRT-PCR (n = 6 or 8). *$p < 0.05$, ***$p < 0.001$ (Mann-Whitney U-test). **f** and **g** Expression of TDP-43 lacking nuclear localisation signal (TDP-43 dNLS) or TDP-43 C-terminal 25 kDa fragment (TDP-43 CT) does not affect paraspeckles or NEAT1 levels. Representative images of paraspeckles in transfected SH-SY5Y cells (**f**) and their quantiation (**g**, $n = 56$ and $n = 41$ for GFP- and TDP-43 dNLS-expressing cells respectively) are shown. Scale bars are 10 μm in all panels

(TDP-43 dNLS) and a C-terminal TDP-43 fragment corresponding to ~ 25 kDa TDP-43 cleavage product (TDP-43 CT, aa. 191–414), both characterized by predominantly cytoplasmic distribution, were transiently expressed in neuroblastoma cells (Fig. 2f). However, neither paraspeckle numbers nor NEAT1 levels were affected by these cytoplasmic proteins (Fig. 2f and g). TDP-43 dNLS forms cytoplasmic aggregates in a fraction of cells, but their presence also did not affect paraspeckles (Fig. 2g, bottom panel). Finally, in order to recapitulate simultaneous nuclear depletion and cytoplasmic accumulation of TDP-43, we targeted endogenous TDP-43 out of the nucleus while preserving its total cellular levels by CRISPR/Cas9 editing of the endogenous *TARDBP* gene. Cells were transiently transfected with plasmids for expression of two independent guide RNA pairs targeting upstream and downstream sequences encoding NLS of TDP-43 (Additional file 1: Fig. S1 g). For both guide RNA pairs tested, 15–20% transfected cells displayed partial TDP-43 redistribution to the cytoplasm which nevertheless did not enhance paraspeckle assembly (Additional file 1: Fig. S1 h), suggesting that substantial loss of nuclear TDP-43 is required to produce an effect on paraspeckles.

Overall, a decrease in cellular TDP-43 levels results in paraspeckle hyper-assembly.

Compromising miRNA pathway results in enhanced paraspeckle assembly

TDP-43 is known to contribute to miRNA biogenesis at two different levels, enhancing the activity of the Microprocessor in the nucleus and of the Dicer complex in the cytoplasm [32, 33]. Recently, paraspeckles have been shown to contribute to pri-miRNA processing by spatially organizing the Microprocessor and enhancing its processivity [16]. We hypothesised that augmented paraspeckle assembly in cells depleted of TDP-43 might be a compensatory mechanism to counterbalance the effect of TDP-43 loss of function on miRNA processing. If this indeed is true, paraspeckle assembly should be also increased in cells with compromised function of the miRNA pathway. To test this hypothesis, we knocked down three core enzymes of the miRNA pathway, a Microprocessor component Drosha, the pre-miRNA processing ribonuclease Dicer and the RISC endonuclease Ago2, in neuroblastoma cells. In our analysis we also included ADAR1 protein recently reported to promote miRNA processing [34]. Using specific siRNAs, we achieved at least 40% knockdown for each of these genes

(Fig. 3a). Consistent with the major role of Drosha in pri-miRNA processing, its knockdown led to the build-up of pri-miRNAs; both Drosha and TDP-43 knockdown also resulted in significantly diminished levels of select mature miRNAs (Additional file 2: Fig. S2).

RNA-FISH and paraspeckle quantification showed that downregulation each of the above proteins is accompanied by enhanced paraspeckle assembly (Fig. 3b and c) and upregulation of total NEAT1 and NEAT1_2 (Fig. 3d). Another ALS-linked protein, FUS, is structurally and functionally similar to TDP-43 and also plays a role in miRNA biogenesis [35], but it is a core paraspeckle protein required for paraspeckle integrity [8, 23]. As expected from its essential paraspeckle function, FUS depletion resulted in decreased paraspeckle numbers (Fig. 3b and c). Finally, a small molecule inhibitor of RISC loading, suramin [36], was also able to increase NEAT1_2 levels and promote paraspeckle assembly (Fig. 3e).

Thus, interfering with the function of the miRNA pathway causes NEAT1 upregulation and enhanced paraspeckle formation in cultured cells. This may represent one of the mechanisms behind the effect of TDP-43 loss of function on paraspeckles.

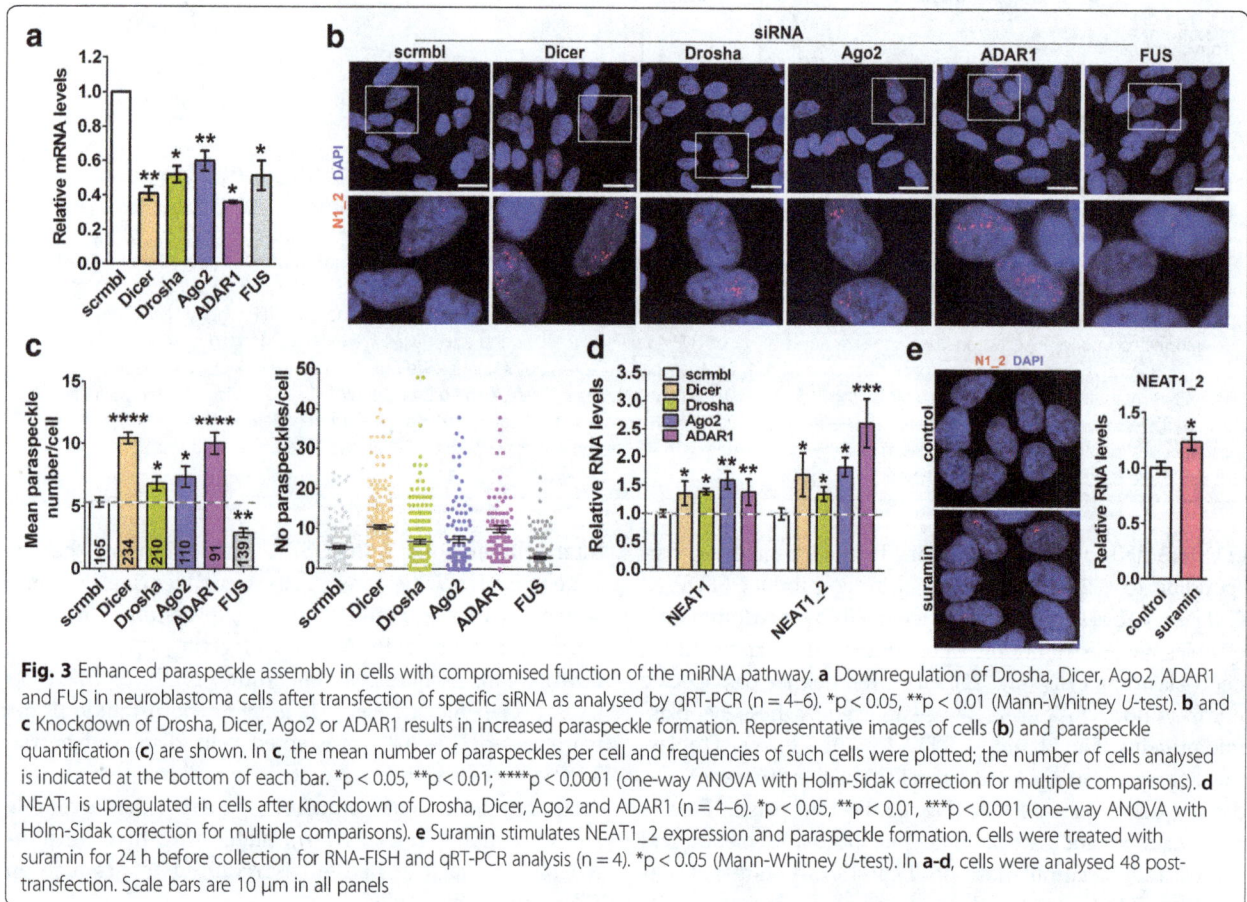

Fig. 3 Enhanced paraspeckle assembly in cells with compromised function of the miRNA pathway. **a** Downregulation of Drosha, Dicer, Ago2, ADAR1 and FUS in neuroblastoma cells after transfection of specific siRNA as analysed by qRT-PCR (n = 4–6). *p < 0.05, **p < 0.01 (Mann-Whitney U-test). **b** and **c** Knockdown of Drosha, Dicer, Ago2 or ADAR1 results in increased paraspeckle formation. Representative images of cells (**b**) and paraspeckle quantification (**c**) are shown. In **c**, the mean number of paraspeckles per cell and frequencies of such cells were plotted; the number of cells analysed is indicated at the bottom of each bar. *p < 0.05, **p < 0.01; ****p < 0.0001 (one-way ANOVA with Holm-Sidak correction for multiple comparisons). **d** NEAT1 is upregulated in cells after knockdown of Drosha, Dicer, Ago2 and ADAR1 (n = 4–6). *p < 0.05, **p < 0.01, ***p < 0.001 (one-way ANOVA with Holm-Sidak correction for multiple comparisons). **e** Suramin stimulates NEAT1_2 expression and paraspeckle formation. Cells were treated with suramin for 24 h before collection for RNA-FISH and qRT-PCR analysis (n = 4). *p < 0.05 (Mann-Whitney U-test). In **a-d**, cells were analysed 48 post-transfection. Scale bars are 10 μm in all panels

Type I IFN signaling is activated in cells depleted of TDP-43 or other miRNA factors and stimulates paraspeckle formation

TDP-43 is known to bind and regulate long transcripts [37], and its loss correlates with accumulation of transcripts prone to form double stranded (ds) RNA [38]. Conspicuously, regulation of cellular response to viral dsRNA is one of the best characterized functions of paraspeckles [14, 39]. Therefore, we considered abnormal accumulation of endogenous dsRNA in TDP-43 depleted cells as another mechanism underlying the effect of TDP-43 loss of function on paraspeckles. Critically, miRNA pathway itself is the biggest cellular source of dsRNA, and its factors Dicer, Drosha and ADAR1 are known to limit the accumulation of transcripts with extensive secondary structure [40–42].

We used J2 antibody, a gold standard for dsRNA detection [43], to study the presence of dsRNA species in cells depleted of TDP-43, Drosha, Dicer or ADAR1. An increase in J2-positive signal was obvious after knockdown of each of these genes (Fig. 4a and b, Additional file 3: Fig. S3a). In contrast, Ago2 or FUS knockdown did not cause dsRNA accumulation (Fig. 4b). J2 antibody was reported to recognise Alu repeats especially well [44]. We next used primers which specifically detect Alu-containing RNAs [45]. Dicer and Drosha but not TDP-43 or ADAR1 knockdown resulted in increased levels of Alu-containing RNAs as measured by qRT-PCR (Fig. 4c) indicating that a different repertoire of dsRNA species accumulate after knockdown of each gene.

The build-up of dsRNA is known to trigger phosphorylation of PKR and eIF2α and activation of type I interferon (IFN) signaling. In cells transfected with TDP-43 siRNA, levels of phosphorylated PKR and eIF2α were elevated (Fig. 4d; Additional file 3: Fig. S3b), and the expression of *IFNB1* and an IFN-stimulated gene (ISG) *CXCL10* was increased (Fig. 4e). Since dsRNA response eventually converges on type I IFNs, we asked whether these cytokines can contribute to paraspeckle response in TDP-43 depleted cells. Firstly, we showed that IFN-beta is the main type I IFN induced by dsRNA in neuroblastoma cells (Additional file 4: Fig. S4a). IFNbeta simulation per se was sufficient to stimulate paraspeckle assembly, although the effect was transient (Fig. 4f). In line with this, ligands of TLR3 (poly(I:C)) and TLR4 (bacterial lipopolysaccharide, LPS) which stimulate IFNbeta expression, but not a TLR2 ligand zymosan which does not affect IFNbeta production, were able to boost NEAT1 expression and paraspeckle assembly (Additional file 4: Fig. S4b-d). Finally, co-transfection of IFNbeta siRNA was sufficient to reduce paraspeckle abundance in cells transfected with TDP-43 siRNA although did not abrogate the hyper-assembly completely (Fig. 4g).

Taken together, these data suggest that endogenous dsRNA accumulation and associated type I IFN response represent one of the mechanisms behind augmented paraspeckle assembly caused by TDP-43 loss of function.

Paraspeckles are protective in cells with compromised miRNA biogenesis and activated dsRNA response

We next examined whether paraspeckles confer protection to cells depleted of TDP-43 or stimulated with exogenous dsRNA. Neuroblastoma cells were transfected with siRNAs targeting TDP-43 or another Microprocessor component Drosha alone or in combination with NEAT1 siRNA. Cytotoxicity was assessed after 36 h using cleaved caspase 3 (CC3) and DNA damage-inducible transcript 3 also known as GADD153 or CHOP, a pro-apoptotic transcription factor [46, 47] as markers of apoptotic cell death. NEAT1 siRNA-mediated knockdown was equally efficient alone and in cells co-transfected with TDP-43 or Drosha siRNA, allowing 60% NEAT1_2 downregulation and loss of paraspeckles in the majority of cells (Fig. 5a and data not shown). We found that while knockdown of TDP-43 or Drosha alone did not result in significant cell death, simultaneous disruption of paraspeckles increased the rates of apoptosis for both genes studied (Fig. 5b and c). Although regulation of dsRNA response by paraspeckles is well documented [14], their ability to modulate dsRNA-induced apoptosis has not been addressed. We transfected cells with scrambled siRNA or NEAT1 siRNA and subsequently exposed them to a synthetic dsRNA analogue poly(I:C). Cultures depleted of paraspeckles had increased CHOP mRNA levels and higher numbers of CC3-positive cells after 8 h and 24 h of poly(I:C) stimulation, respectively (Fig. 5d-f).

How does paraspeckle deficiency promote apoptosis in cells with compromised miRNA biogenesis and activated dsRNA response? A whole class of cytotoxicity-associated IFN-stimulated genes (ISGs) were reported to be negatively regulated by miRNAs [48]. We found that potentially pro-apoptotic ISGs from this class, *STAT1* and *CYCS*, were significantly upregulated in paraspeckle-deficient cells depleted of TDP-43 and Drosha (Fig. 5g). Furthermore, three such ISGs, *STAT1*, *MYD88* and *IFIH1*, were consistently upregulated in NEAT1-depleted cells in the course of poly(I:C) stimulation (Fig. 5h).

Thus, paraspeckles are protective against apoptotic death in cells with compromised miRNA machinery and/or activated dsRNA response.

Cultured human neurons lack paraspeckles but their de novo assembly can be triggered by dsRNA

Normal postmitotic neurons in the brain or spinal cord of adult mice express very low levels of NEAT1_2 isoform and do not form paraspeckles in vivo [21]. However it was not clear whether neurons cultured in vitro

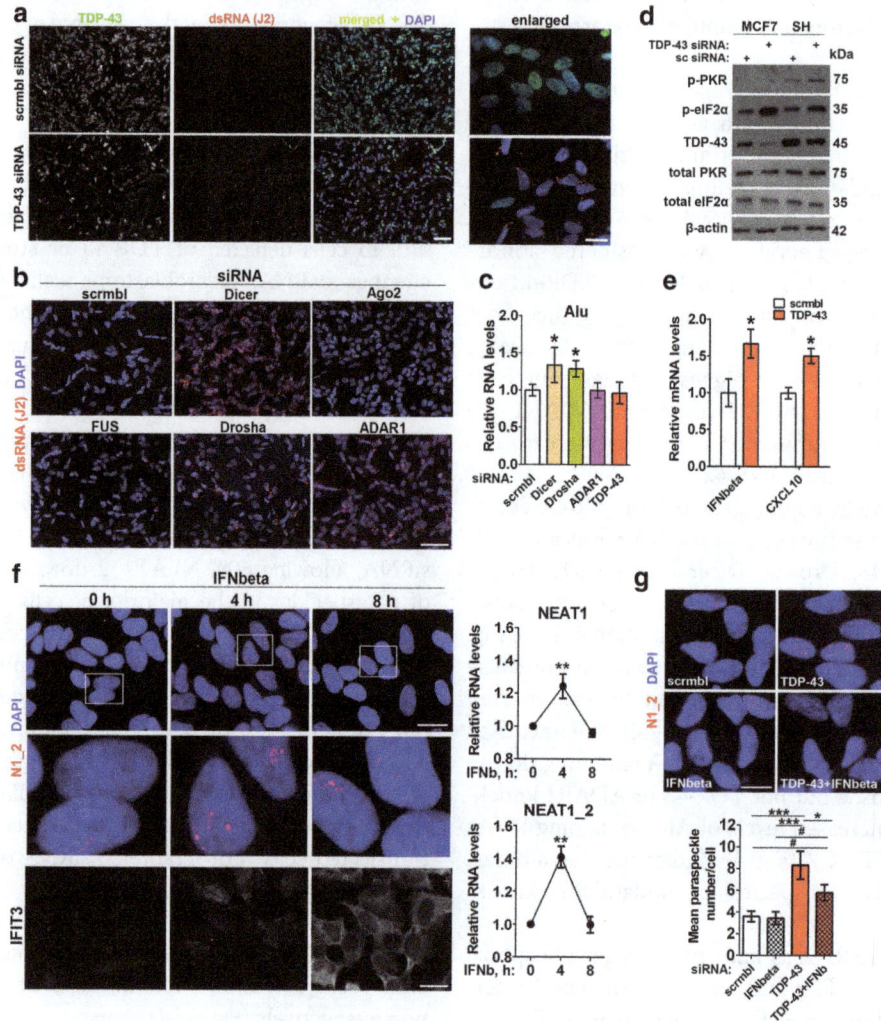

Fig. 4 Endogenous dsRNA response and type I interferon promote paraspeckle hyper-assembly in stable cell lines. **a** and **b** Depletion of TDP-43, Dicer, Drosha, ADAR1 but not Ago2 or FUS causes intracellular build-up of dsRNA. dsRNA was detected by immunocytochemistry using J2 antibody. Representative images of all conditions are shown. Scale bars, 50 and 10 μm for general plane and close-up panels respectively. **c** Levels of Alu-containing RNA as analysed by qRT-PCR using specific primers recognising Alu elements (n = 4). *p < 0.05 (Mann-Whitney U-test). **d** and **e** Markers of activated cellular reponse to dsRNA are upregulated in TDP-43 depleted cells. Levels of phosphorylated PKR and eIF2α were analysed by Western blot (**d**, representative blots are shown) and expression of *IFNB1* and an IFN-stimulated gene *CXCL10* - by qRT-PCR (**e**, n = 6). *p < 0.05 (Mann-Whitney U-test). **f** IFNbeta treatment stimulates NEAT1 expression and paraspeckle formation. NEAT1 levels were measured by qRT-PCR (n = 6). **p < 0.01 (Mann-Whitney U-test). Staining for an IFN-inducible protein IFIT3 was used as a positive control. Scale bar, 10 μm. **g** Simultaneous IFNbeta knockdown partially reverses the effect of TDP-43 depletion on paraspeckles. * and #p < 0.05, ***p < 0.001 (one-way ANOVA with Holm-Sidak correction for multiple comparisons). Scale bar, 10 μm. In all panels, cells were harvested for analysis 48 h post-transfection. Paraspeckles in panels **f** and **g** were visualised by NEAT1_2 RNA-FISH

would acquire and preserve paraspeckles. First, we studied primary hippocampal cultures from newborn mice. While glial cells have readily detectable paraspeckles already at 5 days in vitro, neurons had no sign of paraspeckles even after 14 days in vitro (Fig. 6a). Next we examined paraspeckle assembly during differentiation of human ES cells into motor neurons. Human ES cells lack paraspeckles but they appear during differentiation (days 4–5 into differentiation, trophoblast stage) [49]. Consistent with this study, we started observing paraspeckles in Day 4 neural precursor cells (NPCs), and they were prominent in Day 8

and Day 16 NPCs (Fig. 6b). However, paraspeckles were absent even in immature (Day 23) neurons and onwards (Fig. 6b). In contrast, retinoic acid/BDNF-induced differentiation of SH-SY5Y neuroblastoma cells for 6 days did not affect their ability to form paraspeckles (Additional file 5: Fig. S5), suggesting fundamental differences in the biology of neurons and neuroblastoma-derived neuron-like cells. Thus, disappearance of paraspeckles marks the transition between human NPCs and neurons, whereas de novo paraspeckle assembly is not triggered by in vitro conditions in primary neurons.

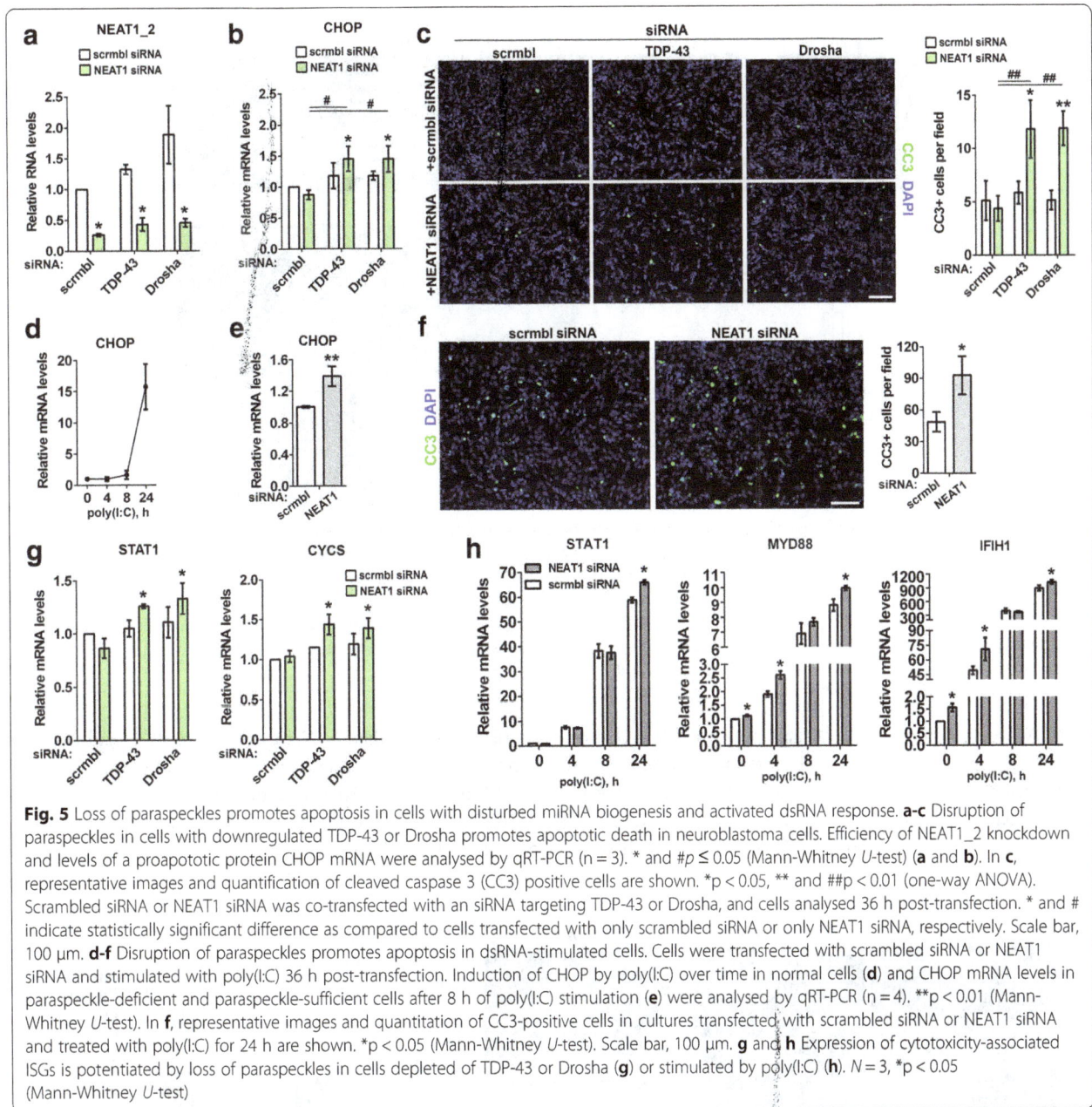

Fig. 5 Loss of paraspeckles promotes apoptosis in cells with disturbed miRNA biogenesis and activated dsRNA response. **a-c** Disruption of paraspeckles in cells with downregulated TDP-43 or Drosha promotes apoptotic death in neuroblastoma cells. Efficiency of NEAT1_2 knockdown and levels of a proapototic protein CHOP mRNA were analysed by qRT-PCR (n = 3). * and #$p \leq 0.05$ (Mann-Whitney U-test) (**a** and **b**). In **c**, representative images and quantification of cleaved caspase 3 (CC3) positive cells are shown. *$p < 0.05$, ** and ##$p < 0.01$ (one-way ANOVA). Scrambled siRNA or NEAT1 siRNA was co-transfected with an siRNA targeting TDP-43 or Drosha, and cells analysed 36 h post-transfection. * and # indicate statistically significant difference as compared to cells transfected with only scrambled siRNA or only NEAT1 siRNA, respectively. Scale bar, 100 μm. **d-f** Disruption of paraspeckles promotes apoptosis in dsRNA-stimulated cells. Cells were transfected with scrambled siRNA or NEAT1 siRNA and stimulated with poly(I:C) 36 h post-transfection. Induction of CHOP by poly(I:C) over time in normal cells (**d**) and CHOP mRNA levels in paraspeckle-deficient and paraspeckle-sufficient cells after 8 h of poly(I:C) stimulation (**e**) were analysed by qRT-PCR (n = 4). **$p < 0.01$ (Mann-Whitney U-test). In **f**, representative images and quantitation of CC3-positive cells in cultures transfected with scrambled siRNA or NEAT1 siRNA and treated with poly(I:C) for 24 h are shown. *$p < 0.05$ (Mann-Whitney U-test). Scale bar, 100 μm. **g** and **h** Expression of cytotoxicity-associated ISGs is potentiated by loss of paraspeckles in cells depleted of TDP-43 or Drosha (**g**) or stimulated by poly(I:C) (**h**). $N = 3$, *$p < 0.05$ (Mann-Whitney U-test)

Finally, we tested whether inhibition of miRNA function, exposure to dsRNA or IFNbeta treatment can initiate paraspeckle formation in neurons. Human Day 40 motor neurons [30] were stimulated with poly(I:C) or treated with suramin or IFNbeta for 24 h. Induction of endogenous IFNbeta and NEAT1 was observed in poly(I:C)-treated neuronal cultures (Fig. 6c), and paraspeckles could be detected in a small fraction of poly(I:C)-stimulated neurons (Fig. 6d). In contrast, neither suramin nor IFNbeta induced paraspeckle assembly in neurons.

Paraspeckle assembly can be promoted by a small molecule enhancer of miRNA biogenesis

Very few chemicals capable of stimulating paraspeckle assembly in cells with pre-existing paraspeckles have been identified so far. Proteasome inhibitors are known to promote NEAT1 synthesis and paraspeckle formation [13], however they are poor candidates as therapeutic molecules for ALS. Enoxacin is a small molecule enhancer of the miRNA pathway which stimulates the activity of the Dicer complex [50, 51]. In doing so, enoxacin increases levels of mature miRNAs thereby depleting

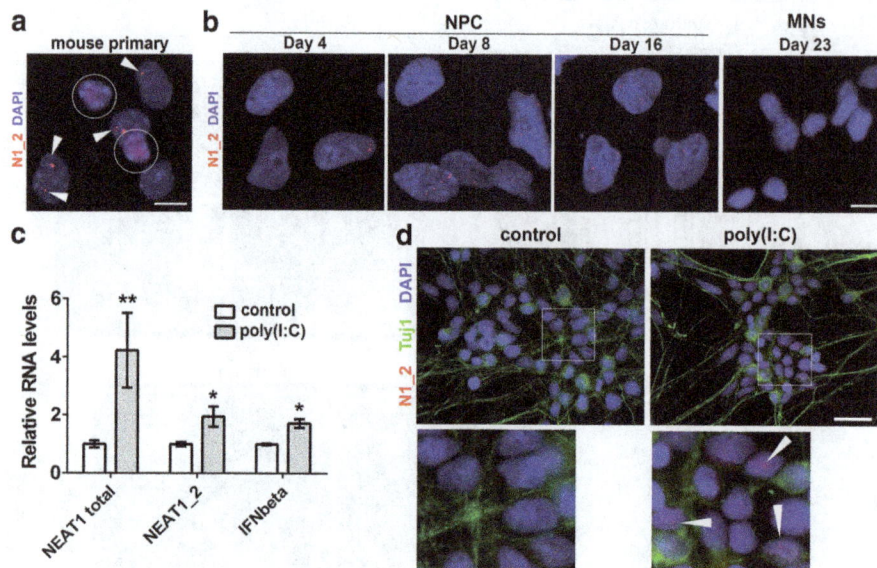

Fig. 6 Post-mitotic neurons lack paraspeckles in vitro, but their assembly can be triggered by dsRNA. **a** Paraspeckles are present in glial cells but not in neurons in murine primary hippocampal cultures. Cultures were analysed at DIV14 by NEAT1_2 RNA-FISH. A representative image is shown. Neuronal nuclei are circled and paraspeckles in glial cells are indicated by arrowheads. **b** Paraspeckles are present in human neural precursor cells (NPCs) but disappear during their differentiation into motor neurons. Cultures were analysed at the indicated time-points by NEAT1_2 RNA-FISH. **c** and **d** Treatment of Day 40 cultures of human motor neurons with poly(I:C) leads to activation of IFN signaling, increased NEAT1 expression (**c**) and paraspeckle assembly in a fraction of cells (**d**, arrowheads). In **c**, gene expression was analysed by qRT-PCR (n = 4). *p < 0.05, **p < 0.01 (Mann-Whitney U-test). Scale bars, 10 μm in **a**, **b** and 20 μm in **d**

miRNA precursors, pri-miRNA and pre-miRNA [51]. Recently, enoxacin been shown to ameliorate pathology in mouse models of ALS [52]. We studied the effect of enoxacin on paraspeckles in neuroblastoma cells. In addition, in our analysis we included HDAC inhibitors which were reported to stimulate NEAT1 expression [53] and two approved ALS therapeutics, riluzole and edaravone.

Treatment with 10 μM enoxacin for 24 h increased NEAT1_2 levels and paraspeckle assembly in neuroblastoma cells (Fig. 7a and b); similar effect on paraspeckles

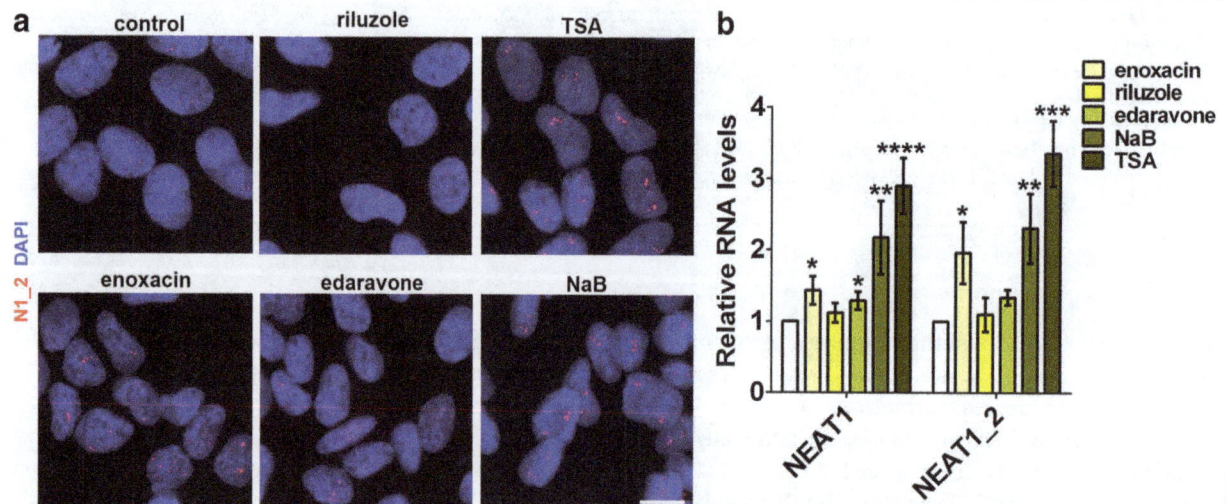

Fig. 7 A small molecule enhancer of miRNA biogenesis stimulates paraspeckle assembly in neuroblastoma cells. **a** and **b** SH-SY5Y cells were treated with enoxacin, riluzole, edaravone and HDAC inhibitors trichostatin A (TSA) and sodium butyrate (NaB), and paraspeckle assembly was assessed by NEAT1_2 RNA-FISH (**a**) and qRT-PCR (n = 4–6, **b**). *p < 0.05, **p < 0.01, ***p < 0.001, ****p < 0.0001 (Kruskal-Wallis test with Dunn's correction for multiple comparisons). Cells were harvested for analysis after 4 h of TSA and NaB treatment (500 nM and 2 mM, respectively) and after 24 h of enoxacin, riluzole and edaravone treatment (all 10 μM). Scale bar, 10 μm

was observed with short (4 h) treatment and with a higher enoxacin dose (Additional file 6: Fig. S6). Global HDAC inhibitors trichostatin A (TSA) and sodium butyrate (NaB) also significantly increased NEAT1_2 levels and led to the formation of large, elongated paraspeckles (Fig. 7a and b). Interestingly, edaravone but not riluzole also promoted paraspeckle biogenesis (Fig. 7a and b). None of the compounds studied was able to trigger de novo paraspeckles in hES cell derived motor neurons.

Discussion

Nuclear bodies spatially organize and modulate various cellular processes [54]. Therefore it is not surprising that these membraneless organelles and their components have been implicated in multiple human diseases. Prominent examples are PML bodies and Gems linked to carcinogenesis and motor neuron degeneration, respectively [55, 56]. Paraspeckles have recently come into the limelight in the ALS field because of the extensive involvement of paraspeckle proteins in ALS pathogenesis. In the present study, we found that paraspeckle assembly in the spinal cord is shared by ALS cases with different aetiology and, as such, a hallmark of the disease. Using cell models, we identified two possible mechanisms which may initiate paraspeckle assembly in the spinal cord cells of the majority of ALS cases – compromised miRNA biogenesis and activated dsRNA response – both downstream of loss of TDP-43 function.

In the CNS, miRNAs are highly abundant and are subject to abnormal regulation in many neurodegenerative diseases, including ALS [57–61]. Levels of mature miRNAs in ALS spinal cord were reported to be globally reduced [52, 57, 62]. This dysregulation is consistent with TDP-43 loss of function in the majority of ALS cases since this protein is a known miRNA biogenesis factor [32]. An important role of paraspeckles in miRNA processing is supported by two recent studies [16, 63]. Thus, paraspeckle hyper-assembly in ALS motor neurons affected by TDP-43 loss of function may serve as one of the mechanisms to compensate for miRNA biogenesis deficiency. We also show that not only compromised function of the miRNA pathway but also its pharmacological enhancement results in paraspeckle hyper-assembly. This suggests that paraspeckles can respond to bi-directional changes in the activity of the miRNA pathway to either compensate for its compromised function or to meet the demand for miRNA precursors when its final step is over-active.

Another function of TDP-43 is acting as a chaperone to control RNA secondary structure [38] and therefore cellular dsRNA response. Paraspeckles are known to respond to exogenous dsRNA (viral and its analogues) [14], and here we show that abnormal accumulation of endogenous dsRNA can also initiate paraspeckle response. Given a significant crosstalk between miRNA and dsRNA response pathways [64], it is not surprising that paraspeckles function as a regulatory platform for both pathways. Although dsRNA response triggered by dysfunction of the miRNA pathway factors is mediated via different molecular sensors, including TLR3 (for Drosha, our unpublished observations), MyD88 (for Dicer) [65] and MDA5/RIG-I (for ADAR1) [66], it eventually converges on type I IFN. In contrast to the previous study [14], we found that IFNbeta treatment alone can stimulate NEAT1 expression and paraspeckle formation. This discrepancy is likely due to the transient effect of IFN treatment on paraspeckles which peaks at the 4-h time-point, whereas in the previous work, the 24 h time-point was examined. It is possible that IFN levels oscillate to maintain the dsRNA response active but at the same time preserve cellular viability [67]. Our in vitro data are consistent with a recent in vivo study demonstrating that TDP-43 knockdown in the adult murine nervous system leads to widespread upregulation of immune and, more specifically, antiviral genes [27]. Loss of TDP-43 function in the nervous system might be sufficient to trigger a chronic neuroinflammatory response.

In a previous study, siRNA-mediated TDP-43 knockdown led to decreased paraspeckle numbers in HeLa cells [8]. One possible explanation for this discrepancy is differences in cellular response to dsRNA and/or differences in the miRNA pathway regulation between the cell lines. Indeed, in the study on TDP-43 functions as an RNA chaperone, dsRNA was shown to be accumulated only in the nucleus of HeLa cells, whereas in neuroblastoma M17 cell line it was mainly cytoplasmic [38], similar to our study. Another possibility is the reliance of paraspeckle assembly on some TDP-43 function(s) specifically in HeLa cells.

Loss of TDP-43 function can explain paraspeckle hyper-assembly in the majority of ALS cases, i.e. almost all sALS cases as well as fALS cases caused by mutations in TARDBP and C9ORF72 genes. Recently, Drosha has been identified as a component of C9orf72 dipeptide inclusions in patient's neurons [68]. Therefore in fALS-C9 cases, loss of function for both TDP-43 and Drosha can jointly contribute to paraspeckle response. In a subset of sALS patients, activation of an endogenous retrovirus (ERV), HERV-K, was reported [69]. Elevated expression of ERVs can initiate dsRNA response [70, 71]. Activation of HERV-K may therefore contribute to paraspeckle hyper-assembly at least in some sALS cases. It still remains to be established whether paraspeckle formation is typical for other fALS cases such as those caused by mutations in genes encoding SOD1, FUS, TBK1 or OPTN and, if so, the underlying mechanisms. Many of ALS proteins function in miRNA and dsRNA metabolism, for example FUS is involved in miRNA biogenesis and miRNA-mediated silencing [35, 72], whereas TBK1 is one of the central factors in dsRNA response and type I IFN signaling. Thus compromised function of these pathways may represent a common mechanism behind paraspeckle response in different ALS cases.

Previously, paraspeckles were shown to be protective against cell death caused by proteasomal inhibition [13]. In current study, we show that paraspeckles confer protection to cells with compromised metabolism of miRNA and activated dsRNA response. Intriguingly, many of miRNA-controlled cytotoxicity-associated ISGs [48] were also reported to be regulated by paraspeckles either by sequestration of transcription factors or by nuclear retention of edited RNAs [14, 49, 73] suggesting a multi-layered control of cellular toxicity by paraspeckles. It should be noted however that the effect of paraspeckle disruption on survival in stable cell lines was small both in this and in the previous [13] report, despite the use of cells completely lacking NEAT1 and hence paraspeckles in the latter study. Such limited effect is in line with the fact that NEAT1 knockout mice do not have an overt phenotype [21] and further supports a modulatory role for paraspeckles in cellular responses (such as miRNA biogenesis, gene expression, RNA retention) which only becomes relevant under stressful/pathophysiological conditions. However, such modulatory activities of paraspeckles might be particularly important for neurons coping with neurodegeneration-inducing stresses.

Conclusions

Paraspeckle hyper-assembly might be broadly neuroprotective in ALS. As a word of caution, however, these data were obtained in stable cell lines with pre-existing paraspeckles. Since normal post-mitotic neurons are free from paraspeckles, the impact of their de novo formation on neuronal metabolism may be much more dramatic than in stable cell lines. For example, it is coupled with changes in the levels of the short NEAT1 isoform with diverse paraspeckle-independent regulatory functions, including modulation of neuronal excitability [74–77]. Further studies, using neurons derived from human stem cells with ablated NEAT1_2 expression and from ALS patients' iPS cells, are required to understand whether paraspeckles are protective for motor neurons in the disease context and in the long-term. This shall help us understand whether, how and when paraspeckles can be targeted for therapeutic purposes.

Additional files

Additional file 1: Figure S1. The effect of TDP-43 dysfunction on paraspeckles, speckles and paraspeckle proteins in MCF7 and SH-SY5Y cells. a and b TDP-43 siRNA-mediated knockdown upregulates NEAT1_2 (a) and enhances paraspeckle assembly (b) in SH-SY5Y cells. Cells were transfected with

scrambled siRNA or Silencer® TDP-43 siRNA and analysed by qRT-PCR ($n = 6$). Mean number of paraspeckles per cell was also quantified using NEAT1_2 RNA FISH. $**p < 0.01$, $***p < 0.001$ (Mann-Whitney U-test in a and Student's t-test in b). c and d Downregulation of TDP-43 using an esiRNA (endoribonuclease-prepared MISSION® esiRNA, c) or shRNA (d) stimulates paraspeckle assembly. The efficiency of knockdown was analysed by TDP-43 immunocytochemistry, and paraspeckle assembly – by NEAT1_2 RNA-FISH. Representative images are shown. Scale bars, 100 μm for left panels and 10 μm for right panels. e Speckles visualised by MALAT1 RNA-FISH are not affected by TDP-43 knockdown. Representative images are shown. Scale bar, 10 μm. f Levels of core paraspeckle proteins NONO, SFPQ and FUS are not affected by TDP-43 knockdown in SH-SY5Y cells. Representative Western blots are shown. g Sequences and positions of gRNAs used for disrupting the NLS of the endogenous TDP-43 protein by CRISPR/Cas9-mediated editing. Two combinations of upstream and downstream gRNA sequences within *TARDBP* gene selected to disrupt the NLS are shown. The sequence encoding for the NLS is given in blue and PAM sites are boxed. h Transient transfection of two combinations of plasmids encoding upstream and downstream gRNAs for targeting the NLS of TDP-43 results in partial redistribution of endogenous TDP-43 but does not lead to enhanced paraspeckle formation. Cells were analysed 72 h posttransfection. Representative images are shown, asterisks indicate cells with cytoplasmic TDP-43 redistribution. Scale bar, 10 μm. In a-f, cells were analysed 48 h post-transfection.

Additional file 2: Figure S2. Drosha or TDP-43 downregulation affects miRNA processing. a Drosha knockdown leads to accumulation of miRNA precursors, pri-miR-17-92a and pri-miR-15a ($n = 4$–6). $**p < 0.01$ (one-way ANOVA with Holm-Sidak correction for multiple comparisons). Note the absence of significant accumulation of these pri-miRNAs in TDP-43 depleted cells, in accord with modulatory rather than essential function of this protein in miRNA processing in the nucleus. b Drosha or TDP-43 knockdown leads to downregulation of mature miRNAs processed from pri-miR-17-92a ($n = 3$). $*p < 0.05$; $**p < 0.01$ (one-way ANOVA with Holm-Sidak correction for multiple comparisons). Note that levels of all three mature miRNAs are significantly decreased in Drosha depleted cells, and TDP-43 knockdown also negatively affects two of the three miRNAs measured.

Additional file 3: Figure S3. Accumulation of dsRNA (a) and increased levels of p-eIF2α (b) in MCF7 cells depleted of TDP-43. Cells were analysed 48 h post-transfection. Scale bars, 100 μm and 10 μm for general plane and close-up panels respectively.

Additional file 4: Figure S4. The effect of IFN-inducing ligands on NEAT1 and paraspeckles. a IFNbeta is robustly induced by poly(I:C) in neuroblastoma cells. Cells were analysed by qRT-PCR after 24 h of poly(I:C) stimulation ($n = 5$). $**p < 0.01$ (Mann-Whitney U-test). b-d TLR3 and TLR4 ligands poly(I:C) and LPS, but not a TLR2 ligand zymosan, trigger IFNbeta response stimulating NEAT1 expression (b) and paraspeckle assembly (c). Cells were treated with poly(I:C), LPS or zymosan for 4 h and analysed by qRT-PCR ($n = 3$ or 4). $*p < 0.05$, $**p < 0.01$. NF-κB nuclear translocation was examined in parallel to confirm the activity of the compounds (d, asterisks indicate cells with nuclear NF-κB). Scale bar, 10 μm.

Additional file 5: Figure S5. Differentiation of human neuroblastoma cells into neuron-like cells does not lead to the loss of paraspeckles. Differentiated SH-SY5Y cells develop extensive neurite network and are uniformly positive for a neuronal marker Tuj 1 (left panel) but preserve their ability to form paraspeckles (right panel). SH-SY5Y cells were induced to differentiate into neuron-like cells using retinoic acid/BDNF and analysed 6 days into differentiation by immunocytochemitry and NEAT1_2 RNA-FISH. Representative images are shown. Scale bars, 100 μm (left panel) and 10 μm (right panel).

Additional file 6: Figure S6. Dose-dependent toxicity of enoxacin, edaravone and riluzole. a SH-SY5Y cells were treated with corresponding doses of compounds for 24 h, and toxicity was assessed using CellTiter Blue® Cell Viability Assay. $*p < 0.05$, $**p < 0.01$, $***p < 0.001$, $****p < 0.0001$ as compared to control (non-treated) cells (Kruskal-Wallis test with Dunn's correction for multiple comparisons). b Enoxacin enhances paraspeckle assembly both with short (4 h) and prolonged (24 h) treatment at a non-toxic concentration of 50 μM. Representative images are shown.

Abbreviations

(F)ISH: (fluorescent) in situ hybridisation; ALS: Amyotrophic lateral sclerosis; dsRNA: double-stranded RNA; FTLD: Frontotemporal lobar degeneration; HDAC: Histone deacetylase; IFN: Interferon; ISG: Interferon-stimulated gene; LPS: Lipopolysaccharide; miRNA: microRNA; NEAT1: Nuclear enriched abundant transcript 1; NPC: Neural precursor cell; poly(I:C): Polyinosinic:polycytidylic acid; TDP-43: TAR DNA-binding protein 43; TSA: Trichostatin A

Acknowledgements

We acknowledge the Sheffield Brain Tissue Bank and London Neurodegenerative Diseases Brain Bank for providing human materials.

Funding

TAS is a recipient of a fellowship from Medical Research Foundation. The study was also funded by Research Grant from Motor Neuron Disease Association to VLB (Buchman/Apr13/6096) and miRNA analysis was supported by the Russian Science Foundation grant (18–15-00357). HA and PD are recipients of Cardiff University/China Council PhD studentship and Erasmus studentship, respectively.

Authors' contributions

TAS conceived research; TAS, HA, MSK, PD, SA, OS and PRH performed experiments; TAS and VLB analysed data; TAS wrote manuscript with input from all authors. All authors read and approved the final version of the manuscript.

Competing interests

The authors declare that they have no competing interests.

Author details

[1]School of Biosciences, Cardiff University, Museum Avenue, Cardiff CF10 3AX, UK. [2]Institute of Physiologically Active Compounds Russian Academy of Sciences, 1 Severniy proezd, Chernogolovka, Moscow Region, Russian Federation142432. [3]The Sheffield Institute for Translational Neuroscience, 385A Glossop Road, Sheffield S10 2HQ, UK.

References

1. Renton AE, Chio A, Traynor BJ. State of play in amyotrophic lateral sclerosis genetics. Nat Neurosci. 2014;17:17–23. https://doi.org/10.1038/nn.3584.
2. DeJesus-Hernandez M, Mackenzie IR, Boeve BF, Boxer AL, Baker M, Rutherford NJ, et al. Expanded GGGGCC hexanucleotide repeat in noncoding region of C9ORF72 causes chromosome 9p-linked FTD and ALS. Neuron. 2011;72:245–56. https://doi.org/10.1016/j.neuron.2011.09.011.
3. Sreedharan J, Blair IP, Tripathi VB, Hu X, Vance C, Rogelj B, et al. TDP-43 mutations in familial and sporadic amyotrophic lateral sclerosis. Science. 2008;319:1668–72. https://doi.org/10.1126/science.1154584.
4. Lattante S, Rouleau GA, Kabashi E. TARDBP and FUS mutations associated with amyotrophic lateral sclerosis: summary and update. Hum Mutat. 2013; 34:812–26. https://doi.org/10.1002/humu.22319.
5. Neumann M, Sampathu DM, Kwong LK, Truax AC, Micsenyi MC, Chou TT, et al. Ubiquitinated TDP-43 in frontotemporal lobar degeneration and amyotrophic lateral sclerosis. Science. 2006;314:130–3. https://doi.org/10.1126/science.1134108.
6. Arai T, Hasegawa M, Akiyama H, Ikeda K, Nonaka T, Mori H, et al. TDP-43 is a component of ubiquitin-positive tau-negative inclusions in frontotemporal lobar degeneration and amyotrophic lateral sclerosis. Biochem Biophys Res Commun. 2006;351:602–11. https://doi.org/10.1016/j.bbrc.2006.10.093.
7. Fox AH, Lamond AI. Paraspeckles. Cold Spring Harb Perspect Biol. 2010;2: a000687. https://doi.org/10.1101/cshperspect. a000687.
8. Naganuma T, Nakagawa S, Tanigawa A, Sasaki YF, Goshima N, Hirose T. Alternative 3′-end processing of long noncoding RNA initiates construction of nuclear paraspeckles. EMBO J. 2012;31:4020–34. https://doi.org/10.1038/emboj.2012.251.
9. West JA, Mito M, Kurosaka S, Takumi T, Tanegashima C, Chujo T, et al. Structural, super-resolution microscopy analysis of paraspeckle nuclear body organization. J Cell Biol. 2016; https://doi.org/10.1083/jcb.201601071.
10. Clemson CM, Hutchinson JN, Sara SA, Ensminger AW, Fox AH, Chess A, et al. An architectural role for a nuclear noncoding RNA: NEAT1 RNA is essential for the structure of paraspeckles. Mol Cell. 2009;33:717–26. https://doi.org/10.1016/j.molcel.2009.01.026.
11. Hennig S, Kong G, Mannen T, Sadowska A, Kobelke S, Blythe A, et al. Prion-like domains in RNA binding proteins are essential for building subnuclear paraspeckles. J Cell Biol. 2015;210:529–39. https://doi.org/10.1083/jcb.201504117.
12. Sunwoo H, Dinger ME, Wilusz JE, Amaral PP, Mattick JS. Spector DL. MEN epsilon/beta nuclear-retained non-coding RNAs are up-regulated upon muscle differentiation and are essential components of paraspeckles. Genome Res. 2009;19:347–59. https://doi.org/10.1101/gr.087775.108.
13. Hirose T, Virnicchi G, Tanigawa A, Naganuma T, Li R, Kimura H, et al. NEAT1 long noncoding RNA regulates transcription via protein sequestration within subnuclear bodies. Mol Biol Cell. 2014;25:169–83. https://doi.org/10.1091/mbc.E13-09-0558.
14. Imamura K, Imamachi N, Akizuki G, Kumakura M, Kawaguchi A, Nagata K, et al. Long noncoding RNA NEAT1-dependent SFPQ relocation from promoter region to paraspeckle mediates IL8 expression upon immune stimuli. Mol Cell. 2014;53:393–406. https://doi.org/10.1016/j.molcel.2014.01.009.
15. Zhang Z, Carmichael GG. The fate of dsRNA in the nucleus: a p54(nrb)-containing complex mediates the nuclear retention of promiscuously A-to-I edited RNAs. Cell. 2001;106:465–75. http://www.ncbi.nlm.nih.gov/pubmed/11525732.
16. Jiang L, Shao C, Wu QJ, Chen G, Zhou J, Yang B, et al. NEAT1 scaffolds RNA-binding proteins and the microprocessor to globally enhance pri-miRNA processing. Nat Struct Mol Biol. 2017;24:816–24. https://doi.org/10.1038/nsmb.3455.
17. Choudhry H, Albukhari A, Morotti M, Haider S, Moralli D, Smythies J, et al. Tumor hypoxia induces nuclear paraspeckle formation through HIF-2alpha dependent transcriptional activation of NEAT1 leading to cancer cell survival. Oncogene. 2015;34:4546. https://doi.org/10.1038/onc.2014.431.
18. Chakravarty D, Sboner A, Nair SS, Giannopoulou E, Li R, Hennig S, et al. The oestrogen receptor alpha-regulated lncRNA NEAT1 is a critical modulator of prostate cancer. Nat Commun. 2014;5:5383. https://doi.org/10.1038/ncomms6383.
19. Adriaens C, Standaert L, Barra J, Latil M, Verfaillie A, Kalev P, et al. p53 induces formation of NEAT1 lncRNA-containing paraspeckles that modulate replication stress response and chemosensitivity. Nat Med. 2016;22:861–8. https://doi.org/10.1038/nm.4135.
20. Nishimoto Y, Nakagawa S, Hirose T, Okano HJ, Takao M, Shibata S, et al. The long non-coding RNA nuclear-enriched abundant transcript 1_2 induces paraspeckle formation in the motor neuron during the early phase of amyotrophic lateral sclerosis. Molecular brain. 2013;6:31. https://doi.org/10.1186/1756-6606-6-31.
21. Nakagawa S, Naganuma T, Shioi G, Hirose T. Paraspeckles are subpopulation-specific nuclear bodies that are not essential in mice. J Cell Biol. 2011;193:31–9. https://doi.org/10.1083/jcb.201011110.
22. Thomas-Jinu S, Gordon PM, Fielding T, Taylor R, Smith BN, Snowden V, et al. Non-nuclear pool of splicing factor SFPQ regulates axonal transcripts required for normal motor development. Neuron. 2017;94:931. https://doi.org/10.1016/j.neuron.2017.04.036.
23. Shelkovnikova TA, Robinson HK, Troakes C, Ninkina N, Buchman VL. Compromised paraspeckle formation as a pathogenic factor in FUSopathies. Hum Mol Genet. 2014;23:2298–312. https://doi.org/10.1093/hmg/ddt622.

24. Chesi A, Staahl BT, Jovicic A, Couthouis J, Fasolino M, Raphael AR, et al. Exome sequencing to identify de novo mutations in sporadic ALS trios. Nat Neurosci. 2013;16:851–5. https://doi.org/10.1038/nn.3412.

25. Kim HJ, Kim NC, Wang YD, Scarborough EA, Moore J, Diaz Z, et al. Mutations in prion-like domains in hnRNPA2B1 and hnRNPA1 cause multisystem proteinopathy and ALS. Nature. 2013;495:467–73. https://doi.org/10.1038/nature11922.

26. Tollervey JR, Curk T, Rogelj B, Briese M, Cereda M, Kayikci M, et al. Characterizing the RNA targets and position-dependent splicing regulation by TDP-43. Nat Neurosci. 2011;14:452–8. https://doi.org/10.1038/nn.2778.

27. Polymenidou M, Lagier-Tourenne C, Hutt KR, Huelga SC, Moran J, Liang TY, et al. Long pre-mRNA depletion and RNA missplicing contribute to neuronal vulnerability from loss of TDP-43. Nat Neurosci. 2011;14:459–68. https://doi.org/10.1038/nn.2779.

28. Kukharsky MS, Quintiero A, Matsumoto T, Matsukawa K, An H, Hashimoto T, et al. Calcium-responsive transactivator (CREST) protein shares a set of structural and functional traits with other proteins associated with amyotrophic lateral sclerosis. Mol Neurodegener. 2015;10:20. https://doi.org/10.1186/s13024-015-0014-y.

29. Cong L, Ran FA, Cox D, Lin S, Barretto R, Habib N, et al. Multiplex genome engineering using CRISPR/Cas systems. Science. 2013;339:819–23. https://doi.org/10.1126/science.1231143.

30. Shelkovnikova TA, Dimasi P, Kukharsky MS, An H, Quintiero A, Schirmer C, et al. Chronically stressed or stress-preconditioned neurons fail to maintain stress granule assembly. Cell Death Dis. 2017;8:e2788. https://doi.org/10.1038/cddis.2017.199.

31. Renton AE, Majounie E, Waite A, Simon-Sanchez J, Rollinson S, Gibbs JR, et al. A hexanucleotide repeat expansion in C9ORF72 is the cause of chromosome 9p21-linked ALS-FTD. Neuron. 2011;72:257–68. https://doi.org/10.1016/j.neuron.2011.09.010.

32. Kawahara Y, Mieda-Sato A. TDP-43 promotes microRNA biogenesis as a component of the Drosha and dicer complexes. Proc Natl Acad Sci U S A. 2012;109:3347–52. https://doi.org/10.1073/pnas.1112427109.

33. Buratti E, De Conti L, Stuani C, Romano M, Baralle M, Baralle F. Nuclear factor TDP-43 can affect selected microRNA levels. FEBS J. 2010;277:2268–81. https://doi.org/10.1111/j.1742-4658.2010.07643.x.

34. Ota H, Sakurai M, Gupta R, Valente L, Wulff BE, Ariyoshi K, et al. ADAR1 forms a complex with dicer to promote microRNA processing and RNA-induced gene silencing. Cell. 2013;153:575–89. https://doi.org/10.1016/j.cell.2013.03.024.

35. Morlando M, Dini Modigliani S, Torrelli G, Rosa A, Di Carlo V, Caffarelli E, et al. FUS stimulates microRNA biogenesis by facilitating co-transcriptional Drosha recruitment. EMBO J. 2012;31:4502–10. https://doi.org/10.1038/emboj.2012.319.

36. Tan GS, Chiu CH, Garchow BG, Metzler D, Diamond SL, Kiriakidou M. Small molecule inhibition of RISC loading. ACS Chem Biol. 2012;7:403–10. https://doi.org/10.1021/cb200253h.

37. Lagier-Tourenne C, Polymenidou M, Hutt KR, Vu AQ, Baughn M, Huelga SC, et al. Divergent roles of ALS-linked proteins FUS/TLS and TDP-43 intersect in processing long pre-mRNAs. Nat Neurosci. 2012;15:1488–97. https://doi.org/10.1038/nn.3230.

38. Saldi TK, Ash PE, Wilson G, Gonzales P, Garrido-Lecca A, Roberts CM, et al. TDP-1, the Caenorhabditis elegans ortholog of TDP-43, limits the accumulation of double-stranded RNA. EMBO J. 2014;33:2947–66. https://doi.org/10.15252/embj.201488740.

39. Ma H, Han P, Ye W, Chen H, Zheng X, Cheng L, et al. The long noncoding RNA NEAT1 exerts Antihantaviral effects by acting as positive feedback for RIG-I signaling. J Virol. 2017;91 https://doi.org/10.1128/JVI.02250-16.

40. White E, Schlackow M, Kamieniarz-Gdula K, Proudfoot NJ, Gullerova M. Human nuclear dicer restricts the deleterious accumulation of endogenous double-stranded RNA. Nat Struct Mol Biol. 2014;21:552–9. https://doi.org/10.1038/nsmb.2827.

41. Heras SR, Macias S, Plass M, Fernandez N, Cano D, Eyras E, et al. The microprocessor controls the activity of mammalian retrotransposons. Nat Struct Mol Biol. 2013;20:1173–81. https://doi.org/10.1038/nsmb.2658.

42. Liddicoat BJ, Piskol R, Chalk AM, Ramaswami G, Higuchi M, Hartner JC, et al. RNA editing by ADAR1 prevents MDA5 sensing of endogenous dsRNA as nonself. Science. 2015;349:1115–20. https://doi.org/10.1126/science.aac7049.

43. Weber F, Wagner V, Rasmussen SB, Hartmann R, Paludan SR. Double-stranded RNA is produced by positive-strand RNA viruses and DNA viruses but not in detectable amounts by negative-strand RNA viruses. J Virol. 2006;80:5059–64. https://doi.org/10.1128/JVI.80.10.5059-5064.2006.

44. Kaneko H, Dridi S, Tarallo V, Gelfand BD, Fowler BJ, Cho WG, et al. DICER1 deficit induces Alu RNA toxicity in age-related macular degeneration. Nature. 2011;471:325–30. https://doi.org/10.1038/nature09830.

45. Marullo M, Zuccato C, Mariotti C, Lahiri N, Tabrizi SJ, Di Donato S, et al. Expressed Alu repeats as a novel, reliable tool for normalization of real-time quantitative RT-PCR data. Genome Biol. 2010;11:R9. https://doi.org/10.1186/gb-2010-11-1-r9.

46. Marciniak SJ, Yun CY, Oyadomari S, Novoa I, Zhang Y, Jungreis R, et al. CHOP induces death by promoting protein synthesis and oxidation in the stressed endoplasmic reticulum. Genes Dev. 2004;18:3066–77. https://doi.org/10.1101/gad.1250704.

47. Matsumoto M, Minami M, Takeda K, Sakao Y, Akira S. Ectopic expression of CHOP (GADD153) induces apoptosis in M1 myeloblastic leukemia cells. FEBS Lett 1996; 395:143–147. doi: 0014–5793(96)01016–2.

48. Seo GJ, Kincaid RP, Phanaksri T, Burke JM, Pare JM, Cox JE, et al. Reciprocal inhibition between intracellular antiviral signaling and the RNAi machinery in mammalian cells. Cell Host Microbe. 2013;14:435–45. https://doi.org/10.1016/j.chom.2013.09.002.

49. Chen LL, Carmichael GG. Altered nuclear retention of mRNAs containing inverted repeats in human embryonic stem cells: functional role of a nuclear noncoding RNA. Mol Cell. 2009;35:467–78. https://doi.org/10.1016/j.molcel.2009.06.027.

50. Melo S, Villanueva A, Moutinho C, Davalos V, Spizzo R, Ivan C, et al. Small molecule enoxacin is a cancer-specific growth inhibitor that acts by enhancing TAR RNA-binding protein 2-mediated microRNA processing. Proc Natl Acad Sci U S A. 2011;108:4394–9. https://doi.org/10.1073/pnas.1014720108.

51. Shan G, Li Y, Zhang J, Li W, Szulwach KE, Duan R, et al. A small molecule enhances RNA interference and promotes microRNA processing. Nat Biotechnol. 2008;26:933–40. https://doi.org/10.1038/nbt.1481.

52. Emde A, Eitan C, Liou LL, Libby RT, Rivkin N, Magen I, et al. Dysregulated miRNA biogenesis downstream of cellular stress and ALS-causing mutations: a new mechanism for ALS. EMBO J. 2015;34:2633–51. https://doi.org/10.15252/embj.201490493.

53. Schor IE, Lleres D, Risso GJ, Pawellek A, Ule J, Lamond AI, et al. Perturbation of chromatin structure globally affects localization and recruitment of splicing factors. PLoS One. 2012;7:e48084. https://doi.org/10.1371/journal.pone.0048084.

54. Misteli T. Higher-order genome organization in human disease. Cold Spring Harb Perspect Biol. 2010;2:a000794. https://doi.org/10.1101/cshperspect.a000794.

55. de The H, Le Bras M, Lallemand-Breitenbach V. The cell biology of disease: acute promyelocytic leukemia, arsenic, and PML bodies. J Cell Biol 2012;198: 11–21. doi: https://doi.org/10.1083/jcb.201112044.

56. Yamazaki T, Chen S, Yu Y, Yan B, Haertlein TC, Carrasco MA, et al. FUS-SMN protein interactions link the motor neuron diseases ALS and SMA. Cell Rep. 2012;2:799–806. https://doi.org/10.1016/j.celrep.2012.08.025.

57. Figueroa-Romero C, Hur J, Lunn JS, Paez-Colasante X, Bender DE, Yung R, et al. Expression of microRNAs in human post-mortem amyotrophic lateral sclerosis spinal cords provides insight into disease mechanisms. Mol Cell Neurosci. 2016;71:34–45. https://doi.org/10.1016/j.mcn.2015.12.008.

58. Freischmidt A, Muller K, Ludolph AC, Weishaupt JH. Systemic dysregulation of TDP-43 binding microRNAs in amyotrophic lateral sclerosis. Acta Neuropathol Commun. 2013;1:42. https://doi.org/10.1186/2051-5960-1-42.

59. Gascon E, Gao FB. The emerging roles of microRNAs in the pathogenesis of frontotemporal dementia-amyotrophic lateral sclerosis (FTD-ALS) spectrum disorders. J Neurogenet. 2014;28:30–40. https://doi.org/10.3109/01677063.2013.876021.

60. Goodall EF, Heath PR, Bandmann O, Kirby J, Shaw PJ. Neuronal dark matter: the emerging role of microRNAs in neurodegeneration. Front Cell Neurosci. 2013;7:178. https://doi.org/10.3389/fncel.2013.00178.

61. Eitan C, Hornstein E. Vulnerability of microRNA biogenesis in FTD-ALS. Brain Res. 2016;1647:105–11. https://doi.org/10.1016/j.brainres.2015.12.063.

62. Campos-Melo D, Droppelmann CA, He Z, Volkening K, Strong MJ. Altered microRNA expression profile in amyotrophic lateral sclerosis: a role in the regulation of NFL mRNA levels. Molecular brain. 2013;6:26. https://doi.org/10.1186/1756-6606-6-26.

63. Bottini S, Hamouda-Tekaya N, Mategot R, Zaragosi LE, Audebert S, Pisano S, et al. Post-transcriptional gene silencing mediated by microRNAs is controlled by nucleoplasmic Sfpq. Nat Commun. 2017;8:1189. https://doi.org/10.1038/s41467-017-01126-x.

64. Heyam A, Lagos D, Plevin M. Dissecting the roles of TRBP and PACT in double-stranded RNA recognition and processing of noncoding RNAs. Wiley Interdiscip Rev RNA. 2015;6:271–89. https://doi.org/10.1002/wrna.1272.

65. Tarallo V, Hirano Y, Gelfand BD, Dridi S, Kerur N, Kim Y, et al. DICER1 loss and Alu RNA induce age-related macular degeneration via the NLRP3 inflammasome and MyD88. Cell. 2012;149:847–59. https://doi.org/10.1016/j.cell.2012.03.036.

66. Mannion NM, Greenwood SM, Young R, Cox S, Brindle J, Read D, et al. The RNA-editing enzyme ADAR1 controls innate immune responses to RNA. Cell Rep. 2014;9:1482–94. https://doi.org/10.1016/j.celrep.2014.10.041.

67. Ruggieri A, Dazert E, Metz P, Hofmann S, Bergeest JP, Mazur J, et al. Dynamic oscillation of translation and stress granule formation mark the cellular response to virus infection. Cell Host Microbe. 2012;12:71–85. https://doi.org/10.1016/j.chom.2012.05.013.

68. Porta S, Kwong LK, Trojanowski JQ, Lee VM. Drosha inclusions are new components of dipeptide-repeat protein aggregates in FTLD-TDP and ALS C9orf72 expansion cases. J Neuropathol Exp Neurol. 2015;74:380–7. https://doi.org/10.1097/NEN.0000000000000182.

69. Li W, Lee MH, Henderson L, Tyagi R, Bachani M, Steiner J, et al. Human endogenous retrovirus-K contributes to motor neuron disease. Sci Transl Med. 2015;7:307ra153. https://doi.org/10.1126/scitranslmed.aac8201.

70. Hurst TP, Magiorkinis G. Activation of the innate immune response by endogenous retroviruses. J Gen Virol. 2015;96:1207–18. https://doi.org/10.1099/jgv.0.000017.

71. Chiappinelli KB, Strissel PL, Desrichard A, Li H, Henke C, Akman B, et al. Inhibiting DNA methylation causes an interferon response in Cancer via dsRNA including endogenous retroviruses. Cell. 2016;164:1073. https://doi.org/10.1016/j.cell.2015.10.020.

72. Zhang T, Wu YC, Mullane P, Ji YJ, Liu H, He L, et al. FUS regulates activity of MicroRNA-mediated gene silencing. Mol Cell 2018; 69:787–801 e8. doi: https://doi.org/10.1016/j.molcel.2018.02.001.

73. Elbarbary RA, Li W, Tian B, Maquat LE. STAU1 binding 3' UTR IRAlus complements nuclear retention to protect cells from PKR-mediated translational shutdown. Genes Dev. 2013;27:1495–510. https://doi.org/10.1101/gad.220962.113.

74. Barry G, Briggs JA, Hwang DW, Nayler SP, Fortuna PR, Jonkhout N, et al. The long non-coding RNA NEAT1 is responsive to neuronal activity and is associated with hyperexcitability states. Sci Rep. 2017;7:40127. https://doi.org/10.1038/srep40127.

75. Li R, Harvey AR, Hodgetts SI, Fox AH. Functional dissection of NEAT1 using genome editing reveals substantial localisation of the NEAT1_1 isoform outside paraspeckles. RNA. 2017; https://doi.org/10.1261/rna.059477.116.

76. Zhang F, Wu L, Qian J, Qu B, Xia S, La T, et al. Identification of the long noncoding RNA NEAT1 as a novel inflammatory regulator acting through MAPK pathway in human lupus. J Autoimmun. 2016;75:96–104. https://doi.org/10.1016/j.jaut.2016.07.012.

77. West JA, Davis CP, Sunwoo H, Simon MD, Sadreyev RI, Wang PI, et al. The long noncoding RNAs NEAT1 and MALAT1 bind active chromatin sites. Mol Cell. 2014;55:791–802. https://doi.org/10.1016/j.molcel.2014.07.012.

5

Counteracting roles of MHCI and CD8$^+$ T cells in the peripheral and central nervous system of ALS SOD1^{G93A} mice

Giovanni Nardo[1*†] (iD), Maria Chiara Trolese[1†], Mattia Verderio[1], Alessandro Mariani[2], Massimiliano de Paola[2], Nilo Riva[3], Giorgia Dina[3], Nicolò Panini[4], Eugenio Erba[4], Angelo Quattrini[3] and Caterina Bendotti[1]

Abstract

Background: The major histocompatibility complex I (MHCI) is a key molecule for the interaction of mononucleated cells with CD8$^+$T lymphocytes. We previously showed that MHCI is upregulated in the spinal cord microglia and motor axons of transgenic SOD1^{G93A} mice.

Methods: To assess the role of MHCI in the disease, we examined transgenic SOD1^{G93A} mice crossbred with β2 microglobulin-deficient mice, which express little if any MHCI on the cell surface and are defective for CD8$^+$ T cells.

Results: The lack of MHCI and CD8$^+$ T cells in the sciatic nerve affects the motor axon stability, anticipating the muscle atrophy and the disease onset. In contrast, MHCI depletion in resident microglia and the lack of CD8$^+$ T cell infiltration in the spinal cord protect the cervical motor neurons delaying the paralysis of forelimbs and prolonging the survival of SOD1^{G93A} mice.

Conclusions: We provided straightforward evidence for a dual role of MHCI in the peripheral nervous system (PNS) compared to the CNS, pointing out regional and temporal differences in the clinical responses of ALS mice. These findings offer a possible explanation for the failure of systemic immunomodulatory treatments and suggest new potential strategies to prevent the progression of ALS.

Keywords: Amyotrophic lateral sclerosis, SOD1G93A mice, Neuroinflammation, MHCI, CD8+ T cells, Motor neuron, Peripheral nervous system

Background

Amyotrophic lateral sclerosis (ALS) is the most common neuromuscular disorder, affecting individuals from all ethnic backgrounds, with an incidence of 2–3 cases per 100,000 individuals per year [1, 2]. The pathology, causing a progressive motor neuron (MN) loss and muscle denervation, results in progressive paralysis and death, usually due to respiratory failure [1, 2]. The average patient's lifespan ranges between 2 and 5 years after diagnosis [2].

Genetic factors contribute to the disease in 10% of all ALS cases corresponding to the familial form [3]. Although more than 30 genes have been associated with

familial ALS yet, transgenic mice overexpressing mutant human Cu/Zn dependent SOD1 (mSOD1) are currently the animal model that best mimics some phenotypical and pathological features of both familial and sporadic ALS [2, 4]. There is growing evidence of a prominent role of the immune system in the pathogenesis and progression of ALS [5–9].

Adaptive and innate immune cell infiltrate the CNS of ALS patients [10] and in the CNS [6–8] and peripheral nervous system (PNS) of mSOD1 mice [11, 12] at different stages of the disease. The role of immunity is multifaceted with different cell types influencing the disease progression and the same cell type having a positive or negative effect depending on the disease stage [9]. This may explain why immunosuppressive treatments used in different clinical trials were not effective and in some cases even detrimental [13, 14]. For example, CD4$^+$ T cells, in

* Correspondence: giovanni.nardo@marionegri.it

†Giovanni Nardo and Maria Chiara Trolese contributed equally to this work.

[1]Laboratory of Molecular Neurobiology, Department of Neuroscience, IRCCS - Istituto di Ricerche Farmacologiche Mario Negri, Via La Masa 19, 20156 Milan, Italy

Full list of author information is available at the end of the article

particular, CD4+-FoxP3 T cells, are recruited to the sites of damage in mSOD1 mice to protect MNs by maintaining an anti-inflammatory milieu during the early stable phase of the disease [7, 15]. In contrast, CD8+ T-cells (cytotoxic T lymphocytes; CTLs) infiltrating the CNS of ALS patients and mSOD1 mice [8, 10, 16, 17] have been classically considered detrimental for MNs. This is because CTLs are antigen-specific effector cells that express the ligand for Fas (FasL) [18] and MNs expressing ALS-linked SOD1 mutations showed enhanced susceptibility to Fas-mediated death in vitro [19, 20]. Moreover, mSOD1 mice with homozygous loss-of-function FasL mutation present a reduced MN loss and prolonger life expectancy [21]. These data indicate that CTLs may contribute to exacerbating the neuromuscular damage, but this hypothesis has never been adequately verified in mSOD1 mice.

We previously found that the immunoproteasome and the major histocompatibility complex I (MHCI), responsible for the generation and presentation of antigen peptides to CTLs, respectively, were highly expressed in the spinal cord and peripheral motor axons of mSOD1 mice [11, 22–25]. Surprisingly, MHCI signaling and CTLs infiltrates were higher in the periphery of mice with slower denervation and progression of disease than mouse with fast disease progression [11, 22]. We therefore hypothesized that the extent of expression of MHCI and CTLs infiltration in the PNS might influence the variability in disease progression in mSOD1 mice, suggesting a potential protective role of the MHCI-related process [5, 11, 26].

Song et al. [27] also showed that the sustained expression of MHCI in MNs protects them from ALS astrocyte–induced toxicity and delays disease progression in mSOD1 mice. However, it was not been addressed whether the protective action of MHCI in vivo was independent of the interaction with the CTLs. Therefore, we investigated if the depletion of MHCI-dependent CTLs activity in mSOD1 mice had a detrimental or beneficial effect on MN viability and disease progression. For this purpose, we produced C57SOD1^{G93A} mice defective for MHCI cell-surface expression and CTLs.

This lack resulted in acceleration of the motor onset due to the increase of hindlimb muscle denervation. However, the MN somata were protected in the spinal cord especially at the cervical level resulting in significant delay in the forelimbs impairment which led to an extension of survival. This suggested that the activation of MHCI in the PNS of ALS mice is an early protective response directed to the preservation of muscle innervation and motor function. Whereas, in the CNS the interaction of microglia expressing MHCI with CD8+ T cells accelerates MN death and reduces the overall survival of SOD1^{G93A} mice.

Methods

Animals

C57BL6.129P2-B2mtm1Unc/J (stock no: 002087; Jackson Laboratories) females were crossed with C57BL/6JSOD1^{G93A} (stock no: 002726; Jackson Laboratories) male mice, expressing approximately 20 copies of human mutant SOD1 with a Gly93Ala substitution to obtain transgenic mice null for the β2m subunit. Female mSOD1 mice with or without β2m and the corresponding NTG littermates were used for the analysis. Procedures involving animals and their care were conducted according to the Mario Negri institutional guidelines. The Institute adheres to the principles set out in the following laws, regulations, and policies governing the care and use of laboratory animals: Italian Governing Law (D.lgs 26/2014; Authorisation n.19/2008-A issued March 6, 2008 by Ministry of Health); Mario Negri Institutional regulations and Policies providing internal authorisation for personsconducting animal experiments (Quality Management System Certificate- UNI EN ISO 9001:2008 - Reg. N° 6121); the NIH Guide for the Care and Use of Laboratory Animals (2011 edition) and EU directives and guidelines (EEC Council Directive 2010/63/UE). The Statement of Compliance (Assurnace) with the Public Health Service (PHS) Policy on Human Care and Use of Laboratory Animals has been recently reviewed (9/9/2014) and will expire on September 30, 2019 (Animal Welfare Assurnace #A5023–01). Mice were maintained at a temperature of 22 ± 2 °C with a relative humidity $55 \pm 10\%$ and 12 h of light / dark cycle. Food (standard pellets) and water were supplied ad libitum.

Disease progression and survival

Disease progression was monitored bi-weekly, starting from ten weeks of age, in SOD1^{G93A} transgenic mice wild-type and knockout for β2 microglobulin, and their respective NTG littermates,. Body weight and paw grip strength were recorded for each session, as previously described [28]. The Paw Grip Endurance (PaGE) test involved placing the mouse on the wire-lid of a conventional housing cage. For this analysis, the mice are placed on a horizontal grid at about 30 cm from the table and the tail is gently pulled until they grasp the grid with their fore and hind paws. The lid is then gently turned upside down and the latency time of the mouse to fall on the table is recorded for a maximum of 90 s. Each mouse is given up to three attempts and the longest latency is recorded. The onset of hindlimb force deficit is considered when the mice showed the first signs of impairment (latency less than 90 s) in PaGE test. The disability onset is when the mouse for the first time is unable to perform the PaGE test. The mice are euthanized when they are unable to right themselves within ten seconds after being placed on each side according to the institutional ethical committee guidelines. The age at the euthanasia was considered as time of survival.

Disease duration was calculated as the difference in days between the onset of hindlimb impairment and the age of death. Days of survival after the onset of disability is the difference in days between the age when the animal is entirely unable to perform the PaGE test and the age at euthanasia. All tests were done by the same operator blinded to the mouse genotype.

Immunohistochemistry

Spinal cord and sciatic nerve and muscles were processed as previously described [22]. Briefly, mice were perfused with Tyrodes's buffer, followed by Lana's fixative (4% formalin and 0.4% picric acid in 0.16 M PBS, pH 7.2) at 20 °C, and tissues were quickly dissected out. The tissue was left in the same fixative for 180 min at 4 °C, rinsed, and stored 24 h in 10% sucrose with 0.1% sodium azide in 0.01 M PSB at 4 °C for cryoprotection, before mounting in optimal cutting temperature compound (OCT).

Unless otherwise specified, the following primary antibodies and staining were used: rat anti-MHC class I ER-HR 52 clone (1:100; Abcam); mouse anti-GFAP (1:2500; Millipore); rabbit anti-NF200 (1:200; Sigma-Aldrich); mouse anti-vimentin (1:250; Millipore); mouse anti-phosphorylated neurofilament H (Smi31; 1:5000; Sigma); Neurotrace conjugated with Alexa-647 (1:500; Invitrogen); goat anti p75^{NTR} (1:200; Santa Cruz Biotech). Alexa- 488, 594 and 647 secondary antibodies (Invitrogen) were used with a dilution of 1:500. All immunohistochemistry was done following an indirect immunostaining protocol.

Spinal cord immunohistochemistry was done on free-floating sections (30 µm), then mounted on glass slides (Waldemar Knittle) with 1:1 PBS 0.1 M: glycerol. Longitudinal sections of sciatic and radial nerves (14 µm) were treated directly on poly-lysine objective slides (VWR International) as described below, then mounted with 1:1 PBS 0.1 M: glycerol. Fluorescence-labeled samples were analyzed under a sequential scanning mode to avoid bleed-through effects with an IX81 microscope equipped with a confocal scan unit FV500 with three laser lines: Ar-Kr (488 nm), He-Ne red (646 nm), and He-Ne green (532 nm) (Olympus, Tokyo, Japan) and a UV diode using a 10X objective (zoom 1,5×).

Motor neuron impairment

The number of MNs was determined on serial sections (one every ten sections) from lumbar spinal cord segments L2-L5 and cervical spinal cord segments C1-C8 for each mouse. The sections were stained with cresyl violet to detect the Nissl substance of neuronal cells. A total of 12 serial sections were acquired with a CCD color camera (Color View III; Soft Imaging System GmbH) at 10X, using AnalYSIS software (Soft Imaging Systems GmbH, ver. 3.2) and neuron areas were analyzed with Fiji software

(Image J, U. S. National Institutes of Health, Bethesda, Maryland, USA). Only neuronal somas with an area ≥ 400 µm^2 were considered for quantitative analysis of MN numbers.

MN impairment was evaluated on serial sections from lumbar and cervical spinal cord segments for each mouse. Six sections per animal were acquired under the laser scanning confocal microscope (Olympus, Tokyo, Japan) using a 20X objective, and analyzed using Fiji software (Image J, U. S. National Institutes of Health, Bethesda, Maryland, USA) to determine the percentage of MNs with an area ≥ 400 µm^2 (identified by Neurotrace) immunostained with Smi31.

Immunohistochemical analysis of MHCl, GFAP, and p75^{NTR} in sciatic and radial nerves

After 0.1 M PBS perfusion, radial and sciatic nerves were dissected out from the same animal and mounted in OCT. Serial longitudinal sections (14 µm) were collected on poly-lysine objective slides (VWR International). For each slice, fluorescence fields were taken the laser scanning confocal microscope (Olympus, Tokyo, Japan). The mean grey value of the immunoreactivity was assessed through Fiji (Image J, U. S. National Institutes of Health, Bethesda, Maryland, USA) for each section in the analysis.

Muscle denervation and endplates

Tibialis anterior and *triceps brachii* were dissected out, and snap-frozen in isopentane cooled in liquid nitrogen. 20-µm serial longitudinal cryosections were collected on poly-lysine objective slides (VWR International). Five serial sections (average ~ 70 NMJs) per animal were analyzed. Muscle sections were stained with anti-synaptic vesicle protein (SV2; 1:100; Developmental Studies Hybridoma Bank), mouse anti-neurofilament 165 kDa (2H3; 1:50; Developmental Studies Hybridoma Bank), followed by 647 anti-mouse secondary antibody (1:500; Invitrogen). α-Bungarotoxin coupled to Alexa Fluor 488 (1:500) (Invitrogen) was then added and left for 2 h at room temperature.

Innervation analysis was performed directly. Images of all genotypes for the innervation analysis were obtained with an Olympus virtual slide system VS110 (Olympus, Center Valley, PA, USA) at 40X-magnification. Images for endplate size analyses were captured with an epifluorescence microscope system (Axio Imager M1 Upright microscope, Zeiss) at 40× magnification with Q-capture software. The percentage of neuromuscular innervation was quantified in OlyVIA (Olympus) on the basis of the overlay between neurofilament (SV2/2H3) staining and α-BTX labeled endplates. Endplates were quantified as occupied when there was any neurofilament staining overlying the endplate and as vacant when there was no overlay. Endplate area was determined using Fiji software (ImageJ, National Institutes of Health). Endplates were manually outlined, and the area was measured. Diaphragm: after excision, tissues were stretch over silicone rubber to make it taut, using insect pins, in a glass 100 mm Petri dish, fixed in 4% paraformaldehyde for 4 h and stored 24 h in 30% sucrose with 0.1% sodium azide in 0.01 M PSB at 4 °C for cryoprotection. After this, connective tissue was cleaned off using a stereomicroscope and the right and left muscle areas were cut into pieces before mounting in OCT; 20-μm serial longitudinal cryosections were collected on poly-lysine objective slides (VWR International). At least five serial sections per animal were analyzed. Muscle sections were stained with anti-Synaptophysin (1:100; Synaptic system), followed by 488 anti-mouse secondary antibody (1:500; Invitrogen). α-Bungarotoxin coupled to Alexa Fluor 594 (1:1000) (Invitrogen) was then added and left for 15′ at room temperature. For each slice, consecutive fluorescence fields along the z-axis were taken using the laser scanning confocal microscope (Olympus, Tokyo, Japan) using a 20X objective (zoom 2×) at 0.43 μm intervals Denervation was analysed using Imaris 7.4.2 (Bitplane). The colocalization channel between Synaptophysin and BTX immunostaining was produced for each Z-stack. Then, rendering in iso-surfaces was done on the colocalization and BTX channels, and the ratio in voxels (μm^3) was calculated.

Morphometric analysis of muscles and sciatic nerves

Tibialis anterior muscles were dissected out and snap-frozen in isopentane cooled in liquid nitrogen. Muscle fiber architecture and composition were analyzed by hematoxylin and eosin (H&E) and nicotinamide adenine dinucleotide tetrazolium reductase (NADH-TR) staining. Serial transverse cryosections (12 μm) from the mid-belly region of the tibialis anterior muscle were mounted on poly-lysine objective slides (VWR International). For H&E staining, sections were air-dried and fixed in 4% paraformaldehyde solution for 5′, washed in water and stained with hematoxylin (Merck) for 5′. After bluing, sections were stained with 0.5% eosin solution (Merck) containing 1% acetic acid for 10′ and washed. After dehydration in a graded series of alcohol (70, 90, 100%) and clearing in 100% xylene, sections were mounted with DPX compound (Sigma Aldrich). For NADH staining, sections were air-dried then incubated at 37 °C for 30′ in Tris-HCl buffer (50 mM, pH 7.4) containing 0.4 mg/mL β-NAD reduced disodium salt hydrate (Sigma-Aldrich, St. Louis, MO, USA, 0.71 mg/mL buffer solution) and 1 mg/mL nitro blue tetrazolium (Sigma-Aldrich, 0.29 mg/mL buffer solution). After staining, sections were fixed with 4% paraformaldehyde, dehydrated in a graded series of alcohol (70, 90, 100%), cleared in 100% xylene and finally mounted with DPX compound (Sigma Aldrich). For both applications,

images were acquired with a CCD color camera (Color View III; Soft Imaging System, GmbH), using AnaliSYS software (Soft Imaging Systems, GmbH, ver. 3.2) at 10X and 20X-magnification for H&E and NADH staining, respectively.

Muscle fiber CSA, number, and density were analyzed with Fiji (Image J, U. S. National Institutes of Health, Bethesda, Maryland, USA) as previously described [29]. Briefly, a grid of rectangular sampling fields was outlined on the muscle slice profile. To ensure that every part of the slice had an equal chance of being sampled, a systematic random sampling procedure was applied considering rectangular field placed at a fixed distance from each other using the "Grid" function in Fiji. Respectively, four and two serial cryosections for each mouse were analyzed for H&E and NADH. For the morphometric analysis of axons, sciatic nerve samples were fixed with 4% PFA and 2% glutaraldehyde in 0.12 M PBS and post-fixed with 1% OsO4 in 0.12 M cacodylate buffer, dehydrated in graded series of ethanol, and embedded in epoxy resin (Fluka). Coronal semithin sections (1 um), were stained with 0.1% toluidine blue in 0.12 M phosphate buffer. The images were acquired with an Olympus virtual slide system VS110 (Olympus, Center Valley, PA, USA) at 20X-magnification. Diameter and caliber of axons were assessed through Fiji (Image J, U. S. National Institutes of Health, Bethesda, Maryland, USA) on three serial sections per animal with the same procedure described above.

Flow cytometric analysis

At 70, 123 and 140 d 25 μL of whole blood were collected in EDTA 10 mM and Polybrene 0.125% from the submandibular plexus of anesthetized mice. Samples were incubated with 600 μL ACK lysing buffer (Lonza) to lyse red blood cells. After centrifugation (1,4 rcf at 4 °C for 7 min), the ACK solution was removed, and the pellet was washed twice with cold PBS + 1% FBS (FACS buffer). The pellet was then incubated for 30 min at 4 °C in the dark in 100 μL of FACS buffer with the following primary monoclonal antibodies: FITC-labeled rat anti-mouse CD3ε (BD Pharmingen), Cy5.5-labeled rat anti-mouse CD8 α-chain (BD Pharmingen); APC-labeled rat anti mouse CD4 α-chain (BD Pharmingen). Each flow cytometric analysis was run on at least 10,000 cells on a Gallios flow cytometer (Beckman Coulter) equipped with 488, and 638 nm lasers and the data were analyzed using Kaluza software.

Western blot

After deep anesthesia, mice were decapitated and sciatic nerve and muscles were rapidly dissected, frozen on dry ice and stored at − 80 °C. The samples were powdered in liquid nitrogen then homogenized by sonication in ice-cold homogenization buffer (Tris HCl pH 8 50 mM, NaCl 150 mM, EGTA pH 8.5 mM, MgCl2 1.5 mM, Triton x-100 1%, anhydrous glycerol 10%, NaF 50 mM,

NaPP 10 mM, Na$_3$VO$_4$ 10 mM, PMSF 0,1 mg/mL, leupeptin 0,02 mg/mL, aprotinin 0.02 mg/mL, DTT 1 mM), centrifuged at 13000 rpm for 15 min at 4 °C and the supernatants were collected and stored at – 80 °C.

Equal amounts of total protein homogenates were loaded on polyacrylamide gels and electroblotted onto PVDF membrane (Millipore) as previously described [22]. Membranes were immunoblotted with the following primary antibodies: mouse anti β-actin (1:30000; Chemicon); mouse anti Importin β; (1:5000; Millipore); mouse anti β^{III}-tubulin (1:1000; Millipore); rabbit anti ERK (1:1000; Santa Cruz Biotech); mouse anti phospho-ERK (1:1000; Santa Cruz Biotech); rabbit anti NF200 (1:1000; Sigma-Aldrich); mouse anti GFAP (1:10000; Millipore); goat anti p75^{NTR} (1:1000; Santa Cruz Biotech); rabbit anti S100β (1:200; Sigma Aldrich); rabbit anti AChR-α7 (1:100; Millipore); rabbit anti NCAM (1:2000; Millipore); mouse anti GAPDH (1:10.000; Millipore); mouse anti MBP (1:1000; R&D); followed by HRP-conjugated secondary antibodies (Santa Cruz) and developed with Luminata Forte Western Chemiluminescent HRP Substrate (Millipore) on the Chemi-Doc XRS system (Bio-Rad). Densitometric analysis was done with Progenesis PG240 v2006 software (Nonlinear Dynamics). Immunoreactivity (IR) was normalized to β-actin, GAPDH or to the total amount of protein detected by red Ponceau (Sigma Aldrich) as previously published [22]. When necessary, more than one membrane was analysed as follows: i) an internal standard (IS) representing the mix of all the samples in the experiment was loaded on each gel; ii) membranes were acquired at the same time; iii) the immunoreactivity of each sample was further normalized to the immunoreactivity of the IS.

Real-time PCR

Tissues (spinal cords, sciatic nerves, and muscles) were freshly collected and immediately frozen on dry ice after mouse perfusion with 0.1 M PBS. The total RNA from spinal cord was extracted using the Trizol method (Invitrogen) and purified with PureLink RNA columns (Life Technologies). For fibrous tissues (sciatic nerve and muscles), the RNeasy® Mini Kit (Qiagen) was used. RNA samples were treated with DNase I and reverse transcription was done with a High Capacity cDNA Reverse Transcription Kit (Life Technologies). For Real-time PCR we used the Taq Man Gene expression assay (Applied Biosystems) following the manufacturer's instructions, on cDNA specimens in triplicate, using 1X Universal PCR master mix (Life Technologies) and 1X mix containing specific receptor probes. The following probes were used for the real-time PCR: CD8 alpha receptor (CD8; Mm01182107_g1; Life Technologies); CD4 alpha receptor (CD4; Mm00442754_m1); Forkhead box P3 (FoxP3; Mm00475162_m1); cholinergic receptor nicotinic, gamma subunit (CHRNG; Mm00437419_m1; Life Technologies); insulin growth factor 1 (Igf1; Mm00439560_m1); Interferon-γ

(Ifnγ; Mm01168134_m1; Life Technologies) monocytes chemoattract protein-1 (Ccl2; Mm00441242_m1; Life Technologies); CD68 (Cd68; Mm03047343_m1; Life Technologies); interleukin 1β (Il-1β; Mm01268569_m1; Life Technologies); interleukin 23 (Il-23; Mm00519943_m1; Life Technologies). Relative quantification was calculated from the ratio between the cycle number (Ct) at which the signal crossed a threshold set within the logarithmic phase of the given gene and that of the reference β-actin gene (4310881E; Life Technologies). Mean values of the triplicate results for each animal were used as individual data for $2^{-\Delta\Delta Ct}$ statistical analysis.

In vitro analysis of motor neuron loss and microglia activation in primary co-cultures

Primary cultures were obtained from the spinal cord of 13-day-old (E13) NTG+/+ or NTG–/– mouse embryos, as previously described [30]. Briefly, ventral horns were dissected from spinal cords, exposed to DNAse and trypsin (Sigma-Aldrich) and centrifuged with a bovine serum albumin (BSA) cushion. Cells obtained at this step were a mixed neuron/glia population and were centrifuged (800 g for 15 min) through a 6% iodixanol (OptiPrep™; Sigma-Aldrich) cushion for motor neuron enrichment. A sharp band (motor neuron-enriched fraction) at the top of the iodixanol cushion and a pellet (glial fraction) were obtained. The glial feeder layer was prepared by plating the glial fraction at a density of 25,000 cells/cm^2 into flasks already pre-coated with poly-L-lysine (Sigma-Aldrich). Flasks containing confluent mixed glial cultures were shaken overnight at 275 rpm in incubators to obtain purified microglia cultures. The supernatants containing microglial cells from NTG+/+ or NTG–/– mouse embryos were collected and seeded at a density of 40,000 cells/cm^2 in 24-well plates for mRNA expression analysis or added (10% of the astrocyte number) to astrocyte cultures the day before MN sowing. NTG+/+ astrocyte-enriched cultures were obtained by treating the glial cultures from which microglia had been harvested with 60 mmol/L L-leucine methyl ester (Sigma-Aldrich) for 90 min. To prepare a feeder layer for "sandwich" co-cultures, astrocytes were collected and seeded at a density of 25,000 cells/cm^2 into 12-well plates.

To establish neuron/glia cocultures, the NTG+/+ motor neuron-enriched fraction (from the iodixanol-based separation) was seeded at a density of 10,000 cells/cm^2 onto mature glial layers composed of mixed glial cells (NTG+/+ astrocyte plus NTG+/+ or NTG–/– microglia).

Culture treatments: Primary cultures were exposed to 1 µg/mL LPS (from Escherichia coli 0111:B4) on the fifth-sixth day in vitro (5–6 DIV) for 24 h. Cultures maintained with normal medium served as the control condition. As reported below, MN viability was assessed by counting SMI32-positive cells in each treatment condition, and microglia activation was analyzed considering different cell morphology parameters and the gene expression of pro-inflammatory cytokines. Immunocytochemical and immunofluorescent Assays: cells were fixed with 4% paraformaldehyde and permeabilized by 0.2% Triton X-100 (Sigma-Aldrich). Staining was carried out by overnight incubation with the primary antibody, followed by incubation with an appropriate fluorescent secondary antibody for immunofluorescence (Dy-light; Rockland Immunochemicals). Double staining was done by overnight incubation of the cultures separately with each primary antibody. In each experiment, some wells were processed without the primary antibody to verify the specificity of the staining. Primary antibodies were: mouse anti-nonphosphorylated neurofilament H (SMI32, 1:1000; Covance). Appropriate fluorescent secondary antibodies conjugated to different fluorochromes were used at 1:1000 dilution. Pictures of stained cells were obtained with an Olympus virtual slide system VS110 (Olympus, Center Valley, PA, USA) at 10X-magnification, and images were analyzed with Fiji (Image J, U.S. National Institutes of Health).

MN viability: The viability of MNs was assayed by counting SMI32-positive cells with typical morphology (triangular shape, single well-defined axon) and intact axons and dendrites, considering five non-overlapping 2×12-mm fields (total area analysed: about 30% of each well). This number was normalized to the mean of SMI32-positive cells counted in the appropriate control wells. Microglia activation: to determine the activation status of NTG+/+ or NTG−/− immunocompetent cells after LPS treatment, mixed neuron/glia cocultures were examined by immunocytochemistry with rabbit anti Iba-1 (1:200; Wako), while purified cultures of microglia were analyzed for the gene expression of pro-inflammatory cytokines (IL-23 and IL-1β). Images of Iba-1-positive cells were obtained with an Olympus virtual slide system VS110 (Olympus, Center Valley, PA, USA) at 100X magnification, and the morphological parameters (cell area and circularity) were measured with Fiji (Image J, U.S. National Institutes of Health) considering from four to eight non-overlapping stereological 2×12-mm fields. For mRNA analysis, we harvested microglia cell cultures and extracted the mRNA following the approach described in the "Real-time PCR" section.

Statistical analysis

GraphPad v7.03 (GraphPad Software) was used. The Mantel-Cox log rank test was used for comparing disease onset and survival between groups. Paw Grip Strength and body weight were analyzed by repeated measures ANOVA with Sidak's post analysis. The unpaired t-test was used to compare differences between two groups. One-way ANOVA with Tukey's post analysis was used to compare differences between more than two groups. Further details are provided in the captions.

Results

The lack of MHCI and CTLs accelerates the symptoms onset but extends the survival in mSOD1 mice

Mice homozygous for the $\beta 2m^{tm1Unc}$ targeted mutation (B6.129P2-$\beta 2m^{tm1Unc}$/J mice) lacking $\beta 2m$ produce minimal, if any, MHCI presentation on the cell surface [31]. They have no mature CD8$^+$ T cells and do not present CD8$^+$ T cell-mediated toxicity [31, 32]. We crossed female mice homozygous lacking $\beta 2m$ with C57SOD1^{G93A} transgenic male mice and examined their F1 progeny (Fig. 1a). To accurately assess the level of CD8$^+$ T cells in SOD1^{G93A} mice, we did a longitudinal FACS analysis on the peripheral blood of SOD1$^{G93A}\beta 2M^{-/-}$ (**G93A−/−**) mice, SOD1$^{G93A}\beta 2M^{+/+}$ (**G93A+/+**) mice and relative non-transgenic (NTG) littermates (**NTG+/+; NTG−/−**) during the disease progression (70 d = presymptomatic, 123 d = motor onset; 140 d = symptomatic stage). Blood CD3$^+$-CD8$^+$ lymphocytes in G93A+/+ mice at age 123 and 140, but not 70 d, were significantly lower than in NTG littermates (Fig. 1b, c). In contrast, the expression level of the CD8α receptor in the lumbar spinal cord of the same G93A+/+ mice at 123 and 140 d was significantly higher than in NTG littermates, and the same was found in the cervical spinal cord of G93A+/+ mice at 140 d (Fig. 1d). This agrees with the possible recruitment of these cells in the CNS from the systemic circulation. However, both NTG and mSOD1 mice lacking MHCI/CTLs (**NTG−/−; G93A−/−**) had negligible hematogenous CD3$^+$-CD8$^+$ lymphocyte counts at all time-points (Fig. 1b, c), with complete depletion of CD8α receptor mRNA in the spinal cord (Fig. 1d).

We next evaluated the blood levels of CD4 T+ cells in both G93A+/+ and G93A−/− mice and relative controls. In keeping with the literature [31], we found that Ntg$^{-/-}$ and G93A$^{-/-}$ mice compensated for the lack of CD8+ T cells by increasing the blood expression of CD3$^+$-CD4$^+$ lymphocytes with respect to Ntg+/+ and G93A+/+, at all time-points considered (Additional file 1: Figure S1a, b). However, this did not translate in a higher infiltration of CD4$^+$ T cells within the spinal cord since no difference was found in the levels of the CD4 receptor, FoxP3 and FoxP3/CD4 ratio between G93A+/+ and G93A$^{-/-}$ mice at both 123 d and 140 d (Additional file 1: Figure S1c-f).

Next, we investigated the effects of MHCI and CTL depletion on motor performance and disease progression in mSOD1 mice and NTG littermates. NTG−/− mice did not show any general health problems or alteration in motor function in comparison with **NTG+/+** mice during the entire duration of the experiment (Fig. 2a). However, G93A−/− mice had earlier onset of paw grip strength impairment about ten days sooner than G93A+/+

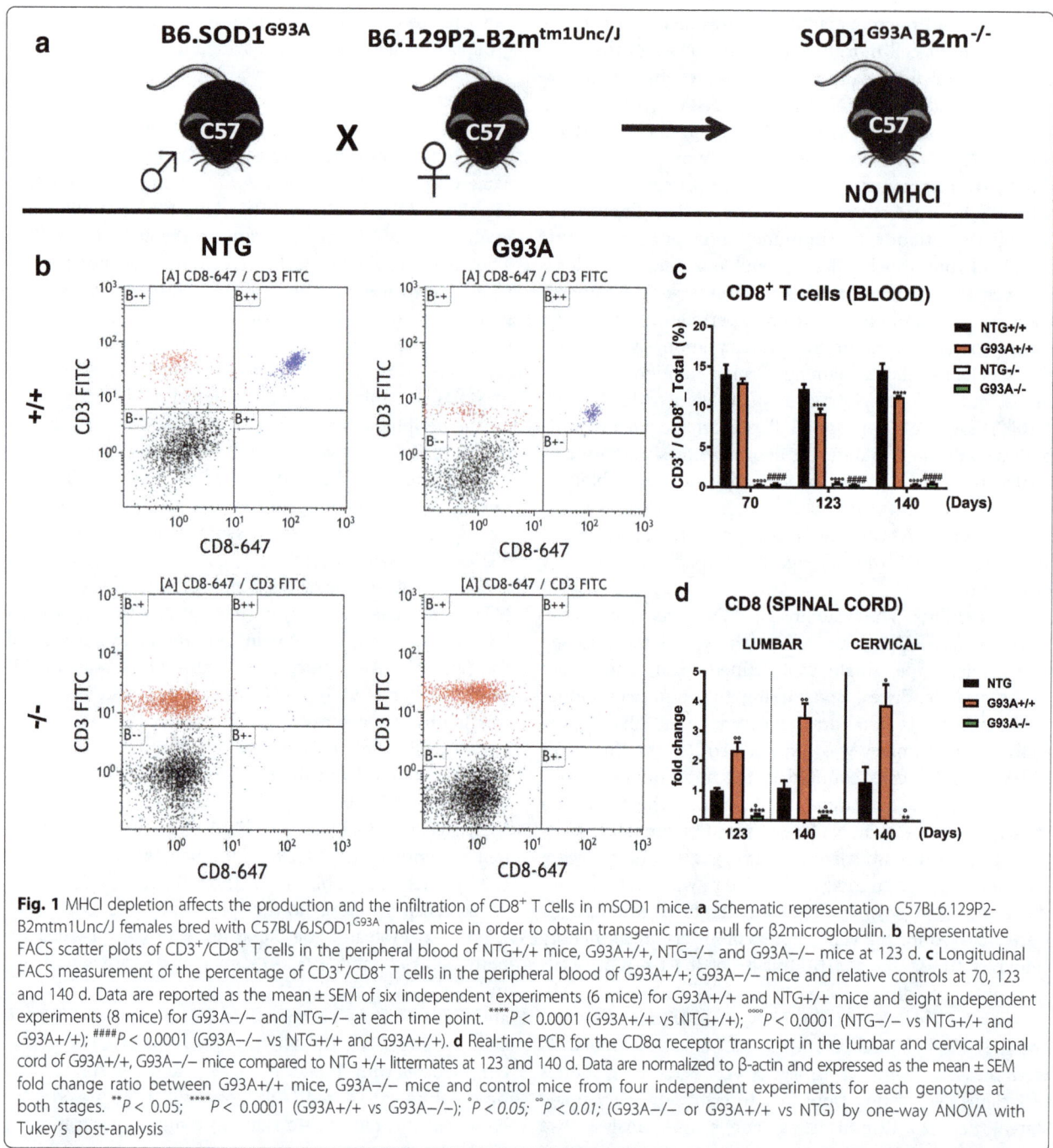

Fig. 1 MHCI depletion affects the production and the infiltration of CD8[+] T cells in mSOD1 mice. **a** Schematic representation C57BL6.129P2-B2mtm1Unc/J females bred with C57BL/6JSOD1[G93A] males mice in order to obtain transgenic mice null for β2microglobulin. **b** Representative FACS scatter plots of CD3[+]/CD8[+] T cells in the peripheral blood of NTG+/+ mice, G93A+/+, NTG−/− and G93A−/− mice at 123 d. **c** Longitudinal FACS measurement of the percentage of CD3[+]/CD8[+] T cells in the peripheral blood of G93A+/+; G93A−/− mice and relative controls at 70, 123 and 140 d. Data are reported as the mean ± SEM of six independent experiments (6 mice) for G93A+/+ and NTG+/+ mice and eight independent experiments (8 mice) for G93A−/− and NTG−/− at each time point. [****]$P < 0.0001$ (G93A+/+ vs NTG+/+); [°°°°]$P < 0.0001$ (NTG−/− vs NTG+/+ and G93A+/+); [####]$P < 0.0001$ (G93A−/− vs NTG+/+ and G93A+/+). **d** Real-time PCR for the CD8α receptor transcript in the lumbar and cervical spinal cord of G93A+/+, G93A−/− mice compared to NTG +/+ littermates at 123 and 140 d. Data are normalized to β-actin and expressed as the mean ± SEM fold change ratio between G93A+/+ mice, G93A−/− mice and control mice from four independent experiments for each genotype at both stages. [**]$P < 0.05$; [****]$P < 0.0001$ (G93A+/+ vs G93A−/−); [°]$P < 0.05$; [°°]$P < 0.01$; (G93A−/− or G93A+/+ vs NTG) by one-way ANOVA with Tukey's post-analysis

mice (Fig. 2b). The age at the onset of muscle weakness was 114.1 ± 6.2 d in G93A−/− mice compared with 121.2 ± 7 d in SOD1[G93A]β2M[+/−] (**G93A+/−**) and 123.2 ± 7 d in G93A+/+ ($P < 0.0022$ by Mantel-Cox log-rank test) (Fig. 2b). The double genetically modified mice showed no difference in body weight loss compared to G93A+/+ and G93A+/− transgenic mice during disease progression (data not shown). Despite the earlier muscle impairment in G93A −/− mice the disease progressed more slowly than G93A +/+ mice toward complete inability to remain attached to

the grid with all four limbs. This time point was defined as the onset of disability and in G93A−/− mice it was 5.8 d later than in G93A+/+ mice ($p = 0.075$) (Fig. 2c). This delay may be attributed to the ability of G93A−/− mice to stay clung longer to the grid with the forelimbs (Additional file 2: Video S1).

Interestingly, G93A−/− mice lived respectively 17 and 10 d longer than G93A+/+ mice and G93A+/− mice ($P < 0.0001$). The G93A+/− mice also survived of 6 d longer than G93A+/+ mice ($P < 0.015$). The average

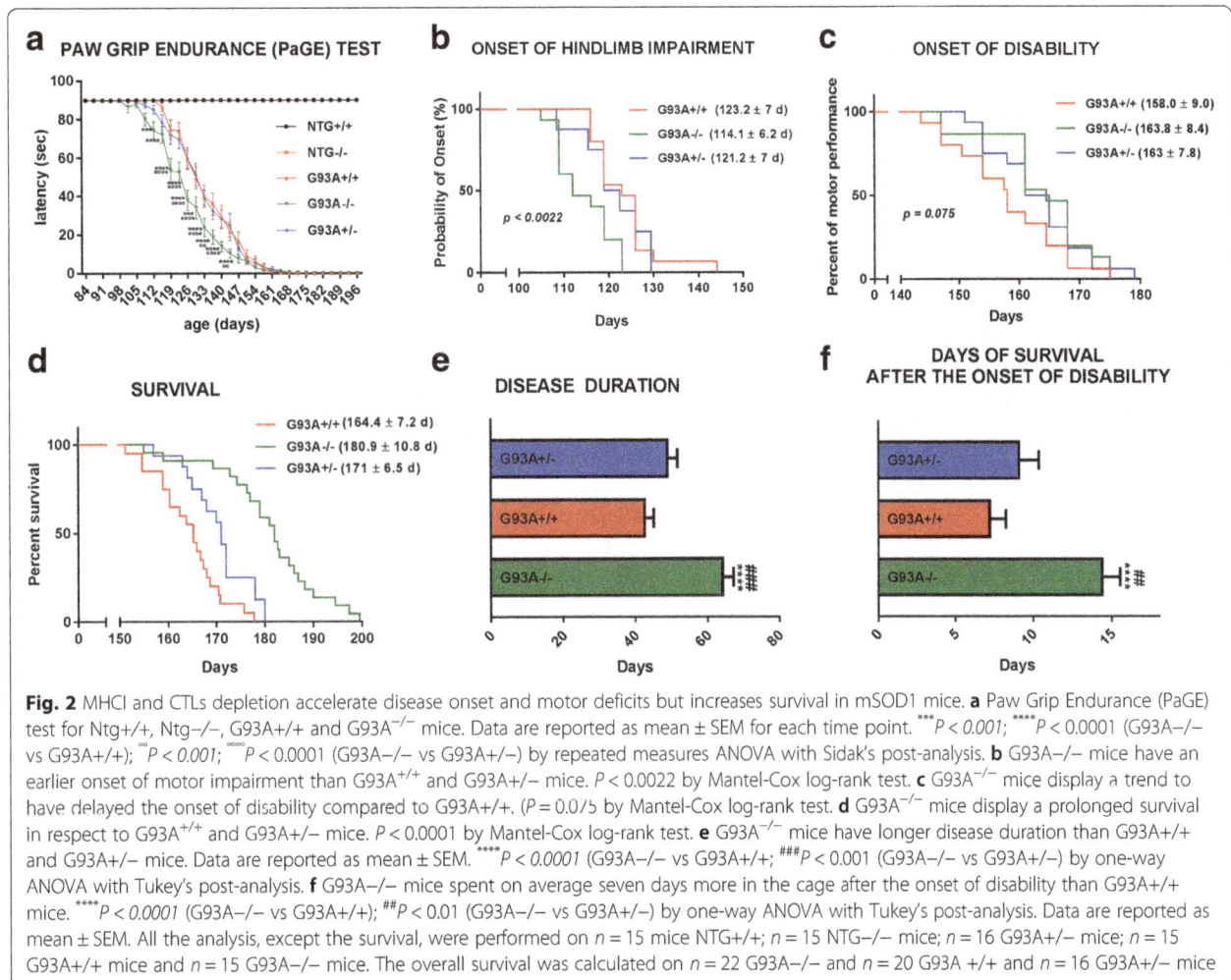

Fig. 2 MHCl and CTLs depletion accelerate disease onset and motor deficits but increases survival in mSOD1 mice. **a** Paw Grip Endurance (PaGE) test for Ntg+/+, Ntg–/–, G93A+/+ and G93A$^{-/-}$ mice. Data are reported as mean ± SEM for each time point. $^{***}P < 0.001$; $^{****}P < 0.0001$ (G93A–/– vs G93A+/+); $^{\infty}P < 0.001$; $^{\infty\infty\infty}P < 0.0001$ (G93A–/– vs G93A+/–) by repeated measures ANOVA with Sidak's post-analysis. **b** G93A–/– mice have an earlier onset of motor impairment than G93A$^{+/+}$ and G93A+/– mice. $P < 0.0022$ by Mantel-Cox log-rank test. **c** G93A$^{-/-}$ mice display a trend to have delayed the onset of disability compared to G93A+/+. ($P = 0.075$ by Mantel-Cox log-rank test. **d** G93A$^{-/-}$ mice display a prolonged survival in respect to G93A$^{+/+}$ and G93A+/– mice. $P < 0.0001$ by Mantel-Cox log-rank test. **e** G93A$^{-/-}$ mice have longer disease duration than G93A+/+ and G93A+/– mice. Data are reported as mean ± SEM. $^{****}P < 0.0001$ (G93A–/– vs G93A+/+); $^{###}P < 0.001$ (G93A–/– vs G93A+/–) by one-way ANOVA with Tukey's post-analysis. **f** G93A–/– mice spent on average seven days more in the cage after the onset of disability than G93A+/+ mice. $^{****}P < 0.0001$ (G93A–/– vs G93A+/+); $^{##}P < 0.01$ (G93A–/– vs G93A+/–) by one-way ANOVA with Tukey's post-analysis. Data are reported as mean ± SEM. All the analysis, except the survival, were performed on $n = 15$ mice NTG+/+; $n = 15$ NTG–/– mice; $n = 16$ G93A+/– mice; $n = 15$ G93A+/+ mice and $n = 15$ G93A–/– mice. The overall survival was calculated on $n = 22$ G93A–/– and $n = 20$ G93A +/+ and $n = 16$ G93A+/– mice

ages (±SD) at death were respectively 164.4 ± 7.2, 171 ± 6.5 and 180.9 ± 10.8 d in the G93A+/+, G93A+/– and G93A–/– mice (Fig. 2d). Thus, the disease in G93A–/– mice lasted significantly longer (64 ± 10.6 d) than in G93A+/+ (42.5 ± 7.3 d, $P < 0.0001$) and in G93A+/– (51.8 ± 9.6 days, $P < 0.001$) mice (Fig. 2e). In agreement with the institutional ethical committee guidelines, the ALS mice must be euthanized when they are unable to right themselves within 10 s after being placed on each side. Given that in mSOD1 mice hindlimbs underwent earlier paralysis, this ability is mainly due to the strength of the forepaws (Additional file 3: Video S2, Additional file 4: Video S3, Additional file 5: Video S4). These results suggest that in G93A–/– mice, while the function of the posterior paws is impaired earlier than in G93A+/+ mice, the preserved function of the forelimbs attenuated the progression of the disease and prolonged the animal ability to stay prone compared to **G93A+/+** mice (Additional file 6: Video S5). Thus, **G93A–/–** mice survived seven and five d more after the onset of disability than **G93A +/+** mice ($P < 0.0001$) and **G93A+/–** mice ($p < 0.01$), respectively (Fig. 2f).

We therefore thoroughly investigated the hindlimb neuromuscular system [lumbar spinal cord, sciatic nerves, *Tibialis Anterior* (TA), *Gastrocnemius* (GC)] of G93A+/+ and G93A–/– mice at two time points during the progression of the disease, namely 123 d and 140 d, corresponding respectively to the onset of the hindlimb motor deficit and the advanced symptomatic stage of G93A+/+ mice. Intentionally, G93A+/+ and G93A–/– mice were examined at the same age and not at the same disease stage, to correlate the difference of clinical phenotype with the potential mechanisms involved.

The forepaw neuromuscular system [cervical spinal cord, radial nerves and *Triceps brachii* (TB) muscles] was examined only at the 140 d due to the delayed involvement during the disease course in ALS mice [33, 34].

The lack of MHCl and CTLs promotes motor neuron survival

We examined whether the more severe hindlimb pathology in G93A–/– mice was related to a higher MN death than in G93A+/+ mice. Large MNs with a cell body area of ≥ 400 μm^2 were quantified after Nissl stain-ing in the lumbar spinal cord. Thus only the large α-MNs, the most vulnerable to cell death in ALS, were quantified [35]. Surprisingly, there was a partial, al-though non-significant, protection of MN in the lumbar spinal cord of G93A−/− compared to G93A+/+ litter-mates at 123 d but not at 140 d (Fig. 3a, b, d). Moreover, MNs in the cervical spinal cord were significantly pro-tected in G93A−/− mice at 140 d compared to G93A+/+ littermates (Fig. 3c, e). Cervical MNs also preserved their function, as demonstrated by the reduced accumulation of phosphorylated neurofilaments in their perikarya, a marker of neuronal dysfunction and degeneration [24]. In fact, only 4.6% of MNs accumulated SMI-31

(phosphorylated neurofilaments) in their soma in G93A−/− mice, while 23.1% were recordered in G93A+/+ mice (Additional file 1: Figure S2a, b). The same evaluation on the lumbar spinal cord at 123 d did not show a significant difference between G93A+/+ and G93A−/− mice (Additional file 1: Figure S2a, c).

The lack of MHCI-mediated interaction between microglia and CTLs reduces the inflammation in the spinal cord

We reported that microglia express high levels of MHCI in the lumbar spinal cord of C57SOD1^{G93A} mice [22, 26]. Microglia is the principal antigen-presenting cell and is one of the leading culprits in the non-cell autonomous MN death in ALS [36, 37]. Since induced MHCI in

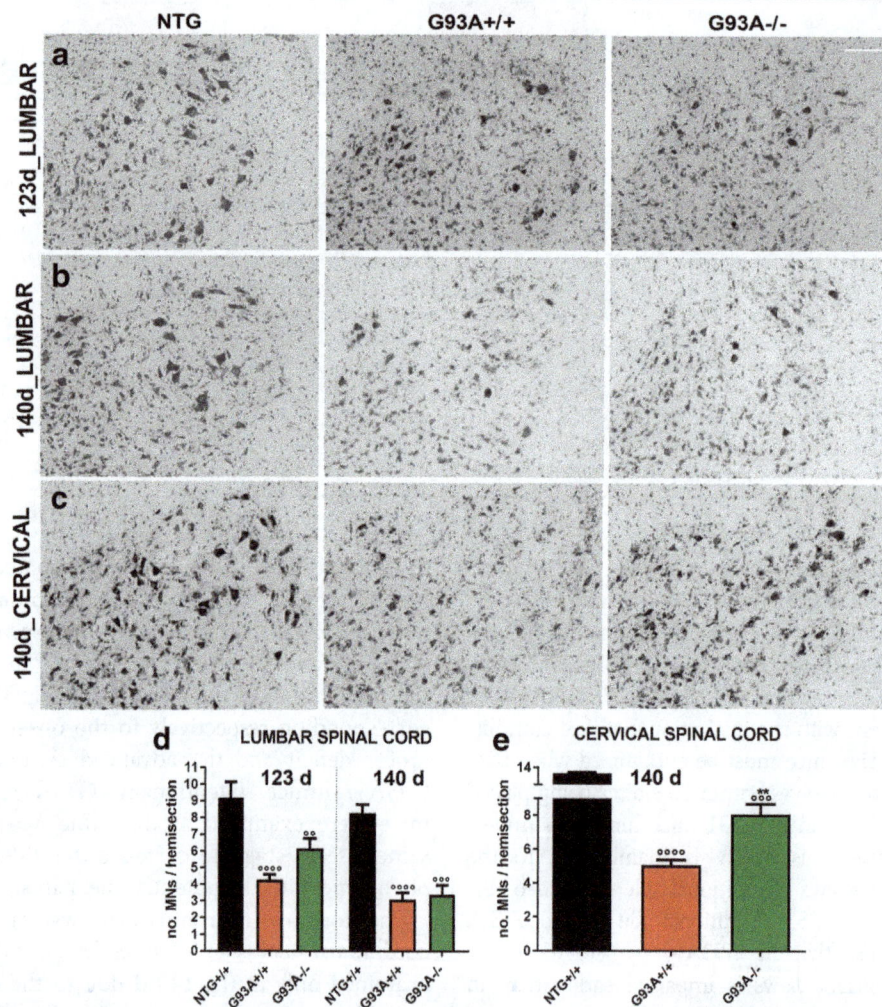

Fig. 3 MHCI and CTLs depletion promotes motor neuron survival in mSOD1 mice. **a, b** Representative Nissl-stained lumbar spinal cord sections of NTG; G93A+/+ and G93A−/− mice at 123 d. **c** Representative Nissl stained lumbar and cervical spinal cord sections of NTG; G93A+/+ and G93A −/− mice at 140 d. Bar, 50 μm. **d, e** Motor neuron counts. Data are expressed as mean ± SEM of MNs ($\geq$ 400 μm^2) per hemisection. At 123 d, four, seven and seven independent experiments were analyzed for NTG, G93A+/+ and, G93A−/− mice, respectively. At 140 d, three, five and five independent experiments were analyzed for NTG, G93A+/+ and, G93A−/− mice, respectively. At 140 d, for the cervical spinal cord, three, five and five independent experiments were analyzed for NTG, G93A+/+ and, G93A−/− mice, respectively. $^{ooo}P < 0.001$; $^{oooo}P < 0.0001$ (G93A+/+; G93A−/− vs NTG); $^{**}P < 0.001$ (G93A−/− vs G93A+/+) by one-way ANOVA with Tukey's post analysis

reactive microglia contributes to the activation and recruitment of CD8$^+$ T cells [38, 39], we examined wether the lack of interaction between microglia and CD8$^+$ T cells reduced inflammation in the CNS of transgenic mice and protected aginst MN loss. At 123 d, the activation of CD68$^+$-microglia was lower in the lumbar spinal cord G93A–/– mice than in G93A+/+ littermates. This difference disappeared at 140 d (Fig. 4a, b, e). MHCI-labeled microglia was also observed in the ventral portion of the

cervical spinal cord of G93A+/+ mice at 140 d (Fig. 4c). Thus, a significant reduction of CD68$^+$-microglia was also observed in the cervical spinal cord of 140 d old G93A–/– compared to G93A+/+ mice (Fig. 4d, i). The decrease of CD68$^+$ microglia in both lumbar and cervical spinal cords at respectively 123 d and 140 d was confirmed by the lower levels of CD68 mRNA in G93A–/– mice than in G93A+/+ mice (Additional file 1: Figure S3a, b). No difference was instead found in reactive atrocytosis between

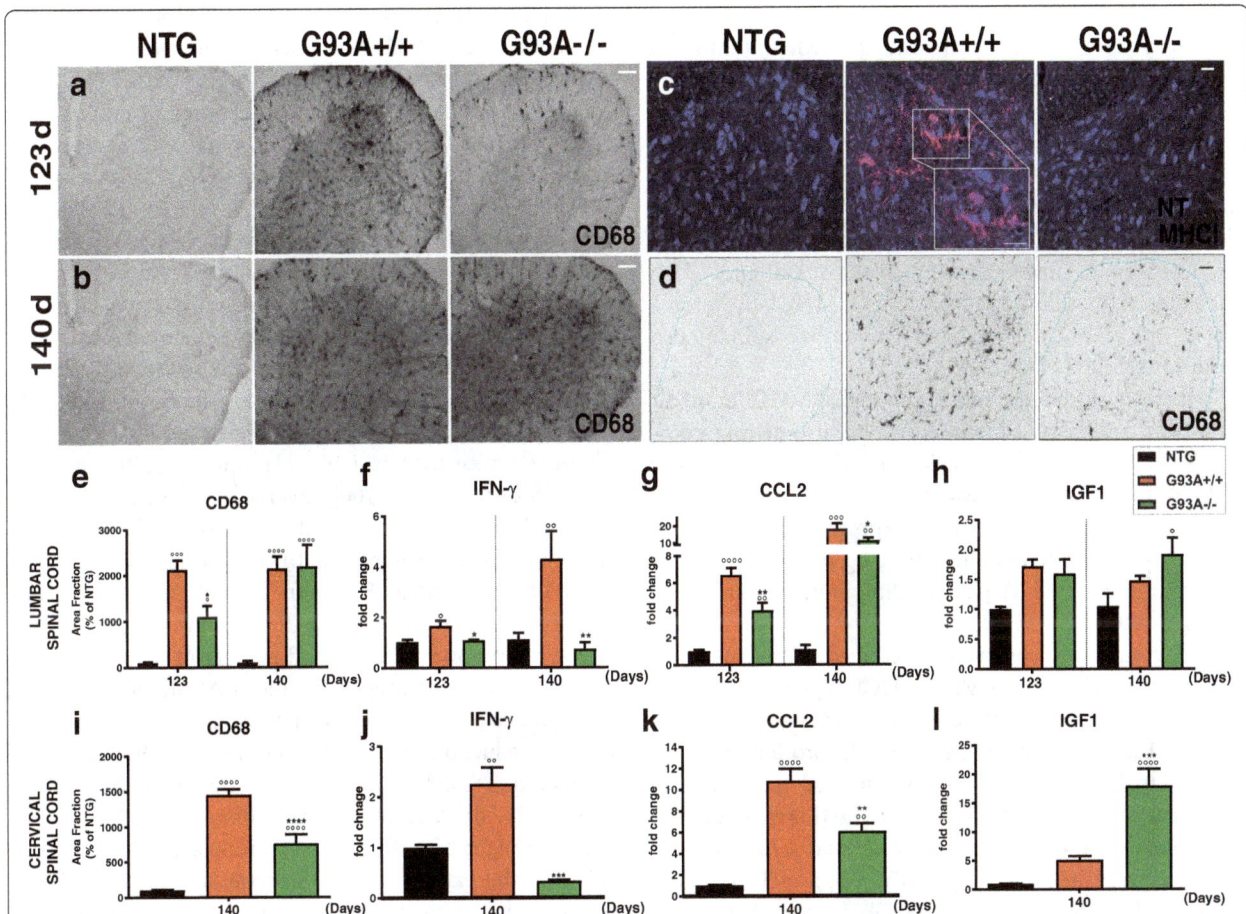

Fig. 4 MHCI depletion reduces the inflammation in the lumbar and cervical spinal cord of mSOD1 mice during the disease course. a, b DAB immunostaining for CD68 in the lumbar spinal cord of NTG; G93A+/+ and G93A–/– mice at 123 and 140 d. Bar, 50 μm. c Immunofluorescence staining for MHCI (purple) and motor neurons (neuro-trance, NT; blue) in the cervical spinal cord of NTG; G93A+/+ and G93A–/– mice at 140 d. The inset shows a magnification of MHCI-labeled microglia surrounding MNs. The images are representative of at least four sections from two independent experiments from each genotype. Bar, 50 μm; Inset Bar: 50 μm. d Immunofluorescence staining for CD68 in the cervical spinal cord of NTG; G93A+/+ and G93A–/– mice at 140 d. Bar, 50 μm (e, i) Quantification of CD68 staining in (e) lumbar and (i) cervical spinal cord hemisections of G93A+/+, G93A–/– mice compared to NTG+/+ littermates at 123 and 140 d. Data are expressed as mean ± SEM (four serial sections for each animal). At 123 d, four, six and four independent experiments were analyzed for NTG, G93A+/+ and, G93A–/– mice, respectively. At 140 d, in cervical and lumbar spinal cord, four independent experiments were analyzed for each genotype. f-h Real-time PCR for Ifn-γ, Ccl2 and Igf1 transcripts in the lumbar spinal cord of G93A+/+, G93A–/– mice compared to NTG+/+ littermates at 123 and 140 d. Data are normalized to β-actin and expressed as the mean ± SEM fold change ratio between G93A+/+ mice, G93A–/– mice and controls from four independent experiments for each genotype. j-l Real-time PCR for Ifn-γ, Ccl2 and Igf1 transcripts in the cervical spinal cord of G93A+/+, G93A–/– mice compared to NTG+/+ littermates at 140 d. Data are normalized to β-actin and expressed as the mean ± SEM fold change ratio between G93A+/+, G93A–/– and controls mice from four independent experiments for each genotype. $^*P < 0.05$; $^{**}P < 0.01$; $^{***}P < 0.001$; $^{****}P < 0.0001$; (G93A+/+ vs G93A–/–); $^°P < 0.05$; $^{°°}P < 0.01$; $^{°°°}P < 0.001$; $^{°°°°}P < 0.0001$ (G93A–/–; G93A+/+ vs NTG) by one-way ANOVA with Tukey's post-analysis

G93A−/− mice and G93A+/+ littermates in both lumbar and cervical spinal cord as assessed by GFAP immunohisto-chemistry and western blot (Additional file 1: Figure S4a-d).

We then examined whether the reduced CD68$^+$ microglia activation in both segments of the spinal cord from G93A−/− mice was accompanied by any change in the inflammatory environment compared to G93A +/+ mice, by measuring the expression levels of Ccl2, Ifn-γ, and Igf1 transcripts. We found that the increase of Ifn-γ and Ccl2 in G93A+/+ mice was significantly reduced by the lack of MHCI/CTLs in the lumbar and cervical spinal cord at both 123 and 140 d (Fig. 4f-k). In contrast, Igf1 was remarkably upregulated in the cervical spinal cord of G93A−/− mice compared to G93A+/+ mice at 140 d while no relevant differences were found in the lumbar spinal cord of mice during the disease progression (Fig. 4h, l). Notably, gliosis and inflammation (see Ccl2; Ifnγ; Igf1mRNA levels) are lower in the cervical than in the lumbar spinal cord of G93A+/+ mice at 140d, further indicating the delayed compromise of the upper versus the lower segment of the spinal cord. This correlates with a lower activation of MHCI by micro-glia in the cervical compared to lumbar spinal cord (Additional file 1: Figure S5a-c).

To further address the role of microglial MHCI in medi-ating MN death, we established an in vitro setting com-posed by cocultures of microglia derived from NTG+/+ or NTG−/− mice added to wild-type (NTG+/+) astrocytes and MNs. These cocultures were exposed to an inflamma-tory load by 24 h treatment with 1 μg/mL LPS that it is known to induce the MHCI signaling in microglia / mac-rophages [40, 41].

As a result, we observed a reduced LPS-dependent MN death in co-cultures with MHCI depleted microglia (NTG−/−) compared to control NTG+/+ microglia ($p < 0.05$; Fig. 5a, b). Interestingly, after the pro-inflammatory load, microglia from NTG−/− mice showed reduced mor-phological activation (detected as decreased area and circu-larity) and lower transcription of Il-23 and Il1β mRNA if compared to NTG+/+ microglia (Fig. 5c-g). qRT-PCR ana-lysis in the lumbar spinal cord of G93A−/− mice showed sig-nificant reductions in the transcription of Il-23 and Il-1β compared to G93A+/+ at both 123 and 140 d (Fig. 5h, j). These findings suggest that microglia deprived of MHCI is less sensitive to pro-inflammatory stimuli and become less neurotoxic.

Our data cumulatively point to a shift to an anti-inflammatory environment in the lumbar and cer-vical spinal cord of G93A−/− mice during the disease course suggesting that the MN preservation, particularly in the cervical spinal cord, is due to a lack of interaction between microglia and CTLs. But, why do G93A −/− mice suffer earlier muscle strength impairment than G93A +/+ mice? To address this, we focused on the peripheral compartment of the MNs: the nerves and neuromuscular junctions.

Lack of MHCI and CTLs anticipates the denervation atrophy of hindlimb muscles while delaying that of forelimb muscles and diaphragm

Denervation atrophy of muscles is an early event in ALS pathology [42], so we examined whether the more severe motor function impairment in G93A−/− mice was corre-lated with earlier denervation atrophy of hindlimbs and forelimbs muscles.

At 123 d, NMJs in the TA showed more marked de-nervation in G93A−/− mice with only 45 ± 7.1% remaining innervated compared to 72 ± 3.6 in G93A+/+ mice (Fig. 6a, b). At 140 d, no difference in denervation were observed in the two mSOD1 mice with respectively 18,2 ± 7.4% and 19,8 ± 4.3% of the NMJs remaining in-nervated in G93A−/− and G93A+/+. At 123 d, the mRNA levels of fetal AChR-γ, a marker of NMJ denerv-ation [43], were significantly more upregulated in G93A−/− than in G93A+/+ TA muscles than in the NTG mice (Fig. 6c). In addition, immunoblot analysis on TA homoge-nates indicate greater expression of the neuronal AChR-α7 subunit and the neural cell adhesion molecule (NCAM), two markers of disused or denervated muscles [44, 45], in G93A−/− mice than in G93A+/+ mice (Additional file 1: Figure S6a-c). Finally, S100β was markedly higher in the TA of G93A−/− mice at 123 d than in NTG littermates (Additional file 1: Figure S7a, b) suggesting a reduced pro-liferation of terminal Schwann cells (TSCs) at terminal motor axons [46]. In view of the positive correlation be-tween the number of TSCs and the size of the AChR clus-ter [47], next we examined the mean AChR cluster area in TA muscles of both mSOD1 mice at 123 d. We identified a specific reduction in the endplate area of G93A−/− mice compared to G93A+/+ and NTG+/+ mice (Additional file 1: Figure S7c, d). Measurements of hindlimb (TA and GC) muscle weight of both transgenic mouse models perfectly reflected the extent of their denervation. At 123 d, G93A −/− mice had greater hindlimb muscle wasting than G93A +/+ mice. G93A−/− mice had weight losses of respectively 66.4 ± 2.5% and 61.4 ± 8% for the GC and TA; G93A +/+ mice had a loss of 48.9 ± 5.3% for the GC and 36.2 ± 2.7% for the TA (Fig. 7a-c). At 140 d, the weight of both TA and GC had fallen further in G93A+/+ mice while in G93A−/− mice it remained unchanged (Fig. 7a-c).

We also confirmed the atrophy of the hindlimbs of G93A −/− mice compared to G93A+/+ mice at 123 d by stereologi-cal analysis on transverse sections of TA from mSOD1 mice. First we found a reduction in the mean of muscle fiber cross-sectional area in the TA of G93A−/− mice (Additional file 1: Figure S8a, b). This was reflected in a lar-ger number of fibers with a small diameter (1–1000 μm) and

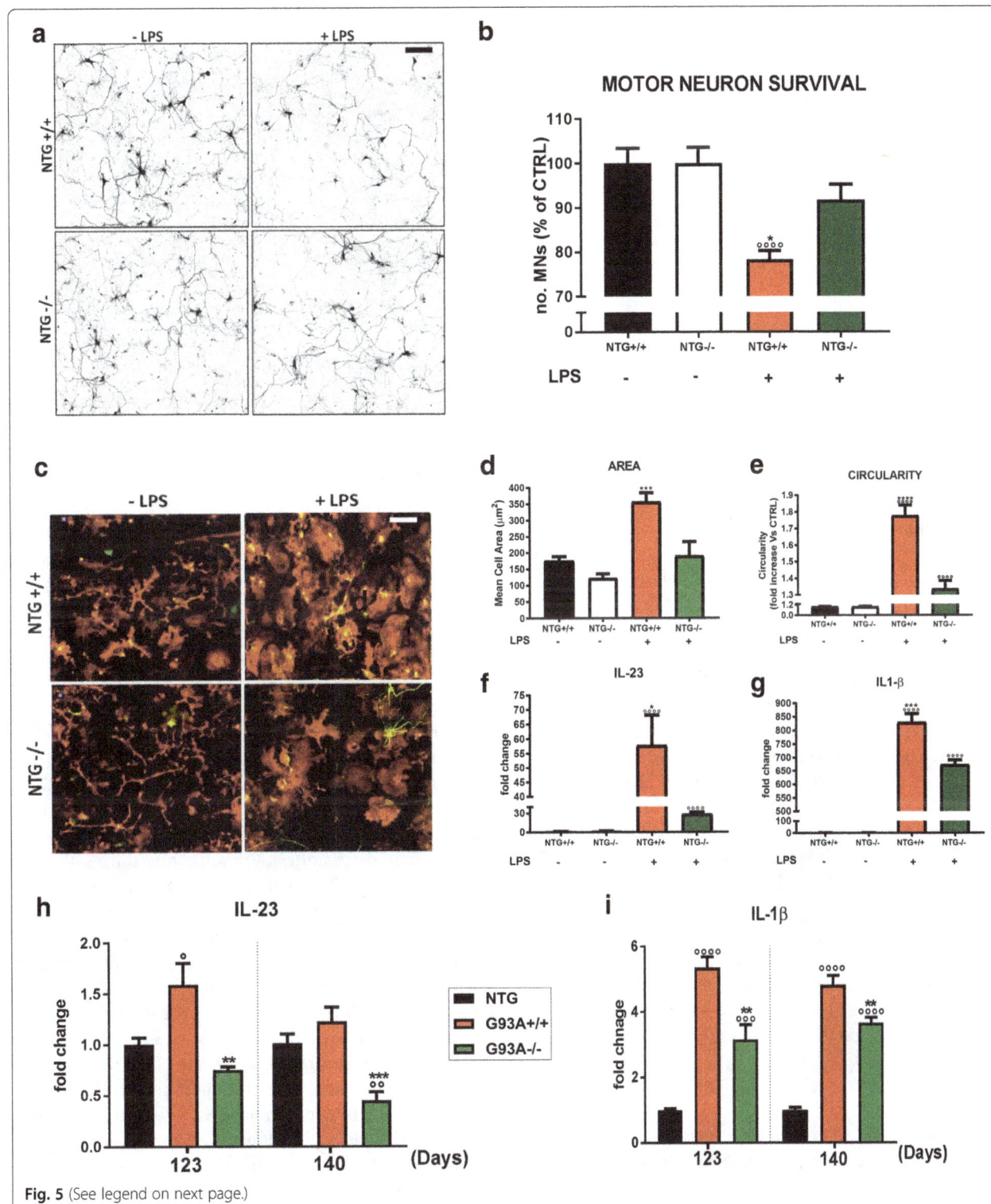

Fig. 5 (See legend on next page.)

fewer large-diameter fibers (2000–6000 um) (Additional file 1: Figure S8a, c).

To examine the composition of muscle fibers (glycolytic versus oxidative) at 123 d, we employed NADH staining on transverse sections of TA of both transgenic mice groups compared to NTG+/+ mice. This indicted lower density and a smaller percentage of Type IIb fast-fatigable muscle fibers in the hindlimb muscles of G93A−/− (5 ± 2.8%) compared to G93A+/+ (26 ± 5%) mice (Additional file 1: Figure S6d-f). We next looked at the level of innervation of muscles whose activity is directly controlled by the cervical spinal cord. Surprisingly, NMJs in the TB showed the opposite situation to the TA. Denervation was reduced in G93A−/− mice with 68.7 ± 9.2% of the NMJs remaining innervated compared to only 32 ± 1% of G93A+/+ mice (Fig. 6d, e). In keeping with this, the mRNA levels of fetal AChRγ were less upregulated in the TB of G93A−/− mice than in G93A+/+ mice than in NTG mice (Fig. 6f). Besides, in both transgenic mouse models at 140 d there was a weight loss of 41.3 ± 6.5% in G93A−/− mice compared to 52.8 ± 3.2% in G93A+/+ mice (Fig. 7d, e). We also examined the degree of denervation of the diaphragm of both transgenic mice compared to NTG mice. While in G93A+/+ mice the diaphragm innervation was ~ 30% lower, in G93A−/− mice the effect was much smaller with no significant variation with NTG mice (Additional file 1: Figure S9a-c).

Lack of MHCI and CTLs severely affects the structure of motor axons innervating hindlimb muscles in the course of the disease

Other groups and we have demonstrated that lumbar MNs, after acute injury or chronic disease like in mSOD1 mice activate the expression of MHCI which is rapidly transported into the peripheral axons. Here, it plays a role in the regeneration of motor axons and the stabilization of the NMJs [11, 26, 27, 48]. To clarify the mechanisms underlying this process, we examined the

sciatic nerves of G93A−/− and G93A+/+ mice during the progression of disease.

Immunoblot and immunohistochemical analysis on sciatic nerves showed lower levels of neurofilaments with high molecular weight (200kD) in motor axons (Fig. 8a-c) and a marked reduction in the expression of tubulin β^III (Fig. 8d, e) and importin β (Fig. 8d, f) at both 123 d and 140 d in G93A−/− mice compared to G93A+/+ mice. This indicates that the lack of MHCI exacerbate the progressive structural [49, 50] and functional [51, 52] alterations of peripheral motor axons of G93A mice.

Schwann cells (SCs) are the first-line response to the peripheral damage. They phagocytize the myelin debris and produce the chemotactic signals necessary for correct regeneration [53, 54]. To assess the ability of SCs to respond to stress during ALS progression, we investigated the level of activation of ERK, GFAP, and vimentin in the sciatic nerves of both mSOD mice during the disease progression. These three proteins are essential for the proliferation of the SCs after nerve damage [52–60]. Starting from 123 d, G93A+/+ mice had higher levels of GFAP (Fig. 9a, b, e), the phosphorylated form of ERK (Fig. 9a, c) and vimentin (Fig. 9f) than NTG mice. In contrast, in the sciatic nerves of G93A−/− mice, this response was not present, and the levels of these three markers were even lower than in the NTG mice at both 123 and 140 d. These results suggest substantial impairment in SCs proliferation in G93A−/− mice [59, 60]. However, this does not affect SC de-differentiation as the levels of p75^NTR were markedly increased in sciatic nerves of both mSOD1 mice during disease progression (Fig. 6a, d) [53]. Notably, the basal levels of GFAP (Additional file 1: Figure S10a, b); p-ERK (Additional file 1: Figure S10a, c) and vimentin (Fig. 9f) in the sciatic nerves of NTG−/− mice were much lower than in the NTG+/+ mice, indicating that MHCI signaling may have a direct effect on the proliferation of SCs even in the absence of stressful stimuli.

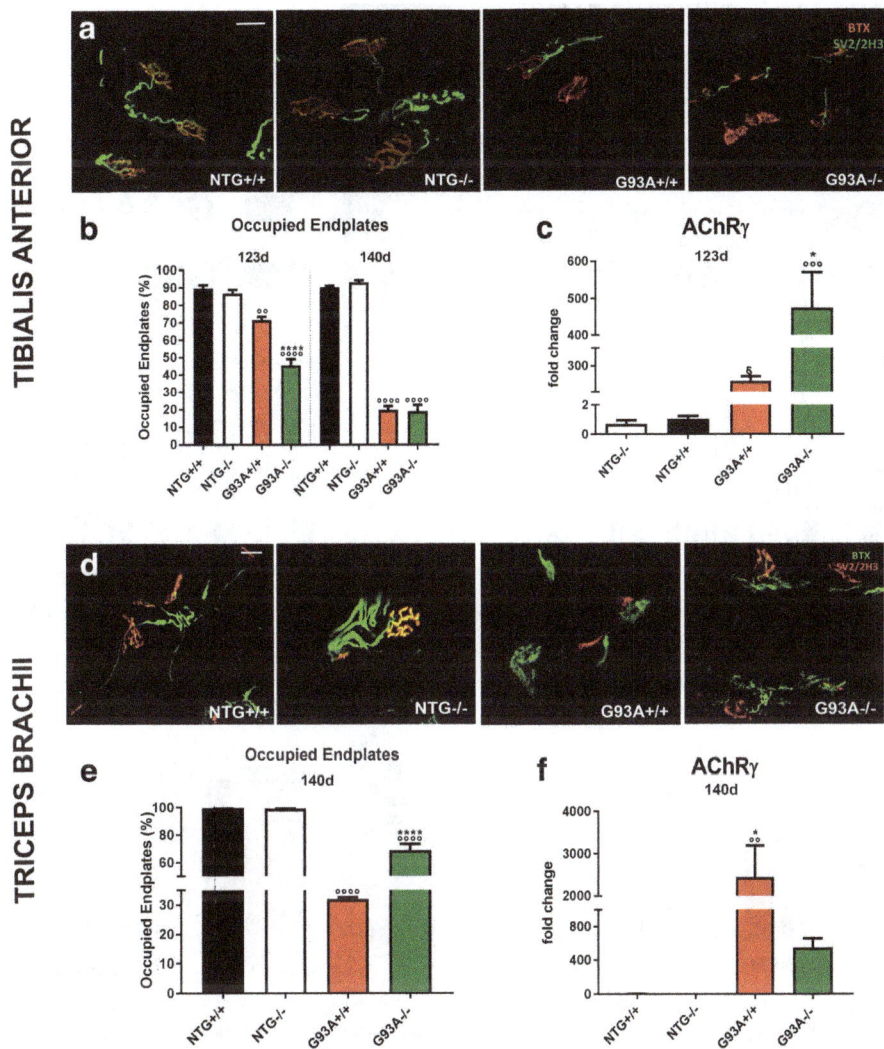

Fig. 6 MHCI and CTLs depletion accelerates the denervation of tibialis anterior but delays that of triceps brachii muscle in SOD1 mutant mice. **a** Analysis of muscle denervation on tibialis anterior (TA) muscle of both, G93A+/+, G93A−/− mice and corresponding NTG littermates at 123 d and 140 d. α-Bungarotoxin (BTX, red) was used to identify the postsynaptic domain, synaptic vesicle glycoprotein 2A (SV2, green) + neurofilament (2H3, green) were used to identify presynaptic terminals. Bar, 20 μm. **b** For each mouse group, the percentage of occupied endplates (~ 70 bungarotoxin positive endplates randomly taken) was calculated. Data are reported as mean ± SEM of four independent experiments for each genotype at 123d and from three independent experiments for each genotype at 140 d. $^{****}P < 0.0001$ (G93A+/+ vs G93A) $^{∞∞}P < 0.01$; $^{∞∞∞}P < 0.001$ (G93A+/+ or G93A−/− vs NTG+/+ and NTG−/−) by two-way ANOVA with Sidak's post-analysis. **c** Real-time PCR for AChR-γ transcript in the TA muscles of G93A+/+, G93A−/− mice compared to the corresponding NTG littermates. Data are normalized to β-actin and expressed as the mean ± SEM fold change ratio between G93A+/+ mice, G93A−/− mice and relative controls from four independent experiments for each genotype. $^{*}P < 0.05$ (G93A−/− vs G93A+/+); $^{∞∞∞}P < 0.001$ (G93A−/− vs NTG+/+; NTG−/−); $^{§}P < 0.05$ (G93A+/+ vs NTG+/+ and NTG−/−). **d** Analysis of muscle denervation on triceps brachii (TB) muscle of G93A+/+ and G93A−/− mice compared to corresponding NTG littermates at 140 d. α-Bungarotoxin (BTX, green) was used to identify the postsynaptic domain, synaptic vesicle glycoprotein 2A (SV2, green) + neurofilament (2H3, red) were used to identify presynaptic terminals. Bar, 20 μm. For each mouse group, the percentage of occupied endplates (~ 70 bungarotoxin positive end plates randomly chosen) was calculated. **e** Data are reported as mean ± SEM. Four, three, three and three independent experiments were analyzed for G93A−/−, G93A+/+, NTG+/+ and NTG−/− mice, mice, respectively. $^{****}P < 0.0001$; (G93A−/− vs G93A+/+); $^{∞∞∞}P < 0.0001$ (G93A+/+ or G93A−/− vs NTG+/+ and NTG−/−) by One-way ANOVA with Tukey's post-analysis. **f** Real-time PCR for AChR-γ transcript in the TB muscles of G93A+/+, G93A −/− mice and the corresponding NTG littermates. Data are normalized to β-actin and expressed as the mean ± SEM fold change ratio between G93A+/+, G93A−/− mice and relative controls from four independent experiments for each genotype. $^{*}P < 0.05$ (G93A−/− vs G93A+/+); $^{∞∞}P < 0.001$ (G93A+/+ vs NTG+/+; NTG−/−)

We next assess the motor axonal structure by a stereological analysis of semithin transverse sections of SNs at the advanced stage of the disease. We first investigated the morphology of the motor axons of G93A−/− and G93A+/+ mice reporting an overall disorganization of the axonal structure in G93A−/− mice (Fig. 10a-c). In

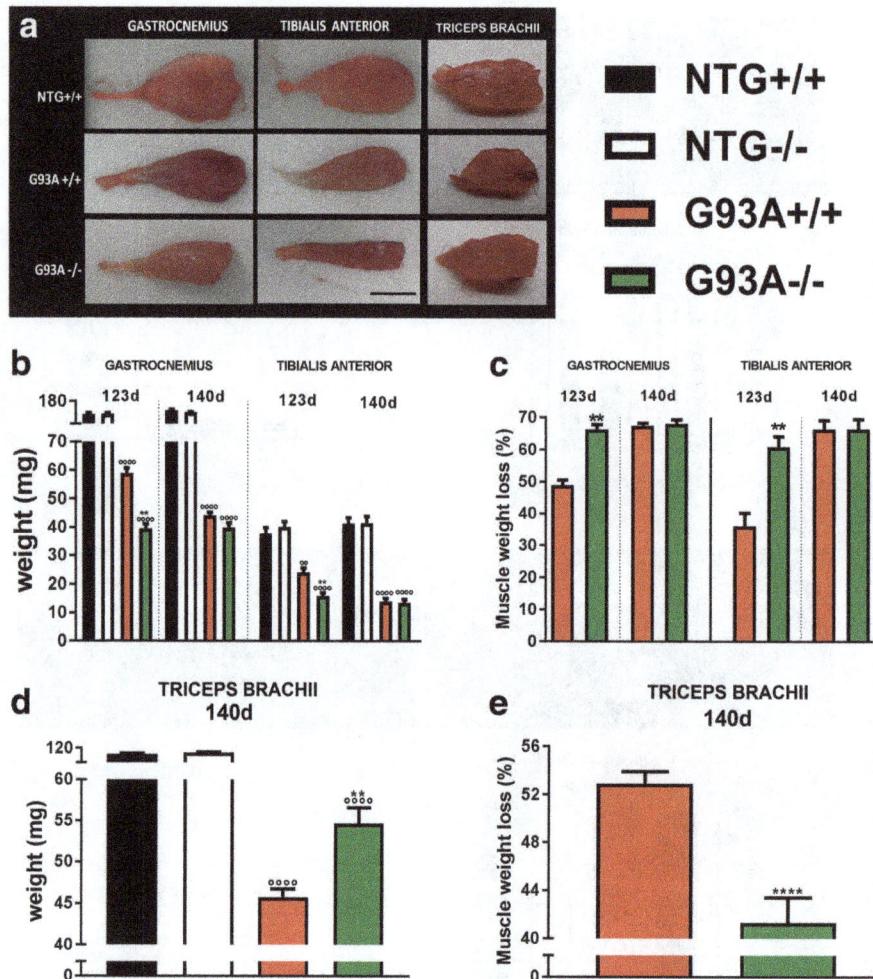

Fig. 7 MHCI and CTLs depletion accelerate hindlimb muscle atrophy in SOD1 mutant mice but delays that of triceps brachii muscles in SOD1 mutant mice. (**a**) Representative images of the gastrocnemius, tibialis anterior and triceps brachii muscles showing increased muscle atrophy of hindlimbs muscles in G93A-/- mice at 123 d, but less weight loss of triceps brachii at 140 d compared to G93A+/+ mice; Bar, 0.5 cm. (**b**) Muscle wasting was calculated by measuring of the gastrocnemius and tibialis anterior muscle weight of G93A-/- and G93A+/+ mice compared to relative NTG littermates (NTG+/+; NTG-/-). At 123 d, six, eight, nine and nine GC muscles and six, eight, eight and ten TA muscles were analyzed for NTG+/+, NTG-/-, G93A+/+ and G93A-/- mice, respectively. At 140 d, 11, 14, ten and 16 GC muscles and 11, 14, 16 and 16 TA muscles were analyzed for NTG+/+, NTG-/-, G93A+/+ and G93A-/- mice, respectively. Percent muscle atrophy in (**c**) was calculated relative to NTG mice. (**d**) Triceps brachii muscle wasting was calculated by measurement of the muscle weight of G93A+/+ and G93A-/- mice compared to relative NTG littermates (NTG+/+; NTG-/-) at 140 d. Six, seven, ten and ten independent experiments were analyzed for NTG+/+, NTG-/-, G93A+/+ and G93A-/-, respectively. The percentage of muscle atrophy in (**e**) was calculated relative to corresponding NTG mice. Data are presented as mean ± SEM of three independent experiments for G93A+/+ mice and four independent experiments for G93A-/- mice. $^*P < 0.05$; $^{**}P < 0.01$ (G93A+/+ vs G93A-/); $^{oooo}P < 0.0001$

fact, there was a larger reduction in the number of rounde fibers (convexity between 0.9 and 1) and a greater increase in the number of fibers with an irregular shape (convexity between 0.0 and 0.6) in sciatic nerves of G93A–/– mice compared to G93A+/+ mice (Fig. 10d). In addition, we identified a significant reduction in the percentage of motor axons with a larger diameter (≥ 10 μm; myelinated axons) in the sciatic nerve of G93A–/– mice in comparison to G93A+/+ mice (Fig. 10e). To evaluate the status of myelination of each nerve fiber we measured the *g-ratio* (ratio between the axon diameter and the fiber diameter) in both G93A+/+

and G93A–/– mice identifyng a specific increase in the sciatic nerves G93A–/– mice (Fig. 10f). In addition, we found lower levels of the four isoforms (21 kD; 18.5 kD; 17.2 kD; 14 kD) of the myelin basic protein (MBP) in thes ciatic nerves of G93A–/– mice compared to G93A+/+ mice (Additional file 1: Figure S11a, b).

Lack of MHCI and CTLs does not affect the cervical spinal nerves at the advanced disease stage

While MN loss was similar (– 67%) in the cervical and lumbar spinal cord in G93A+/+ mice at the symptomatic stage (140 d), the muscle wasting occurred earlier

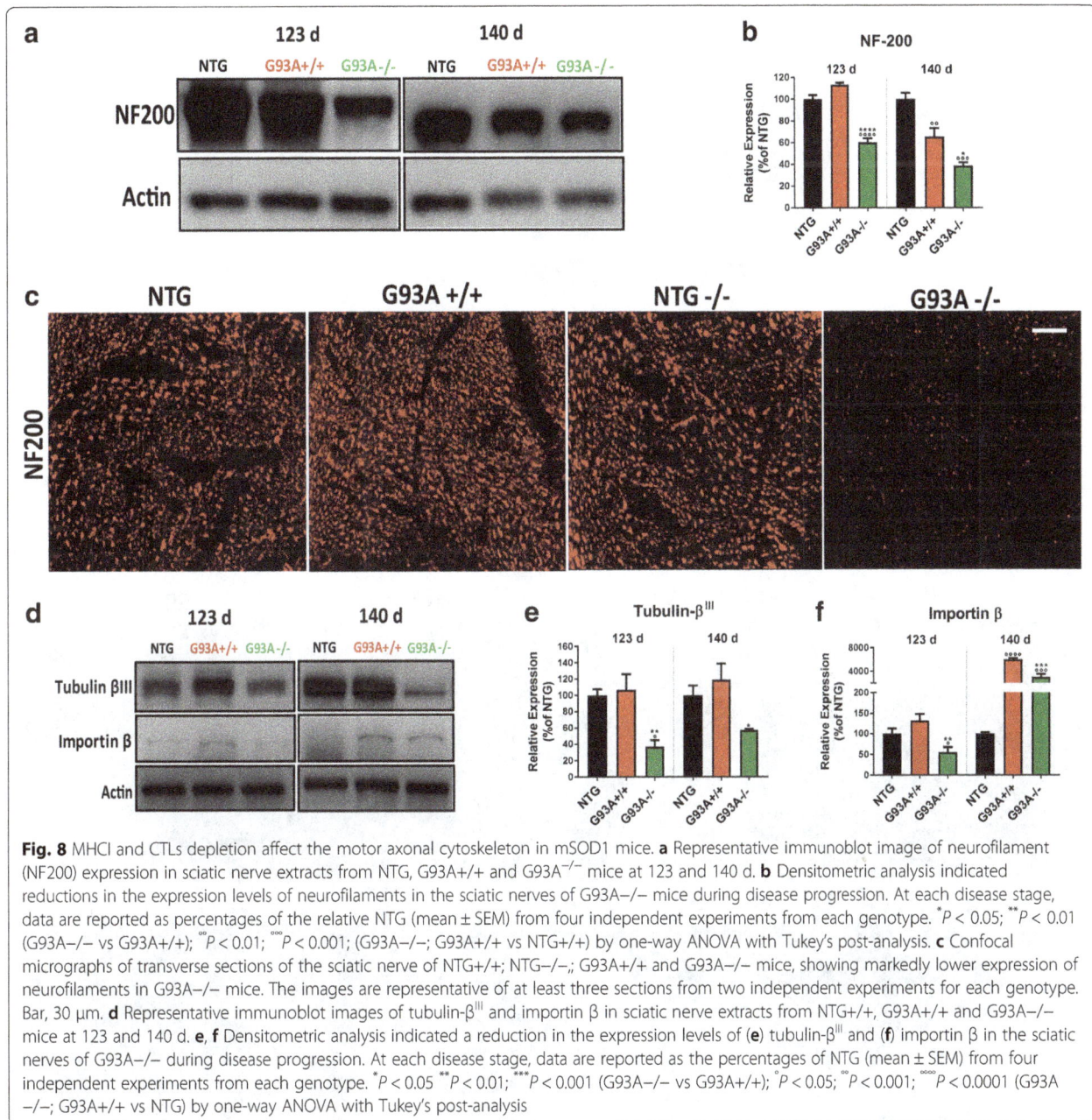

Fig. 8 MHCI and CTLs depletion affect the motor axonal cytoskeleton in mSOD1 mice. **a** Representative immunoblot image of neurofilament (NF200) expression in sciatic nerve extracts from NTG, G93A+/+ and G93A$^{-/-}$ mice at 123 and 140 d. **b** Densitometric analysis indicated reductions in the expression levels of neurofilaments in the sciatic nerves of G93A–/– mice during disease progression. At each disease stage, data are reported as percentages of the relative NTG (mean ± SEM) from four independent experiments from each genotype. $^*P < 0.05$; $^{**}P < 0.01$ (G93A–/– vs G93A+/+); $^{oo}P < 0.01$; $^{ooo}P < 0.001$; (G93A–/–; G93A+/+ vs NTG+/+) by one-way ANOVA with Tukey's post-analysis. **c** Confocal micrographs of transverse sections of the sciatic nerve of NTG+/+; NTG–/–; G93A+/+ and G93A–/– mice, showing markedly lower expression of neurofilaments in G93A–/– mice. The images are representative of at least three sections from two independent experiments for each genotype. Bar, 30 μm. **d** Representative immunoblot images of tubulin-β^{III} and importin β in sciatic nerve extracts from NTG+/+, G93A+/+ and G93A–/– mice at 123 and 140 d. **e, f** Densitometric analysis indicated a reduction in the expression levels of (**e**) tubulin-β^{III} and (**f**) importin β in the sciatic nerves of G93A–/– during disease progression. At each disease stage, data are reported as the percentages of NTG (mean ± SEM) from four independent experiments from each genotype. $^*P < 0.05$ $^{**}P < 0.01$; $^{***}P < 0.001$ (G93A–/– vs G93A+/+); $^{o}P < 0.05$; $^{oo}P < 0.001$; $^{ooo}P < 0.0001$ (G93A –/–; G93A+/+ vs NTG) by one-way ANOVA with Tukey's post-analysis

and more severely in hindlimbs (TA and GC) than fore-limbs (TB). At 140 d, the TA and GC of G93A+/+ mice showed weight loss of respectively 67.5 ± 2.6% and 66.3 ± 11.1% compared to 52.8 ± 3.2% in the TB (Fig. 11d). Interestingly, unlike for the sciatic nerves, no or little activation was observed for MHCI (Fig. 11a, e) or stress-related proteins such as GFAP (Fig. 11b, f) and p75^{NTR} (Fig. 11c, g) in radial nerves of G93A+/+ mice at 140 d. However, at the end stage of the disease the levels of all these proteins were significantly increased in the radial nerve even if at a lower extent with respect to the sciatic nerve. (Additional file 1: Figure S12 a-d). This could explain why in mSOD1 mice the disease

progression starts from the hindlimbs and only in a second time involves the forepaws. In addition, these data suggest that the activation of MHCI in the periphery is proportional to the degree of damage.

Discussion

Adaptive immunity, associated with MHCI and infiltrating CTLs, is increasingly recognized as critical in the pathogenesis of many neuroinflammatory diseases, including ALS [5, 22, 26, 27, 61]. Data on CTL infiltration in the damaged area of the brain and spinal cord of ALS patients [10, 17] and mouse models [12, 15] suggest that these cells contribute to MN death. However, the role of the MHCI

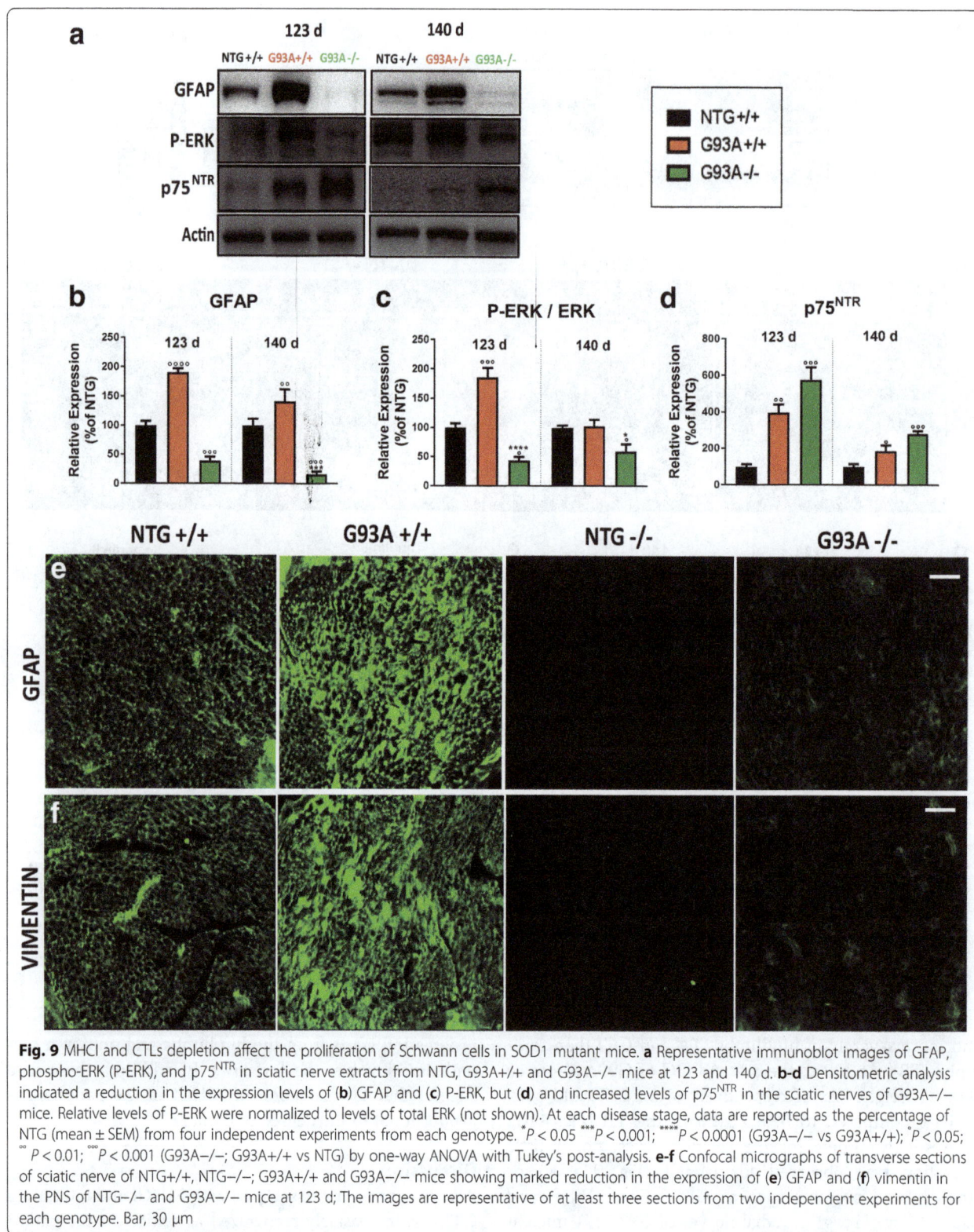

Fig. 9 MHCI and CTLs depletion affect the proliferation of Schwann cells in SOD1 mutant mice. **a** Representative immunoblot images of GFAP, phospho-ERK (P-ERK), and p75^{NTR} in sciatic nerve extracts from NTG, G93A+/+ and G93A−/− mice at 123 and 140 d. **b-d** Densitometric analysis indicated a reduction in the expression levels of (**b**) GFAP and (**c**) P-ERK, but (**d**) and increased levels of p75^{NTR} in the sciatic nerves of G93A−/− mice. Relative levels of P-ERK were normalized to levels of total ERK (not shown). At each disease stage, data are reported as the percentage of NTG (mean ± SEM) from four independent experiments from each genotype. $^*P < 0.05$ $^{***}P < 0.001$; $^{****}P < 0.0001$ (G93A−/− vs G93A+/+); $^{°}P < 0.05$; $^{°°}P < 0.01$; $^{°°°}P < 0.001$ (G93A−/−; G93A+/+ vs NTG) by one-way ANOVA with Tukey's post-analysis. **e-f** Confocal micrographs of transverse sections of sciatic nerve of NTG+/+, NTG−/−; G93A+/+ and G93A−/− mice showing marked reduction in the expression of (**e**) GFAP and (**f**) vimentin in the PNS of NTG−/− and G93A−/− mice at 123 d; The images are representative of at least three sections from two independent experiments for each genotype. Bar, 30 μm

signlling in the disease pathogenesis is still controversial [5, 26]. Here we provide new information in support of a dual role of the MHCI pathway in the CNS and the PNS over the course of the disease in mSOD1 mice.

We found that the ubiquitary removal of MHCI and depletion of CD8$^+$ T cells brought forward the onset of hindlimb force impairment and paralysis in mSOD1 mice due to increased denervation atrophy of hindlimb

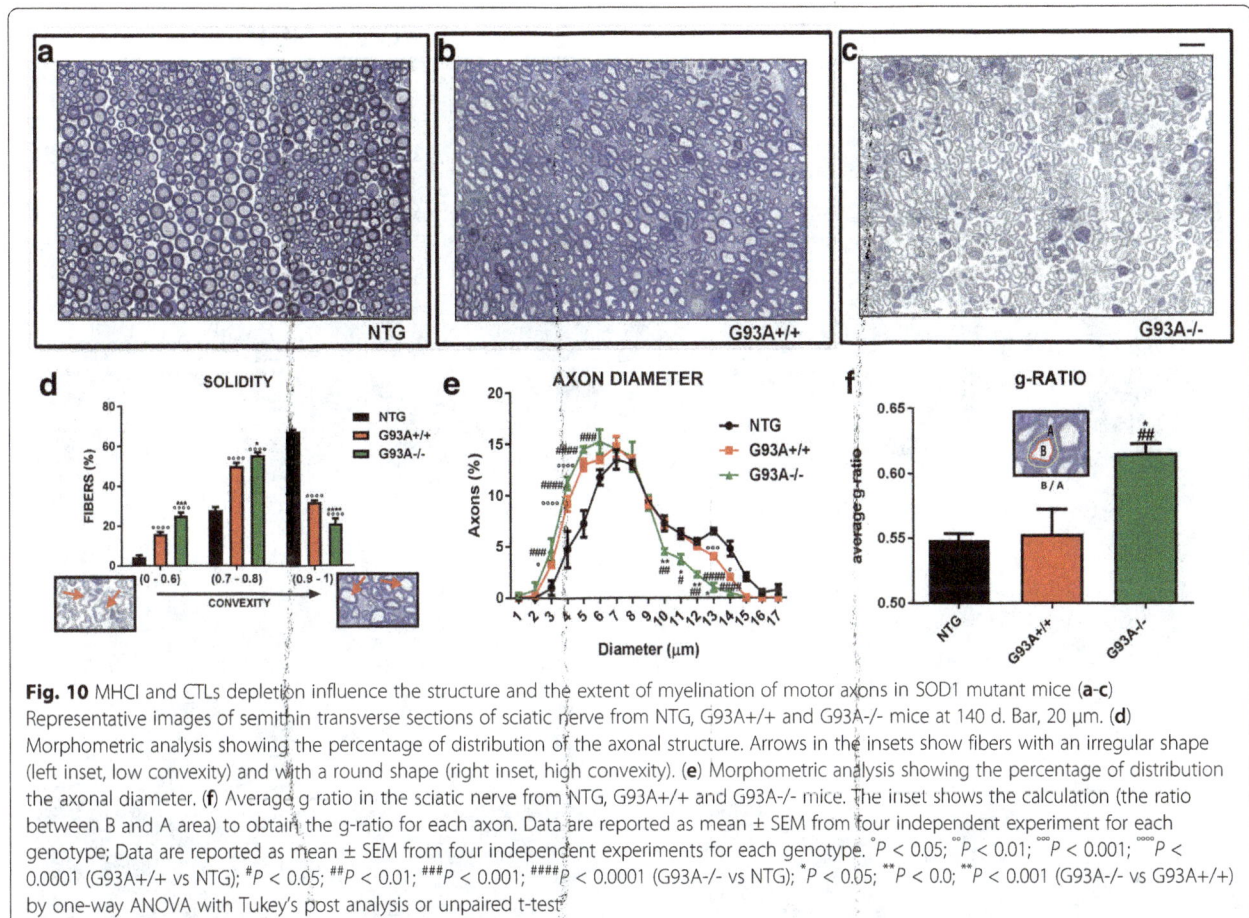

Fig. 10 MHCI and CTLs depletion influence the structure and the extent of myelination of motor axons in SOD1 mutant mice (**a-c**) Representative images of semithin transverse sections of sciatic nerve from NTG, G93A+/+ and G93A-/- mice at 140 d. Bar, 20 μm. (**d**) Morphometric analysis showing the percentage of distribution of the axonal structure. Arrows in the insets show fibers with an irregular shape (left inset, low convexity) and with a round shape (right inset, high convexity). (**e**) Morphometric analysis showing the percentage of distribution the axonal diameter. (**f**) Average g ratio in the sciatic nerve from NTG, G93A+/+ and G93A-/- mice. The inset shows the calculation (the ratio between B and A area) to obtain the g-ratio for each axon. Data are reported as mean ± SEM from four independent experiment for each genotype; Data are reported as mean ± SEM from four independent experiments for each genotype. $^*P < 0.05$; $^{**}P < 0.01$; $^{***}P < 0.001$; $^{****}P < 0.0001$ (G93A+/+ vs NTG); $^\#P < 0.05$; $^{\#\#}P < 0.01$; $^{\#\#\#}P < 0.001$; $^{\#\#\#\#}P < 0.0001$ (G93A-/- vs NTG); $^*P < 0.05$; $^{**}P < 0.0$; $^{**}P < 0.001$ (G93A-/- vs G93A+/+) by one-way ANOVA with Tukey's post analysis or unpaired t-test.

muscles. In contrast, the forelimb muscles and diaphragm were less denervated in G93A-/- mice, in line with the significant protection of MNs in the cervical spinal cord. This resulted in the prolonged ability of the G93A-/- mouse to bring-back prone with the front paws when placed on its side, despite complete paralysis of the hindlimbs, with a consequent later euthanasia than G93A+/+ mice.

This result contrasts with the study from Staats et al. [62] reporting a shorter survival of β2m-/- SOD1G93A mice compared with the β2m+/- SOD1G93A mice. However, the authors did not observe any increase of CD8 gene expression in the spinal cord of mSOD1 mice suggesting that CTLs did not infiltrate the CNS during the disease progression. We have not explanation for this since there are clear evidence of CD8+ T cells infiltration in spinal cord of ALS patients and mSDO1 mice [8, 10, 16, 17].

Furthermore, while we used a large cohort of female mice (according to the standard operating procedures for preclinical animal research in ALS/MND [63]), the number of mice examined in Staats' work varied between eight and thirteen without indications of gender balancing within the experimental groups although it is

well known the sexual dimorphism in the pathology of SOD1G93A mice [64]. All together this evidence may explain the discrepancy of results in the overall survival of β2m-/- SOD1G93A mice.

MHCI signaling and CD8+ T cells infiltration in the PNS enhance the connections of motor axons with hindlimb muscles during the progression of the disease

Our study has strengthened our hypothesis that the specific activation of the MHCI in the sciatic nerves of mSOD1-related ALS mice at disease onset is instrumental in facilitating axonal preservation and maintaining hindlimb muscle innervation, with a positive impact on the early stage of the disease [5, 11, 26]. This partially agrees with Song et al. [27] who recently showed that the specific induction of MHCI in MNs delayed the disease onset and prolong the survival of mSOD1 mice. While they focused mainly on the role of neuronal MHCI overexpression in the CNS in relation to the astrocytes-neuron interaction, little attention was paid to the role of MHCI in the PNS.

We previously showed that 129SvSOD1^{G93A} mice, with faster disease progression and a rapid hindlimb denervation, were unable to activate an MHCI-dependent

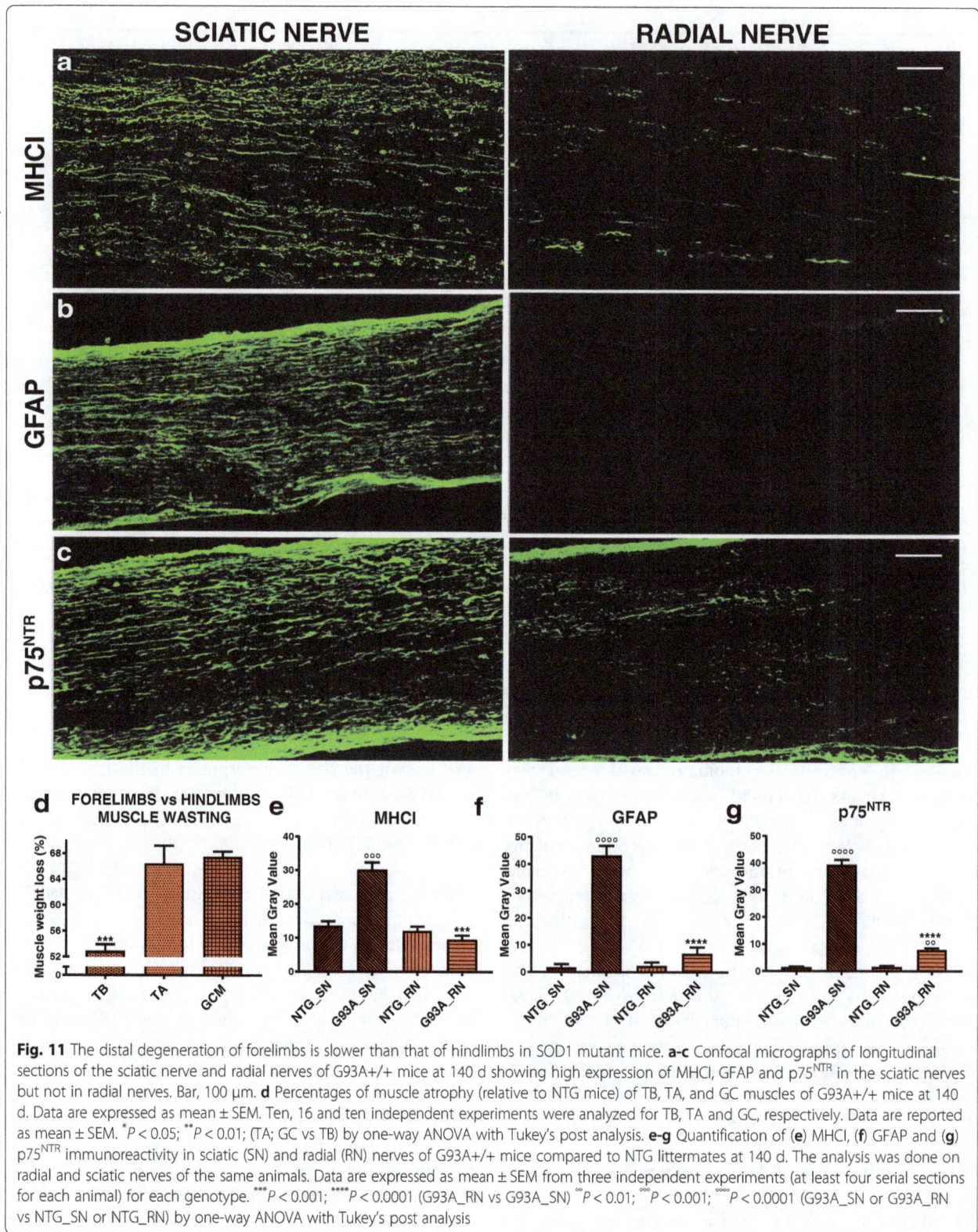

Fig. 11 The distal degeneration of forelimbs is slower than that of hindlimbs in SOD1 mutant mice. **a-c** Confocal micrographs of longitudinal sections of the sciatic nerve and radial nerves of G93A+/+ mice at 140 d showing high expression of MHCI, GFAP and p75^{NTR} in the sciatic nerves but not in radial nerves. Bar, 100 μm. **d** Percentages of muscle atrophy (relative to NTG mice) of TB, TA, and GC muscles of G93A+/+ mice at 140 d. Data are expressed as mean ± SEM. Ten, 16 and ten independent experiments were analyzed for TB, TA and GC, respectively. Data are reported as mean ± SEM. $^*P < 0.05$; $^{**}P < 0.01$; (TA; GC vs TB) by one-way ANOVA with Tukey's post analysis. **e-g** Quantification of (**e**) MHCI, (**f**) GFAP and (**g**) p75^{NTR} immunoreactivity in sciatic (SN) and radial (RN) nerves of G93A+/+ mice compared to NTG littermates at 140 d. The analysis was done on radial and sciatic nerves of the same animals. Data are expressed as mean ± SEM from three independent experiments (at least four serial sections for each animal) for each genotype. $^{***}P < 0.001$; $^{****}P < 0.0001$ (G93A_RN vs G93A_SN) $^{oo}P < 0.01$; $^{ooo}P < 0.001$; $^{oooo}P < 0.0001$ (G93A_SN or G93A_RN vs NTG_SN or NTG_RN) by one-way ANOVA with Tukey's post analysis

adaptive immune response in their motor axons, while the slow-progressor C57SOD1^{G93A} mice had a robust increase of MHCI and CTL infiltration in their sciatic nerves [11]. Here we demonstrate that the lack of MHCI activation and CTL infiltration in the PNS of mSOD1 mice destabilizes the peripheral motor axons, which progressively lose their cytoarchitecture and function, exacerbating the denervation of hindlimb muscles. This is accompanied by altered function and proliferation of SCs, preventing the establishment of a favorable environment for collateral re-innervation [53]. To obtain efficient nerve regeneration after damage mature SCs have to dedifferentiate, proliferate, and provide this favorable environment for axonal sprouting [53]. A defect in one of these functions, that imply continuous rearrangement of the cytoskeleton, may result in defective remyelination of motor axons. After axonal damage, both GFAP and Vimentin are upregulated to ensure the efficient cytoskeleton rearrangement necessary for the de-differentiation and proliferation of SCs [65–67]. While GFAP (and the relative activation of ERK) is essential to initiate the proliferation of SCs, Vimentin is involved in sustaining this process until its completion [59]. Accordingly, depletion of GFAP, Vimentin or both delays axonal regeneration and motor recovery after peripheral nerve damage [55, 57, 59, 60]. Here we showed that while G93A+/+ mice strongly activated GFAP and vimentin starting from the disease onset, MHCI depletion affected the basal level of vimentin, GFAP and ERK phosphorylation in the PNS of NTG −/− mice and, as a consequence, their level of activation in pathological conditions. As a result, G93A−/− mice showed a progressive and marked reduction of myelinated fibers in sciatic nerves in addition to a remarked alteration of axonal cytoarchitecture.

These findings suggest that MHCI signaling directly influences the architecture of the sciatic nerve so that MHCI activation in addition to CTLs infiltration in the PNS preserve the quality of connections between motor axons and hindlimb muscles during the disease progression. This scenario resembles that previously reported in experimental mouse models of axon remyelination in which the proliferation and differentiation of precursor cells were accompanied by immune cells infiltration [68]. For example, the depletion or pharmacological inhibition of T-cells following toxin- or virus- induced demyelination leads to an impairment of remyelination [69, 70]. Besides, Bombeiro et al. [71] recently showed that boosting the immune response by early adoptive transfer of activated WT lymphocytes three days after axonal injury improved motor recovery in WT and RAG-KO mice. Overall, these data support the hypothesis that the activation of an immune response in the PNS is essential to promote the targeted destruction of defective motor fibers to create a growth-permissive milieu for sprouting of new neurites [54].

Distal forelimb pathology is delayed in SOD1G93A mice

Early studies of mSOD1 mice reported that the mice first developed hindlimb tremors, then progressive hindlimb weakness with rapidly deteriorating gait, eventually culminating in paralysis of one or both hindlimbs [34, 72, 73]. Forelimb function remains comparatively spared in ALS mice throughout disease progression [34] indicating a different susceptibility of this motor unit. The delayed forelimb motor weakness in ALS mice was partially explained by Beers et al. [74] showing an augmented protective immune response in the cervical spinal cord. In keeping with this, we found how the gliosis and the overall inflammation (including the extent of MHCI activation by microglia) are attenuated in the cervical spinal cord of G93A+/+ mice compared to the lumbar spinal cord during the disease progression.

Here we also showed that muscle atrophy is more significant in GC and TA than in TB of mSOD1 mice. This is possibly because of different patterns of cellular metabolism and cytoskeletal derangements of the forelimb and hindlimb muscles [75].

We also found that the radial nerves of mSOD1 mice were less susceptible to stress than the sciatic nerves of the same mice. This is in line with Clark et al. [33], showing that at late symptomatic stage (140 d) in forelimbs of mSOD1 mice (with the same backround of the present study), axonal (fragmentation, branching) and NMJ (denervation, fragmentation, and beading) alterations are irrilevant if compared to hindlimb which suggests regional differences in the pathogenic mechanisms underlying the disease. In fact, we did not find any activation of MHCI in radial nerves of mSOD1 mice compared to sciatic nerves at the symptomatic disease stage. However, MHCI is activated at the end-stage of disease with levels similar to those observed in the sciatic nerves at 140 d indicating that the induction of MHCI depends directly on the extent of peripheral stress. In conclusion, data from this work and the literature suggest that the differences in inflammation between the two spinal cord segments of ALS mice, after the initiation of disease, is partially due to the stress related signals that MNs and axons receive from the corresponding skeletal muscle targets. In fact, we previously showed an opposite response to a common early down-regulation of complex I in the two muscles type of SOD1G93A mice with earlier metabolic changes and cytoskeletal derangements of the hindlimbs than forelimbs muscle [75]. This agrees with the evidence that hindlimb muscles are more susceptible to alterations in energy production than forelimb muscles [76].

Therefore we assume that MHCI signaling is essential to preserve the quality of the connections of motor axons with rapidly degenerating hindlimb muscles, independently from MN loss. This could explain the earlier motor onset in G93A−/− mice. In contrast, the denervation atrophy of forelimbs is mainly dependent on the health status of the MN cell body in the cervical spinal cord.

MHCI activation by microglia and CD8+ T cells infiltration in the spinal cord are detrimental to motor neuron survival

The role of the inflammatory response in the PNS stands in stark contrast to that of the CNS, where the reaction of nearby cells is mainly associated with inhibitory scar formation, quiescence, and degeneration/apoptosis [54]. Activated microglia in the CNS can cross-present antigen and stimulate the cytotoxic activity of naive CD8+ T cells in a proteasome- and TAP-dependent manner [38, 39]. CD8+ T cells progressively infiltrate the spinal cord of SOD1^{G93A} mice [8, 15]. However, the consequences of these events have never been investigated in ALS mice. Here we report that microglia depleted of MHCI are less sensitive to pro-inflammatory stimuli and this, in addition to the lack of CTL infiltration in the CNS, resulted in less inflammation that led to the preservation of MNs in the spinal cord of SOD1^{G93A} mice. In fact, despite the earlier motor onset, G93A−/− mice showed no difference in lumbar MN loss compared to G93A+/+ mice. Moreover, the cervical MNs of these mice were significantly preserved at the advanced stage of the disease in comparison to G93A

+/+ mice. These findings comply with our previous evidence showing that rapidly progressing mSOD1 mice had a lower MHCI-dependent adaptive immune response, higher hindlimb muscle denervation but a similar lumbar MN loss than slowing progressing mSOD1 mice [11, 28]. Recently, Komine et al. [77] reported that CTLs may not be the main modulator of MHCI-mediated inflammation since their reduction through anti-CD8 antibody did not influence the disease progression of mSOD1 mice. This study lack of a detailed the evaluation of histological signatures (MN loss, inflammation, denervation atrophy) so that we ignore if the inhibition of CTLs infiltration is really ineffective on the disease progression of mSOD1 mice. In fact, we still need to understand why CD8+ T cell infiltration within the spinal cord is remarkably elicited in mSOD1 mice. Given that in Komine et al. [77] spinal cord microglia still express MHCI, it is possible that other unknown mechanisms compensate for the reduction of CTLs. Alternatively, the remaining number of CTLs after the inhibition (~ 1000) could be still able to induce a response. Further studies are necessary to disentangle this issue. Nevertheless, our data clearly showed that the lack of MHCI expression by microglia reduces the pro-inflammatory response in vitro and in vivo.

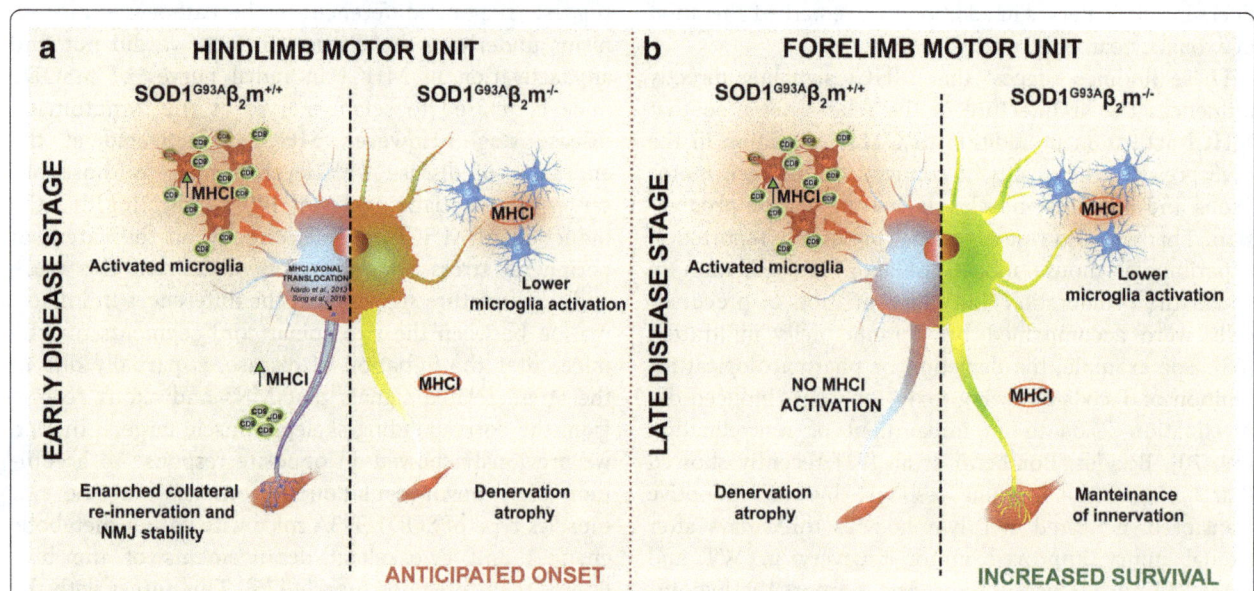

Fig. 12 The lack of MHCI signaling anticipated the onset of disease but increase the overall survival of mSOD1 mice. Schematic representation of (**a**) hindlimb and (**b**) forelimb motor unit of SOD1^{G93A}B2m$^{+/+}$ (G93A +/+) and SOD1^{G93A}B2m$^{−/−}$ (G93A−/−) mice at early and late disease stages. **a** The interaction of MHCI and CTLs in the PNS is essential to preserve the quality of the connections of motor axons with rapidly degenerating hindlimb muscles, independently from MN loss. This could explain the earlier motor onset in G93A−/− mice. These animals, while partially preserving MNs (due the lack of MHCI-mediated interaction of microglia and CTLs), are not able to activate the neuroprotective stress MHCI signalling in the PNS. This lead to an earlier denervation atrophy of hindlimb muscles. **b** In the cervical nerves, the extent of stress is not such as to cause an activation of MHCI signalling in the PNS of G93A+/+ mice. As a consequence, the denervation atrophy of forelimbs is mainly dependent on the health status of the MN cell body in the cervical spinal cord. In G93A−/− mice, the lack of MHCI-mediated interaction of microglia and CTLs results in lower inflammation and higher protection of MNs. Accordingly, the greater functionality of forelimbs causes these mice survive more than G93A+/+ mice

Conclusions

This study illustrates ALS as a complex disease defined by specific pathogenesis in the CNS and PNS and counteracting responses in the lumbar and cervical motor units. We showed that in the lumbar spinal cord motor units of mSOD1 mouse, MN loss is secondary to NMJ destruction and muscle denervation, which are accelerated in the absence of peripheral MHCI activation and CTL infiltration (Fig. 12a). In contrast, in the cervical spinal cord motor units the degree of muscle denervation atrophy is mainly dependent on the viability of MN cell bodies. In this case, the MHCI-dependent interaction between CTLs and microglia plays a crucial role in triggering the neuroinflammation that leads to MN degeneration (Fig. 12b).

Accordingly, a strategy aimed at activating MHCI signaling in the periphery during the early disease stages may be useful to maintaining axonal integrity and maximal connectivity with the muscle, providing a functional reserve for surviving MNs and slowing the disease progression.

In parallel, the inhibition of the MHCI-dependent interaction between CD8$^+$ T cells and microglia within the CNS should attenuates the inflammation, prevents MN loss and increases the overall survival.

The failure of non-targeted anti-inflammatory and anti-immune therapies in clinical trials [13, 14] shows up our incomplete knowledge of the dynamic changes that occur during the disease progression and indirectly supports reconsideration of the immune system in ALS. We expect that better understanding of the molecular mechanisms underlying the immune response in transgenic ALS mice should help in finding new approaches for promoting MN survival, axonal regeneration and muscle innervation in ALS patients.

Additional files

Additional file 1: Figure S1. MHCI depletion affect the number of CD3+ / CD4+ T cells but not their extent of infiltration in the spinal cord during the disease progression. **Figure S2.** MHCI depletion reduces the impairment of the cervical motor neurons in mSOD1 mice. **Figure S3.** MHCI depletion lowered the CD68 mRNA levels in the spinal cord of mSOD1 mice. **Figure S4.** MHCI depletion did not affect the extent of astrocytosis in the cervical and the lumbar spinal cord of G93A+/+ mice. **Figure S5.** MHCI expression is lower in the cervical than in the lumbar spinal cord of G93A+/+ mice. **Figure S6.** MHCI depletion accelerates denervation of hindlimb muscles in mSOD1mice. **Figure S7.** MHCI depletion inhibits the proliferation of the terminal Schwann cells and the size of AChR clusters in SOD1 mutant mice. **Figure S8.** MHCI depletion accelerates the atrophy of hindlimbs muscles in SOD1 mutant mice. **Figure S9.** MHCI depletion preserves the diaphragm innervation in SOD1 mutant mice. **Figure S10.** GFAP and phospho-ERK expression are reduced in the sciatic nerve of NTG-/- mice. **Figure S11.** Myelin basic protein isoforms are markedly dwonregulated in the sciatic nerve of G93A-/- mice at 140 d. **Figure S12.** Regional and temporal differences defines the disease progression of mSOD1 mice.

Additional file 2: Video S1. G93A–/– mice use forelimbs during the last sessions of the PaGE test. An example of a G93A–/– mouse at 154 d mainly using its forelimbs to remain clinging to the grid.
Additional file 3: Video S2. SOD1^{G93A} mice at the endstage use forelimbs to pass the survival test. An example of SOD1^{G93A} mice at 168 d using the forelimbs to wrap themselves around in prone position.
Additional file 4: Video S3. SOD1^{G93A} mice at the endstage use forelimbs to pass the survival test. An example of SOD1^{G93A} mice at 168 d using the forelimbs to wrap themselves around in prone position.
Additional file 5: Video S4. SOD1^{G93A} mice at the endstage use forelimbs to pass the survival test. An example of SOD1^{G93A} mice at 170 d using the forelimbs to wrap themselves around in prone position.

Additional file 6: Video S5. G93A–/– mice have better forelimb activity than G93A+/+ mice during the last disease stages. Examples of G93A–/– mice showing good forelimb function on the grid compared to G93A+/+ mice that struggled or could not stay in prone position on the grid, with clear atrophy of at least one anterior paw (Additional file 5: Video S4).

Abbreviations

AChR: Acetyl choline receptor; ALS: Amyotrophic lateral sclerosis; CTLs: Cytotoxic T lymphocytes; G93A–/–: SOD1^{G93A}β2M$^{-/-}$; G93A +/+: SOD1^{G93A}β2M$^{+/+}$; GC: *Gastrocnemius*; MHCI: Major histocompatibility complex I; MN: Motor neuron; NMJ: Neuro muscular junction; NTG: Non transgenic; NTG–/–: Non transgenic β2M$^{-/-}$; NTG+/+: Non transgenic β2M$^{+/+}$; PNS: Peripheral nervous system; SC: Schwann cells; SN: Sciatic nerve; SOD1: Cu/Zn superoxIde dismutase; TA: *Tibialis Anterior*; TB: *Triceps Brachii*; TSC: Terminal Schwann cell

Acknowledgements

We thank Prof. Stanley H. Appel (Methodist Neurological Institute, Huston, Texas) for the critical reading of the manuscript and the useful suggestions. A special thank to Dr. Alessandro Di Bartolo and Dr. Gabriela Bortolanca Chiarotto for their help to in vitro and in vivo analysis and to Matteo Sironi and Alessandro Soave for the artwork of the Fig. 11.

Funding

This work was mainly supported by the Thierry Latran Foundation (TLF) together with the Motor Neurone Disease Association (MNDA), the "Amici del Mario Negri" Association, Regione Lombardia under Institutional Agreement no. 14501, the "Translating molecular mechanisms into ALS risk and patient's well-being" (TRANS-ALS) - Regione Lombardia (no. 2015–0023), and the European Community's (FP7/2007–2013) under grant EuroMOTOR (no. 259867). The MTC's fellowship is kindly supported by Prof. Ennio Galante.

Authors' contributions

MCT recruited mouse tissues, did the behavioral, immunohistochemical, biomolecular and biochemical analysis of spinal cord, sciatic nerves and muscles of transgenic mice with the help of GN and MV, under the supervision of GN. GD and NR did the IHC of sciatic nerves under the supervision of AQ. NP did the longitudinal FACS analysis of CD8$^+$ T cells under the supervision of EE. AM produced and treated the primary cell cultures and acquired the images under the supervision of MdP. GN did the in vitro morphometric analysis of microglia and MN loss. GN and MCT designed the experiments under the supervision of CB. GN and CB wrote the manuscript. All authors have read and approved the final version of the manuscript.

were conducted. The corresponding author have obtained informed consent from all participants in the study.

Competing interests
The authors declare that they have no competing interests.

Author details
[1]Laboratory of Molecular Neurobiology, Department of Neuroscience, IRCCS - Istituto di Ricerche Farmacologiche Mario Negri, Via La Masa 19, 20156 Milan, Italy. [2]Laboratory of Analytical Biochemistry, Department of Environmental Health Sciences, IRCCS - Istituto di Ricerche Farmacologiche Mario Negri, Via La Masa 19, 20156 Milan, Italy. [3]Neuropathology Unit, Department of Neurology, INSPE- San Raffaele Scientific Institute, Dibit II, Via Olgettina 48, 20132 Milan, Italy. [4]Laboratory of Cancer Pharmacology Department of Oncology, Flow Cytometry Unit, IRCCS – Istituto di Ricerche Farmacologiche Mario Negri, via La Masa 19, 20156 Milan, Italy.

References
1. Hardiman O, Al-Chalabi A, Chio A, Corr EM, Logroscino G, Robberecht W, Shaw PJ, Simmons Z, van den Berg LH. Amyotrophic lateral sclerosis. Nat Rev Dis Primers. 2017;3:17085.
2. Zarei S, Carr K, Reiley L, Diaz K, Guerra O, Altamirano PF, Pagani W, Lodin D, Orozco G, Chinea A. A comprehensive review of amyotrophic lateral sclerosis. Surg Neurol Int. 2015;6:171.
3. Chia R, Chio A, Traynor BJ. Novel genes associated with amyotrophic lateral sclerosis: diagnostic and clinical implications. Lancet Neurol. 2018;17:94–102.
4. Nardo G, Trolese MC, Tortarolo M, Vallarola A, Freschi M, Pasetto L, Bonetto V, Bendotti C. New insights on the mechanisms of disease course variability in ALS from mutant SOD1 mouse models. Brain Pathol. 2016;26:237–47.
5. Nardo G, Trolese MC, Bendotti C. Major histocompatibility complex I expression by motor neurons and its implication in amyotrophic lateral sclerosis. Front Neurol. 2016;7:89.
6. Appel SH, Beers DR, Henkel JS. T cell-microglial dialogue in Parkinson's disease and amyotrophic lateral sclerosis: are we listening? Trends Immunol. 2010;31:7–17.
7. Beers DR, Henkel JS, Zhao W, Wang J, Appel SH. CD4+ T cells support glial neuroprotection, slow disease progression, and modify glial morphology in an animal model of inherited ALS. Proc Natl Acad Sci U S A. 2008;105: 15558–63.
8. Chiu IM, Chen A, Zheng Y, Kosaras B, Tsiftsoglou SA, Vartanian TK, Brown RH Jr, Carroll MC. T lymphocytes potentiate endogenous neuroprotective inflammation in a mouse model of ALS. Proc Natl Acad Sci U S A. 2008;105: 17913–8.
9. Zhao W, Beers DR, Appel SH. Immune-mediated mechanisms in the pathoprogression of amyotrophic lateral sclerosis. J Neuroimmune Pharmacol. 2013;8:888–99.
10. Holmoy T. T cells in amyotrophic lateral sclerosis. Eur J Neurol. 2008;15:360–6.
11. Nardo G, Trolese MC, de Vito G, Cecchi R, Riva N, Dina G, Heath PR, Quattrini A, Shaw PJ, Piazza V, Bendotti C. Immune response in peripheral axons delays disease progression in SOD1(G93A) mice. J Neuroinflammation. 2016;13:261.
12. Chiu IM, Phatnani H, Kuligowski M, Tapia JC, Carrasco MA, Zhang M, Maniatis T, Carroll MC. Activation of innate and humoral immunity in the peripheral nervous system of ALS transgenic mice. Proc Natl Acad Sci U S A. 2009;106:20960–5.
13. Khalid SI, Ampie L, Kelly R, Ladha SS, Dardis C. Immune modulation in the treatment of amyotrophic lateral sclerosis: a review of clinical trials. Front Neurol. 2017;8:486.
14. McCombe PA, Henderson RD. The role of immune and inflammatory mechanisms in ALS. Curr Mol Med. 2011;11:246–54.
15. NBeers DR, Henkel JS, Zhao W, Wang J, Huang A, Wen S, Liao B, Appel SH. Endogenous regulatory T lymphocytes ameliorate amyotrophic lateral sclerosis in mice and correlate with disease progression in patients with amyotrophic lateral sclerosis. Brain. 2011;134:1293–314.
16. Chiu IM, Morimoto ET, Goodarzi H, Liao JT, O'Keeffe S, Phatnani HP, Muratet M, Carroll MC, Levy S, Tavazoie S, et al. A neurodegeneration-specific gene-expression signature of acutely isolated microglia from an amyotrophic lateral sclerosis mouse model. Cell Rep. 2013;4:385–401.
17. Sta M, Sylva-Steenland RM, Casula M, de Jong JM, Troost D, Aronica E, Baas F. Innate and adaptive immunity in amyotrophic lateral sclerosis: evidence of complement activation. Neurobiol Dis. 2011;42:211–20.
18. Peter ME, Budd RC, Desbarats J, Hedrick SM, Hueber AO, Newell MK, Owen LB, Pope RM, Tschopp J, Wajant H, et al. The CD95 receptor: apoptosis revisited. Cell. 2007;129:447–50.
19. Raoul C, Buhler E, Sadeghi C, Jacquier A, Aebischer P, Pettmann B, Henderson CE, Haase G. Chronic activation in presymptomatic amyotrophic lateral sclerosis (ALS) mice of a feedback loop involving Fas, Daxx, and FasL. Proc Natl Acad Sci U S A. 2006;103:6007–12.
20. Raoul C, Estevez AG, Nishimune H, Cleveland DW, deLapeyriere O, Henderson CE, Haase G, Pettmann B. Motoneuron death triggered by a specific pathway downstream of Fas. Potentiation by ALS-linked SOD1 mutations. Neuron. 2002;35:1067–83.
21. Petri S, Kiaei M, Wille E, Calingasan NY, Flint Beal M. Loss of Fas ligand-function improves survival in G93A-transgenic ALS mice. J Neurol Sci. 2006; 251:44–9.
22. Nardo G, Iennaco R, Fusi N, Heath PR, Marino M, Trolese MC, Ferraiuolo L, Lawrence N, Shaw PJ, Bendotti C. Transcriptomic indices of fast and slow disease progression in two mouse models of amyotrophic lateral sclerosis. Brain. 2013;136:3305–32.
23. Bendotti C, Marino M, Cheroni C, Fontana E, Crippa V, Poletti A, De Biasi S. Dysfunction of constitutive and inducible ubiquitin-proteasome system in amyotrophic lateral sclerosis: implication for protein aggregation and immune response. Prog Neurobiol. 2012;97:101–26.
24. Cheroni C, Marino M, Tortarolo M, Veglianese P, De Biasi S, Fontana E, Zuccarello LV, Maynard CJ, Dantuma NP, Bendotti C. Functional alterations of the ubiquitin-proteasome system in motor neurons of a mouse model of familial amyotrophic lateral sclerosis. Hum Mol Genet. 2009;18:82–96.
25. Cheroni C, Peviani M, Cascio P, Debiasi S, Monti C, Bendotti C. Accumulation of human SOD1 and ubiquitinated deposits in the spinal cord of SOD1G93A mice during motor neuron disease progression correlates with a decrease of proteasome. Neurobiol Dis. 2005;18:509–22.
26. Chiarotto GB, Nardo G, Trolese MC, França MC Jr, Bendotti C, Rodrigues de Oliveira AL. The Emerging Role of the Major Histocompatibility Complex Class I in Amyotrophic Lateral Sclerosis. Int J Mol Sci. 2017;18(11).
27. Song S, Miranda CJ, Braun L, Meyer K, Frakes AE, Ferraiuolo L, Likhite S, Bevan AK, Foust KD, McConnell MJ, et al. Major histocompatibility complex class I molecules protect motor neurons from astrocyte-induced toxicity in amyotrophic lateral sclerosis. Nat Med. 2016;22:397–403.
28. Marino M, Papa S, Crippa V, Nardo G, Peviani M, Cheroni C, Trolese MC, Lauranzano E, Bonetto V, Poletti A, et al. Differences in protein quality control correlate with phenotype variability in 2 mouse models of familial amyotrophic lateral sclerosis. Neurobiol Aging. 2015;36:492–504.
29. Geuna S, Tos P, Guglielmone R, Battiston B, Giacobini-Robecchi MG. Methodological issues in size estimation of myelinated nerve fibers in peripheral nerves. Anat Embryol (Berl). 2001;204:1–10.
30. De Paola M, Mariani A, Bigini P, Peviani M, Ferrara G, Molteni M, Gemma S, Veglianese P, Castellaneta V, Boldrin V, et al. Neuroprotective effects of toll-like receptor 4 antagonism in spinal cord cultures and in a mouse model of motor neuron degeneration. Mol Med. 2012;18:971–81.
31. Koller BH, Marrack P, Kappler JW, Smithies O. Normal development of mice deficient in beta 2M, MHC class I proteins, and CD8+ T cells. Science. 1990; 248:1227–30.
32. Zijlstra M, Bix M, Simister NE, Loring JM, Raulet DH, Jaenisch R. Beta 2-microglobulin deficient mice lack CD4-8+ cytolytic T cells. Nature. 1990;344: 742–6.
33. Clark JA, Southam KA, Blizzard CA, King AE, Dickson TC. Axonal degeneration, distal collateral branching and neuromuscular junction architecture alterations occur prior to symptom onset in the SOD1(G93A) mouse model of amyotrophic lateral sclerosis. J Chem Neuroanat. 2016;76:35–47.
34. Bruijn LI, Becher MW, Lee MK, Anderson KL, Jenkins NA, Copeland NG, Sisodia SS, Rothstein JD, Borchelt DR, Price DL, Cleveland DW. ALS-

linked SOD1 mutant G85R mediates damage to astrocytes and promotes rapidly progressive disease with SOD1-containing inclusions. Neuron. 1997;18:327–38.

35. Friese A, Kaltschmidt JA, Ladle DR, Sigrist M, Jessell TM, Arber S. Gamma and alpha motor neurons distinguished by expression of transcription factor Err3. Proc Natl Acad Sci U S A. 2009;106:13588–93.

36. Gerber YN, Sabourin JC, Rabano M, Vivanco M, Perrin FE. Early functional deficit and microglial disturbances in a mouse model of amyotrophic lateral sclerosis. PLoS One. 2012;7:e36000.

37. Weydt P, Yuen EC, Ransom BR, Moller T. Increased cytotoxic potential of microglia from ALS-transgenic mice. Glia. 2004;48:179–82.

38. Jarry U, Jeannin P, Pineau L, Donnou S, Delneste Y, Couez D. Efficiently stimulated adult microglia cross-prime naive CD8+ T cells injected in the brain. Eur J Immunol. 2013;43:1173–84.

39. Beauvillain C, Donnou S, Jarry U, Scotet M, Gascan H, Delneste Y, Guermonprez P, Jeannin P, Couez D. Neonatal and adult microglia cross-present exogenous antigens. Glia. 2008;56:69–77.

40. MacAry PA, Lindsay M, Scott MA, Craig JI, Luzio JP, Lehner PJ. Mobilization of MHC class I molecules from late endosomes to the cell surface following activation of CD34-derived human Langerhans cells. Proc Natl Acad Sci U S A. 2001;98:3982–7.

41. Rangaraju S, Raza SA, Pennati A, Deng Q, Dammer EB, Duong D, Pennington MW, Tansey MG, Lah JJ, Betarbet R, et al. A systems pharmacology-based approach to identify novel Kv1.3 channel-dependent mechanisms in microglial activation. J Neuroinflammation. 2017;14:128.

42. Fischer LR, Culver DG, Tennant P, Davis AA, Wang M, Castellano-Sanchez A, Khan J, Polak MA, Glass JD. Amyotrophic lateral sclerosis is a distal axonopathy: evidence in mice and man. Exp Neurol. 2004;185:232–40.

43. Dobrowolny G, Aucello M, Musaro A. Muscle atrophy induced by SOD1G93A expression does not involve the activation of caspase in the absence of denervation. Skelet Muscle. 2011;1:3.

44. Tsuneki H, Salas R, Dani JA. Mouse muscle denervation increases expression of an alpha7 nicotinic receptor with unusual pharmacology. J Physiol. 2003; 547:169–79.

45. Covault J, Sanes JR. Neural cell adhesion molecule (N-CAM) accumulates in denervated and paralyzed skeletal muscles. Proc Natl Acad Sci U S A. 1985; 82:4544–8.

46. Fujiwara S, Hoshikawa S, Ueno T, Hirata M, Saito T, Ikeda T, Kawaguchi H, Nakamura K, Tanaka S, Ogata T. SOX10 transactivates S100B to suppress Schwann cell proliferation and to promote myelination. PLoS One. 2014;9:e115400.

47. Song Y, Panzer JA, Wyatt RM, Balice-Gordon RJ. Formation and plasticity of neuromuscular synaptic connections. Int Anesthesiol Clin. 2006;44:145–78.

48. Thams S, Brodin P, Plantman S, Saxelin R, Karre K, Cullheim S. Classical major histocompatibility complex class I molecules in motoneurons: new actors at the neuromuscular junction. J Neurosci. 2009;29:13503–15.

49. Fuller HR, Mandefro B, Shirran SL, Gross AR, Kaus AS, Botting CH, Morris GE, Sareen D. Spinal muscular atrophy patient iPSC-derived motor neurons have reduced expression of proteins important in neuronal development. Front Cell Neurosci. 2015;9:506.

50. Lee S, Shea TB. The high molecular weight neurofilament subunit plays an essential role in axonal outgrowth and stabilization. Biol Open. 2014;3:974–81.

51. Perry RB, Doron-Mandel E, Iavnilovitch E, Rishal I, Dagan SY, Tsoory M, Coppola G, McDonald MK, Gomes C, Geschwind DH, et al. Subcellular knockout of importin beta1 perturbs axonal retrograde signaling. Neuron. 2012;75:294–305.

52. Rossi F, Gianola S, Corvetti L. Regulation of intrinsic neuronal properties for axon growth and regeneration. Prog Neurobiol. 2007;81:1–28.

53. Jessen KR, Mirsky R. The repair Schwann cell and its function in regenerating nerves. J Physiol. 2016;594:3521–31.

54. Gaudet AD, Popovich PG, Ramer MS. Wallerian degeneration: gaining perspective on inflammatory events after peripheral nerve injury. J Neuroinflammation. 2011;8:110.

55. Berg A, Zelano J, Pekna M, Wilhelmsson U, Pekny M, Cullheim S. Axonal regeneration after sciatic nerve lesion is delayed but complete in GFAP- and vimentin-deficient mice. PLoS One. 2013;8:e79395.

56. Tsuda Y, Kanje M, Dahlin LB. Axonal outgrowth is associated with increased ERK 1/2 activation but decreased caspase 3 linked cell death in Schwann cells after immediate nerve repair in rats. BMC Neurosci. 2011;12:12.

57. Keller AF, Gravel M, Kriz J. Live imaging of amyotrophic lateral sclerosis pathogenesis: disease onset is characterized by marked induction of GFAP in Schwann cells. Glia. 2009;57:1130–42.

58. Agthong S, Kaewsema A, Tanomsridejchai N, Chentanez V. Activation of MAPK ERK in peripheral nerve after injury. BMC Neurosci. 2006;7:45.

59. Triolo D, Dina G, Lorenzetti I, Malaguti M, Morana P, Del Carro U, Comi G, Messing A, Quattrini A, Previtali SC. Loss of glial fibrillary acidic protein (GFAP) impairs Schwann cell proliferation and delays nerve regeneration after damage. J Cell Sci. 2006;119:3981–93.

60. Perlson E, Hanz S, Ben-Yaakov K, Segal-Ruder Y, Seger R, Fainzilber M. Vimentin-dependent spatial translocation of an activated MAP kinase in injured nerve. Neuron. 2005;45:715–26.

61. Cebrian C, Loike JD, Sulzer D. Neuronal MHC-I expression and its implications in synaptic function, axonal regeneration and Parkinson's and other brain diseases. Front Neuroanat. 2014;8:114.

62. Staats KA, Schonefeldt S, Van Rillaer M, Van Hoecke A, Van Damme P, Robberecht W, Liston A, Van Den Bosch L. Beta-2 microglobulin is important for disease progression in a murine model for amyotrophic lateral sclerosis. Front Cell Neurosci. 2013;7:249.

63. Ludolph AC, Bendotti C, Blaugrund E, Chio A, Greensmith L, Loeffler JP, Mead R, Niessen HG, Petri S, Pradat PF, et al. Guidelines for preclinical animal research in ALS/MND: a consensus meeting. Amyotroph Lateral Scler. 2010;11:38–45.

64. McGoldrick P, Joyce PI, Fisher EM, Greensmith L. Rodent models of amyotrophic lateral sclerosis. Biochim Biophys Acta. 2013;1832:1421–36.

65. Gillen C, Gleichmann M, Spreyer P, Muller HW. Differentially expressed genes after peripheral nerve injury. J Neurosci Res. 1995;42:159–71.

66. Thomson CE, Griffiths IR, McCulloch MC, Kyriakides E, Barrie JA, Montague P. In vitro studies of axonally-regulated Schwann cell genes during Wallerian degeneration. J Neurocytol. 1993;22:590–602.

67. Neuberger TJ, Cornbrooks CJ. Transient modulation of Schwann cell antigens after peripheral nerve transection and subsequent regeneration. J Neurocytol. 1989;18:695–710.

68. Franklin RJ, Kotter MR. The biology of CNS remyelination: the key to therapeutic advances. J Neurol. 2008;255(Suppl 1):19–25.

69. Bieber AJ, Kerr S, Rodriguez M. Efficient central nervous system remyelination requires T cells. Ann Neurol. 2003;53:680–4.

70. Begolka WS, Haynes LM, Olson JK, Padilla J, Neville KL, Dal Canto M, Palma J, Kim BS, Miller SD. CD8-deficient SJL mice display enhanced susceptibility to Theiler's virus infection and increased demyelinating pathology. J Neuro-Oncol. 2001;7:409–20.

71. Bombeiro AL, Santini JC, Thome R, Ferreira ER, Nunes SL, Moreira BM, Bonet IJ, Sartori CR, Verinaud L, Oliveira AL. Enhanced immune response in immunodeficient mice improves peripheral nerve regeneration following axotomy. Front Cell Neurosci. 2016;10:151.

72. Gurney ME, Pu H, Chiu AY, Dal Canto MC, Polchow CY, Alexander DD, Caliendo J, Hentati A, Kwon YW, Deng HX, et al. Motor neuron degeneration in mice that express a human cu,Zn superoxide dismutase mutation. Science. 1994;264:1772–5.

73. Wong PC, Pardo CA, Borchelt DR, Lee MK, Copeland NG, Jenkins NA, Sisodia SS, Cleveland DW, Price DL. An adverse property of a familial ALS-linked SOD1 mutation causes motor neuron disease characterized by vacuolar degeneration of mitochondria. Neuron. 1995;14:1105–16.

74. Beers DR, Zhao W, Liao B, Kano O, Wang J, Huang A, Appel SH, Henkel JS. Neuroinflammation modulates distinct regional and temporal clinical responses in ALS mice. Brain Behav Immun. 2011;25:1025–35.

75. Capitanio D, Vasso M, Ratti A, Grignaschi G, Volta M, Moriggi M, Daleno C, Bendotti C, Silani V, Gelfi C. Molecular signatures of amyotrophic lateral sclerosis disease progression in hind and forelimb muscles of an SOD1(G93A) mouse model. Antioxid Redox Signal. 2012;17:1333–50.

76. Rosser BW, Norris BJ, Nemeth PM. Metabolic capacity of individual muscle fibers from different anatomic locations. J Histochem Cytochem. 1992;40:819–25.

77. Komine O, Yamashita H, Fujimori-Tonou N, Koike M, Jin S, Moriwaki Y, Endo F, Watanabe S, Uematsu S, Akira S, et al. Innate immune adaptor TRIF deficiency accelerates disease progression of ALS mice with accumulation of aberrantly activated astrocytes. Cell Death Differ. 2018; [Epub ahead of print]

6

Identification and therapeutic modulation of a pro-inflammatory subset of disease-associated-microglia in Alzheimer's disease

Srikant Rangaraju[1*†] (iD), Eric B. Dammer[2†], Syed Ali Raza[1], Priyadharshini Rathakrishnan[3], Hailian Xiao[1], Tianwen Gao[1], Duc M. Duong[2], Michael W. Pennington[4], James J. Lah[1], Nicholas T. Seyfried[1] and Allan I. Levey[1]

Abstract

Background: Disease-associated-microglia (DAM) represent transcriptionally-distinct and neurodegeneration-specific microglial profiles with unclear significance in Alzheimer's disease (AD). An understanding of heterogeneity within DAM and their key regulators may guide pre-clinical experimentation and drug discovery.

Methods: Weighted co-expression network analysis (WGCNA) was applied to existing microglial transcriptomic datasets from neuroinflammatory and neurodegenerative disease mouse models to identify modules of highly co-expressed genes. These modules were contrasted with known signatures of homeostatic microglia and DAM to reveal novel molecular heterogeneity within DAM. Flow cytometric validation studies were performed to confirm existence of distinct DAM sub-populations in AD mouse models predicted by WGCNA. Gene ontology analyses coupled with bioinformatics approaches revealed drug targets and transcriptional regulators of microglial modules predicted to favorably modulate neuroinflammation in AD. These guided in-vivo and in-vitro studies in mouse models of neuroinflammation and neurodegeneration (5xFAD) to determine whether inhibition of pro-inflammatory gene expression and promotion of amyloid clearance was feasible. We determined the human relevance of these findings by integrating our results with AD genome-wide association studies and human AD and non-disease post-mortem brain proteomes.

Results: WGCNA applied to microglial gene expression data revealed a transcriptomic framework of microglial activation that predicted distinct pro-inflammatory and anti-inflammatory phenotypes within DAM, which we confirmed in AD and aging models by flow cytometry. Pro-inflammatory DAM emerged earlier in mouse models of AD and were characterized by pro-inflammatory genes (Tlr2, Ptgs2, Il12b, Il1b), surface marker CD44, potassium channel Kv1.3 and regulators (NFkb, Stat1, RelA) while anti-inflammatory DAM expressed phagocytic genes (Igf1, Apoe, Myo1e), surface marker CXCR4 with distinct regulators (LXRα/β, Atf1). As neuro-immunomodulatory strategies, we validated LXRα/β agonism and Kv1.3 blockade by ShK-223 peptide that promoted anti-inflammatory DAM, inhibited pro-inflammatory DAM and augmented Aβ clearance in AD models. Human AD-risk genes were highly represented within homeostatic microglia suggesting causal roles for early microglial dysregulation in AD. Pro-inflammatory DAM proteins were positively associated with neuropathology and preceded cognitive decline confirming the therapeutic relevance of inhibiting pro-inflammatory DAM in AD.

Conclusions: We provide a predictive transcriptomic framework of microglial activation in neurodegeneration that can guide pre-clinical studies to characterize and therapeutically modulate neuroinflammation in AD.

Keywords: Microglia, Macrophage, Alzheimer's disease, Network analysis, Kv1.3, Potassium channel, Amyloid, Neuroinflammation

* Correspondence: Srikant.rangaraju@emory.edu
†Equal contributors
[1]Department of Neurology, Emory University, Atlanta, GA 30322, USA
Full list of author information is available at the end of the article

Background

Microglia represent innate immune cells of the CNS that play important disease-modifying roles in neurodegeneration including Alzheimer's disease (AD) [1–4]. The importance of microglia-mediated neuroinflammation in neurodegeneration has been confirmed by genetic studies that identified several immune gene polymorphisms as risk factors for AD [5–8]. Data from mouse models have suggested dual roles for microglia in AD: pro-inflammatory functions that promote neurotoxicity and amyloid β (Aβ) accumulation, opposed by amyloid-clearing and neuroprotective functions [3, 4]. Recent transcriptomics studies have shown that homeostatic microglia gradually adopt a unique phagocytic disease-associated microglia (DAM) phenotype in neurodegenerative disease, chronic neuroinflammatory states as well as advanced aging [9–12]. While single-cell transcriptomic studies have not clarified molecular or functional heterogeneity within DAM [9], meta-analyses and network-based approaches applied to deeper bulk microglial transcriptomes have indicated greater diversity within microglia in neurodegeneration [10, 13]. Based on analysis of microglial transcriptomic data, the transcriptional signature of "primed" microglia from neurodegenerative disease brains is suggestive of increased phago-lysosome, oxidative phosphorylation and antigen-presentation functions [12, 13]. Trem2, a myeloid protein involved in microglial survival and proliferation, regulates a checkpoint necessary for DAM and deletion of Trem2 prevents microglial accumulation around Aβ plaques and leads to additional neuritic damage [6, 14–17]. These findings suggest that DAM may be protectively geared towards more effective phagocytosis and clearance of pathological protein aggregates in neurodegenerative disorders. However, global microglial depletion in AD mouse models resulted in a protective effect on synaptic health, independent of amyloid β [18, 19]. These emphasize the immense complexity of microglial functional roles in neurodegeneration [20], and support the existence of distinct pro-inflammatory functional states within DAM. A recent network analysis of bulk transcriptomes identified distinct microglial co-expression networks (or modules) which when applied to re-analyze microglial single-cell RNAseq data [9, 10] identified novel interferon-related and lipopolysaccharide (LPS)-related co-expression modules and previously unappreciated microglial sub-populations, in addition to DAM in neurodegeneration models [10]. This highlights the value of integrating deeper bulk transcriptomic findings with single cell data to maximize the chances of identifying cellular heterogeneity within a cell population.

A comprehensive understanding of key regulators, markers and drug targets of homeostatic, pro-inflammatory and anti-inflammatory microglial subtypes could provide novel biological insights and facilitate target nomination and prioritization of immunomodulatory therapeutic approaches in AD [21, 22]. In this study, we applied weighted correlation network analysis (WGCNA) to existing transcriptomic microarray datasets obtained from purified CD11b[+] CNS immune cells spanning neuroinflammatory and neurodegenerative disease states [15, 22, 23] to first identify distinct modules of co-expressed microglial genes that are associated with AD pathology. We then mapped these AD-specific gene modules to existing microglial single-cell RNAseq data to determine whether WGCNA modules represented distinct microglial populations and to further identify molecular heterogeneity within DAM [9]. Gene member and ontological analyses of modules coupled with bioinformatics approaches (connectivity map analysis) revealed specific drug targets and transcriptional regulators of AD-specific microglial modules (LXRα/β for anti-inflammatory DAM and Kv1.3 for pro-inflammatory DAM) as well as flow cytometric markers for each DAM subtype. Flow cytometric studies informed by WGCNA results confirmed distinct pro-inflammatory and anti-inflammatory subpopulations and suggested additional heterogeneity within DAM in aging and the 5xFAD model of AD pathology [24]. In-vivo pharmacologic studies using LXRα/β agonists and Kv1.3 channel inhibitors were then performed to determine whether modulation of pro- and anti-inflammatory DAM gene expression, proportions of DAM subsets and Aβ plaque pathology in 5xFAD mice could be achieved. Finally, we determined the relevance of homeostatic and DAM modules in human AD by integrating our findings with existing AD genome-wide associated studies (GWAS) as well as a human post-mortem brain proteomes from AD and non-disease controls.

Methods

Reagents

ShK-223 peptide was synthesized and folded as previously described [25]. The IC_{50} of ShK-223 for Kv1.3 channels is 25 ± 14 pM, > 10,000 times more selective for Kv1.3 channels as compared to neuronal Kv1.1 and Kv1.2 channels [25]. ShK-223 used for in-vitro at 100 nM concentration and 100 µg/kg for in-vivo (IP) injections in mice [26]. A validated fluorescein-conjugated ShK analog (ShK-F6CA) was used to detect functional cell surface Kv1.3 channels in microglia (Peptides International (Louisville, Kentucky) [26, 27]. LPS was obtained from Sigma Aldrich (Cat. #L4391, *Escherichia coli* 0111:B4). LXRα/β agonist T0901317 was obtained from Cayman Chemicals (Cat# 71810) and dissolved in DMSO and was diluted in saline prior to administration.

Flow cytometric and immunohistochemistry antibodies

Monoclonal fluorophore-conjugated antibodies used for flow cytometry were obtained from BD Biosciences (CD11b-APC-Cy7, CD45-PeCy7, CD11c-BV421, CD274-

APC, CD69-APC, CD44-PeCy7 or FITC, CD184-PE, CD3e-FITC, Ly-6c-PE, Ly-6G-APC) and BioLegend (CD8a-BV785, CD45-PerCP, and ENPP1-BV421). For immunohistochemistry, rabbit anti-Iba1 monoclonal antibody (Abcam # ab178846) was used at 1: 500 dilution. Rat anti-mouse LAMP1 monoclonal Ab was obtained from the Hybridoma Bank (Cat # 1D4B) and used at 1: 250 dilution. Mouse anti-CD68 monoclonal Ab (Abcam # ab955) was used at 1: 200 dilution. To identify amyloid plaques, anti-Aβ monoclonal 4G8 (Aβ 17–42) antibody (Signet Cat # 9220–02) was used at 1: 1000 dilution. Secondary anti-mouse, anti-goat and anti-rabbit antibodies (Jackson labs and Sigma-Aldrich) were used for immunohistochemistry. In immunofluorescence studies, Rhodamine-conjugated donkey anti-rat IgG (1: 500), Alexa-488-conjugated goat anti-rabbit (1: 500), and DyLight 405-conjugated donkey anti-mouse (1: 500) were used as secondary antibodies. Fluorescent-labeled Aβ$_{42}$ fibrils for immunofluorescence studies were prepared as described below and FITC filter was used to observe Aβ fluorescence.

Primary microglial isolation

Adult C57BL6 mice, age-matched female 5xFAD mice were euthanized and brains were isolated following rapid cold saline cardiac perfusion and CNS immune cells were isolated as previously described [26, 28]. Briefly, brains were minced over a 40 µm cell strainer and single cell suspensions were washed in PBS in a centrifuge for 5 min at 800×g at room temperature. Supernatants were discarded and cell pellets re-suspended in 6 mL of 37% stock isotonic Percoll (SIP) solution (90% Percoll + 10% 10X HBSS) per brain. The cell suspension was transferred into 15 mL conical tubes and 2 mL of 70% SIP slowly under laid. Then on top of the 37% layer, 2 mL of 30% SIP was slowly layered. The established gradient was then centrifuged for 25 min at 800×g with zero deceleration at 20 °C. Floating myelin in the top layer was then removed and a Pasteur pipette used to carefully collect 3 mL from the 70–37% interphase without disturbing the 70% layer. Cells were then washed × 3 in 10 mL cold PBS and the pellets comprising of CNS immune cells were then re-suspended in 100 µL of the appropriate buffer.

Microglial Aβ42 phagocytosis assay

The ability of acutely isolated CNS mononuclear cells from wild type, LPS-treated and age-matched 5xFAD mice to phagocytose fluorescent-labeled Aβ fibrils ex-vivo was assessed by a flow cytometric assay. Fluorescent-labeled Aβ42 fibrils were prepared by co-incubating unlabeled and Hilyte488-labeled Aβ42 required unlabeled Aβ42 (Anaspec Cat # AS-60479-01) at a 1:4 ratio. Purified Aβ42 was first linearized in 10% w/v NH$_4$OH and re-lyophilized

to reduce any preexisting aggregates. 0.5 mg of unlabeled lyophilized Aβ42 was then reconstituted to 150 µM by adding 1 mM NaOH, bath sonicated for 10 min followed by addition of 10X buffer (100 mM sodium phosphate, pH 7.1) to bring the final pH to 7.4. 410.64 µL of that aliquot was added to 0.1 mg of HiLyte-488 Aβ42 to achieve a total of 200 µM Aβ42 solution. The sample was incubated in dark at room temperature for 5–7 days before being transferred to 4 °C. Phagocytosis of fluorescent-labeled Aβ42 fibrils (fAβ42-HiLyte488) was performed by incubating acutely isolated CNS immune cells (pretreated ex-vivo with ShK-223 at 100 nM or vehicle) with the reagent at 2.5 µM for 30 min at 37 °C in a 5% CO$_2$ humidified incubator. The cells were then washed with cold PBS and labeled with fluorophore-conjugated CD11b (CD11b-APC-Cy7, BD Biosciences Cat # 557657) and CD45 (CD45-PerCP, BioLegend Cat # 103130) for 30 min at 4 °C. This was followed by washing with cold flow cytometry buffer prior to flow cytometry [29, 30]. Compensation experiments were performed prior to performing the phagocytosis assay using compensation beads. Before sample data acquisition, unstained sample was run (without fAβ42-HiLyte488) and then positive control was run at low speed to allow for voltage level adjustment considering the high intensity of Aβ42 fluorescence in Alexa-488 channel. For phagocytosis assay using flow cytometry, CNS immune cells were first gated for live cells using FSC/SSC gating followed by gating for singlets using FSC-A/FSC-H. Following selection of singlets, CD11b and CD45 gating was used to identify CD11b$^+$, CD11b$^+$CD45^{low} and CD11b$^+$CD45^{high} populations after which phagocytosis was assessed in each group using the second peak of Aβ fluorescence as recently described [31]. We have found that Cytochalasin D inhibits the second peak of fluorescence in this assay, suggesting that the first peak represent nonspecific binding of Aβ42 to cells while the second peak represents true uptake in an actin-dependent manner [31].

Animals

Female C57BL/6 J and female 5xFAD mice used for the studies were housed in the Department of Animal Resources at Emory University under standard conditions with no special food/water accommodations. Institutional Animal Care and Use Committee approval was obtained prior to in-vivo work and all work was performed in strict accordance with the Guide for the Care and Use of Laboratory Animals of the National Institutes of Health. Adult mice were given intraperitoneal LPS injections (10 µg/dose × 4 daily doses) to induce acute neuroinflammation [26, 32]. If ≥25% of weight loss was observed, animals were euthanized. In some experiments, 5xFAD mice received i.p. doses of T0901317 (30 mg/kg) twice a week for 2 weeks.

GEO datasets, microarray normalization, and batch correction

Microarray transcriptomic datasets were obtained from the genomics data repository Gene Expression Omnibus (GEO). Microarray transcriptome datasets of FACS-purified microglia from 8.5 mo old WT ($n = 5$), TREM2 $-/-$ ($n = 4$), 5xFAD (n = 5) and TREM2 $^{-/-}$/5xFAD ($n = 6$) mice were obtained from GEO (GSE65067). GEO dataset GSE49329 provided microarray data from murine microglia treated in-vitro with PBS (control), LPS or IL4 ($n = 9$ arrays). These two disparate Affymetrix platform datasets were RMA normalized using the affy package RMA function, combined, and corrected for batchwise artefacts using WT and PBS-treated microglia as comparable control features and other samples as experimental features across the 2 batches specified as such to the ComBat algorithm loaded from the R SVA package. Unique batch-corrected array features representing gene-level expression were then selected using a filter to retain features with maximum variance across the 29 samples using the WGCNA collapseRows function. Notably, the array annotations for mogene 1.0 database package were downloaded as of September 2015, and this package version is provided to make results, in particular the intersection of common genes across the arrays, reproducible. Existing RNAseq microglial transcriptomes were not included due to lower depth of coverage and inability to sufficiently overcome batch effects when combining microarray and RNAseq transcriptomes.

Agilent microarray data from microglia isolated from WT and APP/PS1 mice ($n = 7$ each) were obtained as a subset of the samples in GEO dataset GSE74615. Agilent green (Cy3) and red (Cy5) channels were background corrected according to the normexp method in limma::backgroundCorrect() function, [33] then quantile-normalized. Genes expressed on average at greater than 400% of the 95th percentile intensity of negative control probes were considered as expressed. $Log_2(Cy5/Cy3)$ signals were calculated and a histogram calculation of shift from 0 was used to center the Gaussian of intensities across the 2 channels. Then WGCNA::collapseRows was applied as above, and astrocyte-specific measurements ($n = 8/22$) were removed. 16,721 gene symbols shared between the expressed genes measured on Affymetrix and Agilent platforms were found and the corrected, normalized, log2-transformed expression values for each platform were combined into a single matrix and subjected to a second pass of SVA::comBat(). The batch-corrected, adjusted datasets were then used for WGCNA. R code is provided online, via synapse.org (https://www.synapse.org/#!Synapse:syn10934660).

In a separate replication analysis, transcript count data from 64 purified microglial medium-throughput sequencing (Nanostring) studies (GEO dataset GSE101689) were obtained from supplemental data [16] which were log2-transformed (0 counts set to 0.5) and batch-corrected using ComBat and assumption of common samples across batches represented by WT or PBS/sham treated mice, considering EAE, LPS, APP/PS1 and SOD datasets as separate batches. Three hundred and sixty-nine genes that were identified across all datasets without any missing data were used for WGCNA as described below. Effectiveness of batch correction was confirmed by comparing the consistency of geometric mean of batch-corrected counts for the 6 pre-determined housekeeping genes in different Nanostring nCounter assays.

WGCNA

The R package WGCNA was used to construct a co-expression network using normalized and batch-corrected data of the 43 microarray-measured samples just described using a previously published approach [34]. A threshold power of 10 was chosen since it was the smallest threshold that resulted in a scale-free R^2 fit of 0.8. The network was created using WGCNA::blockwiseModules() function, in a single block (maxBlockSize > 16,721). Briefly, this function calculated topologic overlap (TO) with bicor correlation function, then genes were hierarchically clustered using 1-TO (dissTOM) as the distance measure. Initial module assignments were determined by using dynamic tree-cutting, using default parameters except deepSplit = 2, mergeCutHeight =0.20, minModulesize = 40, pamStage = TRUE, and pamRespectsDendro = TRUE), but genes were allowed to be reassigned to modules with better correlation if $p < 0.05$ for those correlations. The network type was signed, so that anticorrelated genes were not assigned to the same module. Resulting 19 modules or groups of co-expressed genes ranging in size from 2165 genes (turquoise) to 75 genes (lightyellow) were used to calculate the eigengenes (MEs; or the 1st principal component of the module). MEs were correlated with different biological traits including AD (model), LPS-treated and IL4-treated. R code is provided online via synapse.org (https://www.synapse.org/#!Synapse:syn10934660).

In the validation WGCNA, scale free topology was achieved with beta (power) set at 11.5, and other blockwiseModules() function parameters were deepSplit = 4, minModulesize = 3, mergeCutHeight = 0.12, pamStage = TRUE, pamRespectsDentro = TRUE, reassignThresh = 0.05. Over-representation analysis (ORA) was performed with in an house custom script testing for hypergeometric overlap of gene symbol membership in modules across the derivation and nanostring (validation) networks using the fisher.test() function, with one-tailed sensitivity for overrepresentation of module membership, i.e. using alternative = "greater" parameter.

viSNE plots

WGCNA network gene-level k_{ME} values (gene expression correlation to the module eigengene for the module to which each gene belonged) were used to cull the measured gene list to genes with $k_{ME} > 0.65$ and membership in any of 8 modules of particular interest. Then, normalized, corrected array log2 expression data was row-normalized to set the sample average (row mean) for each gene to zero. Rtsne R package Rtsne Barnes-Hut-Stochastic Neighbor Embedding (SNE) function was then applied to the culled 43-dimension data matrix of genes, reducing it to a 2-dimensional projection for each gene [35] vi-SNE output points representing genes were then colored by the WGCNA module membership of each gene. In another version of the projection, membership of the DAM-microglial genes and Homeostatic microglial genes were also mapped onto the identical vi-SNE projection points. DAM and Homeostatic genes were defined based on published single cell RNAseq data. DAM-specific genes were defined as ≥4-fold higher expression in DAM cells while Homeostatic genes were defined as ≥4-fold higher expression in Homeostatic microglia as compared to DAM cells [9]. R code is provided online via synapse.org (https://www.synapse.org/#!Synapse:syn10934660).

MAGMA GWAS target module over-representation analysis

MAGMA for AD IGAP GWAS targets ($N = 50,000$ patients) and subsequent over-representation analysis for module membership of GWAS target-genes using stat-mod function permutation was performed as previously published [34]. MAGMA script output for gene-wise p-values for AD and other conditions for which GWAS SNPs have been reported selected from the UCSC Genome Browser GWAS track are provided with the R code online at synapse.org (https://www.synapse.org/#!Synapse:syn10934660).

In-vitro assays of fAβ42 degradation and reactive oxygen species production by microglia

Bv2 microglia were maintained in Dulbecco's modified Eagle Medium (with 10% FBS). For in-vitro experiments, Bv2 cells were grown on glass cover slips, loaded with fluorescent Aβ42 fibrils and cultured up to 72 h. At different time points 0.5, 6, 16, 24, 48 and 72 h, the BV2 microglia were fixed for 15 min, washed gently with PBS, permeabilized and mounted in Vectashield hard set mounting medium containing DAPI followed by image acquisition. In separate experiments, Bv2 microglia were first loaded with fluorescent Aβ42 for 1 h, washed × 3, and incubated with 100 nM of ShK-223 and then maintained in culture for 0.5, 6, 16, 24, 48 and 72 h. At each time point, cells were fixed, washed, permeabilized with 1X Permeabilization buffer (eBioscience Cat # 00–8333-

56) and then washed with PBS. This was followed by incubation with blocking buffer (10% normal horse serum in PBS) for 30 min and incubation with rat anti-mouse LAMP1 monoclonal antibody and then the appropriate fluorophore-conjugated secondary antibody. This was then followed by image acquisition for co-localization analyses. Co-localization analysis was performed using the co-localization threshold plugin in ImageJ (Fiji image analysis software Version 1.51n). Green and Red channel images at each time point were converted to gray-scale in FIJI, and co-localization threshold plugin was applied to the region of interest that was limited to one cell at a time.

Immunofluorescence microscopy

Double antigen immunofluorescence for Aβ and Iba1 in slides from ShK-223 and PBS treated mice involved antigen retrieval with 45% formic acid for 5 min followed by heating in microwave for 10 min in 10 mM citric acid (pH 6.0) solution. This was followed by similar blocking steps as outlined above and then overnight incubation in anti-Aβ (4G8) and anti-Iba1 primary antibodies. DyLight 405-conjugated donkey anti-mouse IgG (1: 500) and Alexa-Fluor488-conjugated goat anti-rabbit IgG (1: 500) were used as secondary antibodies. Single antibody controls for each channel were used to optimize settings. Fluorescent images were obtained with a fluorescence microscope (Microscope: Olympus BX51 and Camera: Olympus DP70) using FITC, PE and DAPI filters and the images were processed for further analyses. Immunofluorescence microscopy was also performed for assessment of LAMP-1 and fAβ42 co-localization in mature phago-lysosomes in BV2 microglia. LAMP1 was labeled with rat anti-mouse LAMP1 monoclonal primary antibody followed by anti-rat Rhodamine-conjugated IgG (1: 500). The Bv2 cells on coverslips from each time point after being immunostained were mounted in Vectashield hard set mounting medium containing DAPI and at least 10 images per condition, each in triplicate (acquired at 40× magnification), were collected.

Flow cytometric studies

Freshly isolated CNS immune cells were labeled for CD11b, CD45, CD11c, CD44, CD184 (CXCR4), CD69 and CD274 using well characterized fluorophore-conjugated monoclonal antibodies. Kv1.3 channels expression on cell surface was assessed using fluorescein-conjugated ShK analog as stated above. Compensation experiments were run using compensation beads prior to sample data acquisition using previously published protocols [26]. FSC/SSC gating was used to establish live cell population followed by FSC-A/FSC-H gating to gate for single cells. CD11b and CD45 were then used to identify and gate for CD11b⁺CD45^{low} and CD11b⁺CD45^{high} populations with the criterion for level of CD45^{high} set on the basis of CD45 expression in CD11b-CD3 + CD45^{high} lymphocyte population. CD11b$^+$CD45^{low} and CD11b$^+$CD45^{high} gating strategy was also employed for the ex-vivo phagocytosis assay. In separate experiments, CNS immune cells and splenocytes were also labeled for Ly6c and Ly6G using fluorophore-conjugated antibodies.

Immunohistochemistry

For all these studies, three sagittal brain sections (one from each treatment group and from WT mice) from equivalent regions were placed on each slide to control for any heterogeneity in staining. Paraffin embedded sections of brains obtained from mice from the ShK-223 treatment trial were de-paraffinized in Histoclear and rehydrated, incubated in 90% formic acid for 10 min, washed in buffer, blocked with 3% hydrogen peroxide and 10 μg/ml of Avidin for 30 min and then blocked in 10% normal horse serum prepared in Tris-buffered saline (TBS) for 30 min followed by overnight incubation with primary anti-Aβ42 (4G8) antibody. Sections were rinsed in TBS and then incubated in the appropriate biotin-conjugated secondary antibody before incubation for an hour in Vectastain Elite ABC in accordance with manufacturer's instructions. This was followed by diaminobenzidine as per instructions by manufacturer. Counterstaining of slides was achieved with hematoxylin. Microscopy was performed with an Olympus Light microscope (Olympus, Center Valley, PA).

Long-term ShK-223 treatment trial

Adult female 5xFAD mice aged 3 mo were treated intraperitoneally twice a week until 6 mo of age with PBS or ShK-223 (dose 100 μg/kg), $n = 10$ each and also age-matched 5 female C57BL/6 mice were included in the study. At 6 mo, neurobehavioral testing including Fear conditioning and Morris Water Maze was performed. The mice were euthanized, brains isolated and the brains were utilized for immunohistochemistry studies.

Transient transfection of HEK293 cells

HEK293 cells were maintained in DMEM with 10% FBS. Transient transfections with either pRC/CMV vector or pRC/CMV-mKv1.3 (a kind gift from Dr. Heike Wulff, UC Davis) or sham were performed for 24 h using 1 μg of plasmid DNA per well. Experiments were performed in biological triplicates.

Aβ quantitation in paraffin-embedded mouse brains

Images from slides labeled for Aβ42 from the 6 mo 5xFAD mice following their 3 mo intraperitoneal treatment with PBS or ShK-223 were used for ImageJ analysis to determine Aβ42 plaque load and size. The images of the hippocampal region, cortex and diencephalon underwent background

subtraction, then color deconvolution based on hematoxylin/DAB stains and then conversion to binary images, followed by a blinded measurement of Aβ density per region of interest using ImageJ. Plaque size as square pixels was also measured using a defined minimum threshold of 200 square pixels which excluded Aβ labeling outside of plaques.

Reverse transcriptase quantitative PCR

CNS immune cells isolated from age-matched C57BL6 mice treated with four once daily intraperitoneal doses of sterile PBS, ShK-223 (100 μg/kg), LPS (20 μg/dose) or co-administered LPS + ShK-223 ($n = 3$/group) were washed in PBS containing RNAase inhibitors and used for RT-qPCR using our published protocols [26]. For total RNA extraction from cells, 1 mL Trizol was added to the cells, the pellets were homogenized in the Trizol by repetitive pipetting and incubated for at least 1 h at room temperature. Then, 0.2 mL of chloroform per 1 mL of Trizol was added and incubated for 2–3 min followed by centrifugation at 12000 x g for 15 min at 4 °C to obtain an upper colorless aqueous phase, an interphase and a lower red phenol chloroform phase. RNA in the aqueous phase was transferred to other tubes. 0.5 mL of 100% iso-propranolol was added to the aqueous phase per 1 mL of Trizol used and the mixture was incubated for 10 min and centrifuged at 12000 x g for 10 min at 4 °C. The pellet was washed with 1 mL of 75% ethanol per 1 mL of Trizol used (initial homogenization) and the RNA pellet was air dried and reconstituted in RNase-free water followed by incubation in a heat block set at 55–60 °C for 10–15 min. RNA concentrations were then determined via Nanodrop. RNA was reverse transcribed to cDNA using a high capacity cDNA reverse transcription kit (Ambion). Real time PCR was performed on a 7500 Fast RT-PCR instrument (Applied Biosystems) using cDNA, TaqMan PCR Master Mix (Applied Biosystems), and gene-specific TaqMan probes (Applied Biosystems) against Kcnj2 (Mm00434616_m1), Nceh1 (Mm00626772_m1), Timp2 (Mm00441825_m1), Il1B (Mm00434228_m1), Ptgs2 (Mm00478374_m1), Tmem119 (Mm00525305_m1), and Hprt (Mm03024075_m1) which was used as the 'housekeeping gene.' For each RNA sample, each primer set was run in triplicate. Gene expression was normalized to the internal control HPRT for primary microglia and relative expression calculated for each gene using the $2\Delta\Delta C_T$ method after normalizing to the control [36].

Identification of transcriptional regulators and connectivity map analysis for potential perturbagens

Connectivity map is an online library of cellular signatures from various human cell types that catalogs transcriptional responses to chemical, genetic, and disease perturbation (perturbagens) which can be used to probe relationships between diseases, cell physiology, and therapeutics (https://clue.io/about#cmap) [37]. We used this approach to identify perturbagens likely to result in a desired transcriptional profile. The perturbagens most likely to reproduce the desired transcriptional effect are identified using a summary score (range – 100 to + 100).

Human BLSA brain samples and fisher exact test analyses for module overlap

The patient and pathological characteristics of the 47 post-mortem BLSA samples used for proteomics and the methods for tandem-mass-tag quantitative proteomics, subsequent analyses and WGCNA are available online (https://www.synapse.org/#!Synapse:syn11209141) and will be published subsequently. WGCNA identified 50 protein in this study and the correlations between module expression and neuropathological traits (BRAAK and CERAD) were investigated. A hypergeometric two-tailed Fisher's exact test was used to determine significant overlap between the mouse microglial transcriptomic modules and BLSA proteome modules [34].

Other statistical considerations

Graphpad Prism (Ver. 5), Cytoscape (Ver. 3.5.1) and SPSS (Ver. 22) were used to create graphs and perform statistical analyses. All data are shown as mean ± SEM. For experiments with > 2 groups, one way ANOVA was performed to detect differences across groups and post-hoc pairwise comparisons were performed using Tukey's HSD test. Statistical significance was set at p value ≤0.05 for all experiments unless specified separately.

Results

Co-expression network analysis of microglial gene expression reveals a landscape of diverse and functionally distinct microglial activation states in AD mouse models

Data from 43 existing GEO microarray transcriptomes of CD11b$^+$ microglia including primary mouse microglia treated in-vitro with M1-like activating stimulus LPS (M1-like) or M2-like stimulus IL4, and from WT, TREM2$^{-/-}$, 5xFAD, TREM2$^{-/-}$/5xFAD and APP/PS1 mice were batch-corrected and normalized to adjust for differences in microarray platforms (Fig. 1a) [15, 22, 23]. WGCNA of normalized expression data (16,721 genes) identified 19 modules of highly co-expressed genes (Fig. 1b-c, Additional file 8: Figure S1, Additional file 1: Table S1) including modules significantly upregulated following in-vitro LPS or IL4 treatment, representing the M1-M2 paradigm of in-vitro activation (Fig. 1c). We also identified two modules that were upregulated (Magenta and Yellow) and one that was down-regulated (Blue) across AD models (Fig. 1c-d). Within these three AD modules, we observed enrichment of pro-inflammatory genes in the Magenta module (Ptgs2, Il12b, Tlr2, Hif1a, Cd69, Il1b, Cxcl16 and Irg1) and anti-

inflammatory and phagocytic genes in the Yellow module (Igf1, Dpp7, Apoe, Spp1, Cd200r4 and Lpl) [38] while the Blue module contained several homeostatic microglial genes (Tmem119, P2ry12, Mtss1 and Tgfbr1, Fig. 2d) [39].

Gene ontology (GO) analyses of key module members (Additional file 8: Figure S2, Additional file 2: Table S2) revealed that the Blue module was enriched for cytoplasmic proteins governing homeostatic functions (macromolecule biosynthesis and cellular metabolic processes). The Yellow module was enriched for cytoplasmic proteins involved in carbohydrate and lipid metabolism, cholesterol efflux, antigen presentation, oxido-reductase activity and senescence/autophagy and in contrast, the Magenta module was enriched for pro-inflammatory functions including immune signaling, cell proliferation, adhesion, antigen presentation, calcium influx and cytokine production. Pathway analyses of key members of AD modules identified transcriptional regulators (Additional file 8: Figure S3, Additional file 3: Table S3) including RelA, Stat1, p53 and Nfkb1 for Magenta, Lxrα/β and Atf-1 for Yellow and Cebpα and Foxo3a for Blue modules. These observations agree with known anti-inflammatory and Aβ-clearing effects of LXRα/β agonists in AD models [40–42] as well as the role of Cebpα in regulating PU.1 which maintains microglial quiescence [43]. These patterns of module expression across various traits and their enriched ontologies and transcriptional regulators suggest that the Magenta module is an AD-associated pro-inflammatory module, the Yellow module is an AD-associated anti-inflammatory module/pro-phagocytic and the Blue module is a homeostatic microglial module while other M1/M2-like modules are not relevant to AD pathology.

We also applied a modification of t-distributed stochastic neighbor embedding (viSNE) to normalized expression data to represent all genes in 2 or 3 dimensional space allowing for better appreciation of gene and gene cluster inter-relatedness (Fig. 2a) [35]. By layering WGCNA modules onto viSNE results, we confirmed strong agreement between viSNE clusters and WGCNA modules and observed that both pro-inflammatory (Magenta) and anti-inflammatory (Yellow) modules are closely related but are very distinct from the homeostatic (Blue) module. By representing viSNE results in 3D (Additional file 8: Figure S4, Additional file 9), we observed that homeostatic microglia may reach AD-associated states (Magenta or Yellow modules) via at least 3 distinct pathways (Additional file 8: Figure S4, Additional file 9) including a pro-inflammatory pathway (lower band) comprising of LPS-upregulated modules, a second potentially anti-inflammatory pathway (middle band) containing LPS-downregulated/IL4-upregualted modules and a third possible pathway of microglial activation (upper band). These findings support the application of network-based

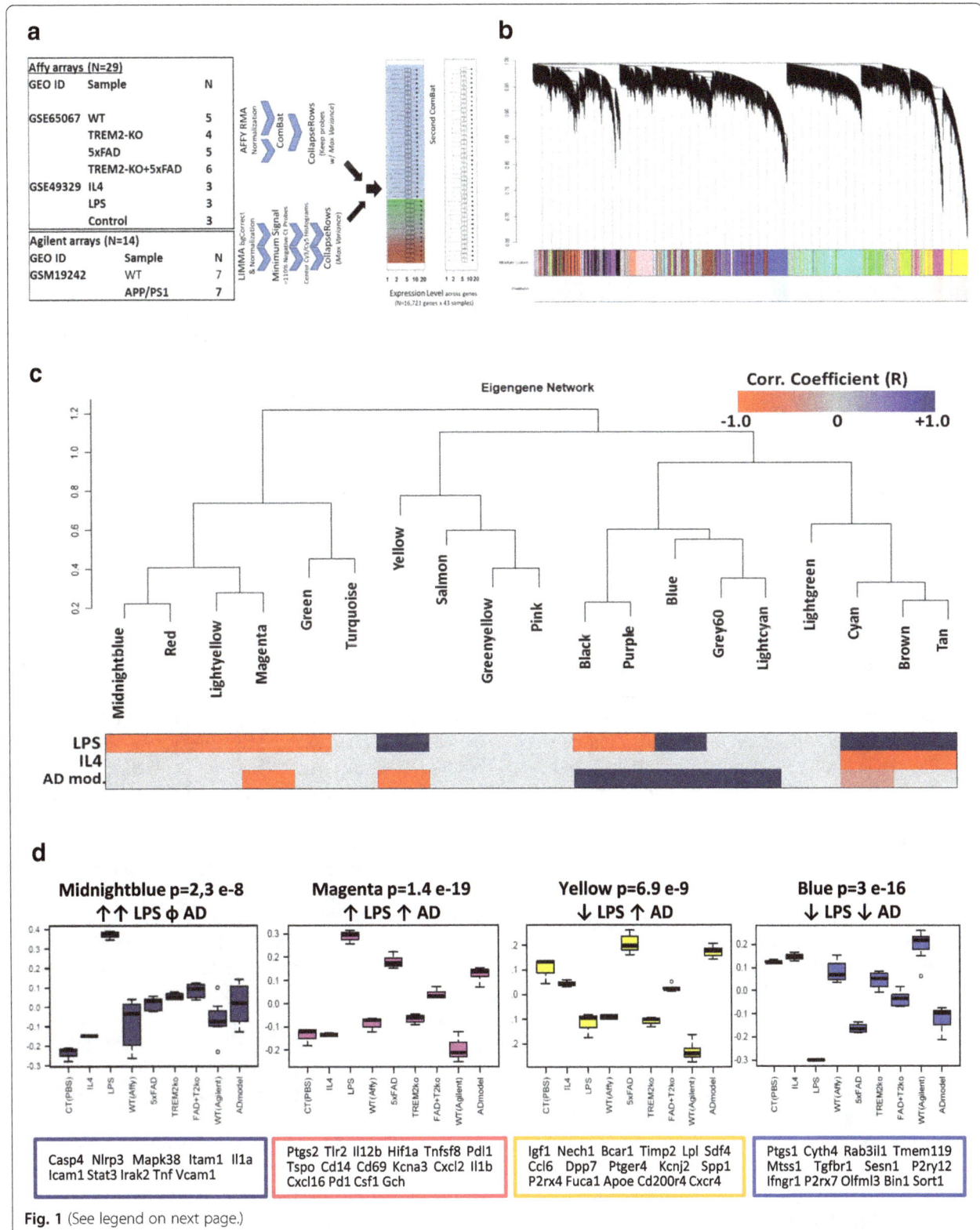

Fig. 1 (See legend on next page.)

(See figure on previous page.)
Fig. 1 WGCNA of mouse microglial transcriptome identifies co-expression modules with distinct AD pathology-associated inflammatory profiles. **a** Three transcriptomic microarray datasets containing 43 arrays derived from CD11b$^+$ mouse microglia were normalized, batch-corrected and used in a WGCNA meta-analysis. Datasets included microglia polarized in-vitro to M1-like (LPS) or M2-like (IL4) states, acutely isolated microglia from WT, 5xFAD, Trem2−/− and 5xFAD/Trem2−/− mice, and from WT and APP/PS1 transgenic mice. **b** WGCNA identified 19 distinct modules (networks) of highly co-expressed genes (See Additional file 1: Table S1). **c** Cluster dendrogram showing the 19 microglial modules and trait correlations with inflammatory status (LPS or IL4) and AD pathology (5xFAD or APP/PS1 vs. wild-type). **d** Comparison of expression of module eigengene for 4 modules of interest, across treatment conditions/traits (Hub gene members are shown in descending order of module membership or k_{ME})

analyses of population-level transcriptomic data to delineate distinct microglial phenotypes, providing a framework demonstrating relatedness and interconnectivity of microglial sub-profiles.

To determine the validity of our results, we performed an external validation of WGCNA using existing microglial transcriptomic studies (Nanostring, $n = 64$ samples, 369 common genes per sample) of purified microglia isolated from WT and aging mice (2 mo–17 mo) as well as from mouse models of neuroinflammation (LPS treatment, experimental autoimmune encephalomyelitis [EAE]) and neurodegeneration (APP/PS1 model of AD pathology and SOD1-G39A transgenic model of motor neuron disease) [16]. We obtained 19 modules in this analysis and an assessment of module overlap between derivation and validation network analyses using overrepresentation analysis (ORA) identified modules in the validation network that were equated to Blue, Magenta and Yellow modules identified in the derivation network (Fig. 3b). Specifically, validation modules M6 and M7 represented the derivation Blue module (common hub genes Cx3cr1, P2ry12, Sall1, Csf1r and Tmem119), validation module M3 represented the derivation Magenta module (common hub gene Tlr2 and Cxcl16) and validation module M4 represented the derivation Yellow module (common hub genes Apoe, Spp1, Axl). The discernment of these validation modules across various traits in an independent expression dataset were consistent with observations in the derivation study (Fig. 3c), confirming the overall validity and generalizability of our WGCNA findings.

Microglial modules upregulated in AD represent distinct pro-inflammatory and anti-inflammatory phenotypes within DAM

Differences in gene co-expression may indicate common upstream regulation, functional relatedness and/or restriction to same cell type or cellular compartment [34, 44]. We hypothesized that the three AD modules (Magenta, Yellow, Blue) represent transcriptomic signatures of distinct microglial sub-populations. Since single-cell RNAseq of microglia from AD mouse models has confirmed the presence of homeostatic and DAM populations [9], we

mapped known DAM and homeostatic signature genes to modules identified by WGCNA (Fig. 2b, Additional file 8: Figure S4) and found that DAM genes were highly represented in both pro-inflammatory (Magenta) and anti-inflammatory (Yellow) AD modules, whereas homeostatic genes mapped to Blue and Purple modules (Fig. 2b, Additional file 8: Figure S4, Additional file 10). These observations confirm that modules identified by WGCNA using cell population data, represent homeostatic and DAM sub-populations previously identified by single-cell RNAseq and that other non-AD modules also represent distinct microglial activation states. Remarkably, we resolved DAM into two related yet functionally divergent profiles of which the Magenta module represents a novel pro-inflammatory subset.

Since both DAM modules were closely related (Fig. 2b), we hypothesized that bottleneck genes present at the Yellow/Magenta inter-modular interface with dual module membership may exist. Accordingly, we identified 35 bottleneck genes (Additional file 8: Figure S5) which mapped to this interface and had strong membership ($k_{ME} \geq 0.75$) in both modules. Further characterization of these inter-modular bottlenecks could identify immune checkpoints that determine phenotypic switching between pro- and anti-inflammatory profiles. Trem2, a known immune checkpoint that regulates the transition of homeostatic microglia to DAM [9], had moderate-level membership (k_{ME} 0.45) to a module closely related to the anti-inflammatory Yellow module while the binding partner of Trem2, Tyrobp (Dap12), was a hub gene in the Yellow module [15, 17]. Since Trem2 regulates microglial survival, proliferation, effector functions [6, 15, 17] and a checkpoint in the origin of DAM in AD [9], we asked whether distinct DAM profiles emerge upstream or downstream of the Trem2 checkpoint. Our WGCNA results showed that Trem2 deletion in 5xFAD mice resulted in downregulation of both pro-inflammatory and anti-inflammatory DAM modules while upregulating the homeostatic module (Fig. 1d and Additional file 8: Figure S6) suggesting that both pro-inflammatory (Magenta) and anti-inflammatory (Yellow) modules co-emerge downstream of Trem2 but represent related yet functionally divergent pro- and anti-inflammatory profiles within DAM.

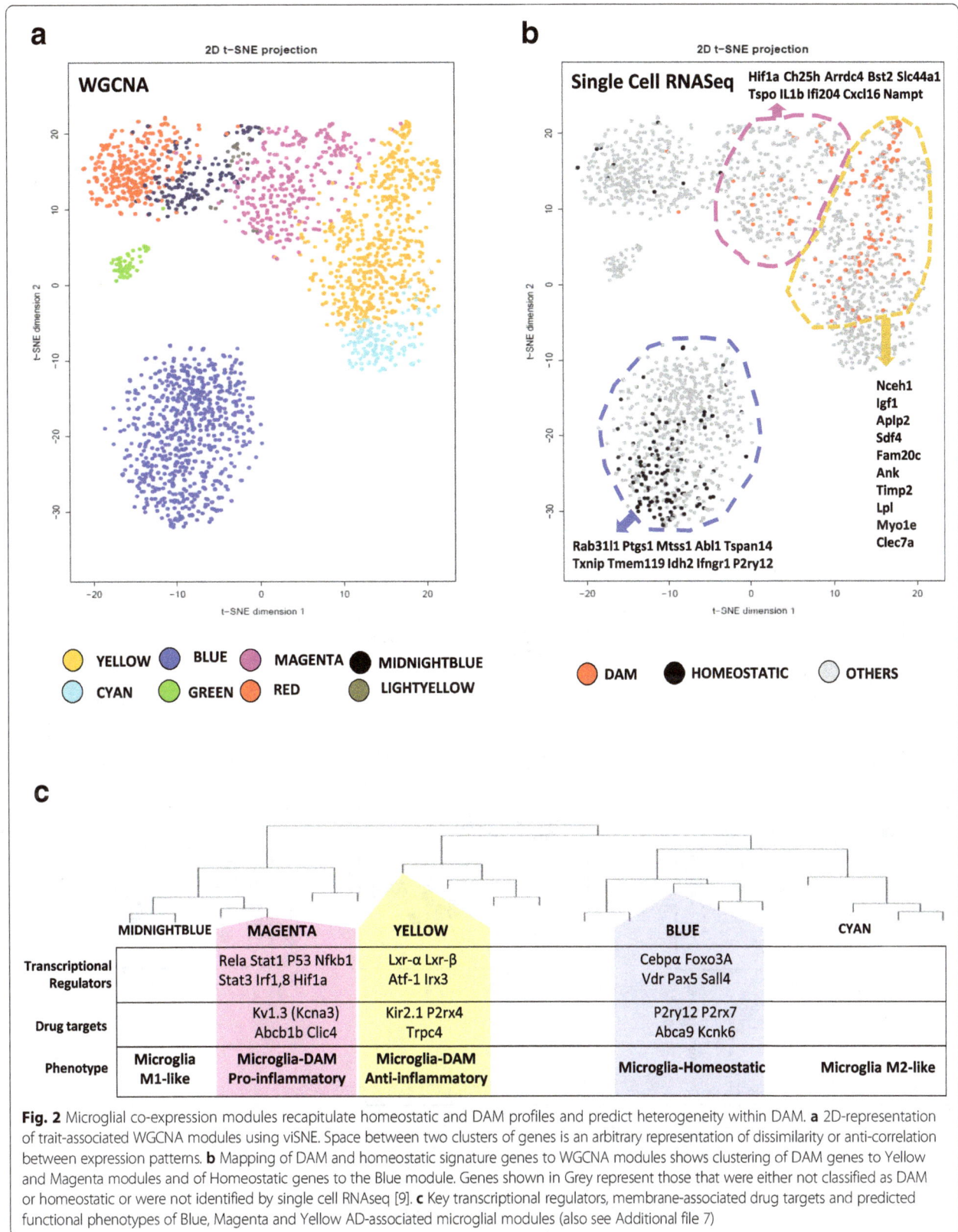

Fig. 2 Microglial co-expression modules recapitulate homeostatic and DAM profiles and predict heterogeneity within DAM. **a** 2D-representation of trait-associated WGCNA modules using viSNE. Space between two clusters of genes is an arbitrary representation of dissimilarity or anti-correlation between expression patterns. **b** Mapping of DAM and homeostatic signature genes to WGCNA modules shows clustering of DAM genes to Yellow and Magenta modules and of Homeostatic genes to the Blue module. Genes shown in Grey represent those that were either not classified as DAM or homeostatic or were not identified by single cell RNAseq [9]. **c** Key transcriptional regulators, membrane-associated drug targets and predicted functional phenotypes of Blue, Magenta and Yellow AD-associated microglial modules (also see Additional file 7)

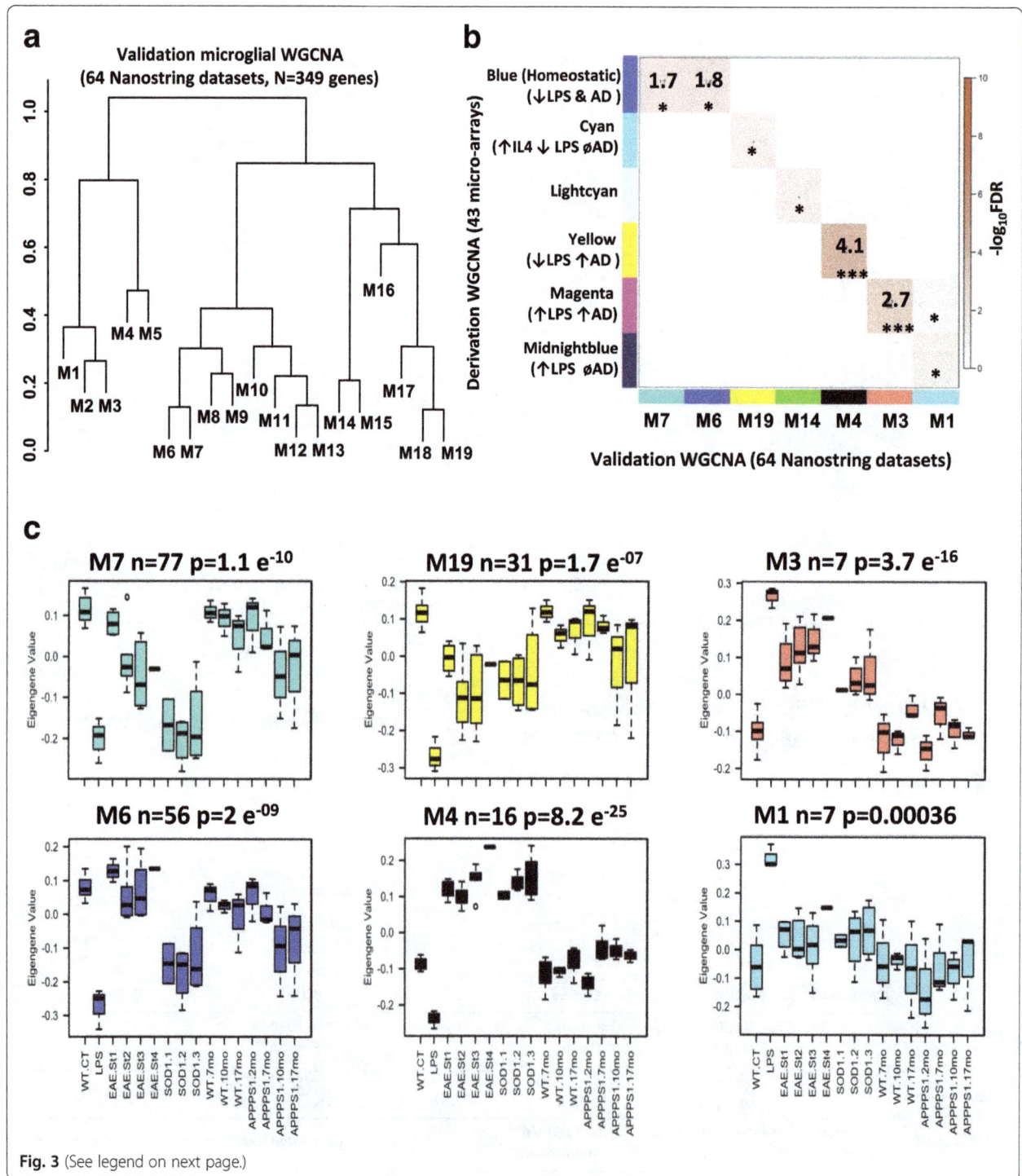

Fig. 3 (See legend on next page.)

Fig. 3 Replication co-expression analysis of microglial transcriptomic datasets across neuroinflammatory and neurodegenerative disease models. **a** Cluster dendrogram summarizing results of validation WGCNA performed using 64 existing Nanostring purified microglial transcriptomic datasets (369 genes in common across all conditions). Datasets included aging WT and APP/PS1 models (age range 2–17 mo, $n = 24$), WT and SOD1-G93A transgenic mice ($n = 13$), control and various stages of EAE in mice ($n = 21$) and WT and intra-cerebral LPS-treated WT mice ($n = 6$). Expression data were first batch-corrected followed by WGCNA to identify modules of highly co-expressed genes. **b** Module over-representation analysis (ORA) of derivation (43 microglial arrays, y-axis) and validation WGCNA (64 microglial Nanostring transcriptomic datasets, x-axis) studies. Module overlap was assessed by Fisher-exact test and the negative $\log_{10}$ transformed false discovery rate (FDR) for overlap is indicated by color intensity. Validation modules are numbered (M1–19) while derivation modules are indicated by the original color scheme. **c** Module eigengene expression and trajectories of change in module expression across various traits in the Nanostring co-expression dataset. Validation modules highlighted here were chosen based on strength of overlap from the over-representation analysis. M6 and M7 are representative of the Blue homeostatic derivation module. M4 is representative of the Yellow anti-inflammatory derivation module while M3 is representative of the Magenta pro-inflammatory derivation module. M1 is representative of LPS-induced Midnightblue derivation module while M19 is representative of the IL4-upregulated Cyan derivation module

Confirmation of pro-inflammatory and anti-inflammatory DAM profiles in AD mouse models

To confirm the presence of distinct pro-inflammatory and anti-inflammatory DAM subsets resolved by co-expression analyses, we performed flow cytometric studies of acutely isolated CNS immune cells from adult WT and 5xFAD mice to determine whether surface markers exclusive to pro-inflammatory and anti-inflammatory DAM modules distinguish distinct sub-populations within DAM [9]. Genes with known cell surface expression and module specificity ($k_{ME} \geq 0.75$ for one and ≤ 0.5 for the other, Fig. 4a) included CXCR4 (anti-inflammatory/Yellow module); and CD44, CD274, CD45 and Kv1.3 (pro-inflammatory/Magenta module). CD11c (*Itgax*) was chosen as a general marker of DAM based on existing single-cell RNAseq and confirmatory studies in human brain [9, 45].

In 6–8 mo old 5xFAD mice, CD11c⁺ DAM were more abundant in 5xFAD (≈50%) as compared to WT (< 10%) CD11b⁺ CNS immune cells, Fig. 4b). Pro-inflammatory DAM markers (CD44, CD45, CD274) and the anti-inflammatory DAM marker (CXCR4) were also increased in CD11c⁺ DAM in 5xFAD mice (Fig. 4c). While DAM from 5xFAD and WT mice had similar CD44, CD274 and CXCR4 surface expression, CD45 was much higher in DAM from 5xFAD mice. In 5xFAD CNS CD11b⁺CD11c⁺ DAM, we confirmed the presence of exclusively CD44⁺, exclusively CXCR4⁺, CD44⁺CXCR4⁺ double positive as well as CD44⁻CXCR4⁻ populations (Fig. 4d). These DAM subsets were then further studied in WT and 5xFAD mice across various age groups (6–12 mo). Aging resulted in increased proportions of CD44⁻CXCR4⁺ and CD44⁺CXCR4⁺ DAM while CD44⁺CXCR4⁻ DAM increased significantly at 9 mo of age and decreased by 12 mo of age (Fig. 4e). Double-negative CD44⁻CXCR4⁻ showed a modest but significant age-associated decline in both WT and 5xFAD mice. While the trajectories of change in all DAM subsets were similar in WT and 5xFAD mice, all age-related changes were augmented in 5xFAD DAM (Fig. 4e). Majority of DAM did not express high levels of either CD44 or CXCR4 suggesting that any additional complexity within

DAM may not have been revealed by our flow cytometry panel. Recent profiling of microglia by mass cytometry [46, 47] identified several subsets of resident myeloid cells in the naive mouse brain including CD14^high, CXCR4^high, CCR5^high, CD115 (Csf1r)^high as well as MHC-II^high CD44^high subsets [47], although proportions of these subsets in AD models is unknown. Interestingly, several of these markers were hub genes of homeostatic microglia (Cx3cr1, CD115/Csf1r, CCR5), pro-inflammatory DAM (CD14, CD44) and anti-inflammatory DAM (CXCR4) modules in our WGCNA. Collectively, our results confirm distinct subsets within DAM in accordance with network-based predictions and highlight previously unappreciated phenotypic diversity within microglia. Distinct age-dependent trajectories of pro- and anti-inflammatory DAM also suggest that aging influences the balance between DAM activation states, linking aging with other determinants of AD pathogenesis.

Identification of drug targets for inhibiting pro-inflammatory DAM and augmenting anti-inflammatory DAM profiles

To identify therapeutic approaches to specifically inhibit pro-inflammatory DAM and promote anti-inflammatory DAM gene expression, we performed an analysis using the connectivity map (CMAP) repository of transcriptional responses in human cells [37]. From our WGCNA results, we identified 85 pro-inflammatory DAM-specific and 145 anti-inflammatory DAM-specific genes as transcriptional signatures of each DAM module (Fig. 5a) and performed CMAP analysis to identify chemical and genetic perturbagens predicted to inhibit pro-inflammatory and augment anti-inflammatory DAM gene expression (Fig. 5b), the desired profile of an ideal neuro-immunomodulatory therapy in AD. We identified several therapeutic candidate drug classes including statins, opioid receptor agonists and inhibitors of Syk/Flt3, Vegfr, Jnk and Rock pathways (Fig. 5c). Perturbagens predicted to result in the opposite less desirable phenotype (increased pro-inflammatory and decreased anti-inflammatory DAM gene expression) were also identified (Fig. 5d), possibly representing effects of environmental exposures that increase AD risk.

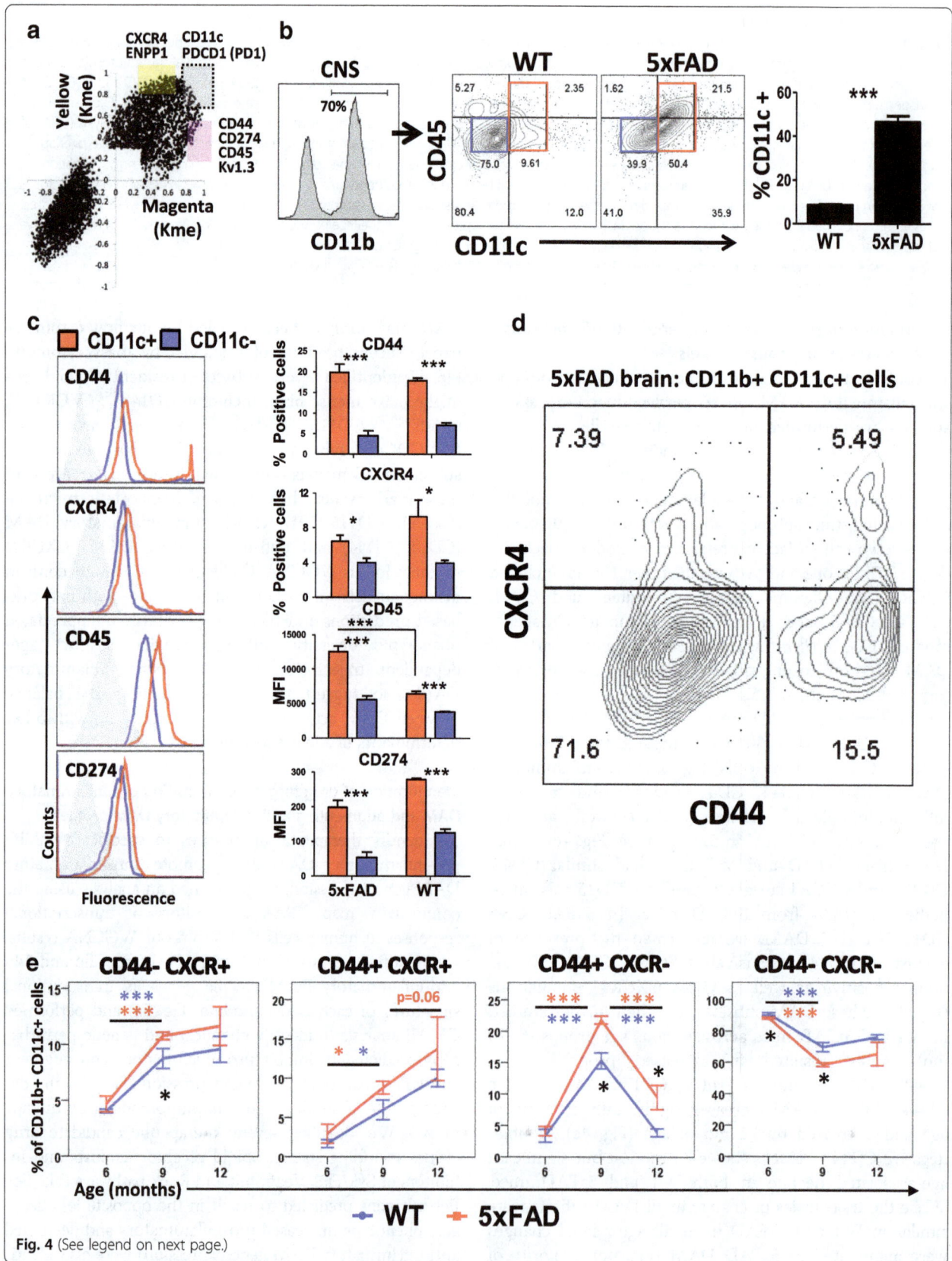

Fig. 4 (See legend on next page.)

(See figure on previous page.)
Fig. 4 Flow cytometric phenotyping of microglia using pro- and anti-inflammatory DAM markers. **a** Selection of potential flow cytometric markers for Magenta (pro-inflammatory) and Yellow (anti-inflammatory) DAM modules in acutely isolated WT and 5xFAD microglia. Criteria included k_{ME} ≥ 0.75 for one module, ≤0.5 for the other module and predominant cell membrane localization. Yellow module: Cxcr4 (CD184); DAM-phenotype: CD11c and Pdcd11 (PD1); Magenta module: CD44, CD274 (PDL1), CD45 and Kv1.3. Cell surface functional Kv1.3 channel expression was detected by ShK-F6CA, a fluorescein-conjugated Kv1.3 channel blocker that selectively binds to Kv1.3 channels. **b** Acutely isolated CNS immune cells were gated for live cells (FSC/SSC) and then for single cells (using FSC-A/FSC-H) followed by CD11b positivity. CD11c was used as a marker of DAM based on prior RNAseq studies. CD11c$^+$ DAM were gated as shown and proportions of CD11c$^+$ DAM in CD11b$^+$ CNS immune cells were compared between WT and 5xFAD mice (n = 6 mice/group, age 6–8 mo). **c** Comparison of pro-inflammatory DAM (CD44, CD45 and CD274) and anti-inflammatory DAM (CXCR4) specific markers within CD11c$^+$ DAM in 5xFAD and WT mice (n = 6/group, age 6–8 mo). Grey histogram represents isotype control. **d** Flow cytometric phenotyping of CD11b$^+$ cells in mouse brain based on CD44 and CXCR4 expression. **e** Changes in proportions of DAM subsets in aging WT and in aging 5xFAD mouse brains (n = 4 mice/group/time point). Pairwise and group-wise comparisons and significant differences are highlighted. Levels of significance: *p < 0.05, **p < 0.01, ***p < 0.005. Colored markers indicate within group comparisons (Red: 5xFAD, Blue: WT) while Black markers indicate inter-group differences (WT vs. 5xFAD)

We also searched homeostatic and DAM modules for genes encoding membrane-associated transporters and receptors since these are more likely to represent drug targets. We identified transmembrane receptors/transporter genes (Additional file 4: Table S4) that met at least 2 of the following criteria: (1) confirmed expression and function in microglia/macrophages, (2) existing drug modulators, and (3) relevance to neurological diseases. These included K$^+$ channel Kv1.3 (Kcna3), multi-drug-resistance protein Abcb1b and chloride transporter Clic4 in the pro-inflammatory DAM module; K$^+$ channel Kir2.1 (Kcnj2), purinergic channel P2rx4 and transient receptor potential channel Trpc4 in the anti-inflammatory DAM module; and purinoceptors P2ry12 and P2rx7 and two-pore K$^+$ channel Kcnk6 in the homeostatic module. Our pathway analyses also identified transcriptional regulators of pro-inflammatory DAM (NFkB and RelA) and anti-inflammatory DAM (LXRα/β and Atf1). Based on these *in-silico* findings, we prioritized in-vivo target validation studies in 5xFAD models using an activator of LXRα/β to promote anti-inflammatory DAM and a selective blocker of Kv1.3 channels to inhibit pro-inflammatory DAM responses.

Promotion of anti-inflammatory DAM and Aβ phagocytosis by LXRα/β agonists in AD mouse models

Agonists of LXRα/β, predicted to specifically promote anti-inflammatory DAM gene expression in our network analysis, have anti-inflammatory and protective effects in AD models [40, 41]. Therefore, we hypothesized that an agonist of LXRα/β pathways should increase the proportions of anti-inflammatory DAM cells as well as promote the ability of microglia to phagocytose Aβ in the 5xFAD mouse model of AD. We treated 10–12 mo old 5xFAD mice with the LXR agonist T0901317 (or vehicle) using a twice-weekly i.p. dosing regimen for 2 weeks [40, 41] (Fig. 6a-c), after which acutely isolated CD11b$^+$ CNS immune cells were immunophenotyped. This late time point of disease in 5xFAD mice was chosen since majority of microglia adopt the DAM profile [9]. Treatment with T0901317 did not

impact total numbers of CD11b$^+$ CNS immune cells, proportions of CD45^{high} CNS-infiltrating immune cells, proportions of CD11c$^+$ DAM in the brain, or peripheral CD11b$^+$CD45$^+$ splenocytes (data not shown). However, within DAM, we observed nearly two-fold increase in proportions of CXCR4$^+$CD44$^-$ (anti-inflammatory DAM) as well as CXCR4$^+$CD44$^+$ cells, while CXCR4$^-$CD44$^+$ (pro-inflammatory DAM) cells were unaltered (Fig. 6d-e).

To further determine whether augmentation of anti-inflammatory DAM is associated with increased phagocytic properties, we performed ex-vivo phagocytosis assays using acutely isolated CNS immune cells (from vehicle-treated or T0901317-treated mice) which were incubated with fluorophore-conjugated fibrillar Aβ42 followed by flow-cytometric measurement of Aβ uptake. As compared to vehicle-treated microglia, T0901317 treated mouse microglia demonstrated higher fibrillar Aβ42 phagocytosis (Fig. 6f). In summary, we observed specific augmentation of anti-inflammatory DAM as well as overall augmentation of Aβ phagocytosis by an agonist of LXRα/β, consistent with our network-based predictions and with known Aβ-lowering effects of LXRα/β agonists in AD models [42].

Validation of Kv1.3 channels as specific regulators of pro-inflammatory DAM responses and neuropathology in AD mouse models

We also identified Kv1.3 channels as ideal therapeutic targets to inhibit pro-inflammatory DAM and possibly promote anti-inflammatory DAM responses [26, 48, 49]. Kv1.3 channels regulate effector functions of pro-inflammatory activated microglia [26, 50–52] and are highly expressed by microglia surrounding Aβ plaques in AD [48]. Kv1.3 channel blockade by the small molecule Pap1 was also found to mitigate Aβ deposition and improve neurobehavioral measures in AD mouse models [49]. However, it is unclear whether Kv1.3 channels are indeed specifically expressed by pro-inflammatory DAM in AD. Furthermore, the only class of Kv1.3 channel blockers that has successfully completed phase Ib studies in humans for psoriasis (ShK analogs) has

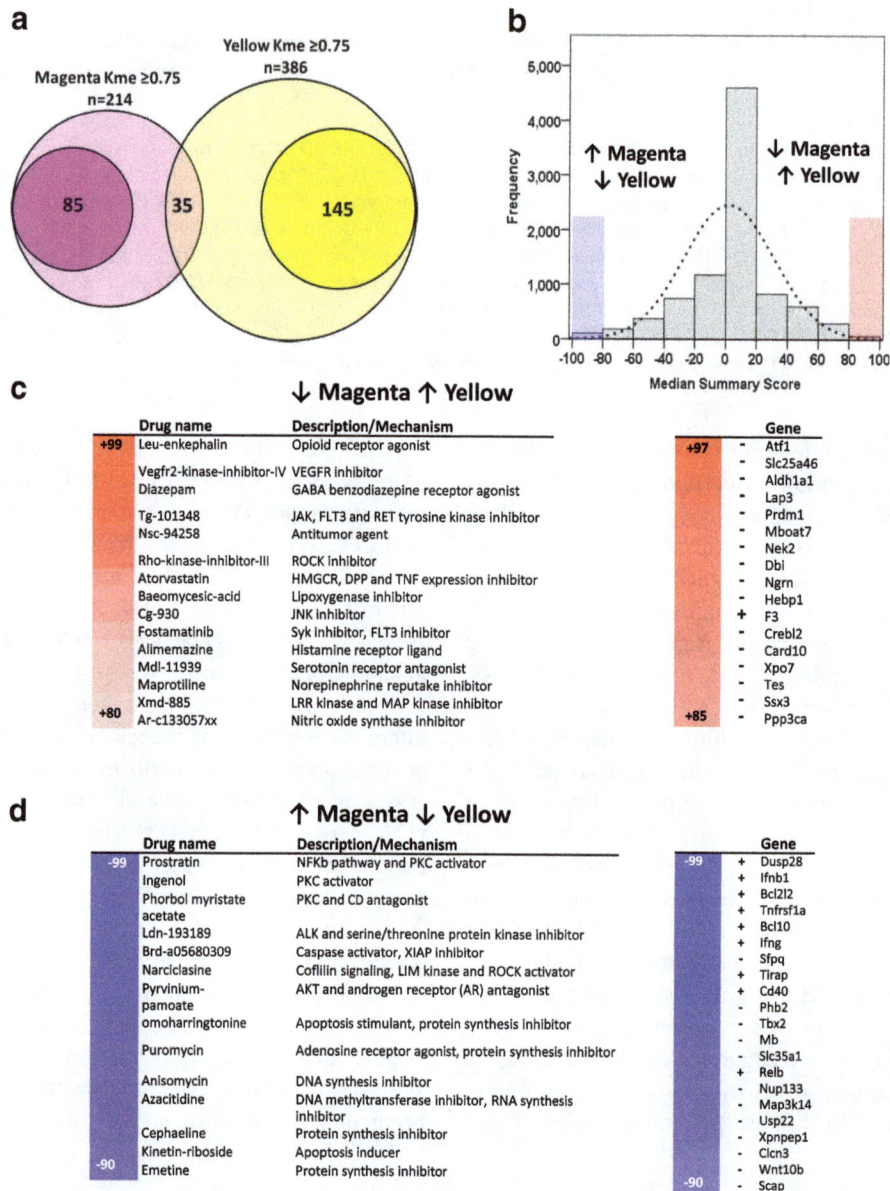

Fig. 5 CMAP analysis pro-inflammatory and anti-inflammatory DAM genes reveals genetic and chemical perturbagens as selective modulators. **a** Venn diagram representing exclusive members and dual members of Magenta and Yellow microglial modules. **b** Distribution of perturbagens from connectivity map (CMAP) analysis based on a median summary score (range − 100 to + 100) that represents likelihood of the perturbagen resulting in the desired transcriptional profile. **c, d** For these analyses, the desired transcriptional profile was upregulation of anti-inflammatory and down-regulation of pro-inflammatory module expression. A summary score ≥ + 90 typically indicates a high likelihood of achieving the desired profile (c, ↓Magenta/pro-inflammatory ↑Yellow/anti-inflammatory) while a score ≤ − 90 indicates likelihood of the opposite transcriptional profile (d, ↑Magenta/pro-inflammatory ↓Yellow/anti-inflammatory). The most significant chemical perturbagens (existing drugs) and genetic perturbagens (gene suppression or over-expression) are shown

not been tested in pre-clinical models of AD pathology [53, 54]. To address these knowledge gaps regarding Kv1.3 as a therapeutic target in AD, we performed flow cytometric studies to determine the pattern of Kv1.3 channel expression in 5xFAD and aging mice and tested the in-vivo efficacy of the ShK analog ShK-223 in acute neuroinflammatory and AD mouse models. ShK-223 was selected due

to its improved stability and > 10,000-fold selectivity for Kv1.3 channels over neuronal Kv channels [53, 54].

To detect functional cell-surface Kv1.3 channels expressed on acutely isolated CNS immune cells, we used a validated flow-cytometric approach [26, 27] in which cells are incubated with a fluorescent Kv1.3 blocker ShK-F6CA which selectively binds to functional Kv1.3 channels. In

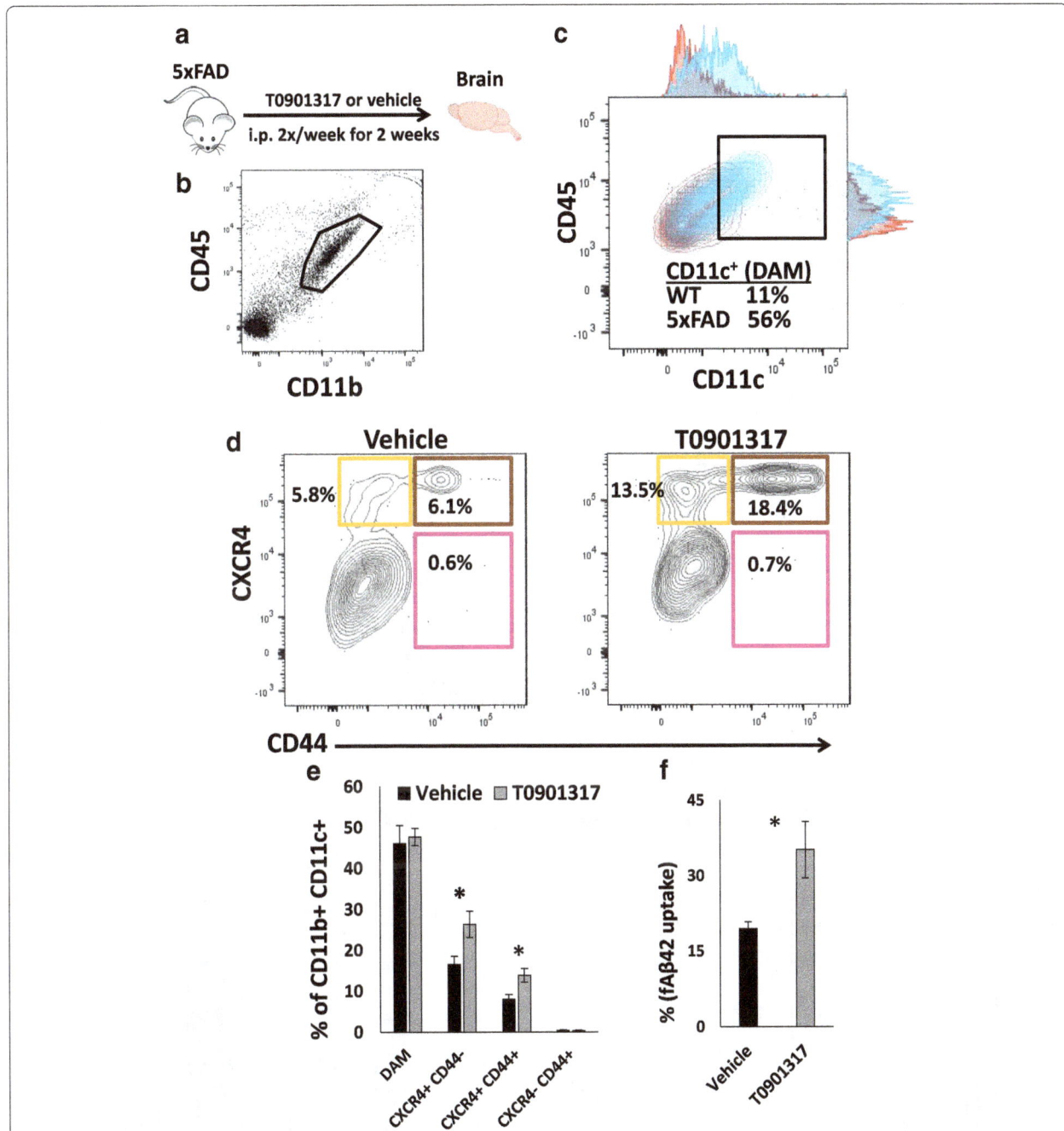

Fig. 6 Agonists of liver-X-receptor (LXR) α/β signaling promote anti-inflammatory DAM and Aβ phagocytic activity in microglia. **a** Experimental design: 6–7 mo 5xFAD mice (females, n = 4/group) received either vehicle (20% DMSO) or a LXR α/β agonist T0901317 (30 mg/kg i.p. daily × 2 weeks) after which acutely isolated CNS immune cells were assessed for flow cytometric immuno-phenotyping as well as flow cytometric assays of fluorescent fibrillar Aβ. **b, c** CD11b⁺CD45^low CNS immune cells were assessed for CD11c expression. A comparison of CD11c expression in 5xFAD mice (blue) and WT mice (red) is shown. Gating threshold for CD11c is shown in (**c**). **d, e** A comparison of CD44 and CXCR4 expression profiles within CD11c⁺ DAM acutely isolated from vehicle-treated or T0901317-treated 5xFAD mice. Relative proportions of each subset (of all CD11b⁺CD45^lowCD11c⁺ DAM) are shown. Yellow represents anti-inflammatory DAM, Magenta represents pro-inflammatory DAM and Brown represents double positive cells. A quantitative analysis of various subsets of CD11c + DAM in vehicle-treated and T0901317-treated mice is shown in (**e**). **f** Comparison of ability of acutely isolated CD11b⁺CD45^low microglia (from vehicle-treated and T0901317-treated mice) to phagocytose fluorescent Aβ42 fibrils. *$p < 0.05$, **$p < 0.01$, ***$p < 0.005$

HEK293 cells, we confirmed that ShK-F6CA binding was only seen in cells transfected with pcDNA3.1-Kv1.3 but not with empty vector (Fig. 7a). Within subpopulations of CD11b⁺CD45^low microglia, we confirmed that surface expression of Kv1.3 was higher in exclusively CD44⁺ microglia (pro-inflammatory DAM) cells as

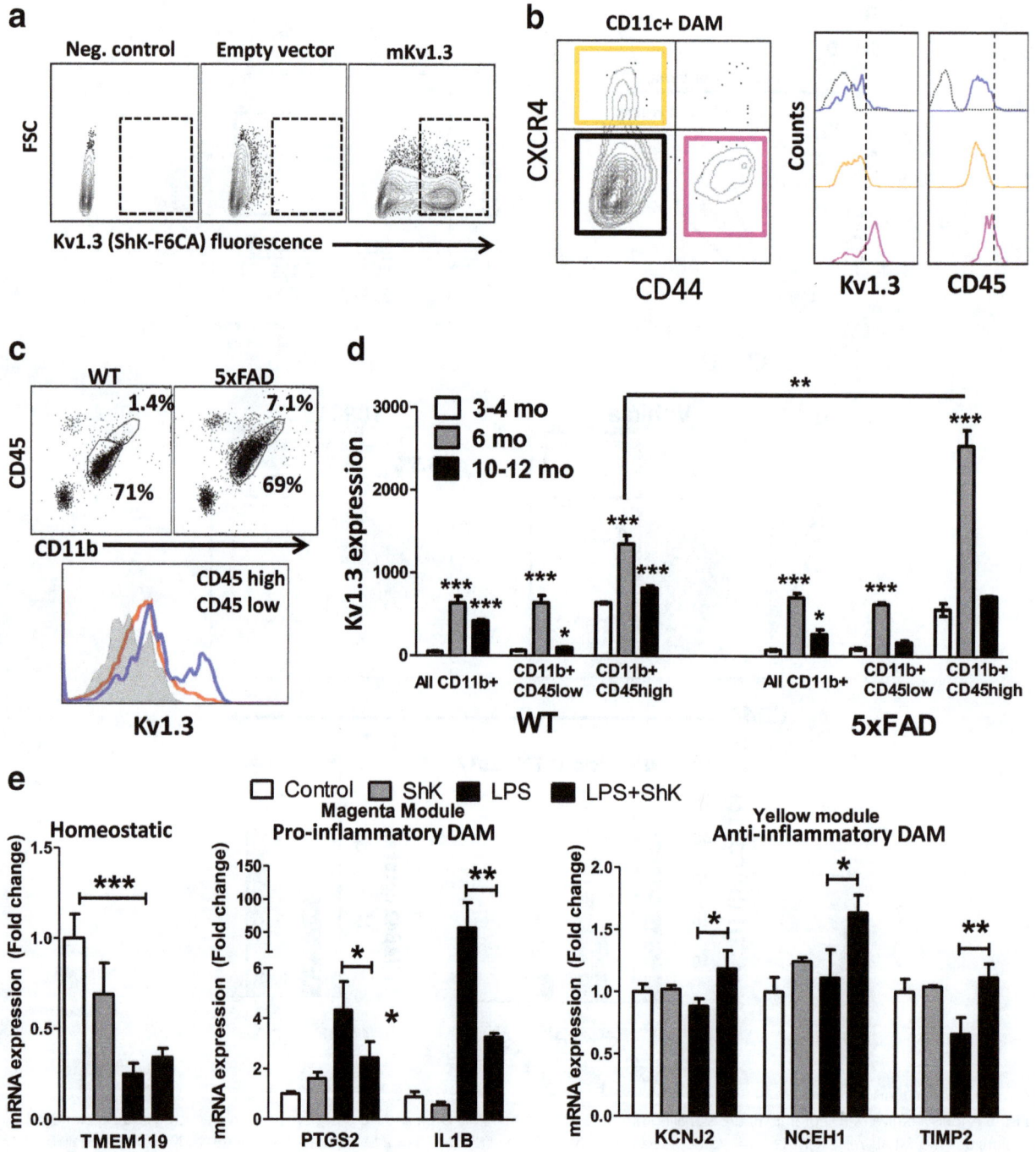

Fig. 7 (See legend on next page.)

(See figure on previous page.)
Fig. 7 Kv1.3 channels are expressed by pro-inflammatory DAM and regulate pro-inflammatory DAM genes. **a** Confirmation of specificity of flow cytometric assay of functional Kv1.3 channels: HEK293 cells were transiently transfected with 1 μg of pRC/CMV (empty vector) or pRC/CMV-mKv1.3 (mouse Kv1.3) after which ShK-F6CA was added (final concentration 100 nM) × 30 min, followed by flow cytometry (3 independent experiments were performed). Electrophysiological confirmation of Kv1.3 current expression was performed by whole-cell patch clamp (data not shown). **b** Expression of Magenta module markers Kv1.3 and CD45 in subsets of CD11c$^+$ DAM in 5xFAD mice (Homeostatic: CD44$^-$CXCR4$^-$, Magenta/pro-inflammatory-DAM: CD44$^+$CXCR4$^-$, Yellow/anti-inflammatory-DAM: CXCR4$^+$CD44$^-$ and double-positive CD44$^+$CXCR4$^+$ DAM) in adult 5xFAD mice ($n = 5$ mice, age 6–8 mo). Grey histogram represents isotype control (for CD45) or negative control (unlabeled cells for ShK-F6CA). **c** Gating of CNS immune cells based on CD11b and CD45 into CD11b$^+$CD45^{low} (resident microglia) and CD11b$^+$CD45^{high} subpopulations (Top). Kv1.3 surface expression in CD45^{high} and CD45^{low} subsets of CD11b$^+$ cells, is shown below. **d** Comparison of Kv1.3 expression in CD45^{low} and CD45^{high} subsets of CD11b$^+$ CNS immune cells in 3 age groups of WT and 5xFAD mice ($n = 3$ mice/group/time point. Post-hoc statistical tests: $*p < 0.05$, $**p < 0.01$, $***p < 0.005$. **e** Comparison of gene expression in acutely isolated CNS immune cells isolated from 6 mo WT mice treated with saline, ShK-223, LPS or LPS + ShK-223 (4 daily i.p. doses, $n = 3$/group). Selected module markers: Homeostatic: *Tmem119*, Pro-inflammatory DAM: *Il1b*, *Ptgs2*; Anti-inflammatory DAM: *Kcnj2*, *Nceh1*, *Timp2*

compared to homeostatic microglia (CD11b$^+$CD11c$^-$ or CD11c$^+$CD44$^-$CXCR4$^-$) or exclusively CXCR4$^+$ microglia (anti-inflammatory DAM) (Fig. 7b). Using the traditional approach of classifying CD11b$^+$ CNS immune cells into CD45^{low} (microglia) and CD45^{high} (activated microglia or peripherally derived CNS-infiltrating macrophages) subpopulations, we found a greater proportion of CD45^{high} cells in 5xFAD mice (Fig. 7c) and as we previously reported [26], Kv1.3 channel expression was highest in CD45^{high} CNS immune cells. In 5xFAD compared to WT mice, Kv1.3 channels were strongly upregulated by CD11b$^+$CD45^{high} CNS immune cells. Maximal Kv1.3 upregulation by CD45^{low} and CD45^{high} CD11b$^+$ immune cells was observed at 6 mo of age, after which Kv1.3 expression decreased (Fig. 7d) a finding that is supported by published electrophysiological data [49].

Next, we performed in-vivo studies to determine whether Kv1.3 channel inhibition by ShK-223 can inhibit pro-inflammatory DAM and augment anti-inflammatory DAM gene expression in the model of acute neuroinflammation induced by low dose systemic LPS administration [26, 54]. We found that ShK-223 treatment inhibited LPS-induced upregulation of proinflammatory genes (Ptgs2, Il1b) and augmented expression of anti-inflammatory DAM genes (Kcnj2, Nceh1, Timp2) without affecting LPS-induced suppression of homeostatic gene Tmem119 (Fig. 7e). The ability of systemic ShK-223 to modulate microglial function in this model indirectly supports its CNS bioavailability.

To determine whether pro-inflammatory DAM inhibition by Kv1.3 blockade promotes Aβ phagocytic activity, we acutely isolated CNS immune cells from untreated and LPS-treated WT and age-matched 6 mo old 5xFAD mice and exposed them to fluorescent Aβ42 fibrils in the presence or absence of ShK-223. ShK-223 augmented phagocytic capacity in WT CD11b$^+$ immune cells, and a more robust augmentation was seen in the CD45^{high} subset of CD11b$^+$ cells, the same subset that also highly expresses Kv1.3 channels (Fig. 8a). No effect of ShK-223 was seen in CD11b$^+$CD45^{high} cells in 5xFAD mice, although these

already had a very high baseline level of phagocytic activity suggesting saturation. In a separate experiment, 5xFAD mice (age 6 months) received i.p. ShK-223 for 30 days, after which acutely isolated CD11b$^+$ CNS immune cells were assessed for Aβ phagocytosis. We observed that ShK-223 treatment resulted in an overall augmentation of Aβ phagocytosis (Fig. 8b). Despite effective uptake, Aβ clearance by microglia in AD may be ineffective despite phagocytic uptake [55]. Therefore, we tested the effect of Kv1.3 blockade on fAβ42 compartmentalization into mature Lamp1-positive phago-lysosomes. BV2 microglia were loaded with fluorescent Aβ fibrils, subsequently washed and cultured with or without ShK-223 for 72 h. ShK-223 significantly increased Lamp1 and Aβ co-localization at 16 and 24 h time points (Additional file 8: Figure S7).

To determine whether long-term Kv1.3 channel blockade by ShK-223 results in lower burden of Aβ in 5xFAD mice, we initiated intra-peritoneal treatments with ShK-223 at 3 mo of age and continued therapy until 6 mo when 5xFAD mice, in our experience, show robust Aβ deposition and neuroinflammation without neuronal loss or neurobehavioral deficits. This time point was chosen as it represents an optimal therapeutic window for neuro-immunomodulation in humans with AD pathology. Following 3 mo of ShK-223 therapy, we observed significantly lower Aβ plaque burden (Fig. 8c-d) in the hippocampus, smaller Aβ plaque size (Fig. 8e) compared to sham-treated mice as well as decreased Iba1-immunoreactivity around Aβ plaques (Fig. 8f-g). To determine whether this observed decrease in microgliosis was a result of ShK-223's effect of lower Aβ burden rather than a direct effect on microglial activation, we assessed Iba1 immunoreactivity in peri-plaque microglia and found that ShK-223 treatment was associated with lower Iba1 positivity around Aβ plaques even after accounting for differences in plaque size (Fig. 8h). Overall, these results show that Kv1.3 blockade can inhibit pro-inflammatory DAM gene expression and promote anti-inflammatory DAM gene expression while promoting phagocytic Aβ clearance, a protective function of DAM in AD.

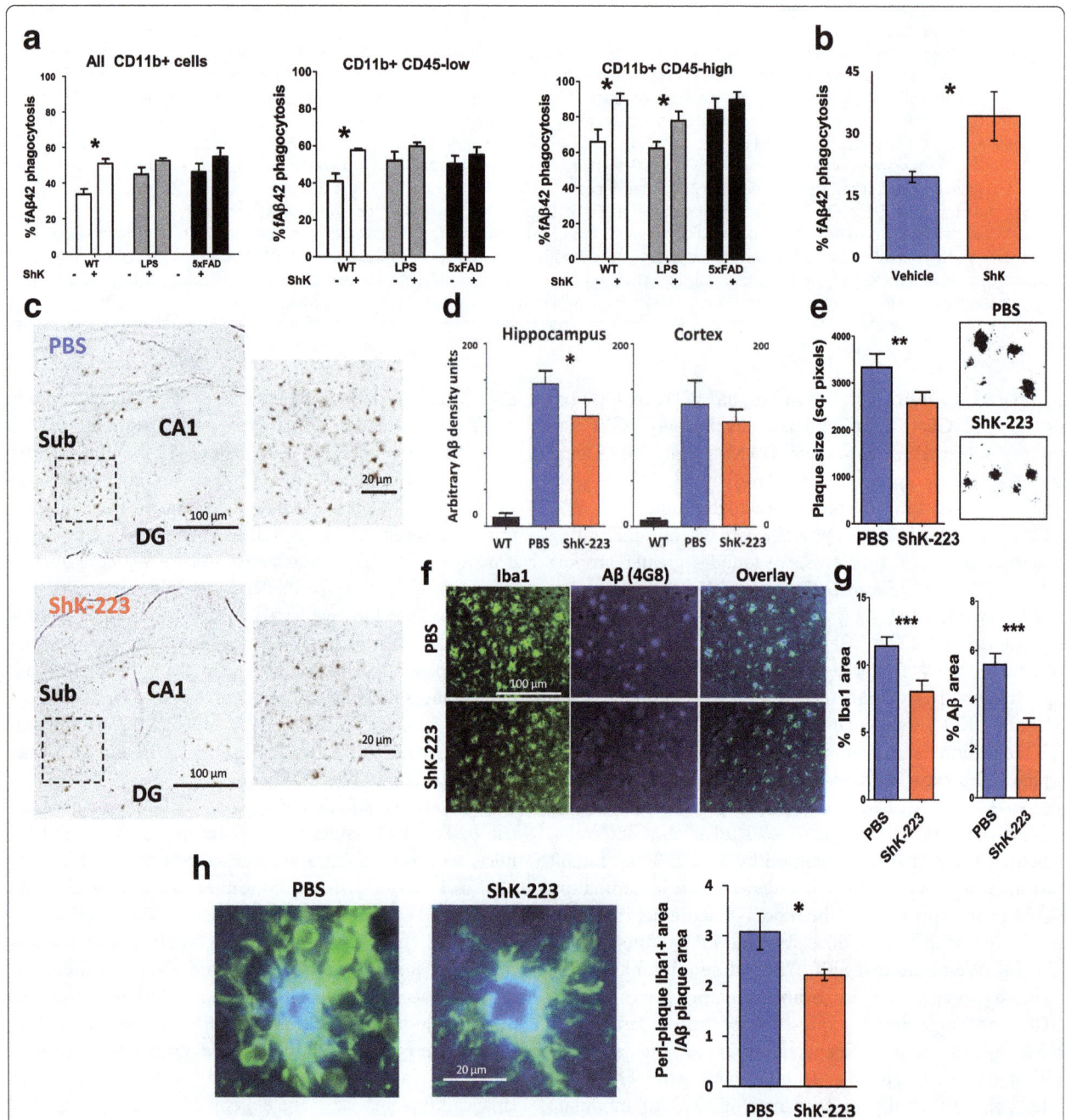

Fig. 8 Kv1.3 channel blockade promotes Aβ phagocytosis and limits amyloid β burden in 5xFAD mice. **a** Comparison of ex-vivo phagocytosis of fluorescent Aβ42 fibrils by acutely isolated CNS CD11b[+] cells from WT (sham-treated or LPS-treated for 4 days) and 5xFAD mice (age 6–8 mo, $n = 4$ mice/group). Cells were loaded with fluorescent fibrillar Aβ42 in the presence of either sham or ShK-223 (100 nM) for 1 h prior to labeling with anti-CD11b and anti-CD45 antibodies. **b** Comparison of ex-vivo phagocytic capacity for fluorescent Aβ42 fibrils by acutely isolated CNS CD11b[+] cells from sham-treated or ShK-223-treated 5xFAD mice ($n = 4$/group). ShK-223 was administered twice a week (i.p., 100 μg/kg) in this study. **c-g** In this study of ShK-223 in 5xFAD mice, mice were treated with PBS or ShK-223 (100 μg/kg) between 3 and 6 mo ($n = 10$ mice/group) and brains were fixed for immunohistochemistry. **c** Comparison of hippocampal Aβ plaques in PBS-treated (top) and ShK-223-treated (bottom) mice (Right: Higher magnification image). **d** Quantification of Aβ plaque burden in the hippocampus and frontal cortex. **e** Comparison of hippocampal (subiculum) Aβ plaque size in PBS- and ShK-223-treated mice. **f, g, h** Immunofluorescence images showing Iba1 (Green) and Aβ (Blue) immunoreactivities in the hippocampus of PBS- and ShK-223-treated mice. **g** Quantitative analyses of Iba1 expression (% area) and Aβ plaque burden. **h** Quantitative analysis of peri-plaque Iba1 immunoreactivity comparing PBS- and ShK-223-treated mice. 5–8 plaques of relatively similar size were selected from each mouse and Iba1[+] area was normalized to the plaque area and compared across groups. *$p < 0.05$, **$p < 0.01$, ***$p < 0.005$

Genetic and pathological links of microglia subtypes in human AD brain

To investigate the relevance of homeostatic, pro- and anti-inflammatory DAM signatures in human AD, we first determined whether the AD-associated microglial modules identified in mice were enriched for known AD genetic risk factors identified by GWAS in humans. Although GWAS of AD patients has identified causative immune gene polymorphisms in AD [34, 56, 57], the aspects of CNS immune responses regulated by AD-associated GWAS hits have not been clarified. From 1234 AD-risk associated genes identified using Multi-marker Analysis of GenoMic Annotation (MAGMA) of GWAS in late-onset AD [34, 56], we found that AD-associated GWAS hits were highly enriched in the homeostatic (Blue) module (Fig. 9a, $p = 0.005$). Genes with strong AD associations and high module memberships within the homeostatic module included Bin1, Cnn2, Picalm and Sorl1 (Fig. 9b). The selective enrichment of AD risk genes in homeostatic microglia suggests that perturbations in homeostatic microglial functions such as immune surveillance are causally implicated in late-onset AD. Although AD GWAS genes were not specifically enriched in the pro- and anti-inflammatory DAM modules, several AD-associated genes were also identified in the anti-inflammatory Yellow module (Apoe, Hla-dqa1) as well as the pro-inflammatory Magenta module (Ms4a4e, Hla-dqb1 and Treml2) (Fig. 9c-d, Additional file 5: Table S5, Additional file 6: Table S6).

Next, we determined whether homeostatic microglial and DAM proteins are expressed in human AD brain and whether their expression is associated with AD pathology. We interrogated a quantitative proteomics dataset (47 post-mortem human brains from the Baltimore Longitudinal Study of Aging) in which WGCNA identified distinct AD-associated protein modules (https://www.synapse.org/#!Synapse:syn11209141). In this dataset from 20 clinical AD, 14 asymptomatic (pre-clinical) AD and 13 non-disease controls, 5084 of 6532 gene symbols were present in our mouse microglial network. Among these, we identified genes with at least moderate membership ($k_{ME} \geq 0.50$) to mouse microglial modules and then determined the overlap between mouse microglial WGCNA modules and human brain protein modules. Anti-inflammatory DAM and pro-inflammatory DAM module members overlapped (FDR < 10%) with human protein modules (M2, M4, M35, un-adjusted p-values < 0.01) that were also positively associated with Braak and CERAD neuropathological grades in human AD (Fig. 9e) [58]. We also found 67 hub genes (Fig. 9f) of mouse microglial modules ($k_{ME} \geq 0.90$) within the human brain proteome which predominantly mapped to homeostatic, pro- and anti-inflammatory DAM mouse microglial modules. Using an aggregate expression of hub genes to represent overall expression

of each module in human brain, we found that upregulation of the pro-inflammatory DAM module preceded clinical diagnosis of AD while the anti-inflammatory DAM module was upregulated modestly only in cases with symptomatic AD (Fig. 9g) while the homeostatic module showed less robust increase with AD progression. Normalized expression data of the top 3 pro-inflammatory DAM hub genes (CD44, Cst2 and Nampt) identified in the human brain proteome are shown in Fig. 9h, demonstrating a gradual increase in expression with accumulating AD pathology. These genomic and proteomic validation studies suggest a causal role for early dysregulation of microglial homeostatic mechanisms in AD and confirm the expression of both pro- and anti-inflammatory DAM modules in human AD and suggest the emergence of pro-inflammatory DAM in pre-clinical and therapeutically meaningful stages of AD.

Discussion

A comprehensive understanding of molecular and functional characteristics and regulators of microglial phenotypes in AD is critical to developing effective neuro-immunomodulatory therapies. By integrating comprehensive network analyses of microglial transcriptomic datasets with validation studies, we have developed a framework of microglial activation states in AD (Fig. 10) that allowed us to predict and confirm molecularly distinct and functionally divergent pro-inflammatory and anti-inflammatory profiles within DAM in AD mouse models, both of which emerge down-stream of the Trem2 immune checkpoint [9]. While pro-inflammatory DAM are characterized by higher expression of CD44, CD45 and Kv1.3 channels and are regulated by NFkB, Stat1 and RelA pathways, anti-inflammatory DAM are characterized by CXCR4 expression and regulated by LXRα/β. Using CD44 and CXCR4 as surface markers of pro-inflammatory and anti-inflammatory DAM respectively, flow-cytometric validation studies confirmed the existence of distinct subsets of exclusive CD44+ and CXCR4+, double-positive as well as double-negative DAM subsets, each with distinct age-dependent trajectories of change that were accentuated in the 5xFAD model of AD pathology. As predicted by our microglial transcriptional framework, we also found that promotion of anti-inflammatory DAM and inhibition of pro-inflammatory DAM were achievable via LXR agonism and Kv1.3 channel inhibition. We also found that pro-inflammatory DAM proteins are increased in human AD at pre-clinical stages and are positively associated with tau and neurofibrillary tangle pathology, emphasizing the therapeutic relevance of our findings.

By targeting decreased pro-inflammatory DAM and increased anti-inflammatory DAM as the desired effects of ideal immuno-modulatory strategies in AD, we used CMAP to identify and prioritize several classes of existing

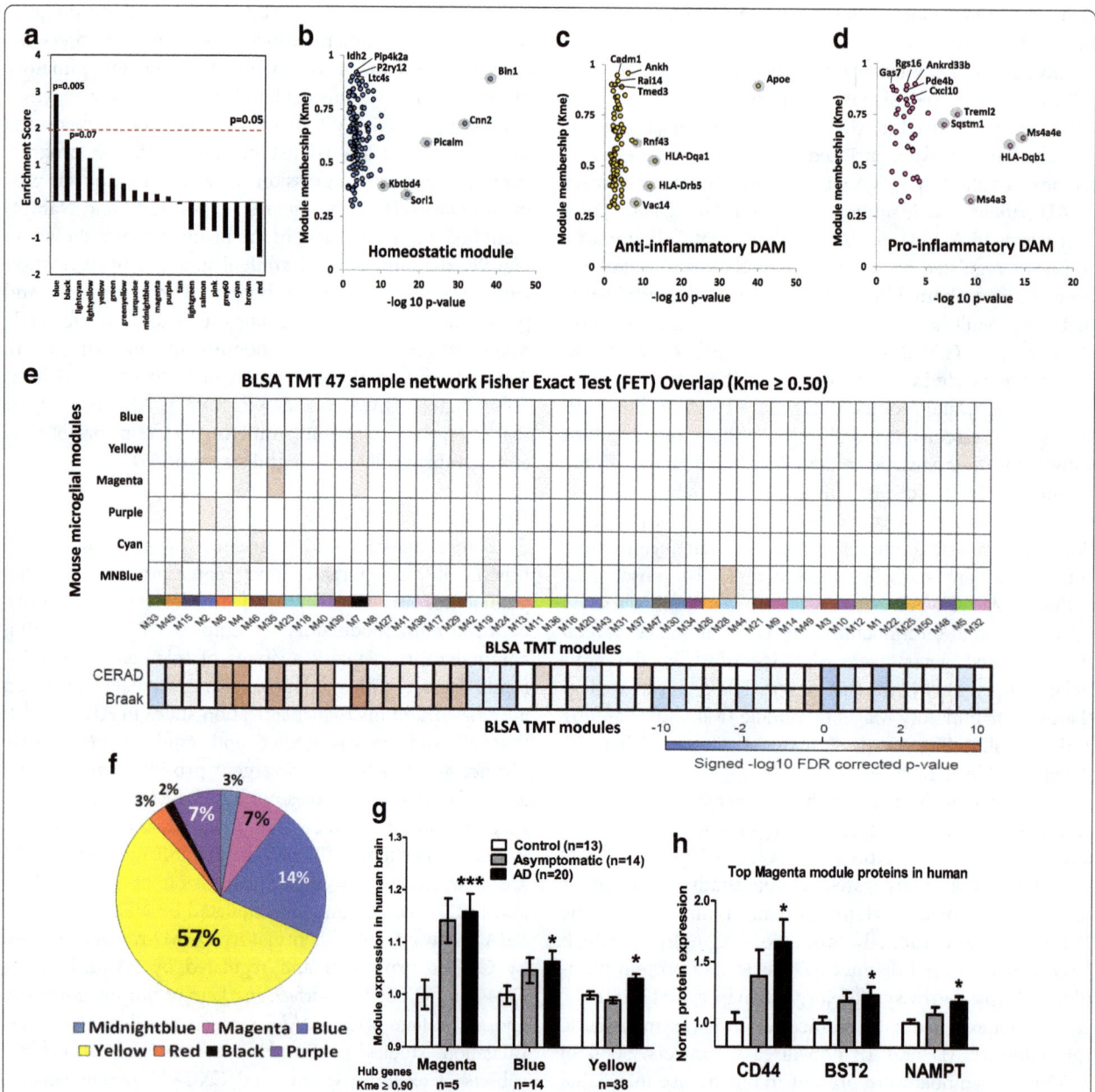

Fig. 9 Identification of AD-risk genes as key members of homeostatic, pro-inflammatory DAM and anti-inflammatory DAM modules. **a** Enrichment analysis of GWAS-identified AD risk genes in mouse microglial modules (1234 genes identified by MAGMA were used for this analysis [34]). An enrichment score of ≥1.96 (red line) corresponds to significant enrichment (p < 0.05). **b-d** AD GWAS hits specific to (**b**) Blue (homeostatic), (**c**) Yellow (anti-inflammatory DAM) and (**d**) Magenta (pro-inflammatory DAM) modules. Top 5 genes based on strength of disease association (X-axis: -log10 p-value) are highlighted by a gray silhouette and top 5 genes based on module membership (k_ME, Y-axis) are shown (also see Additional file 5: Table S5, Additional file 6: Table S6). **e-h** Analyses performed using quantitative proteomic data obtained from 47 post-mortem human frontal cortices (BLSA, n = 20 confirmed AD cases with cognitive decline, n = 13 controls without any AD pathology and n = 14 cases with AD pathology without cognitive symptoms). **e** Overlap of mouse modules [Blue/homeostatic, Yellow/anti-inflammatory DAM, Magenta/pro-inflammatory DAM, Purple (homeostatic), Cyan (IL4-upregulated module) and Midnightblue (LPS-upregulated module)] with human protein modules by hypergeometric one-tailed Fisher-exact test. Color intensity indicates strength of significance after Benjamini-Hochberg FDR correction. Strongest FDR-corrected p-values (0.075) were seen for overlap between Yellow and Magenta mouse microglial modules with M2 (unadjusted p = 0.0013), M4 (unadjusted p = 0.0014) and M35 (unadjusted p = 0.0014) human proteomic modules. Y-axis: Mouse WGCNA modules; X-axis: Protein BLSA modules. Correlations between BLSA modules with CERAD and Braak neuropathological grades of AD are shown. **f** Distribution of mouse microglial module hub genes (k_ME ≥ 0.90) in human BLSA AD proteome. **g** Comparison of aggregate expression of Magenta, Yellow and Blue mouse microglial modules in control, asymptomatic AD and clinical AD. Modules with ≥5 hub genes (k_ME ≥ 0.8) were included. Median module expression was calculated and compared across groups. **h** Normalized protein expression data of top three proteins from the pro-inflammatory Magenta module (CD44, Bst2 and Nampt) are shown

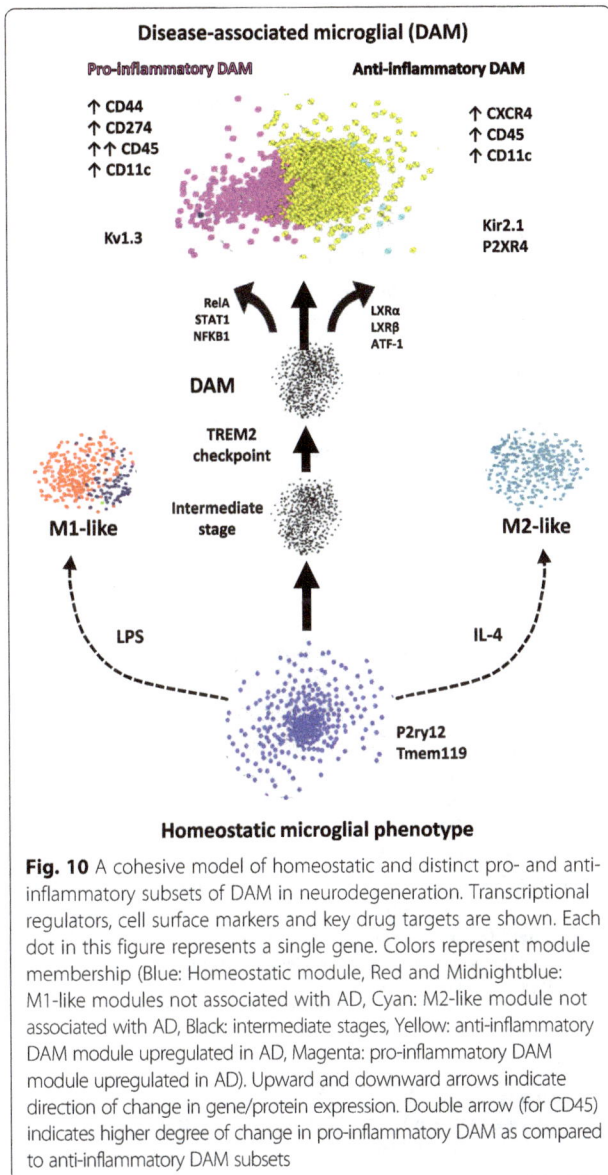

Fig. 10 A cohesive model of homeostatic and distinct pro- and anti-inflammatory subsets of DAM in neurodegeneration. Transcriptional regulators, cell surface markers and key drug targets are shown. Each dot in this figure represents a single gene. Colors represent module membership (Blue: Homeostatic module, Red and Midnightblue: M1-like modules not associated with AD, Cyan: M2-like module not associated with AD, Black: intermediate stages, Yellow: anti-inflammatory DAM module upregulated in AD, Magenta: pro-inflammatory DAM module upregulated in AD). Upward and downward arrows indicate direction of change in gene/protein expression. Double arrow (for CD45) indicates higher degree of change in pro-inflammatory DAM as compared to anti-inflammatory DAM subsets

drugs that can be safely used in humans including statins, Syk inhibitors and norepinephrine reuptake inhibitors that are predicted to selectively inhibit pro-inflammatory DAM while promoting anti-inflammatory DAM. Therefore, our results provide a compelling rationale for testing these existing classes of drugs in human AD preventative trials. We also independently validated blockers of Kv1.3 channels and agonists of the LXRα/β pathway as promising therapeutics in neurodegenerative disorders [42, 49]. Kv1.3 is a voltage-gated K^+ channel that despite low transcript level expression, is highly expressed at the channel level in immune cells where it regulates calcium signaling and effector functions [9, 10, 59]. The homo-tetrameric form of Kv1.3 channels that is susceptible to blockade by ShK analogs (such as ShK-223) is uniquely expressed in the brain by activated microglia while Kv1.3

hetero-tetramers that are resistant to ShK analogs are expressed by some cortical neurons [60, 61]. Kv1.3 channels are highly expressed by pro-inflammatory microglia in mouse models of refractory seizures as well as radiation neurotoxicity and recently, Kv1.3 blockade by Pap1 was shown to have amyloid-lowering and neuroprotective effects in AD mouse models [26, 48, 49, 51, 62, 63]. In our studies, Kv1.3 channel blockade by ShK-223 reduced the expression of pro-inflammatory DAM genes while promoting the expression of anti-inflammatory DAM genes and promoted phagocytic uptake and clearance of Aβ. Kv1.3 channels were also highly upregulated by $CD11b^+CD45^{high}$ CNS immune cells in the 5xFAD brain, consistent with previous findings of increased Kv1.3 expression in microglia in human AD [48]. Our pre-clinical findings using ShK-223 are of translational importance because a Kv1.3-blocking ShK analog (dalazatide or ShK-186) that is very similar to ShK-223, is the only selective Kv1.3 blocker to have successfully completed early phase human studies for systemic autoimmunity [53]. We found that systemically administered ShK-223 can modulate CNS immune responses in both acute neuroinflammatory [26] and chronic neurodegenerative disease models, suggesting its CNS bioavailability, while clearly demonstrating ability to impact neuroimmune responses. In addition to Kv1.3 channels, we also found that an agonist of LXR:RXR nuclear receptor-mediated transcriptional pathway increases the proportions of anti-inflammatory DAM and promotes Aβ phagocytosis by microglia in AD models, providing a novel mechanism for amyloid-lowering effects of LXR agonists in AD mouse models [42].

Beyond these therapeutic implications, our network-based framework of microglial gene profiles, including homeostatic, pro-inflammatory and anti-inflammatory DAM and AD-unrelated activation states, can be applied as a resource to guide target selection, experimental design and development of novel mouse models to study immune mechanisms in neurodegeneration including genetic strategies to achieve conditional microglia subtype-specific gene expression or deletion [64, 65]. For example, if a microglial gene relevant to neurodegeneration at an early stage is to be investigated, it would be most appropriate to use a conditional and cell-specific model, such as the tamoxifen-inducible Cx3cr1 Cre recombinase mouse, since Cx3cr1 is only expressed by homeostatic microglia and is downregulated by DAM [66]. On the other hand, if a pro-inflammatory DAM-specific gene is to be investigated (eg: Ptgs2/Cox2 or Tlr2), an inducible CD11c/Itgax Cre model would be more appropriate since CD11c is specifically upregulated by DAM while Cx3cr1 is downregulated [9]. Development of AD-relevant transgenic mice conditionally lacking or overexpressing pro- or anti-inflammatory DAM genes could help us further understand the roles of these functionally divergent DAM profiles at various stages of AD pathogenesis and aging.

The framework of homeostatic, pro-inflammatory DAM and anti-inflammatory DAM profiles in AD we uncovered has also allowed us to better understand immune consequences of AD risk genes including Bin1, Apoe and Treml2 [56]. Of the top AD-associated genes in the homeostatic module, Bin1 has the highest module membership suggesting a direct role for this gene in regulating homeostatic microglial functions which may be perturbed early in AD. Bin1 is a regulator of endocytosis that is associated with neurofibrillary tangle pathology in AD and is highly expressed in microglia and oligodendrocyte precursors [59]. Unique splicing of Bin1 in microglia and oligodendroglia not seen in neurons or astrocytes has also been suggested [59, 67] and Bin1 has also been identified as a highly abundant microglial protein in a recent microglial proteome [68] although the exact role of Bin1 in homeostatic microglia and in AD pathogenesis remains unclear. In the anti-inflammatory/phagocytic DAM module, Apoe was identified as a hub gene strongly associated with AD risk. This agrees with other lines of evidence confirming the role of Apoe in regulating DAM responses and Aβ-clearance in AD [16, 21]. In the pro-inflammatory DAM module, we identified Treml2 as the gene with highest module membership associated with AD risk. Treml2 has opposing roles to Trem2 in microglia [69], agreeing with the overall concept that pro-inflammatory DAM emerge down-stream of the Trem2 checkpoint after which they may diverge from anti-inflammatory DAM. In addition to these highlighted genes, our transcriptomic network identifies several other AD risk genes as potentially having novel roles in microglial activation and dysfunction in AD, providing a resource for the community and several directions for future investigations.

Conclusion

In summary, our study highlights the value of applying unbiased co-expression analytic approaches to cell population-level transcriptomic data to unravel functionally and molecularly distinct cellular profiles that may not have been detected by single cell profiling studies [10]. By applying WGCNA to pure CD11b$^+$ transcriptomic datasets, we could recapitulate the spectrum of homeostatic microglia and DAM in AD models, in addition to resolving DAM into anti-inflammatory/phagocytic and pro-inflammatory profiles, thereby providing a framework for validation and therapeutic studies. The application of co-expression network analysis to omics data from purified cell populations may allow comprehensive examination and integration of not just transcriptome, but also the proteomic and metabolomic signatures of microglial and adaptive immune responses in aging and neurodegenerative diseases.

Additional files

Additional file 1: Table S1. Mouse microglial transcriptomic modules identified by Weighted Correlation Network Analysis (WGCNA).

Additional file 2: Table S2. Gene Ontology (GO) analyses of Blue, Magenta, Yellow and Midnightblue mouse microglial modules.

Additional file 3: Table S3. Identification of potential transcriptional regulators of mouse microglial modules.

Additional file 4: Table S4. Putative membrane-associated drug targets and regulators of Blue, Magenta, Yellow and Midnightblue microglial transcriptomic modules.

Additional file 5: Table S5. Enrichment analysis of GWAS-identified human AD-risk genes in mouse microglial modules.

Additional file 6: Table S6. Top AD risk genes in Blue, Magenta and Yellow AD-associated microglial modules.

Additional file 7: Table S7. Changes in expression of AD-associated Blue, Magenta and Yellow microglial modules in aging WT and APP/PS1 mice.

Additional file 8: Figure S1, related to Figure 1. Expression of microglial transcriptomic modules identified by WGCNA. **Figure S2,** related to Figure 1. Gene ontology analysis reveals distinct cellular localization and functional profiles of microglial networks in AD. **Figure S3,** related to Figure 1. Identification of transcriptional regulators of AD-associated microglial modules. **Figure S4,** related to Figure 2. A transcriptomic landscape of microglial activation states in AD. **Figure S5,** related to Figure 2. Magenta and Yellow modules likely emerge as distinct subtypes from a common microglial precursor state (Additional file 7: Table S7). **Figure S6,** related to Figure 2. Pro- and anti-inflammatory DAM networks emerge downstream of the Trem2-mediated immune checkpoint in AD. **Figure S7.** ShK-223 promotes compartmentalization of Aβ in mature phagolysosomes.

Additional file 9: 3D viSNE representation of microglial modules. Color is indicative of the respective module color.

Additional file 10: 3D viSNE representation of microglial modules: DAM (Red) and Homeostatic (Black) genes identified by single-cell RNA-seq mapped to WGCNA modules.

Abbreviations
AD: Alzheimer's disease; Aβ: Amyloid beta; DAM: Disease-associated-microglia; LPS: Lipopolysaccharide

Acknowledgements
We thank Dr. Heike Wulff (University of California Davis) for providing us with the mouse Kv1.3 construct.

Funding
Work supported by Emory Alzheimer's Disease Research Center Grant P50 AG025688, American Brain Foundation (SR #28301), Alzheimer's Association (SR #37102), NINDS (K08-NS099474–1), AMP-AD U01 AG046161 and Emory Neuroscience NINDS Core facilities (P30 NS055077).

Authors' contributions
Conceptualization: SR, EBD, SAR and AIL; Methodology: SR, EBD, SAR, NTS, AIL; Investigation: SR, EBD, SAR, DD, PR, TG and HX; Writing-Original draft: SR, EBD, SAR; Writing-Review and Editing: SR, EBD, SAR, AIL, JJL, NTS; Funding Acquisition: SR, AIL, NTS; Resources: MPW, AIL, NTS, JJL; Supervision: SR, AIL, JJL, NTS. All authors read and approved the final manuscript.

Ethics approval

Approval from the Emory University Institutional Animal Care and Use Committee was obtained prior to all animal-related studies (IACUC protocol # 300123).

Competing interests

The authors declare that they have no competing interests.

Author details

[1]Department of Neurology, Emory University, Atlanta, GA 30322, USA. [2]Department of Biochemistry, Emory University, Atlanta, GA 30322, USA. [3]Emory University, Atlanta, GA 30322, USA. [4]Peptides International, Louisville, KY 40269, USA.

References

1. Crotti A, Ransohoff RM. Microglial physiology and pathophysiology: insights from genome-wide transcriptional profiling. Immunity. 2016;44:505–15.
2. Prinz M, Priller J. Microglia and brain macrophages in the molecular age: from origin to neuropsychiatric disease. Nat Rev Neurosci. 2014;15:300–12.
3. Sarlus H, Heneka MT. Microglia in Alzheimer's disease. J Clin Invest. 2017;127:3240–9.
4. Perry VH, Nicoll JA, Holmes C. Microglia in neurodegenerative disease. Nat Rev Neurol. 2010;6:193–201.
5. Villegas-Llerena C, Phillips A, Garcia-Reitboeck P, Hardy J, Pocock JM. Microglial genes regulating neuroinflammation in the progression of Alzheimer's disease. Curr Opin Neurobiol. 2016;36:74–81.
6. Colonna M, Wang Y. TREM2 variants: new keys to decipher Alzheimer disease pathogenesis. Nat Rev Neurosci. 2016;17:201–7.
7. Jonsson T, Stefansson H, Steinberg S, Jonsdottir I, Jonsson PV, Snaedal J, Bjornsson S, Huttenlocher J, Levey AI, Lah JJ, et al. Variant of TREM2 associated with the risk of Alzheimer's disease. N Engl J Med. 2013;368:107–16.
8. Zhang B, Gaiteri C, Bodea LG, Wang Z, McElwee J, Podtelezhnikov AA, Zhang C, Xie T, Tran L, Dobrin R, et al. Integrated systems approach identifies genetic nodes and networks in late-onset Alzheimer's disease. Cell. 2013;153:707–20.
9. Keren-Shaul H, Spinrad A, Weiner A, Matcovitch-Natan O, Dvir-Szternfeld R, Ulland TK, David E, Baruch K, Lara-Astaiso D, Toth B, et al. A unique microglia type associated with restricting development of Alzheimer's disease. Cell. 2017;169:1276–90. e1217
10. Friedman BA, Srinivasan K, Ayalon G, Meilandt WJ, Lin H, Huntley MA, Cao Y, Lee SH, Haddick PCG, Ngu H, et al. Diverse brain myeloid expression profiles reveal distinct microglial activation states and aspects of Alzheimer's disease not evident in mouse models. Cell Rep. 2018;22:832–47.
11. Mathys H, Adaikkan C, Gao F, Young JZ, Manet E, Hemberg M, De Jager PL, Ransohoff RM, Regev A, Tsai LH. Temporal tracking of microglia activation in neurodegeneration at single-cell resolution. Cell Rep. 2017;21:366–80.
12. Chiu IM, Morimoto ET, Goodarzi H, Liao JT, O'Keeffe S, Phatnani HP, Muratet M, Carroll MC, Levy S, Tavazoie S, et al. A neurodegeneration-specific gene-expression signature of acutely isolated microglia from an amyotrophic lateral sclerosis mouse model. Cell Rep. 2013;4:385–401.
13. Holtman IR, Raj DD, Miller JA, Schaafsma W, Yin Z, Brouwer N, Wes PD, Moller T, Orre M, Kamphuis W, et al. Induction of a common microglia gene expression signature by aging and neurodegenerative conditions: a co-expression meta-analysis. Acta Neuropathol Commun. 2015;3:31.
14. Jay TR, Miller CM, Cheng PJ, Graham LC, Bemiller S, Broihier ML, Xu G, Margevicius D, Karlo JC, Sousa GL, et al. TREM2 deficiency eliminates TREM2 + inflammatory macrophages and ameliorates pathology in Alzheimer's disease mouse models. J Exp Med. 2015;212:287–95.
15. Wang Y, Cella M, Mallinson K, Ulrich JD, Young KL, Robinette ML, Gilfillan S, Krishnan GM, Sudhakar S, Zinselmeyer BH, et al. TREM2 lipid sensing sustains the microglial response in an Alzheimer's disease model. Cell. 2015;160:1061–71.
16. Krasemann S, Madore C, Cialic R, Baufeld C, Calcagno N, El Fatimy R, Beckers L, O'Loughlin E, Xu Y, Fanek Z, et al. The TREM2-APOE pathway drives the transcriptional phenotype of dysfunctional microglia in neurodegenerative diseases. Immunity. 2017;47:566–81. e569
17. Wang Y, Ulland TK, Ulrich JD, Song W, Tzaferis JA, Hole JT, Yuan P, Mahan TE, Shi Y, Gilfillan S, et al. TREM2-mediated early microglial response limits diffusion and toxicity of amyloid plaques. J Exp Med. 2016;213:667–75.
18. Spangenberg EE, Lee RJ, Najafi AR, Rice RA, Elmore MR, Blurton-Jones M, West BL, Green KN. Eliminating microglia in Alzheimer's mice prevents neuronal loss without modulating amyloid-beta pathology. Brain. 2016;139:1265–81.
19. Han J, Harris RA, Zhang XM. An updated assessment of microglia depletion: current concepts and future directions. Mol Brain. 2017;10:25.
20. Shemer A, Erny D, Jung S, Prinz M. Microglia plasticity during health and disease: an immunological perspective. Trends Immunol. 2015;36:614–24.
21. Terwel D, Steffensen KR, Verghese PB, Kummer MP, Gustafsson JA, Holtzman DM, Heneka MT. Critical role of astroglial apolipoprotein E and liver X receptor-alpha expression for microglial Abeta phagocytosis. J Neurosci. 2011;31:7049–59.
22. Orre M, Kamphuis W, Osborn LM, Jansen AH, Kooijman L, Bossers K, Hol EM. Isolation of glia from Alzheimer's mice reveals inflammation and dysfunction. Neurobiol Aging. 2014;35:2746–60.
23. Freilich RW, Woodbury ME, Ikezu T. Integrated expression profiles of mRNA and miRNA in polarized primary murine microglia. PLoS One. 2013;8:e79416.
24. Oakley H, Cole SL, Logan S, Maus E, Shao P, Craft J, Guillozet-Bongaarts A, Ohno M, Disterhoft J, Van Eldik L, et al. Intraneuronal beta-amyloid aggregates, neurodegeneration, and neuron loss in transgenic mice with five familial Alzheimer's disease mutations: potential factors in amyloid plaque formation. J Neurosci. 2006;26:10129–40.
25. Pennington MW, Chang SC, Chauhan S, Huq R, Tajhya RB, Chhabra S, Norton RS, Beeton C. Development of highly selective Kv1.3-blocking peptides based on the sea anemone peptide ShK. Mar Drugs. 2015;13:529–42.
26. Rangaraju S, Raza SA, Pennati A, Deng Q, Dammer EB, Duong D, Pennington MW, Tansey MG, Lah JJ, Betarbet R, et al. A systems pharmacology-based approach to identify novel Kv1.3 channel-dependent mechanisms in microglial activation. J Neuroinflammation. 2017;14:128.
27. Beeton C, Wulff H, Singh S, Botsko S, Crossley G, Gutman GA, Cahalan MD, Pennington M, Chandy KG. A novel fluorescent toxin to detect and investigate Kv1.3 channel up-regulation in chronically activated T lymphocytes. J Biol Chem. 2003;278:9928–37.
28. Lee JK, Tansey MG. Microglia isolation from adult mouse brain. Methods Mol Biol. 2013;1041:17–23.
29. Hohsfield LA, Humpel C. Migration of blood cells to beta-amyloid plaques in Alzheimer's disease. Exp Gerontol. 2015;65:8–15.
30. Strauss-Ayali D, Conrad SM, Mosser DM. Monocyte subpopulations and their differentiation patterns during infection. J Leukoc Biol. 2007;82:244–52.
31. Rangaraju S, Raza SA, Li NX, Betarbet R, Dammer EB, Duong D, Lah JJ, Seyfried NT, Levey AI. Differential phagocytic properties of CD45(low) microglia and CD45(high) brain mononuclear phagocytes-activation and age-related effects. Front Immunol. 2018;9:405.
32. Chen Z, Jalabi W, Shpargel KB, Farabaugh KT, Dutta R, Yin X, Kidd GJ, Bergmann CC, Stohlman SA, Trapp BD. Lipopolysaccharide-induced microglial activation and neuroprotection against experimental brain injury is independent of hematogenous TLR4. J Neurosci. 2012;32:11706–15.
33. Ritchie ME, Silver J, Oshlack A, Holmes M, Diyagama D, Holloway A, Smyth GK. A comparison of background correction methods for two-colour microarrays. Bioinformatics. 2007;23:2700–7.
34. Seyfried NT, Dammer EB, Swarup V, Nandakumar D, Duong DM, Yin L, Deng Q, Nguyen T, Hales CM, Wingo T, et al. A multi-network approach identifies protein-specific co-expression in asymptomatic and symptomatic Alzheimer's disease. Cell Syst. 2017;4:60–72. e64
35. Amir el AD, Davis KL, Tadmor MD, Simonds EF, Levine JH, Bendall SC, Shenfeld DK, Krishnaswamy S, Nolan GP, Pe'er D. viSNE enables visualization of high dimensional single-cell data and reveals phenotypic heterogeneity of leukemia. Nat Biotechnol. 2013;31:545–52.
36. Schmittgen TD, Livak KJ. Analyzing real-time PCR data by the comparative CT method. Nat Protocols. 2008;3:1101–8.
37. Lamb J, Crawford ED, Peck D, Modell JW, Blat IC, Wrobel MJ, Lerner J, Brunet JP, Subramanian A, Ross KN, et al. The connectivity map: using gene-expression signatures to connect small molecules, genes, and disease. Science. 2006;313:1929–35.

38. Landel V, Baranger K, Virard I, Loriod B, Khrestchatisky M, Rivera S, Benech P, Feron F. Temporal gene profiling of the 5XFAD transgenic mouse model highlights the importance of microglial activation in Alzheimer's disease. Mol Neurodegen. 2014;9:33.

39. Bennett ML, Bennett FC, Liddelow SA, Ajami B, Zamanian JL, Fernhoff NB, Mulinyawe SB, Bohlen CJ, Adil A, Tucker A, et al. New tools for studying microglia in the mouse and human CNS. Proc Natl Acad Sci U S A. 2016;113:E1738–46.

40. Secor McVoy JR, Oughli HA, Oh U. Liver X receptor-dependent inhibition of microglial nitric oxide synthase 2. J Neuroinflammation. 2015;12:27.

41. Savage JC, Jay T, Goduni E, Quigley C, Mariani MM, Malm T, Ransohoff RM, Lamb BT, Landreth GE. Nuclear receptors license phagocytosis by trem2+ myeloid cells in mouse models of Alzheimer's disease. J Neurosci. 2015;35:6532–43.

42. Riddell DR, Zhou H, Comery TA, Kouranova E, Lo CF, Warwick HK, Ring RH, Kirksey Y, Aschmies S, Xu J, et al. The LXR agonist TO901317 selectively lowers hippocampal Abeta42 and improves memory in the Tg2576 mouse model of Alzheimer's disease. Mol Cell Neurosci. 2007;34:621–8.

43. Ponomarev ED, Veremeyko T, Barteneva N, Krichevsky AM, Weiner HL. MicroRNA-124 promotes microglia quiescence and suppresses EAE by deactivating macrophages via the C/EBP-alpha-PU.1 pathway. Nat Med. 2011;17:64–70.

44. Zhang B, Horvath S. A general framework for weighted gene co-expression network analysis. Stat Appl Genet Mol Biol. 2005;4:1-37. Article17. https://doi.org/10.2202/1544-6115.1128.

45. Kamphuis W, Kooijman L, Schetters S, Orre M, Hol EM. Transcriptional profiling of CD11c-positive microglia accumulating around amyloid plaques in a mouse model for Alzheimer's disease. Biochim Biophys Acta. 1862;2016:1847–60.

46. Korin B, Dubovik T, Rolls A. Mass cytometry analysis of immune cells in the brain. Nat Protoc. 2018;13:377–91.

47. Korin B, Ben-Shaanan TL, Schiller M, Dubovik T, Azulay-Debby H, Boshnak NT, Koren T, Rolls A. High-dimensional, single-cell characterization of the brain's immune compartment. Nat Neurosci. 2017;20:1300–9.

48. Rangaraju S, Gearing M, Jin LW, Levey A. Potassium channel Kv1.3 is highly expressed by microglia in human Alzheimer's disease. J Alzheimers Dis. 2015;44:797–808.

49. Maezawa I, Nguyen HM, Di Lucente J, Jenkins DP, Singh V, Hilt S, Kim K, Rangaraju S, Levey AI, Wulff H, Jin LW. Kv1.3 inhibition as a potential microglia-targeted therapy for Alzheimer's disease: preclinical proof of concept. Brain. 2018;141:596–612.

50. Nguyen HM, Grossinger EM, Horiuchi M, Davis KW, Jin LW, Maezawa I, Wulff H. Differential Kv1.3, KCa3.1, and Kir2.1 expression in "classically" and "alternatively" activated microglia. Glia. 2017;65:106–21.

51. Liu J, Xu C, Chen L, Xu P, Xiong H. Involvement of Kv1.3 and p38 MAPK signaling in HIV-1 glycoprotein 120-induced microglia neurotoxicity. Cell Death Dis. 2012;3:e254.

52. Fordyce CB, Jagasia R, Zhu X, Schlichter LC. Microglia Kv1.3 channels contribute to their ability to kill neurons. J Neurosci. 2005;25:7139–49.

53. Tarcha EJ, Olsen CM, Probst P, Peckham D, Munoz-Elias EJ, Kruger JG, Iadonato SP. Safety and pharmacodynamics of dalazatide, a Kv1.3 channel inhibitor, in the treatment of plaque psoriasis: a randomized phase 1b trial. PLoS One. 2017;12:e0180762.

54. Tarcha EJ, Chi V, Munoz-Elias EJ, Bailey D, Londono LM, Upadhyay SK, Norton K, Banks A, Tjong I, Nguyen H, et al. Durable pharmacological responses from the peptide ShK-186, a specific Kv1.3 channel inhibitor that suppresses T cell mediators of autoimmune disease. J Pharmacol Exp Ther. 2012;342:642–53.

55. Hickman SE, Allison EK, El Khoury J. Microglial dysfunction and defective beta-amyloid clearance pathways in aging Alzheimer's disease mice. J Neurosci. 2008;28:8354–60.

56. de Leeuw CA, Mooij JM, Heskes T, Posthuma D. MAGMA: generalized gene-set analysis of GWAS data. PLoS Comput Biol. 2015;11:e1004219.

57. Sniekers S, Stringer S, Watanabe K, Jansen PR, Coleman JRI, Krapohl E, Taskesen E, Hammerschlag AR, Okbay A, Zabaneh D, et al. Genome-wide association meta-analysis of 78,308 individuals identifies new loci and genes influencing human intelligence. Nat Genet. 2017;49:1107–12.

58. Hyman BT, Phelps CH, Beach TG, Bigio EH, Cairns NJ, Carrillo MC, Dickson DW, Duyckaerts C, Frosch MP, Masliah E, et al. National Institute on Aging-Alzheimer's Association guidelines for the neuropathologic assessment of Alzheimer's disease. Alzheimers Dement. 2012;8:1–13.

59. Zhang Y, Chen K, Sloan SA, Bennett ML, Scholze AR, O'Keeffe S, Phatnani HP, Guarnieri P, Caneda C, Ruderisch N, et al. An RNA-sequencing transcriptome and splicing database of glia, neurons, and vascular cells of the cerebral cortex. J Neurosci. 2014;34:11929–47.

60. Chiang EY, Li T, Jeet S, Peng I, Zhang J, Lee WP, DeVoss J, Caplazi P, Chen J, Warming S, et al. Potassium channels Kv1.3 and KCa3.1 cooperatively and compensatorily regulate antigen-specific memory T cell functions. Nat Commun. 2017;8:14644.

61. Grosse G, Draguhn A, Hohne L, Tapp R, Veh RW, Ahnert-Hilger G. Expression of Kv1 potassium channels in mouse hippocampal primary cultures: development and activity-dependent regulation. J Neurosci. 2000;20:1869–82.

62. Peng Y, Lu K, Li Z, Zhao Y, Wang Y, Hu B, Xu P, Shi X, Zhou B, Pennington M, et al. Blockade of Kv1.3 channels ameliorates radiation-induced brain injury. Neuro-Oncology. 2014;16:528–39.

63. Rangaraju S, Chi V, Pennington MW, Chandy KG. Kv1.3 potassium channels as a therapeutic target in multiple sclerosis. Expert Opin Ther Targets. 2009;13:909–24.

64. Wolf Y, Yona S, Kim KW, Jung S. Microglia, seen from the CX3CR1 angle. Front Cell Neurosci. 2013;7:26.

65. Liu G, Bi Y, Xue L, Zhang Y, Yang H, Chen X, Lu Y, Zhang Z, Liu H, Wang X, et al. Dendritic cell SIRT1-HIF1alpha axis programs the differentiation of CD4+ T cells through IL-12 and TGF-beta1. Proc Natl Acad Sci U S A. 2015;112:E957–65.

66. Wynne AM, Henry CJ, Huang Y, Cleland A, Godbout JP. Protracted downregulation of CX3CR1 on microglia of aged mice after lipopolysaccharide challenge. Brain Behav Immun. 2010;24:1190–201.

67. De Rossi P, Buggia-Prevot V, Clayton BL, Vasquez JB, van Sanford C, Andrew RJ, Lesnick R, Botte A, Deyts C, Salem S, et al. Predominant expression of Alzheimer's disease-associated BIN1 in mature oligodendrocytes and localization to white matter tracts. Mol Neurodegen. 2016;11:59.

68. Sharma K, Schmitt S, Bergner CG, Tyanova S, Kannaiyan N, Manrique-Hoyos N, Kongi K, Cantuti L, Hanisch UK, Philips MA, et al. Cell type- and brain region-resolved mouse brain proteome. Nat Neurosci. 2015;18:1819–31.

69. Zheng H, Liu CC, Atagi Y, Chen XF, Jia L, Yang L, He W, Zhang X, Kang SS, Rosenberry TL, et al. Opposing roles of the triggering receptor expressed on myeloid cells 2 and triggering receptor expressed on myeloid cells-like transcript 2 in microglia activation. Neurobiol Aging. 2016;42:132–41.

7

The Trem2 R47H Alzheimer's risk variant impairs splicing and reduces Trem2 mRNA and protein in mice but not in humans

Xianyuan Xiang[1,2], Thomas M. Piers[3], Benedikt Wefers[4,6], Kaichuan Zhu[4,5], Anna Mallach[3], Bettina Brunner[4], Gernot Kleinberger[1,5], Wilbur Song[7], Marco Colonna[7], Jochen Herms[4,5,8], Wolfgang Wurst[4,5,6,9], Jennifer M. Pocock[3] and Christian Haass[1,4,5*]

Abstract

Background: The R47H variant of the Triggering Receptor Expressed on Myeloid cells 2 (TREM2) significantly increases the risk for late onset Alzheimer's disease. Mouse models accurately reproducing phenotypes observed in Alzheimer' disease patients carrying the R47H coding variant are required to understand the TREM2 related dysfunctions responsible for the enhanced risk for late onset Alzheimer's disease.

Methods: A CRISPR/Cas9-assisted gene targeting strategy was used to generate Trem2 R47H knock-in mice. Trem2 mRNA and protein levels as well as Trem2 splicing patterns were assessed in these mice, in iPSC-derived human microglia-like cells, and in human brains from Alzheimer's patients carrying the TREM2 R47H risk factor.

Results: Two independent Trem2 R47H knock-in mouse models show reduced Trem2 mRNA and protein production. In both mouse models Trem2 haploinsufficiency was due to atypical splicing of mouse Trem2 R47H, which introduced a premature stop codon. Cellular splicing assays using minigene constructs demonstrate that the R47H variant induced abnormal splicing only occurs in mice but not in humans. TREM2 mRNA levels and splicing patterns were both normal in iPSC-derived human microglia-like cells and patient brains with the TREM2 R47H variant.

Conclusions: The Trem2 R47H variant activates a cryptic splice site that generates miss-spliced transcripts leading to Trem2 haploinsufficiency only in mice but not in humans. Since Trem2 R47H related phenotypes are mouse specific and do not occur in humans, humanized TREM2 R47H knock-in mice should be generated to study the cellular consequences caused by the human TREM2 R47H coding variant. Currently described phenotypes of Trem2 R47H knock-in mice can therefore not be translated to humans.

Keywords: Alzheimer's disease, Microglia, Neurodegeneration, TREM2, Pre-mRNA splicing, Human microglia

Background

Microgliosis has long been thought to play a central role in the initiation and progression of Alzheimer's disease (AD) pathology. Indeed, genetic analyses recently revealed risk variants in a number of genes exclusively or at least preferentially expressed in microglia [1–5]. Among these, the gene encoding the triggering receptor

expressed on myeloid cells 2 (TREM2) plays a pivotal role in regulating microglial activity [6–9]. As part of the disease associated signature of microglia (DAM; also called MGnD (microglia neurodegenerative disease)), TREM2 is one of the most upregulated genes when microglia encounter acute injuries within the brain or respond to neurodegenerative disorders such as AD and amyotrophic lateral sclerosis [6, 10]. Moreover, absence of functional TREM2 caused by a gene knockout or certain disease-associated sequence variants, which misfold TREM2 and retain the protein within the endoplasmic reticulum, lock microglia in a homeostatic state and

* Correspondence: christian.haass@mail03.med.uni-muenchen.de
[1]Metabolic Biochemistry, Biomedical Center (BMC), Faculty of Medicine, Ludwig-Maximilians-Universität München, Munich, Germany
[4]German Center for Neurodegenerative Diseases (DZNE) Munich, Munich, Germany
Full list of author information is available at the end of the article

prevent their activation in vivo [7, 11]. As a consequence cellular defense mechanisms such as chemotaxis, prominently visible by the lack of clustering around amyloid plaques, proliferation, phagocytosis of dead cells and amyloid fibrils are all reduced [8, 12, 13]. Furthermore, overexpression of human wild-type (wt) TREM2 in a Trem2 knockout mouse corrects loss-of-function phenotypes [14]. Thus TREM2 is believed to have protective functions. In line with that, TREM2 is upregulated early during disease development. In a study on patients with dominantly inherited AD (DIAN), soluble TREM2 was found to be increased 5 years before onset of clinical symptoms, which may also be interpreted as a protective response [15]. Consistent with this conclusion, lack of functional TREM2 affects amyloid plaque morphology and increases plaque associated neuritic dystrophies [13, 16]. Furthermore, in models of acute neuronal injury such as the cuprizone model, Trem2 activity facilitates clearance of cellular debris and recovery [11, 17, 18]. For tauopathies there are, however, opposing results indicating either protective or detrimental functions [19, 20]. In line with findings in mouse models for amyloid plaque pathology, this may be due to stage specific functions of Trem2.

Mouse models and cellular systems greatly helped to understand the consequences of loss-of-function mutations / haploinsufficiency of TREM2. However, the most important disease variant, namely R47H, which has been shown to increase the risk for late onset AD to a similar extent as the Apo lipoprotein E (ApoE) ε4 allele [3, 4], has been much less investigated. In cultured cells TREM2 R47H reduces ligand binding [8, 21–23]. Consistent with a pivotal role in ligand binding, structural analyses revealed that arginine 47 is required to stabilize a conformation, which is capable to interact with ligands such as ApoE and phosphatidylserine [24]. Furthermore maturation of the R47H variant within the secretory pathway may also be delayed [25]. In line with these findings, expression of human TREM2 R47H in Trem2 knockout mice failed to rescue their phenotypes [14]. These findings may therefore be indicative of a loss-of-function. In fact, very recently CRISPR/Cas9 generated mouse models expressing the R47H variant within the endogenous Trem2 mouse locus revealed a significant loss-of function [26, 27]. Trem2 R47H mice exhibited reduced Trem2 upregulation in microglia, reduced microgliosis, reduced clustering around amyloid plaques and an overall reduction of Trem2 protein [26]. Haploinsufficiency of Trem2 was confirmed by a significant reduction of Trem2 mRNA derived from the mutant allele [26]. Thus heterozygous Trem2 R47H mice appear to phenocopy a heterozygous knockout of Trem2.

We also independently generated Trem2 R47H knock-in mice using the CRISPR/Cas9 technology and reproduced haploinsufficiency of Trem2 in this model.

Moreover, we could demonstrate that reduced mRNA stability due to a splicing error leads to a severe reduction of Trem2 mRNA. However, aberrant splicing was mouse specific and could not be observed in humans. Thus phenotypes associated with the R47H variant inserted into the endogenous mouse locus may not allow conclusions on the cellular mechanisms affected in humans.

Methods
Mice
Animal handling and animal experiments were performed in accordance to local animal laws and housed in standard cages in a specific pathogen-free facility on a 12-h light/dark cycle with ad libitum access to food and water.

Jax Trem2 R47H knock-in mice were purchased from Jackson laboratory. In-house Trem2 R47H knock-in mice were generated using CRISPR/Cas9 technology in C57BL/6 N background. Both strains were housed and bred in the same animal facility. To extract bone marrow, mice were first euthanized by CO_2 followed by cervical dislocation.

Generation of Trem2 R47H knock-in mice
Trem2 R47H knock-in mice (R47H ki mice) were generated by CRISPR/Cas9-assisted gene targeting in zygotes as described previously [28, 29]. Briefly, pronuclear stage zygotes were obtained by mating C57BL/6 N males with superovulated C57BL/6 N females (Charles River). Embryos were then microinjected into the male pronucleus with an injection mix containing 25 ng/µl Cas9 mRNA, 12.5 ng/µl Trem2-specific sgRNA, and 25 ng/µl single-stranded oligodeoxynucleotide (ssODN). Cas9 mRNA was prepared from XbaI-linerized pCAG-Cas9v2-162A by in vitro transcription using the mMESSAGE mMACHINE™ T7 ULTRA Transcription Kit (Thermo Fisher Scientific, #AM1345) and purified using the MEGAclear™ Transcription Clean-Up Kit (Thermo Fisher Scientific, #AM1908). Trem2-specific sgRNA (protospacer: GAAGCACTG GGGGAGACGCA) was prepared by IVT from pBS-T7-sgTrem2 using the MEGAshortscript™ T7 Transcription Kit (Thermo Fisher Scientific, #AM1354) and purified with the MEGAclear™ Transcription Clean-Up Kit. The 130 nt ssODN targeting molecule ssTrem2 R47H (5′- GGGC ATGGCCGGCCAGTCCTTGAGGGTGTCATGTACTTA TGACGCCTTGAAGCACTGGGG**TC**GAC**A**CAA**A**GCC TGGTGTCGGCAGCTGGGTGAGGAGG**G**CCCATGCC AGCGTGTGGTGAGCACACACGGT -3′), comprising the G > A substitution (underlined) and three additional silent mutations (bold), was synthetized by Metabion. After microinjection, zygotes were cultured in KSOM medium until they were transferred into pseudopregnant CD-1 foster animals.

Off-target analysis of Trem2 R47H mice

To identify putative off-target sites of the Trem2-specific sgRNA, the online tool CRISPOR (http://crispor.tefor.net/) [30] was used. Predicted sites with a CFD score > 0.5 and an MIT score > 0.6 were chosen for off-target analysis. For analysis, genomic DNA of wildtype and heterozygous mutant Trem2 R47H mice was isolated and the loci were PCR amplified with primers flanking the putative cut sites. PCR amplicons were subsequently Sanger sequenced using PCR amplification primers and the traces compared to a reference sequence.

Bone marrow derived macrophages culture

Bone marrow derived macrophages (BMDM) were prepared as previously described [31, 32]. Briefly, the bone marrow cells were flushed out using advanced RPMI 1640 (Life Technologies). Cells were differentiated using advanced RPMI 1640 supplemented with 2 mM L-Glutamine, 10% (v/v)) fetal calf serum (FCS), 100 U/ml penicillin, 100 µg/ml streptomycin and 50 ng/ml murine M-CSF (R&D System) for 7 days in non-cell culture treated dishes.

Microglia isolation

Microglia were isolated as previously described with some modification [33]. Wild type and Trem2 R47H ki mice were perfused with cold phosphate buffered saline (PBS). Whole brain without the cerebellum was cut into small pieces and gently homogenized by mechanical dissociation in homogenization buffer (HBSS no calcium, no magnesium, with phenol red; 15 mM HEPES, 0.6% glucose). Homogenized cell suspensions were passed through a 100 µm cell strainer. Cells were pelleted at 300 g for 10 min and the supernatant discarded. To remove myelin, the cell pellets were re-suspended in 22% percoll (GE Healthcare) and centrifuged for 20 min at 900 g (acceleration 4, deceleration 0). Microglia were purified from the pellet using MACS CD11b magnetic beads according to manufacturer's instructions. Briefly, 20 µl CD11b microbeads (Miltenyi) were incubated with cell suspension for 15 min. After incubation, 500 µl MACS buffer were added and cells were passed over a pre-rinsed Miltenyi LS column attached to a magnetic field. The column was washed three times with 500 µl MACS buffer, removed from the magnetic field and CD11b positive cells were washed out in 5 ml of MACS buffer.

Cell lysis and immunoblotting

To detect membrane bound Trem2, membrane fractions were collected as previously described [32]. Briefly, cells were lysed in hypotonic buffer (100 mM Tris-HCl, pH 7.4, 1 mM EDTA, 1 mM EGTA, pH 7.4) freshly supplemented with a protease inhibitors cocktail (Sigma-Aldrich). Membrane fractions were pelleted by centrifugation for 45 min at 16,000 g at 4 °C. Membranes were lysed in STEN lysis buffer (150 mM NaCl, 50 mM Tris-HCl, pH 7.6, 2 mM EDTA, 1% Triton-X 100) on ice for 20 min. Equal amounts of protein were mixed with Laemmli sample buffer supplemented with β mercaptoethanol followed by by SDS-PAGE. Proteins were transferred onto polyvinylidene difluoride membranes (Amersham Hybond P 0.45 PVDF, GE Healthcare Life Science) and blocked in 10% I-BlockTM (Thermo Fisher Scientific) for 1 h. Monoclonal antibody 5F4 (dilution 1:100) [32] was used to detect Trem2.

iPSC generation

Ethical permission for this study was obtained from the National Hospital for Neurology and Neurosurgery and the Institute of Neurology joint research ethics committee (study reference 09/H0716/64). R47H heterozygous fibroblasts were acquired with a material transfer agreement between University College London and University of California Irvine Alzheimer's Disease Research Center (UCI ADRC; M Blurton-Jones). Fibroblast reprogramming was performed by episomal plasmid nucleofection (Lonza) as previously described [34], using plasmids obtained from Addgene (#27077, #27078 and #27080). Nucleofected cultures were transferred to Essential 8 medium (Life Technologies) after 7 days in vitro (DIV) and individual colonies were picked after 25–30 DIV. All iPSCs were maintained and routinely passaged in Essential 8 medium. Karyotype analysis was performed by The Doctors Laboratory (London, UK). Control iPSC lines used in this study are as follows: CTRL1 (kindly provided by Dr. Selina Wray, UCL Institute of Neurology); CTRL2 (SBAD03, Stembancc); CTRL3 (SFC840, Stembancc); CTRL4 (BIONi010-C, EBiSC).

iPSC-derived microglia-like cells (iMG)

Using previously described protocols, iPSC-derived microglia-like cells (iMG) were generated [35, 36].

Day 0: iPSC lines were cultured to 60% confluency in E8 medium on vitronectin-coated 6-well plates. Cells were washed with PBS (w/o Ca2+/Mg2+), followed by trypLE digestion (1 ml/well; 4 min at 37 °C). The solution was added to 4 volumes of PBS (w/o Ca2+/Mg2+), and triturated to a single cell suspension. The suspension was centrifuged for 3 min at 300 g and the cell pellet resuspended in 1 ml EB differentiation medium (Adapted from [36]; EBdiff; Essential 8, 50 ng/ml BMP-4, 50 ng/ml VEGF, 20 ng/ml SCF, and 10 µM Y-27632). Cells were counted, and resuspended in EBDiff medium to a density of 10^5 cells/ml. To generate embryoid bodies (EBs), 100 µl of the suspension was added to 96 well ultra-low attachment round bottom tissue culture plates (Corning), centrifuged at 115 g for 3 min, and transferred to a tissue culture incubator at 37 °C with 5% CO2.

Day 2: 50 μl of EBdiff medium was added to each well.

Day 3: Dense EBs were formed and collected with a P1000 Gilson pipette into a sterile 15 ml tube, and left to settle. The spent EBdiff medium was discarded and 10 ml of myeloid differentiation medium (Mdiff; X-VIVO 15 medium (Lonza), 1X Glutamax (Life Technologies), 100 U Penicillin/Streptomycin (Life Technologies), 50 μM β-mercaptoethanol (Life Technologies), 100 ng/ml MCSF (Peprotech), and 25 ng/ml IL-3 (Cell Guidance Systems)) added. Approximately 150 embryoid bodies (1.5 × 96 well plates) were transferred to a 175 cm2 flask containing a further 20 ml of Mdiff medium.

Day 9–11: Mdiff medium (30 ml) was added, to avoid acidosis, being careful not to disturb the EBs.

Day 26: Cells were collected from the medium for myeloid marker analysis.

Day 33: Once a week, 1/2 of the Mdiff medium/flask containing budded myeloid cells was collected through a 40 μm cell strainer (Falcon, Corning), replacing the collected medium with fresh Mdiff. The myeloid cell suspension was centrifuged for 3 min at 300 g and the cell pellet resuspended in 1 ml microglial differentiation medium (Adapted from [35]; MGdiff; DMEM/F12 HEPES no phenol red, 2% ITS-G (Life Technologies), 1% N2 supplement (Life Technologies), 200 μM mono-thioglycerol (Sigma), 1X Glutamax, 1X NEAA (Life Technologies), 5 μg/ml Insulin (Sigma), 100 ng/ml IL34 (Peprotech), 25 ng/ml MCSF and 5 ng/ml TGFβ1 (Peprotech), filtered through a 0.22 μm syringe filter. Cells were counted and plated in MGdiff, and medium replaced every 3–4 days.

Day 46: MGdiff medium was replaced with microglial maturation medium (MGmat: MGdiff + 100 ng/ml CD200 (Generon), and 100 ng/ml CX3CL1 (Peprotech)) for 4 days to generate iMG.

Isolation of human blood derived-monocytes

Monocytes were obtained from blood through centrifugation with Histopaque (Sigma) to isolate peripheral blood mononuclear cells followed by separation and purification with CD14-conjugated magnetic beads (Miltenyi). Peripheral blood monocytes (PBM) were matured into monocyte-derived macrophages (hMacs) in X-VIVO 15 medium with 1% Glutamax, 100 U Penicillin/Streptomycin, and 100 ng/ml MCSF for 7 days.

Microglia signature gene array

A custom gene array based on published microglial expression data [35, 37–39] was used to confirm a microglial signature in our iMG cultures (TaqMan Array Plate 32 plus Candidate Endogenous Control Genes; Thermo Fisher Scientific). Complementary DNA was generated from iMG, iPSC-derived microglial-like cells [36], and human monocyte-derived macrophages

(hMacs) RNA samples using the High-Capacity RNA-cDNA kit (Life Technologies), according to the manufacturer's instructions. Human primary microglia cDNA was also analyzed as a control sample (ScienCell). Quantitative PCR were conducted on the Mx3000p qPCR system with MxPro qPCR software (Stratagene) using TaqMan Gene Expression Mastermix (Thermo Fisher Scientific). Heat maps were generated with the gplots [40] and d3heatmap [41] packages in R.

Microglial gene signature primer details:

Gene name	Primer ID
18 s rRNA	Hs99999901_s1
GAPDH	Hs99999905_m1
HPRT	Hs99999909_m1
GUSB	Hs99999908_m1
APOE	Hs00171168_m1
C1QA	Hs00706358_s1
C1QB	Hs00608019_m1
ITGAM	Hs00167304_m1
CSF1R	Hs00911250_m1
CX3CR1	Hs01922583_s1
GAS6	Hs01090305_m1
GPR34	Hs00271105_s1
AIF1	Hs00610419_g1
MERTK	Hs01031979_m1
OLFML3	Hs01113293_g1
PROS1	Hs00165590_m1
SALL1	Hs01548765_m1
SLCO2B1	Hs01030343_m1
TGFBR1	Hs00610320_m1
TMEM119	Hs01938722_u1
TREM2	Hs00219132_m1
BIN1	Hs00184913_m1
CD33	Hs01076282_g1
SPI1	Hs02786711_m1
HEXB	Hs01077594_m1
ITM2B	Hs00222753_m1
C3	Hs00163811_m1
A2M	Hs00929971_m1
C1QC	Hs00757779_m1
RGS1	Hs01023772_m1
FTL	Hs00830226_gH
P2RY12	Hs01881698_s1

Immunocytochemistry

Cells were fixed in 4% PFA/sucrose in PBS for 20 min at room temperature (RT), quenched with 50 mM NH4Cl in PBS for 10 min at RT, and permebalized with 0.2% Triton X-100 in PBS for 5 min at RT. Blocking was performed with 5% normal goat serum (NGS) in PBS for 30 min. Primary antibodies were diluted in 5% NGS/PBS and incubated at RT for 2 h, followed by PBS washes and incubation with corresponding secondary antibodies for 1 h at RT in the dark, with gentle rocking. Nuclei were counterstained during mounting using Vectorshield with DAPI (4′, 6-diamidino-2-phenylindol; Vector Labs). Fluorescence microscopy was performed on a Zeiss Axioskop 2 microscope and Axiovison software (Zeiss, v4.8). Confocal microscopy was performed on a Zeiss LSM 710 confocal microscope using Zen software (Zeiss, Version 2012), and all images were processed with Image J1.51 K (https://imagej.nih.gov/ij/). The following antibodies were used: mouse anti-CD68 (1:100, DAKO), rabbit-anti-P2YR12 (1:200, Atlas Antibodies), mouse-anti-β-Actin (1:500, Sigma), mouse-anti-EZR (1:250, Atlas Antibodies), goat anti-rabbit Alexafluor488 (1:500, Life Technologies), goat-anti-mouse Alexafluor568 (1:500, Life Technologies).

Cellular splicing assay

Human and mouse Trem2 genomic fragments encoding exon 1, intron 1, exon 2, and a FLAG tag were synthesized by Integrated DNA Technologies. The following primer sets were used for vector cloning: EcoRV-Hs TREM2-Fw (GGATATCCGGGCAGCGCCTGACATGCCTG) and No tI-Hs TREM2-Rv (ATGCGGCCGCTTAGGATTACAA GGATGACGACGATAAG); HindIII-Mm Trem2 Fw (CC CAAGCTTGGGGCGCCTACCCTAGTCC) and XohvI-Mm Trem2-Rv (CCGCTCGAGCGGCTACTTGTCGTCA TCG). The amplified fragments were digested by EcoRV/ NotI or HindIII/XohI and the digested fragments were inserted into pcDNA3.1 (+) (Invitrogen). The mutations were introduced in the human and mouse minigene using the Quikchange™ site-directed mutagenesis kit (Agilent). The following mutants were generated:

(1) R47H is the G > A variant alone encoding arginine;
(2) R47H^TCA corresponds to sequence variants expressed by the in-house generated Trem2 R47H ki mice (GA > TC, G > A, G > A; also see Fig. 4b);
(3) R47H^AA represents the Trem2 R47H ki mice generated by Jackson Laboratory (G > A, G > A, C > A; also see Fig. 4b);

(4) TC are the silent mutations in in-house generated Trem2 R47H ki mice (GA > TC)
(5) AA are the silent mutations in Jax R47H ki mice (G > A, C > A).
(6) R47H^T represents Trem2 R47H ki mice generated by Cheng Hathaway et al. [26]

For the cellular splicing assay 8×10^5 HEK293 cells were seeded in 6-well plates with Dulbecco's Modified Eagle Medium (Life Technologies) supplemented with GlutaMAX™, 10% (v/v) FCS, 100 U/ml penicillin, 100 µg/ml streptomycin and cultured overnight. Cells were transfected with 3 µg of plasmids to express human or mouse Trem2 minigenes using 6 µl lipofectamine 2000 according the manufacturer's instructions (Thermo Fisher Scientific). Transfected cells were cultured in normal medium for 48 h and collected for RNA extraction using RNeasy Mini Kit (Qiagen) according the manufacturer's instructions. The RNA was used for Reverse transcription polymerase chain reaction (RT-PCR).

Reverse transcription polymerase chain reaction

1 µg of total RNA was transcribed into cDNA using SuperScript IV reverse transcriptase and oligo dT (Thermo Fisher Scientific). 2 µl of cDNA was used as template and amplified by polymerase chain reaction (PCR) with GoTaq DNA polymerase (Promega) according the manufacturer's instructions. The reaction condition and primer sequences are listed in Table 1. The PCR products were loaded into 2% agarose gel with GelRed™ (Biotium) for DNA visualization.

Quantitative real-time polymerase chain reaction

RNeasy Mini Kit (Qiagen) was used for total RNA isolation according the manufacturer's instructions. 1 µg of total RNA was transcribed into cDNA using SuperScript IV reverse transcriptase and oligo dT (Thermo Fisher Scientific). RNA levels of human and mouse Trem2 and Tyrobp were analyzed by Taqman® real-time PCR using the 7500 Fast real-time PCR system (Applied Biosystems). For endogenous controls Gusb (Mm01197698_m1, Thermo Fisher Scientific) and Hsp90ab1 (Mm00833431_g1, Thermo Fisher Scientific) or GUSB (Hs00939627_m1, Thermo Fisher Scientific) and HSP90AB1 (Hs03043878_g1, Thermo Fisher Scientific) were used. Probes that target mouse Trem2 and Tyrobp

Table 1 Primers and PCR conditions used for detecting splice pattern (Forward: Fwd; Reverse: Rev)

Name	Sequence	Reaction condition
MmTrem2 Fwd	GCTCAATCCAGGAGCACAGT	95 °C 1 min; (95 °C 30s, 65 °C 15 s, 72 °C 1 min) *35 cycle; 72 °C 10 min
MmTrem2 Rev	TCTGACACTGGTAGAGGCCC	
HsTREM2 Fwd	GCCTGACATGCCTGATCCTC	95 °C 1 min; (95 °C 30s, 65 °C 15 s, 72 °C 1 min) *35 cycle; 72 °C 10 min
HsTREM2 Rev	AGGACCTTCCTGAGGGTGTC	

are Mm04209424_g1, Mm04209423_g1, Mm01273682_g1, Mm00449152_m1 (Thermo Fisher Scientific). Probes that target human TREM2 and TYROBP are Hs01010 721_m1, Hs01003899_m1, Hs00182426_m1 (Thermo Fisher Scientific). For allele specific mRNA expression custom made primers and probes were designed. The primer pair for mouse Trem2 is: CCTTGAGGGTGTCA TGTACTTAT and TCCCATTCCGCTTCTTCAG. The probes for the mouse wild-type allele and R47H allele are /5HEX/CCTT+G + C + GT + CT + CC/3IABkFQ/ (+, lock nucleic acid) and /56-FAM/CTT + T + G + T + GT + C + GA + C/3IABkFQ/, respectively (Integrated DNA Technologies). The primer pair for human TREM2 is ACAAGTTGTGCGTGCTGA and ATGACTCCATGAA GCACTGG. The probes for the human wild-type allele and the R47H allele are /5HEX/CTT + G + C + GCCT +CC/3IABkFQ/ and /56-FAM/TT + G + T + GC + CT + CC/3IABkFQ/, respectively (Integrated DNA Technologies). The probes and primers were mixed in 1:2 ratios for quantitative PCR reaction.

cDNAs were diluted 1:5 with H$_2$O and 9 μl of diluted cDNA together with 1 μl of primer probe mix, 10 μl of Taqman® master mix (Thermo Fisher Scientific) were used in one 20 μl reaction.

Results

Reduced mRNA and protein level in Trem2 R47H knock-in mice

The rare TREM2 variant rs75932628-T encodes a histidine instead of arginine at position 47 (R47H) and increases the risk for AD around three-fold [3, 4]. The DNA and amino acid sequence around arginine at position 47 is highly conserved across different mammalian species (Fig. 1a and b). To study the impact of this variant on TREM2 function in microglia in vivo we generated Trem2 R47H knock-in mice (R47H ki mice) by introducing a G > A mutation using the CRISPR/Cas9 technology (Fig. 1c). Two silent mutations were additionally introduced (GA > TC) to create a SalI restriction site for genotyping (Fig. 1c). In addition a silent G > A mutation was generated to block the protospacer-adjacent motif (PAM) to allow higher gene editing efficiency (Fig. 1c). The predicted potential off-target sites were analyzed. An off-target event with a Δ10-Indel mutation was identified at an intragenic region on chromosome 11 (Additional file 1: Figure S1, putative off-target #2). The founder mouse was back-crossed to C57BL/6 N, and off-spring with positive Trem2 R47H ki but negative off-target #2 (i.e ID-7-1; ID-7-2; ID-7-4) were used for establishing the mouse line. Expression of total Trem2 mRNA as well as both Trem2 mRNA transcripts (NM_031254.3 and NM_001272078.1), encoding either membrane bound Trem2 or a truncated soluble version were validated in brain. Interestingly, total

Trem2 mRNA including both Trem2 transcripts was significantly reduced in a gene dose-dependent manner, whereas mRNA expression of Tyrobp (NM_011662), the adaptor protein of Trem2 [42], remained unchanged (Fig. 1d). Using allele specific qPCR we confirmed that expression of the R47H allele was selectively reduced compared to the wt allele in heterozygous R47H ki mice (Fig. 1e and Additional file 2: Table S1).

To confirm decreased Trem2 expression on protein level, we purified microglia from wild-type (wt), heterozygous (het), and homozygous (hom) R47H ki mice and performed western blotting of membrane fractions. Membrane-bound Trem2 showed a gene dose-dependent reduction (Fig. 1f).

Reduced Trem2 R47H mRNA and protein expression was further confirmed in bone marrow derived macrophages (BMDM). Consistent with our findings in brain and microglia, mRNA of both Trem2 transcripts decreased in a gene dose dependent manner whereas mRNA of Tyrobp remained unchanged (Fig. 1g). Furthermore, immature and mature Trem2 as well as soluble Trem2 (sTrem2) were also reduced in a gene dose dependent manner (Fig. 1h).

To exclude that reduced Trem2 mRNA and protein expression is artificially caused by the introduction of the three silent mutations, we analyzed Trem2 R47H knock-in mice generated by Jackson laboratory (Jax R47H ki mice). In addition to the target variant R47H, these mice harbor two silent mutations (Fig. 2a). One of the silent mutations is a G > A exchange to block the PAM sequence exactly like in the mice generated within our laboratory. The second silent mutation C > A is only present in the Jax R47H ki mice (Fig. 2a). We investigated Trem2 mRNA and protein levels using homozygous Jax R47H ki mice and their wt counterparts. Again, mRNA from total Trem2 as well as from both transcripts of Trem2 decreased in brains of homozygous ki mice whereas mRNA expression of Tyrobp remained unchanged (Fig. 2b). Western blotting of membrane fractions from BMDM from the Jax R47H ki mice also confirmed a significant reduction of membrane bound and soluble Trem2 (Fig. 2c). Thus reduction of mRNA and protein levels in Trem2 R47H ki mouse was confirmed in two independent mouse models.

Aberrant splicing of exon1/2 in Trem2 R47H knock-in mice

Next we searched for the cellular mechanism responsible for the substantial reduction of the Trem2 R47H mRNA in the two mouse models. Since nonfunctional mRNAs are rapidly removed by mRNA surveillance systems [43], we studied splicing of the first intron which separates exon 2 containing the R47H variant from exon 1 harboring the translation initiation site and upstream

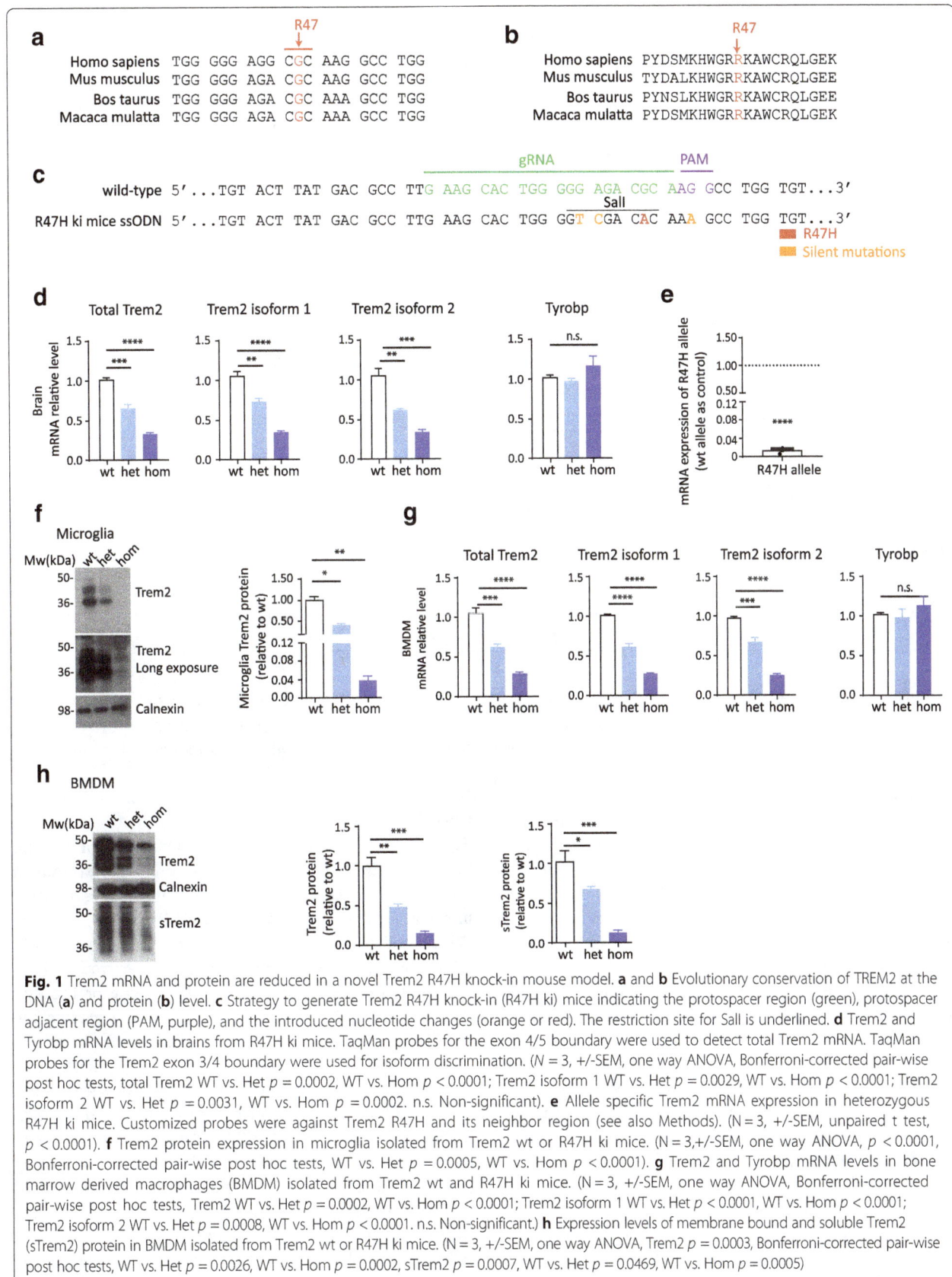

Fig. 1 Trem2 mRNA and protein are reduced in a novel Trem2 R47H knock-in mouse model. **a** and **b** Evolutionary conservation of TREM2 at the DNA (**a**) and protein (**b**) level. **c** Strategy to generate Trem2 R47H knock-in (R47H ki) mice indicating the protospacer region (green), protospacer adjacent region (PAM, purple), and the introduced nucleotide changes (orange or red). The restriction site for SalI is underlined. **d** Trem2 and Tyrobp mRNA levels in brains from R47H ki mice. TaqMan probes for the exon 4/5 boundary were used to detect total Trem2 mRNA. TaqMan probes for the Trem2 exon 3/4 boundary were used for isoform discrimination. (N = 3, +/-SEM, one way ANOVA, Bonferroni-corrected pair-wise post hoc tests, total Trem2 WT vs. Het $p = 0.0002$, WT vs. Hom $p < 0.0001$; Trem2 isoform 1 WT vs. Het $p = 0.0029$, WT vs. Hom $p < 0.0001$; Trem2 isoform 2 WT vs. Het $p = 0.0031$, WT vs. Hom $p = 0.0002$. n.s. Non-significant). **e** Allele specific Trem2 mRNA expression in heterozygous R47H ki mice. Customized probes were against Trem2 R47H and its neighbor region (see also Methods). (N = 3, +/-SEM, unpaired t test, $p < 0.0001$). **f** Trem2 protein expression in microglia isolated from Trem2 wt or R47H ki mice. (N = 3,+/-SEM, one way ANOVA, $p < 0.0001$, Bonferroni-corrected pair-wise post hoc tests, WT vs. Het $p = 0.0005$, WT vs. Hom $p < 0.0001$). **g** Trem2 and Tyrobp mRNA levels in bone marrow derived macrophages (BMDM) isolated from Trem2 wt and R47H ki mice. (N = 3, +/-SEM, one way ANOVA, Bonferroni-corrected pair-wise post hoc tests, Trem2 WT vs. Het $p = 0.0002$, WT vs. Hom $p < 0.0001$; Trem2 isoform 1 WT vs. Het $p < 0.0001$, WT vs. Hom $p < 0.0001$; Trem2 isoform 2 WT vs. Het $p = 0.0008$, WT vs. Hom $p < 0.0001$. n.s. Non-significant.) **h** Expression levels of membrane bound and soluble Trem2 (sTrem2) protein in BMDM isolated from Trem2 wt or R47H ki mice. (N = 3, +/-SEM, one way ANOVA, Trem2 $p = 0.0003$, Bonferroni-corrected pair-wise post hoc tests, WT vs. Het $p = 0.0026$, WT vs. Hom $p = 0.0002$, sTrem2 $p = 0.0007$, WT vs. Het $p = 0.0469$, WT vs. Hom $p = 0.0005$)

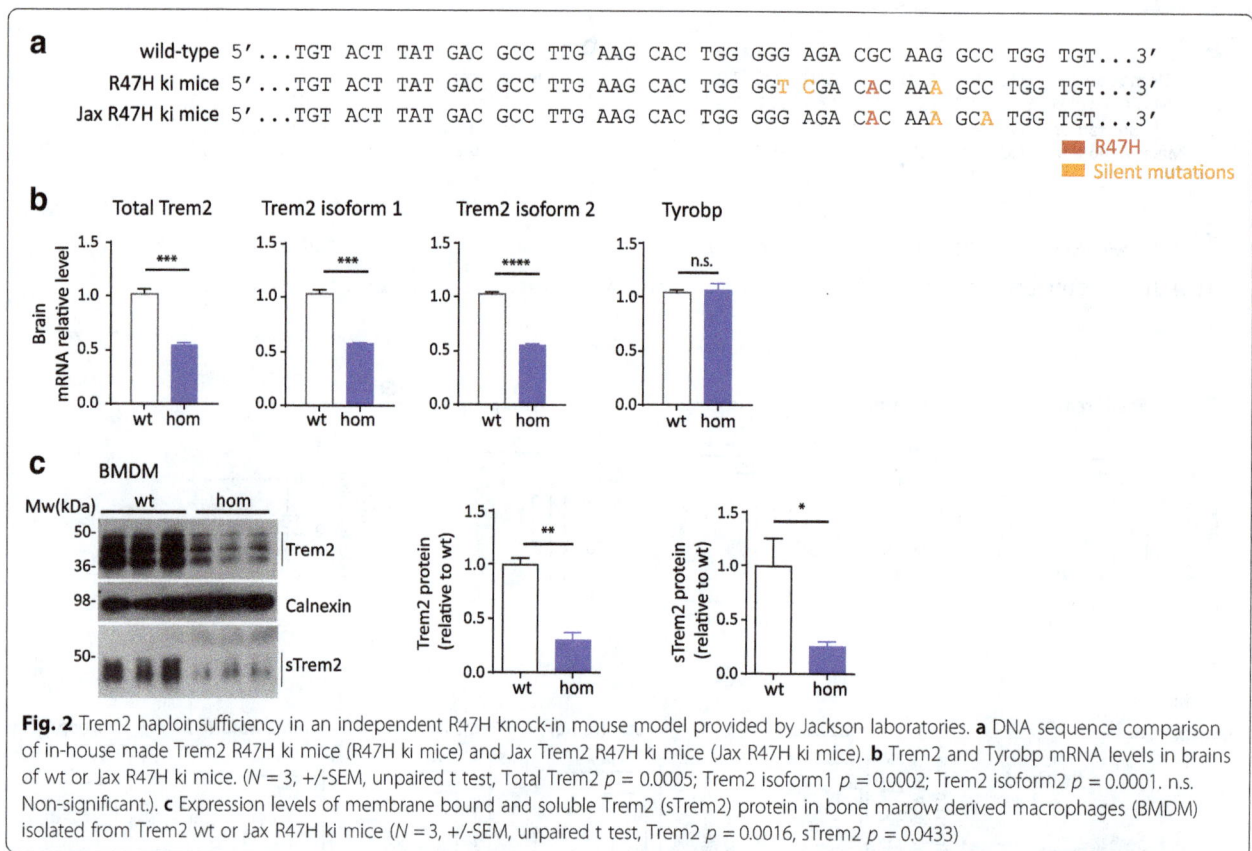

Fig. 2 Trem2 haploinsufficiency in an independent R47H knock-in mouse model provided by Jackson laboratories. **a** DNA sequence comparison of in-house made Trem2 R47H ki mice (R47H ki mice) and Jax Trem2 R47H ki mice (Jax R47H ki mice). **b** Trem2 and Tyrobp mRNA levels in brains of wt or Jax R47H ki mice. ($N = 3$, +/-SEM, unpaired t test, Total Trem2 $p = 0.0005$; Trem2 isoform1 $p = 0.0002$; Trem2 isoform2 $p = 0.0001$. n.s. Non-significant.). **c** Expression levels of membrane bound and soluble Trem2 (sTrem2) protein in bone marrow derived macrophages (BMDM) isolated from Trem2 wt or Jax R47H ki mice ($N = 3$, +/-SEM, unpaired t test, Trem2 $p = 0.0016$, sTrem2 $p = 0.0433$)

untranslated sequences. Using RT-PCR with primer pairs against the 5′ end of exon 1 and the 3′ end of exon 2, we compared the splicing patterns of Trem2 in R47H ki and wt mice (Fig. 3a). A single splicing product of the expected length (465 base pairs) was obtained from wt Trem2 mRNA (Fig. 3b). Surprisingly, an additional smaller splicing product (346 base pairs) was observed in Trem2 R47H heterozygous mice, which was even more abundant in Trem2 R47H homozygous mice (Fig. 3b) while at the same time the larger splicing product was reduced in a gene dose dependent manner (Fig. 3b). This suggests aberrant splicing of Trem2 pre-mRNA derived from the mutant allele. To independently confirm aberrant splicing, we investigated the Jax R47H ki mice described in Fig. 2. Again, we found an additional smaller RT-PCR product in mutant but not wt mice (Fig. 3c). Furthermore, the larger splicing product was reduced in homozygous ki mice (Fig. 3c). Thus aberrant splicing of R47H pre-mRNA occurs in two independent mouse models. DNA sequencing of the splicing products revealed correct splicing of exon 1 and exon 2 in wt mice and to a lesser extent also in the ki mice (Fig. 3d). However, DNA sequencing of the additional shorter RT-PCR product of both mutant mice revealed that 119 base pairs were deleted at the 5′ end of exon 2 (Fig. 3d and Additional file 3: Figure S2). The deletion leads to a frame shift and a premature stop codon in

exon 2 (Fig. 3d), which may lead to nonsense mediated mRNA decay and thus explain the consistent reduction of the mutant mRNA in both mouse models.

The R47H variant does not affect splicing and mRNA levels in humans

To directly compare the splicing pattern of mouse and human TREM2 R47H, we expressed mouse or human TREM2 minigenes containing exon 1, intron 1, and exon 2 in human embryonic kidney 293 cells (HEK 293) (Fig. 4a). To separately investigate the disease causing TREM2 R47H variant and the silent mutations, we introduced the corresponding sequence variants either alone or together (Fig. 4b). Upon expression of the minigene encoding the mouse Trem2 sequence, we observed miss-splicing induced by the R47H variant alone (R47H) (Fig. 4c). Similar aberrant splicing was observed when the two silent mutations of the Jax R47H ki mice were expressed in addition to the R47H variant (R47H^AA), whereas introduction of the two silent mutations alone (AA) did not affect splicing (Fig. 4c). Moreover, when the three silent mutations used to generate our in-house mouse model were combined with the R47H (R47H^TCA), a striking increase of aberrant splicing was observed. When we only introduced the unique TC mutations used to generate our mouse model (TC) we also observed impaired splicing (Fig. 4c),

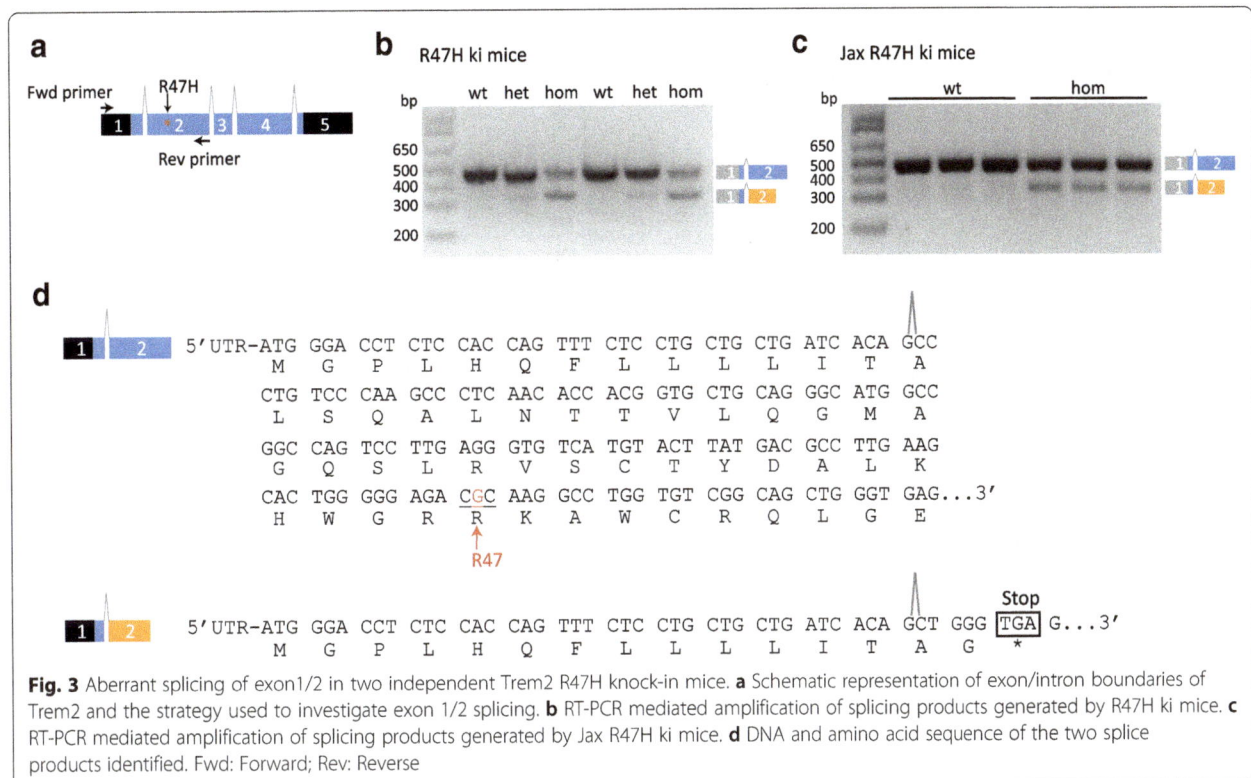

Fig. 3 Aberrant splicing of exon1/2 in two independent Trem2 R47H knock-in mice. **a** Schematic representation of exon/intron boundaries of Trem2 and the strategy used to investigate exon 1/2 splicing. **b** RT-PCR mediated amplification of splicing products generated by R47H ki mice. **c** RT-PCR mediated amplification of splicing products generated by Jax R47H ki mice. **d** DNA and amino acid sequence of the two splice products identified. Fwd: Forward; Rev: Reverse

suggesting that R47H and TC together display synergistic effects on aberrant splicing. This demonstrates that the R47H variant by itself is sufficient to induce aberrant splicing, but enhanced miss-splicing upon the addition of silent mutations implies that this genomic region is very sensitive for splicing errors induced by minor changes within the pre-mRNA sequence. Finally, we also investigated if the mutations introduced into the mouse genome by Cheng-hathaway et al. [26] affect pre-mRNA splicing of Trem2. Very similar to our R47H ki mice and those generated by the Jackson Laboratories, the mutations introduced by Cheng-hathaway and colleagues (R47H^{T}) caused aberrant splicing (Fig. 4c), which is consistent with the haploinsufficiency also observed in this model [26].

To prove if this is also true for human TREM2, we investigated the same TREM2 variants in human minigene constructs (Fig. 4a, b and d). Surprisingly, our results demonstrate that neither the R47H variant alone or in combination with the silent mutations used to generate the ki mouse models affected correct exon1/2 splicing (Fig. 4d). This suggests that only the mouse gene locus is vulnerable for aberrant splicing upon introduction of these sequence variants and implies that the R47H mutation does not affect splicing and mRNA levels in humans.

To provide direct evidence for this prediction, we investigated exon 1/2 splicing in humanized TREM2 mice generated by ectopic expression of the human wt or R47H mutant TREM2 locus in Trem2$^{-/-}$ mice [14]. Using the same RT-PCR strategy as described above (Fig. 3a), we could only detect the correctly spliced exon 1 and 2 but no aberrantly spliced additional products (Fig. 5a).

Similarly, in human induced pluripotent stem cell (iPSC)-derived microglia-like cells (iMG) with the wt TREM2 allele or heterozygous for the TREM2 R47H variant (Additional file 4: Figure S3) we also detected only the correctly spliced exon 1 and 2 (Fig. 5b). Furthermore, no aberrant splicing was detected in AD cases carrying one R47H mutant allele (Fig. 5c). Direct sequencing demonstrated correct exon1/2 splicing in human iMG and in AD cases. Lack of aberrant splicing of human TREM2 R47H is consistent with no reduction of total TREM2 mRNA in iMG with one R47H allele (Fig. 5d). In addition, using allele specific qPCR we confirmed that the expression of the R47H allele is comparable to wt in iMG (Fig. 5e and Additional file 5: Table S2), and in human brain (Fig. 5f and Additional file 5: Table S2). Taken together, aberrant splicing of R47H mutant pre-mRNA is not observed in humans and consequently no haploinsufficiency of TREM2 could be detected.

Discussion

Most functional studies of TREM2 have so far been performed with either total loss-of-function models or by studying the TREM2 T66M mutation [7, 8, 11–13, 19, 20, 44, 45], which is associated with an FTD-like syndrome. Homozygous mice expressing the Trem2 T66M

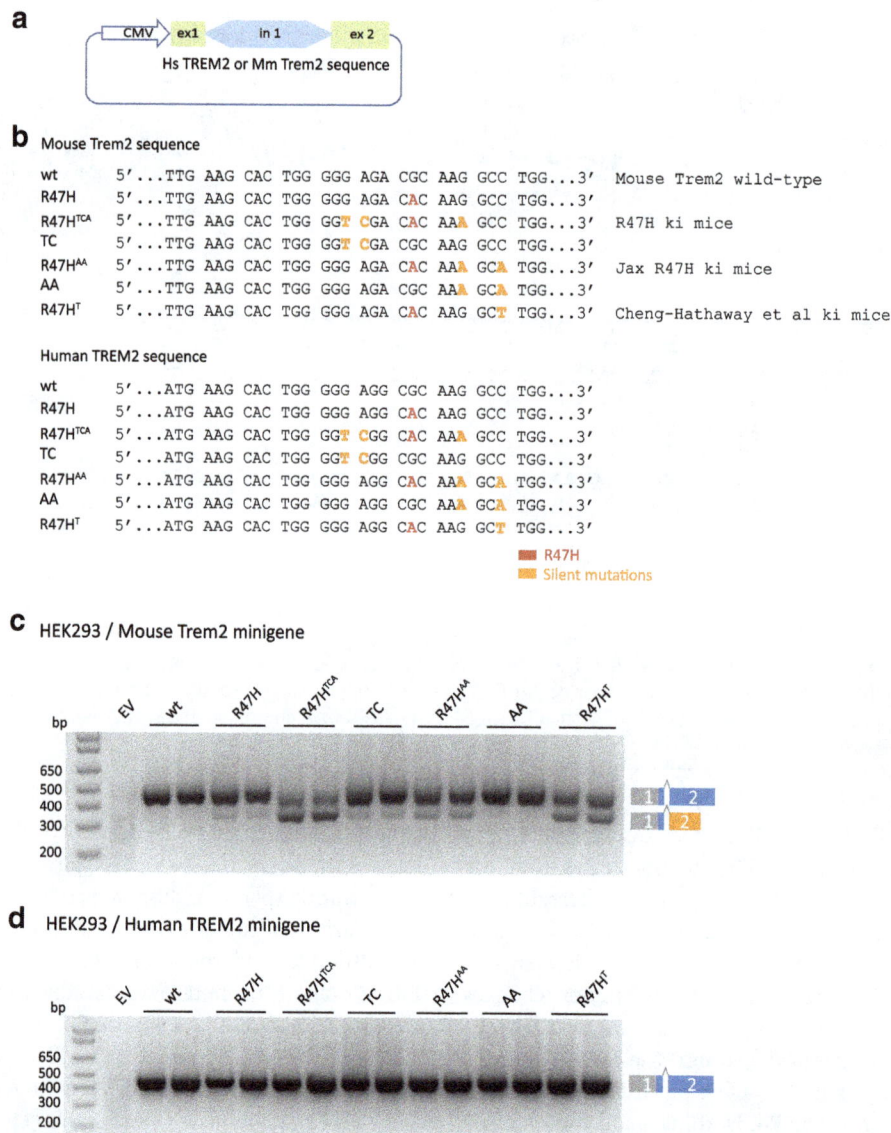

Fig. 4 Aberrant splicing of Trem2 variants containing the R47H mutation with and without additional mutations used to create three different R47H ki mice. **a** The minigene construct used to investigate exon1/2 splicing of the Trem2 variants shown in (**b**). **b** Sequence alignment of Trem2 variants investigated for aberrant splicing. **c** Exon 1/2 splicing of mouse Trem2 variants described in (**b**). **d** Exon 1/2 splicing of human TREM2 variants described in (**b**). Note that only mouse transcripts undergo aberrant splicing. EV: empty vector

variant phenocopy a number of functional deficits also observed upon total loss of the Trem2 encoding gene [11]. These include delayed resolution of inflammation upon lipopolysaccharide stimulation, reduced phagocytic activity, reduced microglial activation during physiological ageing and neurological insults, reduced cerebral blood flow, reduced cerebral brain glucose metabolism, impaired chemotaxis and clustering of microglia around amyloid plaques [11]. However, much less is known about the functional impact of the TREM2 R47H variant, which is associated with a high risk for AD similar to that caused by the ApoE ε4 allele [3, 4, 46]. In vitro

studies suggested reduced binding of Aβ oligomers, ApoE, and phosphatidylserine due to structural alterations in TREM2 [8, 21–24]. Furthermore maturation of the R47H variant within the secretory pathway may also be delayed [25]. Expression of human TREM2 R47H in Trem2 knockout mice failed to rescue the knockout phenotypes again supporting the notion that TREM2 is protective and that TREM2 variants associated with neurodegenerative diseases may cause a loss-of-function [14]. Trem2 R47H knock-in mice expressing this variant under physiological conditions resulted in phenotypes that were compatible with a loss-of function [26]. Cheng-Hathaway et al.

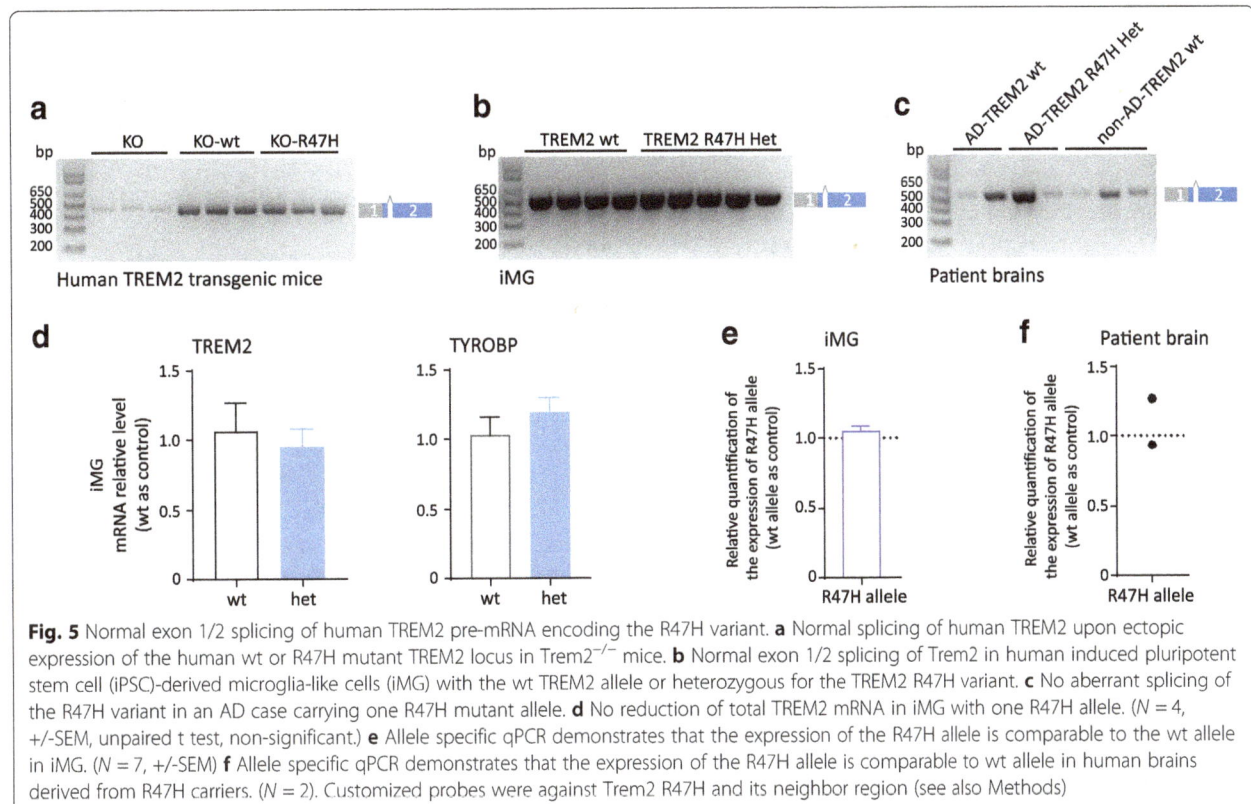

Fig. 5 Normal exon 1/2 splicing of human TREM2 pre-mRNA encoding the R47H variant. **a** Normal splicing of human TREM2 upon ectopic expression of the human wt or R47H mutant TREM2 locus in Trem2$^{-/-}$ mice. **b** Normal exon 1/2 splicing of Trem2 in human induced pluripotent stem cell (iPSC)-derived microglia-like cells (iMG) with the wt TREM2 allele or heterozygous for the TREM2 R47H variant. **c** No aberrant splicing of the R47H variant in an AD case carrying one R47H mutant allele. **d** No reduction of total TREM2 mRNA in iMG with one R47H allele. (N = 4, +/-SEM, unpaired t test, non-significant.) **e** Allele specific qPCR demonstrates that the expression of the R47H allele is comparable to the wt allele in iMG. (N = 7, +/-SEM) **f** Allele specific qPCR demonstrates that the expression of the R47H allele is comparable to wt allele in human brains derived from R47H carriers. (N = 2). Customized probes were against Trem2 R47H and its neighbor region (see also Methods)

reported that Trem2 R47H heterozygous mice showed reduced Trem2 expression in microglia close to amyloid plaques, reduced microglial proliferation, reduced dense core plaques and increased neuritic dystrophy [26]. These phenotypes were associated with reduced Trem2 mRNA expression [26]. Similarly, Sudom et al. reported reduced Trem2 protein expression in brain as well as reduced sTrem2 in plasma from R47H knock-in mice [24]. All together, this suggests that the AD-associated Trem2 R47H variant is also associated with a loss-of-function. However, while the T66M mutation causes a loss-of-function due to retention of the misfolded mutant protein within the endoplasmatic reticulum [11, 25], the R47H mutation appears to cause haploinsufficiency due to reduced mRNA levels [26]. We generated a similar mouse model using the CRISPR/Cas9 technology. Consistent with published findings, our mouse model also showed reduced Trem2 mRNA and protein levels. Furthermore, similar findings were made using an independent mouse generated by Jackson Laboratories. We therefore searched for a joined cellular mechanism, which may be involved in the significant reduction of Trem2 mRNA and protein in both mouse models. Surprisingly, we found that the introduction of the R47H variant by itself but even more so the introduction of additional silent mutations caused aberrant splicing. Direct sequencing of the aberrant splicing product revealed that it lacks 119 base pairs. Close inspection of the sequence of the alternative splice product

revealed that a cryptic splice acceptor site within the exon 2 was activated. This leads to the elimination of parts of exon 2 resulting in a splicing product containing a premature stop codon. It is well known that such aberrant mRNAs are rapidly degraded by nonsense-mediated mRNA decay [47]. Note that the TaqMan probes used for detecting Trem2 mRNA were either bound to exon 3/4 or exon 4/5 boundary (Fig. 1d) thus they detect both the full length functional Trem2 mRNA and the aberrantly spliced shorter variant. Therefore, the apparent degree of reduction for Trem2 mRNA and protein is not equal (Fig. 1d and f). However, we cannot fully exclude the possibility that the R47H variant may also affect mouse Trem2 protein stability.

The mRNA reductions caused by aberrant splicing, which were consistent in two independent mouse models, led us to investigate if aberrant exon 2 splicing in humans also leads to TREM2 haploinsufficiency. We found that TREM2 mRNA levels and splicing patterns were both normal in iPSC-derived human microglia-like cells and in patient brains with the TREM2 R47H variant. Furthermore, cellular splicing assays using minigene constructs demonstrate that the R47H variant induced abnormal splicing only occurs in mice but not in humans. Thus, both the R47H variant as well as additionally introduced silent variants cause a mouse-specific reduction of Trem2 mRNA. Therefore, these findings cannot be translated to humans calling for novel humanized R47H mouse models.

Conclusions

The AD-associated Trem2 R47H variant in combination with silent mutations introduced by the CRISPR/Cas9 technology causes mouse specific aberrant splicing of exon 2, which leads to an alternative Trem2 mRNA containing a premature stop codon. The observed significant reduction of Trem2 mRNA and protein in R47H ki mice is most likely the consequence of nonsense-mediated mRNA decay of the aberrant transcript and is not observed in human systems. Thus, functional data derived from Trem2 R47H knock-in mice cannot be translated to humans.

Additional files

Additional file 1: Figure S1. Off-target analysis of in-house made Trem2 R47H knock-in mice. **a** Sanger-sequencing chromatograms of the Trem2 on-target site and the six putative off target sites of animal Trem2 R47H ki ID-7. Mixed peaks in the Trem2 locus show the correct R47H substitution (CGC > CAC) and the three silent mutations for genotyping purposes. Mixed peaks in traces of site #2 reveal a Δ10-Indel mutation at the putative cut site, indicating a true off target event. Underlined: Protospacer; arrow head: putative cut site; green letters: PAM site on shown strand; red letters: PAM site on complementary strand; yellow: Δ10-Indel mutation. **b** Sanger sequencing results of Trem2 R47H positive off-springs of male ID-7, which was crossed with a C57BL/6 N female. The Δ10-Indel allele was inherited to animals ID-7-3 und ID-7-12 that were excluded from any further breedings and experiments.

Additional file 2: Table S1. Allele specific quantitative PCR for Trem2 R47H knock-in mice

Additional file 3: Figure S2. Sequence of the aberrantly spliced murine Trem2 mRNA. Trem2 gene sequence. Exon in black; intron in green; // indicates splicing sites.

Additional file 4: Figure S3. iMG differentiation and validation. **a** Schematic of the in vitro differentiation of iPSC-derived microglia-like cells (iMG). (i): Human iPSCs are grown in feeder free conditions with no spontaneous differentiation. Scale bar: 250 μm. (ii): Embryoid bodies are formed in the presence of 3 factors SCF, BMP4, and VEGF; Scale bar: 750 μm. (iii): Myeloid cells are generated after culturing with IL3 and MCSF growth factors for 3–4 weeks, then stained for classic myeloid/macrophage markers CD68. Scale bar: 50 μm. (iv): Further differentiation to microglia-like cells that positive for microglial markers P2RY12. Scale bar: 20 μm. (v): Addition of the two final factors (CD200 and CX3CL1) matures the iMG. Scale bar: 20 μm. **b** Heat map showing mRNA expression of a microglial gene signature in iMG, human monocyte-derived macrophages (hMac), human primary microglia (hMG), and iPSC samples. Clear clustering is observed between iMG and hMG.

Additional file 5: Table S2. Allele specific quantitative PCR for iMG and patient brains

Abbreviations

AD: Alzheimer's disease; Aβ: Amyloid β-peptide; BMDM: Bone marrow derived macrophages; HEK293: Human embryonic kidney 293; Hom: Homozygous; iMG: iPSC derived microglia-like cells; iPSC: Induced pluripotent stem cell; ki: Knock-in; PAM: Protospacer-adjacent motif; qPCR: Quantitative polymerase chain reaction; RT-PCR: Reverse transcriptase polymerase chain reaction; sTREM2: Soluble TREM2; TREM2: Triggering receptor expressed on myeloid cell 2; WT: Wild-type; Het: heterozygous

Acknowledgements

The authors thank the Queen Square Brain Bank for access to tissue: this resource is funded in part by the Weston Foundation and the MRC.

Funding

This work was supported by the Deutsche Forschungsgemeinschaft (DFG) within the framework of the Munich Cluster for Systems Neurology (EXC 1010 SyNergy) and the Koselleck Project HA1737/16–1 (to C.H.). This work was funded in part by the German Federal Ministry of Education and Research (BMBF) through the Joint Project HIT-Tau TP2: Grant 01EK1605C to W. W. This work was supported by the Biotechnology and Biological Sciences Research Council (grant number BB/M009513/1) to A.M. and by funding from the Innovative Medicines Initiative 2 Joint Undertaking under grant agreement No 115976 (for T.P to J.P). This Joint Undertaking receives support from the European Union's Horizon 2020 research and innovation programme and EFPIA. This work was funded by NIH grant RF1 AG051485 to M.C.

Authors' contributions

XX designed and conceived the study. XX and CH interpreted the results. CH and XX wrote the manuscript with input from all co-authors. BW and WW generated the Trem2 R47H knock-in mice. GK and BW analyzed potential off-targets. XX, KZ and JH prepared bone marrow and isolated microglia from mice. XX and BB performed RNA analyses and immunoblotting. XX performed RT-PCR, allele specific qPCR and cellular splicing analysis. TP, AM and JP generated the iPSC derived microglia-like cells and performed qPCR on these cells. MC and WS provided the mouse brain samples from humanized TREM2 mice. All authors read and approved the final manuscript.

Ethics approval

All mice were handled according to institutional guidelines approved by the animal welfare and use committee of the government of Upper Bavaria. Ethics committee from Ludwig-Maximilians- University and University College London approved this research project using human tissue.

Competing interests

C.H. collaborates with DENALI Therapeutics and received a speaker honorarium from Novartis and Roche. The other authors declare that they have no competing interests.

Author details

[1]Metabolic Biochemistry, Biomedical Center (BMC), Faculty of Medicine, Ludwig-Maximilians-Universität München, Munich, Germany. [2]Graduate School of Systemic Neuroscience, Ludwig- Maximilians- University Munich, Munich, Germany. [3]Department of Neuroinflammation, Cell Signalling Lab, University College London Institute of Neurology, WC1N 1PJ, London, UK. [4]German Center for Neurodegenerative Diseases (DZNE) Munich, Munich, Germany. [5]Munich Cluster for Systems Neurology (SyNergy), Munich, Germany. [6]Institute of Developmental Genetics, Helmholtz Zentrum München, German Research Center for Environmental Health, Neuherberg, Germany. [7]Department of Immunology and Pathology, Washington University in St. Louis, St. Louis, MO, USA. [8]Center for Neuropathology and Prion Research, Ludwig-Maximilians-Universität München, Munich, Germany. [9]Technische Universität München-Weihenstephan, 85764 Neuherberg/Munich, Germany.

References

1. Sims R, Van Der Lee SJ, Naj AC, Bellenguez C, Badarinarayan N, Jakobsdottir J, et al. Rare coding variants in PLCG2, ABI3, and TREM2 implicate microglial-mediated innate immunity in Alzheimer's disease. Nat Genet. [Internet] 2017;49:1373–84. Available from: https://www.ncbi.nlm.nih.gov/pubmed/28714976.
2. Jiang T, Tan L, Chen Q, Tan MS, Zhou JS, Zhu XC, et al. A rare coding variant in TREM2 increases risk for Alzheimer's disease in Han Chinese. Neurobiol

Aging [Internet]. Elsevier Inc. 2016;42:17.e1–217.e3. Available from: https://doi.org/10.1016/j.neurobiolaging.2016.02.023.

3. Jonsson T, Stefansson H, Steinberg S, Jonsdottir I, Jonsson PV, Snaedal J, et al. Variant of TREM2 associated with the risk of Alzheimer's disease. N Engl J Med. [Internet]. 2013;368:107–16. Available from: http://www.ncbi.nlm.nih.gov/pubmed/23150908.

4. Guerreiro R, Wojtas A, Bras J, Carrasquillo M, Rogaeva E, Majounie E, et al. TREM2 variants in Alzheimer's disease. N Engl J Med [Internet]. 2013;368:117–27. Available from: http://www.nejm.org/doi/abs/10.1056/NEJMoa1211851.

5. Chan G, White CC, Winn P a, Cimpean M, Replogle JM, Glick LR, et al. CD33 modulates TREM2: convergence of Alzheimer loci. Nat. Neurosci. [Internet]. 2015;2015. Available from: https://doi.org/10.1038/nn.4126.

6. Krasemann S, Madore C, Cialic R, Baufeld C, Calcagno N, El Fatimy R, et al. The TREM2-APOE Pathway Drives the Transcriptional Phenotype of Dysfunctional Microglia in Neurodegenerative Diseases. Immunity [Internet]. Elsevier.; 2017;47:566–81.e9. Available from: http://linkinghub.elsevier.com/retrieve/pii/S1074761317303667.

7. Mazaheri F, Snaidero N, Kleinberger G, Madore C, Daria A, Werner G, et al. TREM2 deficiency impairs chemotaxis and microglial responses to neuronal injury. EMBO Rep [Internet] 2017;18:1186–98. Available from: http://embor.embopress.org/lookup/doi/10.15252/embr.201743922.

8. Wang Y, Cella M, Mallinson K, Ulrich JD, Young KL, Robinette ML, et al. TREM2 Lipid Sensing Sustains the Microglial Response in an Alzheimer's Disease Model. Cell [Internet]. Elsevier Inc.; 2015;160:1061–71. Available from: http://linkinghub.elsevier.com/retrieve/pii/S0092867415001270.

9. Ulland TK, Song WM, Huang SCC, Ulrich JD, Sergushichev A, Beatty WL, et al. TREM2 Maintains Microglial Metabolic Fitness in Alzheimer's Disease. Cell [Internet]. Elsevier Inc.; 2017;170:649–63.e13. Available from: https://doi.org/10.1016/j.cell.2017.07.023.

10. Keren-Shaul H, Spinrad A, Weiner A, Matcovitch-Natan O, Dvir-Szternfeld R, Ulland TK, et al. A Unique Microglia Type Associated with Restricting Development of Alzheimer's Disease. Cell [Internet]. Elsevier; 2017;169:1276–90.e17. Available from: https://doi.org/10.1016/j.cell.2017.05.018.

11. Kleinberger G, Brendel M, Mracsko E, Wefers B, Groeneweg L, Xiang X, et al. The FTD-like syndrome causing TREM2 T66M mutation impairs microglia function, brain perfusion, and glucose metabolism. EMBO J [Internet] 2017; 36:1837–53. Available from: http://emboj.embopress.org/lookup/doi/10.15252/embj.201796516.

12. Jay TR, Miller CM, Cheng PJ, Graham LC, Bemiller S, Broihier ML, et al. TREM2 deficiency eliminates TREM2+ inflammatory macrophages and ameliorates pathology in Alzheimer's disease mouse models. J Exp Med [Internet] 2015; 212:287–95. Available from: http://www.jem.org/cgi/doi/10.1084/jem.20142322.

13. Yuan P, Condello C, Keene CD, Wang Y, Bird TD, Paul SM, et al. TREM2 Haplodeficiency in mice and humans impairs the microglia barrier function leading to decreased amyloid compaction and severe axonal dystrophy. Neuron [Internet]. 2016;92:252–64. Available from: https://www.ncbi.nlm.nih.gov/pubmed/27196974.

14. Song WM, Joshita S, Zhou Y, Ulland TK, Gilfillan S, Colonna M. Humanized TREM2 mice reveal microglia-intrinsic and -extrinsic effects of R47H polymorphism. J. Exp. med. [Internet]. 2018;215:745–60. Available from: http://www.ncbi.nlm.nih.gov/pubmed/29321225.

15. Suárez-Calvet M, Araque Caballero MÁ, Kleinberger G, Bateman RJ, Fagan AM, Morris JC, et al. Early changes in CSF sTREM2 in dominantly inherited Alzheimer's disease occur after amyloid deposition and neuronal injury. Sci. Transl. Med. [Internet]. 2016;8:369ra178. Available from: http://www.ncbi.nlm.nih.gov/pubmed/27974666.

16. Wang Y, Ulland TK, Ulrich JD, Song W, Tzaferis JA, Hole JT, et al. TREM2-mediated early microglial response limits diffusion and toxicity of amyloid plaques. J Exp Med [Internet]. 2016;jem.20151948. Available from: http://www.jem.org/lookup/doi/10.1084/jem.20151948.

17. Cantoni C, Bollman B, Licastro D, Xie M, Mikesell R, Schmidt R, et al. TREM2 regulates microglial cell activation in response to demyelination in vivo. Acta Neuropathol. [Internet]. 2015;129:429–47. Available from: http://www.ncbi.nlm.nih.gov/pubmed/25631124.

18. Poliani PL, Wang Y, Fontana E, Robinette ML, Yamanishi Y, Gilfillan S, et al. TREM2 sustains microglial expansion during aging and response to demyelination. J Clin Invest. [Internet]. 2015;125:2161–70. Available from: http://www.ncbi.nlm.nih.gov/pubmed/25893602.

19. Bemiller SM, McCray TJ, Allan K, Formica SV, Xu G, Wilson G, et al. TREM2 deficiency exacerbates tau pathology through dysregulated kinase signaling in a mouse model of tauopathy. Mol Neurodegen. [Internet] 2017;12:1–12. Available from: https://www.ncbi.nlm.nih.gov/pubmed/29037207.

20. Leyns CEG, Ulrich JD, Finn MB, Stewart FR, Koscal LJ, Remolina Serrano J, et al. TREM2 deficiency attenuates neuroinflammation and protects against neurodegeneration in a mouse model of tauopathy. Proc. Natl. Acad. Sci. U. S. A. [Internet]. 2017;114:11524–9. Available from: http://www.pnas.org/lookup/doi/10.1073/pnas.1710311114.

21. Atagi Y, Liu C-C, Painter MM, Chen X-F, Verbeeck C, Zheng H, et al. Apolipoprotein E is a ligand for triggering receptor expressed on myeloid cells 2 (TREM2). J Biol Chem. [Internet] 2015;290:26043–50. Available from: https://www.ncbi.nlm.nih.gov/pubmed/26374899.

22. Yeh FL, Wang Y, Tom I, Gonzalez LC, Sheng M. TREM2 binds to apolipoproteins, including APOE and CLU/APOJ, and thereby facilitates uptake of amyloid-Beta by microglia. Neuron. [Internet] 2016;91:328–40. Available from: https://www.ncbi.nlm.nih.gov/pubmed/27477018.

23. Zhao Y, Wu X, Li X, Jiang L-L, Gui X, Liu Y, et al. TREM2 Is a Receptor for β-Amyloid that Mediates Microglial Function. Neuron [Internet]. 2018;97:1023–31.e7. Available from: http://linkinghub.elsevier.com/retrieve/pii/S0896627318300564.

24. Sudom A, Talreja S, Danao J, Bragg E, Kegel R, Min X, et al. Molecular basis for the loss-of-function effects of the Alzheimer's disease–associated R47H variant of the immune receptor TREM2. J Biol Chem. [internet]. 2018;2:jbc.RA118.002352. Available from: http://www.ncbi.nlm.nih.gov/pubmed/29794134.

25. Kleinberger G, Yamanishi Y, Suárez-Calvet M, Czirr E, Lohmann E, Cuyvers E, et al. TREM2 mutations implicated in neurodegeneration impair cell surface transport and phagocytosis. Sci. Transl. Med. [Internet]. 2014;6:243ra86. Available from: http://www.ncbi.nlm.nih.gov/pubmed/24990881.

26. Cheng-hathaway PJ, Reed-geaghan EG, Jay TR, Casali BT, Bemiller SM, Puntambekar SS, et al. The T rem 2 R47H variant confers loss-of- function-like phenotypes in Alzheimer' s disease. Mol Neurodegen. [Internet] 2018: 1–12. Available from: https://www.ncbi.nlm.nih.gov/pubmed/29859094.

27. Cheng Q, Danao J, Talreja S, Wen P, Yin J, Sun N, et al. TREM2-activating antibodies abrogate the negative pleiotropic effects of the Alzheimer's disease variant TREM2 R47H on murine myeloid cell function. J Biol Chem. [Internet]. 2018;jbc.RA118.001848. Available from: http://www.jbc.org/lookup/doi/10.1074/jbc.RA118.001848.

28. Brandl C, Ortiz O, Röttig B, Wefers B, Wurst W, Kühn R. Creation of targeted genomic deletions using TALEN or CRISPR/Cas nuclease pairs in one-cell mouse embryos. FEBS Open Bio [Internet]. Federation of European Biochemical Societies; 2015;5:26–35. Available from: https://doi.org/10.1016/j.fob.2014.11.009.

29. Wefers B, Bashir S, Rossius J, Wurst W, Kühn R. Gene editing in mouse zygotes using the CRISPR/Cas9 system. Methods [Internet]. Elsevier Inc. 2017;121–122: 55–67. Available from: https://doi.org/10.1016/j.ymeth.2017.02.008.

30. Haeussler M, Schönig K, Eckert H, Eschstruth A, Mianné J, Renaud JB, et al. Evaluation of off-target and on-target scoring algorithms and integration into the guide RNA selection tool CRISPOR. Genome Biol. [Internet] 2016; 17(1):148. Available from: https://doi.org/10.1186/s13059-016-1012-2.

31. Marim FM, Silveira TN, Lima DS, Zamboni DS. A method for generation of bone marrow-derived macrophages from cryopreserved mouse bone marrow cells. PLoS One. [Internet] 2010;5:1–8. Available from: https://www.ncbi.nlm.nih.gov/pubmed/21179419.

32. Xiang X, Werner G, Bohrmann B, Liesz A, Mazaheri F, Capell A, et al. TREM2 deficiency reduces the efficacy of immunotherapeutic amyloid clearance. EMBO Mol. Med. [Internet] 2016;8:992–1004. Available from: https://www.ncbi.nlm.nih.gov/pubmed/27402340.

33. Galatro TF, Vainchtein ID, Brouwer N, Boddeke EWGM, Eggen BJL. Isolation of microglia and immune infiltrates from mouse and primate central nervous system. Methods Mol Biol. [Internet] 2017;1559:333–42. Available from: https://www.ncbi.nlm.nih.gov/pubmed/28063055.

34. Okita K, Matsumura Y, Sato Y, Okada A, Morizane A, Okamoto S, et al. A more efficient method to generate integration-free human iPS cells. Nat methods [Internet]. 2011;8:409–12. Available from: http://www.ncbi.nlm.nih.gov/pubmed/21460823.

35. Abud EM, Ramirez RN, Martinez ES, Healy LM, Nguyen CHH, Newman SA, et al. iPSC-Derived Human Microglia-like Cells to Study Neurological Diseases. Neuron. [Internet] 2017;94:278–293.e9. Available from: https://www.ncbi.nlm.nih.gov/pubmed/28426964.

36. van Wilgenburg B, Browne C, Vowles J, Cowley SA. Efficient, long term production of monocyte-derived macrophages from human pluripotent stem cells under partly-defined and fully-defined conditions. Covas DT, editor. PLoS One. [Internet] 2013;8:e71098. Available from: http://www.ncbi.nlm.nih.gov/pubmed/23951090.

37. Butovsky O, Jedrychowski MP, Moore CS, Cialic R, Lanser AJ, Gabriely G, et al. Identification of a unique TGF-β-dependent molecular and functional

signature in microglia. Nat Neurosci [Internet] 2014;17:131–43. Available from: http://www.pubmedcentral.nih.gov/articlerender.fcgi?artid= 4066672&tool=pmcentrez&rendertype=abstract.

38. Muffat J, Li Y, Yuan B, Mitalipova M, Omer A, Corcoran S, et al. Efficient derivation of microglia-like cells from human pluripotent stem cells. Nat Med. [Internet] 2016;22:1358–67. Available from: https://www.ncbi.nlm.nih. gov/pubmed/27668937.

39. Haenseler W, Sansom SN, Buchrieser J, Newey SE, Moore CS, Nicholls FJ, et al. A highly efficient human pluripotent stem cell microglia model displays a neuronal-co-culture-specific expression profile and inflammatory response. Stem Cell Rep. [Internet] 2017;8:1727–42. Available from: https:// www.ncbi.nlm.nih.gov/pubmed/28591653.

40. CRAN - Package gplots [Internet]. Available from: https://cran.r-project.org/ web/packages/gplots/index.html.

41. R package d3heatmap version 0.6.1.2. Comprehensive R Archive Network (CRAN). Available from: https://cran.r-project.org/web/packages/d3heatmap/ index.html.

42. Bouchon A, Hernández-Munain C, Cella M, Colonna M. A DAP12-mediated pathway regulates expression of CC chemokine receptor 7 and maturation of human dendritic cells. J Exp Med. [Internet] 2001;194:1111–22. Available from: http://www.pubmedcentral.nih.gov/articlerender.fcgi?artid= 2193511&tool=pmcentrez&rendertype=abstract.

43. Isken O, Maquat LE. Quality control of eukaryotic mRNA: safeguarding cells from abnormal mRNA function. Genes Dev. [Internet] 2007;21:1833–56. Available from: https://www.ncbi.nlm.nih.gov/pubmed/17671086.

44. Jay TR, Hirsch AM, Broihier ML, Miller CM, Neilson LE, Ransohoff RM, et al. Disease progression-dependent effects of TREM2 deficiency in a mouse model of Alzheimer's disease. J Neurosci. [Internet] 2017;37:637–47. Available from: http://www.jneurosci.org/content/37/3/637.

45. Wang Y, Ulland TK, Ulrich JD, Song W, Tzaferis JA, Hole JT, et al. TREM2-mediated early microglial response limits diffusion and toxicity of amyloid plaques. J Exp Med. [Internet]. 2016;213:667–75. Available from: http://www. jem.org/lookup/doi/10.1084/jem.20151948.

46. Colonna M, Wang Y. TREM2 variants: new keys to decipher Alzheimer disease pathogenesis. Nat. Rev. Neurosci. [Internet]. Nat Publ Group; 2016;17:201–207. Available from: http://www.nature.com/doifinder/10.1038/nrn.2016.7.

47. Maquat LE. Nonsense-mediated mRNA decay in mammals. J Cell Sci. [Internet] 2005;118:1773–6. Available from: http://jcs.biologists.org/cgi/doi/ 10.1242/jcs.01701.

8

Clinical spectrum and genetic landscape for hereditary spastic paraplegias in China

En-Lin Dong[1†], Chong Wang[1†], Shuang Wu[1†], Ying-Qian Lu[1], Xiao-Hong Lin[1], Hui-Zhen Su[1], Miao Zhao[1], Jin He[1], Li-Xiang Ma[2], Ning Wang[1,3], Wan-Jin Chen[1,3*] and Xiang Lin[1*] (iD)

Abstract

Background: Hereditary spastic paraplegias (HSP) is a heterogeneous group of rare neurodegenerative disorders affecting the corticospinal tracts. To date, more than 78 HSP loci have been mapped to cause HSP. However, both the clinical and mutational spectrum of Chinese patients with HSP remained unclear. In this study, we aim to perform a comprehensive analysis of clinical phenotypes and genetic distributions in a large cohort of Chinese HSP patients, and to elucidate the primary pathogenesis in this population.

Methods: We firstly performed next-generation sequencing targeting 149 genes correlated with HSP in 99 index cases of our cohort. Multiplex ligation-dependent probe amplification testing was further carried out among those patients without known disease-causing gene mutations. We simultaneously performed a retrospective study on the reported patients exhibiting HSP in other Chinese cohorts. All clinical and molecular characterization from above two groups of Chinese HSP patients were analyzed and summarized. Eventually, we further validated the cellular changes in fibroblasts of two major spastic paraplegia (SPG) patients (SPG4 and SPG11) in vitro.

Results: Most patients of ADHSP (94%) are pure forms, whereas most patients of ARHSP (78%) tend to be complicated forms. In ADHSP, we found that SPG4 (79%) was the most prevalent, followed by SPG3A (11%), SPG6 (4%) and SPG33 (2%). Subtle mutations were the common genetic cause for SPG4 patients and most of them located in AAA cassette domain of spastin protein. In ARHSP, the most common subtype was SPG11 (53%), followed by SPG5 (32%), SPG35 (6%) and SPG46 (3%). Moreover, haplotype analysis showed a unique haplotype was shared in 14 families carrying c.334C > T (p.R112*) mutation in *CYP7B1* gene, suggesting the founder effect. Functionally, we observed significantly different patterns of mitochondrial dynamics and network, decreased mitochondrial membrane potential ($\Delta\psi m$), increased reactive oxygen species and reduced ATP content in SPG4 fibroblasts. Moreover, we also found the enlargement of LAMP1-positive organelles and abnormal accumulation of autolysosomes in SPG11 fibroblasts.

Conclusions: Our study present a comprehensive clinical spectrum and genetic landscape for HSP in China. We have also provided additional evidences for mitochondrial and autolysosomal-mediated pathways in the pathogenesis of HSP.

Keywords: Hereditary spastic paraplegias, Clinical features, Mutational spectrum, Heterogeneity, Founder effect, Mitochondria, Autolysosomes

* Correspondence: wanjinchen75@fjmu.edu.cn; linxiang1988@fjmu.edu.cn
†En-Lin Dong, Chong Wang and Shuang Wu contributed equally to this work.
[1]Department of Neurology and Institute of Neurology, The First Affiliated Hospital of Fujian Medical University, Fuzhou 350005, China
Full list of author information is available at the end of the article

Background

Hereditary spastic paraplegias (HSP) refer to a heterogeneous group of rare neurodegenerative disorders. HSP have a variable age at onset (AAO) and are mainly characterized by slow progressive bilateral spasticity and weakness of lower limbs [1]. The estimated prevalence of HSP is about 2–10/100000 in the general population [2]. Clinically, HSP cases are divided into pure and complicated forms. Pure form is characterized by pyramidal signs, associated with isolated spasticity and weakness confined to the lower limbs [3]. These patients rarely need wheel chairs but may use crutches during the disease course, even they usually have normal lifespan [4]. However, additional severe neurological symptoms can be exhibited in the complicated form, such as ataxia, dysarthria, cognitive impairment, mental retardation, epilepsy, peripheral neuropathy, as well as extra-neurological signs like ophthalmoplegia [5]. The functional handicap and lifespan are associated with the full clinical manifestation in complicated form [6].

Genetically, HSP are highly heterogeneous, with 78 spastic paraplegia (SPG) associated loci and more than 60 identified genes [5, 7]. Moreover, at least 20 additional genes have recently been correlated to HSP [5, 6]. HSP can be transmitted with all classical modes of inheritance, including autosomal dominant (AD), autosomal recessive (AR), X-linked or mitochondrial maternal transmission. Autosomal dominant hereditary spastic paraplegia (ADHSP) is the most prevalent form of HSP and accounts for approximately 70% of cases [8]. SPG4 (50%), SPG3A (10%), SPG31 (4.5%) and SPG10 (2.5%) are the most common causes of ADHSP, in decreasing order of prevalence [6]. Autosomal recessive HSP (ARHSP) is the next largest group of HSP. Mutations in the *CYP7B1* (SPG5), *SPG7* (SPG7), *SPG11* (SPG11) and *ZFYVE26* (SPG15) gene are described as the most frequent causes for ARHSP [9, 10]. However, their relative frequencies vary largely depending on the distinct geographical origin.

Membrane trafficking and axonal transport are emerging as potentially main scenario for HSP [4]. The considerable known HSP causative genes encode proteins mainly involved in microtubule dynamics, endoplasmic reticulum morphogenesis, vesicular formation, lipid metabolism and endosomal functions [3, 11]. However, growing evidences revealed that above theories cannot fully explain the etiology of HSP [12]. Identifying the role of responsible genes could have far-reaching effects on patients, as it would reveal the cause of the disease, and help to better understand the correlation between genotypes and phenotypes. With the growing number of causative genes and the complexity of genotypes and phenotypes, it is difficult to achieve a definite genetic diagnosis in many affected individuals using traditional sanger sequencing. To date, comprehensive review of clinical spectrum and genetic landscape in a large cohort of HSP patients have not yet been presented in China.

In the present study, we firstly investigated the causative genes in 99 both ADHSP and ARHSP families in our cohort using the targeted next generation sequencing (NGS) or multiplex ligation-dependent probe amplification (MLPA) approach. We then retrospectively analyzed and summarized the clinical spectrum and genetic landscape in 47 documented families of our cohort, and in 140 confirmed HSP families of other reported cohorts in China. During the course of these studies, we discovered that SPG4 (79%), SPG3A (11%), SPG6 (4%) and SPG33 (2%) were the most frequently found in Chinese ADHSP patients, and were mainly pure forms with wide range AAO. Meanwhile, Chinese ARHSP patients were more complex in clinical terms with early AAO. The major subtypes of ARHSP in decrease order of frequency were SPG11 (53%), SPG5 (32%), SPG35 (6%) and SPG46 (3%). Moreover, we determined that the high prevalence of SPG5 resulted from the founder effect. On these basis, we further conducted functional studies on two major subtypes, SPG4 and SPG11, patients derived fibroblasts to elucidate the pathogenic mechanisms. Overall, these results have provided a new perspective to assess the clinical features, genetic distribution and physiopathology for Chinses HSP patients.

Methods

Subjects recruitment

Subjects participated in our cohort were recruited from the Department of Neurology, First Affiliated Hospital of Fujian Medical University. In total, 99 families fulfilling the clinical diagnostic criteria for HSP were enrolled irrespective of their genetic diagnosis [13]. Patients in other cohort were collected by review of 41 reported studies exhibiting HSP in China (Additional file 1: Table S1). A total of 418 HSP patients from 140 families were included.

In addition, 200 unrelated Chinese individuals without history of spastic paraplegia were selected as the control group.

Targeted NGS and data analysis

Genomic DNA was extracted from peripheral vein blood using a QIAamp DNA Blood Mini Kit (Qiagen, Hilden, Germany) according to the manufacturer's instructions. Targeted NGS panel was designed to cover 149 genes known to be correlated with HSP (Additional file 1: Table S2). The whole exons, along with 20 base pairs of flanking sequences, of targeted genes were enriched with the TruSeq DNA LT Sample Prep Kit v2 (Illumina) according to the manufacturer's standard protocol. DNA libraries were subjected to paired-end sequencing on the Illumina High Seq 3000 platform. After eliminating the low-quality FASTQ sequencing reads by Trim Galore, we mapped the remaining high-quality reads to the human reference genome (UCSC hg19) with Burrows-Wheeler Aligner. The variants were called using Genome Analysis Tool Kit, and were annotated with the annotate variation.

All the variants were further filtered by 1000 Genomes Project (http://phase3browser.1000genomes.org/index.html), Exome Sequencing Project (http://evs.gs.washington.edu/EVS/) and Exome Aggregation Consortium database (http://exac.broadinstitute.org/). The property of variants, either benign or pathogenic, were further analyzed by SIFT (http://sift.jcvi.org), PolyPhen-2 (http://genetics.bwh.harvard.edu/pph2/), and Mutation Taster (http://www.mutationtaster.org). Finally, the pathogenic mutations were compared with the Human Gene Mutation Database (http://www.hgmd.cf.ac.uk/) to determine whether they were known or novel mutations.

Sanger sequencing

Specific primers for amplification of mutations were designed by the Primer 5 software listed in Additional file 1: Table S3. The targeted regions were amplified with polymerase chain reaction (PCR) in a 2720 Thermal Cycler (ABI). After purification, the amplified products were electrophoresed on an ABI 3730XL Automated DNA analyser (PE Applied Biosystems, Foster City, CA) according to standard protocols. The sequencing results were assembled with chromas software.

MLPA testing

MLPA testing was performed in the patients without known disease-causing gene mutations for detection of large deletions or copy number variations. The MLPA analyses were performed according to the manufacturer's protocol using the following SALSA MLPA probemixes: P165-C2 (coverage: *ATL1*, *SPAST*), P211-B4 (coverage: *SPAST*, *NIPA1*), P306-B1 (coverage: *SPG11*) and P213-B2 (coverage: *REEP1*, *SPG7*) (MRC-Holland, Amsterdam, the Netherlands). Data were collected by Genemapper 3.0 (Applied Biosystems, California, USA) and analyzed using Coffalyser software.

Haplotype analysis

Based on the database of Southern Han Chinese in Haplotype Map Project (https://www.ncbi.nlm.nih.gov/variation/tools/1000genomes/), 9 tagSNPs (rs9298109, rs6985116, rs7842714, rs116843046, rs200737038, rs4465006, rs3779869, rs8192906 and rs4367588) were

selected for further haplotype analysis of unrelated SPG5 families. These tagSNPs are linkage to *CYP7B1* gene and spanning ~ 1.5-Mb interval. PCR and sanger sequencing were used to identify the specific genotype of tagSNP. Primers for amplification were listed in Additional file 1: Table S3.

Study on the mutational function in vitro
DNA constructs and cell transfection

The human M1- and M87-spastin cDNAs was prepared as described previously [14]. Briefly, wild-type spastin cDNAs was cloned into the *BamH*I and *Not*I site of the eukaryotic expression vector of pCMV6-Entry, with HA tag at the N terminus. To generate mutagenesis plasmid, the Mut Express II Fast Mutagenesis Kit V2 (Vazyme) was used according to the manufacturer's instructions. The construction was verified by DNA sequencing after ligation, transformation and extraction. The primers for plasmid construct were summarized in Additional file 1: Table S3.

HEK293T cells were cultured in Dulbecco's modified Eagle's medium (DMEM) supplemented with 10% fetal bovine serum (FBS) and maintained at 37 °C under 5% CO_2/air. Transient transfections were performed using Lipofectamine 3000 (Thermo Scientific) for plasmid DNAs.

Primary fibroblasts culture and treatment

Primary fibroblast cell lines were established from skin biopsies with punches (Electron microscopy sciences), obtained from the probands of family F12 of SPG4 and family F4 of SPG11. Fibroblasts were maintained in DMEM supplemented with 20% FBS and 1% penicillin/ streptomycin.

Autophagy was induced by amino acid and serum starvation in Earle's Balanced Salt Solution (Thermo Scientific) for 6 h.

Reverse transcription polymerase chain reaction (RT-PCR) and quantification PCR (qPCR)

Total RNA from leukocytes or fibroblasts were extracted with the TRIzol kit (Invitrogen) according to the manufacturer's instructions. A 0.5-μg aliquot of total RNA was reversely transcribed into cDNA.

RT-PCR was performed in a 2720 Thermal Cycler (ABI), and the resulting products were visualized on 2.5% agarose gels under UV transilluminator (Tanon, China). QPCR were performed with SYBR@Premix EX TaqTM II kit (Takara) and run on an Applied Biosystems Stepone Real-time PCR System. The primers for amplification are listed in Additional file 1: Table S3.

Detection of mitochondrial membrane potential (MMP, Δψm) by JC-1

Fibroblast cells were cultured on glass slide. JC-1 dye solution was added to cells in medium and incubated for 20 min at 37°C (Addition file 1: Table S4), according to the manufacture's recommended protocol. After washing with cold incubation buffer solution, JC-1 staining of mitochondria in live cells was immediately observed using a Leica TCS SP8 confocal system. The wavelength at excitation/emission 525/590 nm was used to assess JC-1 aggregates, and at excitation/emission 488/525 nm was used to assess JC-1 monomer.

Detection of intracellular reactive oxygen species level by DCFH-DA

Reactive oxygen species (ROS) in fibroblasts were detected using a fluorescent probe, 2′7′-dichlorofluorescein diacetate (DCFH-DA). DCFH-DA is hydrolyzed to DCFH, which further be oxidized to fluorescent DCF by intracellular ROS. Briefly, fibroblasts seeded on glass slide were rinsed with $1 \times$ PBS and incubated with DCFH-DA for 20 min at 37°C (Addition file 1: Table S4), according to the manufacture's recommended protocol. After washing with $1 \times$ PBS, DCFH-DA labeled mitochondria in live cells were immediately observed using a Leica TCS SP8 confocal system. The wavelength at 488 nm excitation and 525 nm emission was used to assess DCF.

Measurement of ATP content

ATP content was determined in fibroblasts cell lysates using an ATP bioluminescence assay kit (Addition file 1: Table S4), according to the manufacture's recommended protocol. Measurements were performed in a luminometer (Tecan, Austria). The relative ATP content was recorded as ATP value (nmol) /protein value (mg) ratio.

Immunocytochemistry (ICH) and quantification

The fibroblasts were fixed with 4% paraformaldehyde (10–20 min at room temperature), rinsed three times with 1× PBS (Medicago AB) and incubated in a blocking buffer (10% donkey serum and 0.2% triton X-100 in PBS) for 1 h and then incubated with primary antibodies (Additional file 1: Table S4) overnight in a refrigerator at 4 °C. Fluorescence conjugated secondary antibodies (Thermo Scientific) and DAPI (Sigma) were used at 1:1000 dilution. Images were captured by a Leica TCS SP8 confocal system.

Image-J software (NIH, MD, USA) was used for further quantification of the cell population, particle number, lysosome diameter and fluorescence intensity. Quantification was performed by a person blind to the

experiment and replicated in four random visual fields from three independent experiments.

Western blotting

The cells were harvested in the cell lysis reagent (Sigma) supplemented with a 1% protease inhibitor PMSF (Beyotime) and centrifuged at 13,000 rpm for 20 min at 4 °C. Protein extracts were separated on 12% SDS-PAGE gels and immunoblotted with primary antibodies listed in Additional file 1: Table S4. HRP-conjugated secondary antibodies (1:5000, Santa Cruz) were used to detect primary antibodies and proteins were visualized by chemiluminescence (Millipore).

Statistical analysis

All data were presented as the mean ± SEM. SPSS 16.0 was used for statistical comparisons, and significance was determined using the Student's t-test. Differences were considered statistically significant when the P value was less than 0.05 (*).

Results

NGS targeting 149 genes correlated with HSP was performed in all probands of our cohort. In aggregate, approximately 99.9% target bases were covered by the probe and over 82.3% of bases were covered at greater than 50×, suggesting an accepted threshold for variant calling. After filtering the sequence data down to nonsynonymous or loss-of-function (LOF) variants with allele frequencies less than 1% in the 1000 Genomes, ESP5400 and ExAC, we finally identified 37 novel or known pathogenic variants in both 22 ADHSP and 25 ARHSP families. All these mutations have been confirmed by sanger sequencing and were not detected in 200 ethnically matched controls. Moreover, exon deletion of *SPAST* gene was detected among three SPG4 families by MLPA. With retrospective analysis, 89 ADHSP and 51 ARHSP families in other Chinese cohorts were also included in the present study (Additional file 1: Table S1).

Collectively, a considerable number of ADHSP patients (94%) were pure forms, whereas most ARHSP patients (78%) tended to be complicated forms (Fig. 1a and b). In ADHSP, we found that SPG4 was the most frequent subtype, account for 79% of all cases with causal dominant genes in China (Fig. 1c). SPG4 was followed by SPG3A (11%), SPG6 (4%) and SPG33 (2%). In ARHSP, the most common subtype was SPG11 (53%), followed by SPG5 (32%), SPG35 (6%) and SPG46 (3%) (Fig. 1d). Importantly, some rare subtypes of our cohort patients including SPG8 (1%), SPG28 (1%), SPG30 (1%), SPG43 (1%) and SPG54 (1%) were firstly presented in China.

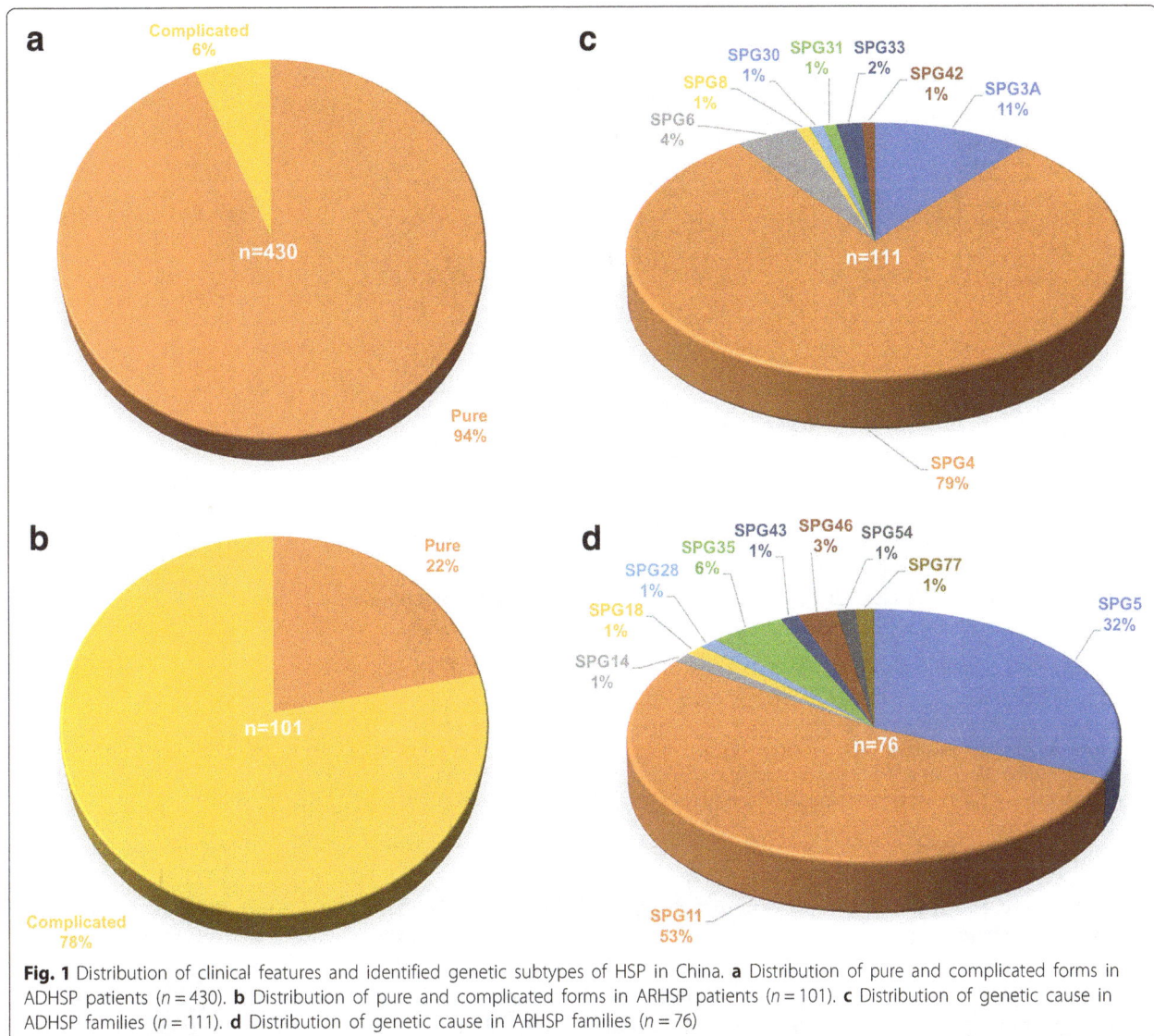

Fig. 1 Distribution of clinical features and identified genetic subtypes of HSP in China. **a** Distribution of pure and complicated forms in ADHSP patients (*n* = 430). **b** Distribution of pure and complicated forms in ARHSP patients (*n* = 101). **c** Distribution of genetic cause in ADHSP families (*n* = 111). **d** Distribution of genetic cause in ARHSP families (*n* = 76)

The clinical features and mutational spectrum in Chinese ADHSP patients

Mutations in SPAST gene cause ADHSP

SPG4 is caused by mutations in *SPAST* gene [15]. The clinical features of Chinese SPG4 patients were summarized in Additional file 1: Table S5. The mean ± SD AAO in these patients was 25.01 ± 15.84 years, ranging from 1 to 62 years old. The mean ± SD disease duration was 17.91 ± 14.98 years. Most cases (93.8%) had the core features of HSP, and were considered as prototypical pure forms. Moreover, peripheral neuropathy was the most common symptom in complicated patients.

Spastin, encoded by *SPAST* gene, contains four functional domains including transmembrane (TM) domain, microtubule interacting and trafficking (MIT) domain, microtubule-binding domain (MTBD), and

AAA (*A*TPases *a*ssociated with diverse cellular *a*ctivities) cassette domain [16]. To date, 46 subtle mutations in *SPAST* gene have been reported in Chinese SPG4 patients (Additional file 1: Table S1). In our cohort, 16 SPG4 families were identified to carry 14 pathogenetic mutations: seven were missense mutations, two were frameshift mutations, one was stop-gain mutation, two were splicing mutations and two were exons deletion (Additional file 2: Figure S1). All of these 58 subtle mutations widely distributed in four domains of spastin protein and mainly located in the AAA cassette (Fig. 2a and b), accounting for up to 78.3%. Except for subtle mutations, 16 kinds of large deletions or duplications of *SPAST* gene have also been detected, of which the exon 11–12 deletion was the most common mode (Fig. 2c). By comparing the frequency, we further discovered that subtle

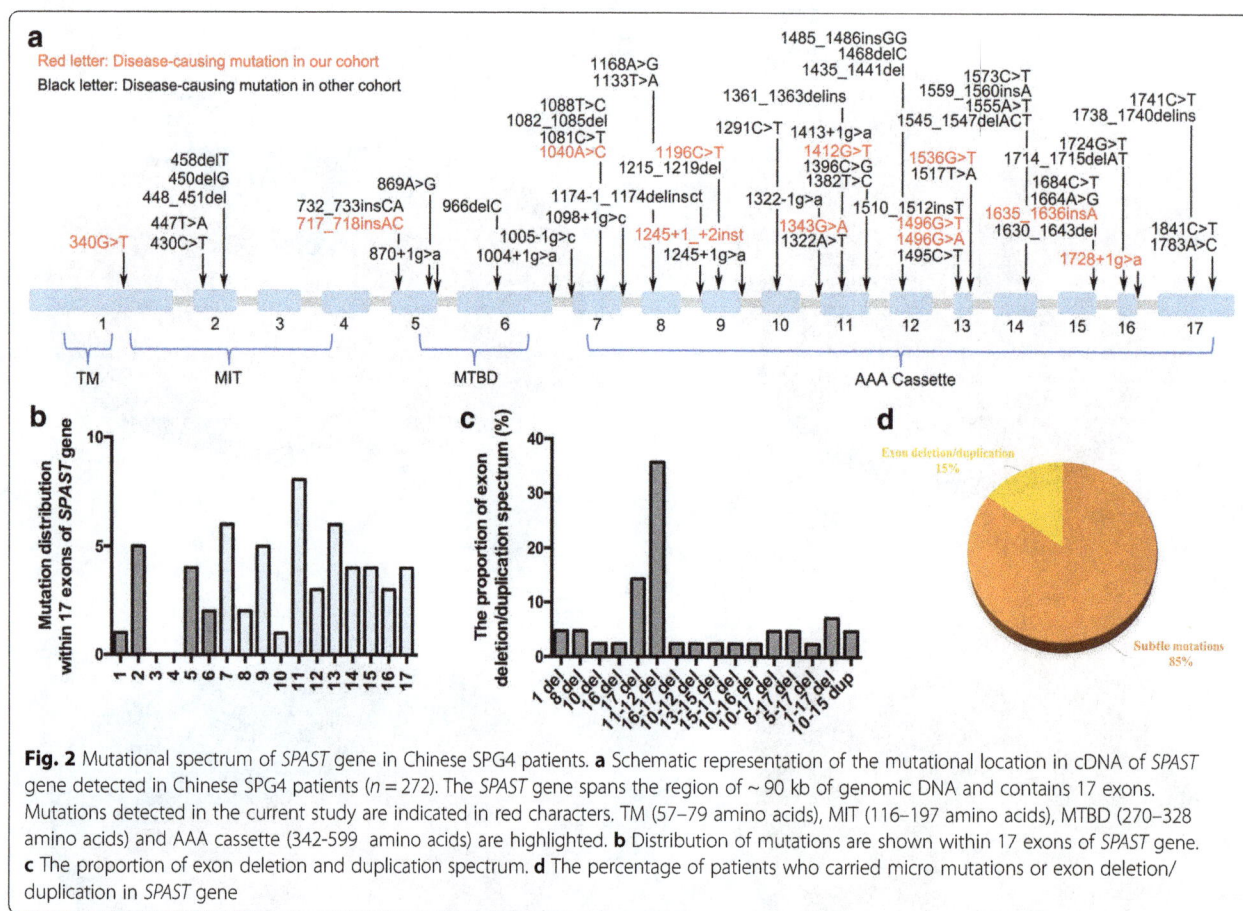

Fig. 2 Mutational spectrum of *SPAST* gene in Chinese SPG4 patients. **a** Schematic representation of the mutational location in cDNA of *SPAST* gene detected in Chinese SPG4 patients (*n* = 272). The *SPAST* gene spans the region of ~ 90 kb of genomic DNA and contains 17 exons. Mutations detected in the current study are indicated in red characters. TM (57–79 amino acids), MIT (116–197 amino acids), MTBD (270–328 amino acids) and AAA cassette (342-599 amino acids) are highlighted. **b** Distribution of mutations are shown within 17 exons of *SPAST* gene. **c** The proportion of exon deletion and duplication spectrum. **d** The percentage of patients who carried micro mutations or exon deletion/duplication in *SPAST* gene

mutations were the much more common (85%) genetic cause for SPG4 (Fig. 2d).

Four novel mutations, c.717_718insAC (p.S243Lfs*12), c.1040A > C (p.Q347P), c.1245 + 1_c.1245 + 2insT and c.1635_1636insA (p.G546Rfs*3) were identified in our cohort. Based on the standards and guidelines for the interpretation of sequence variants [17], p.S243Lfs*12 and p.G546Rfs*3 were considered as both LOF mutations (Additional file 2: Figure S2), which was the very strong evidence for pathogenic effect. To further confirm the pathogenesis of c.1040A > C and c.1245 + 1_c.1245 + 2insT, we studied the functional effect on spastin. As a result of two different initiation codons, two primary isoforms of spastin were synthesized: a full-length isoform called M1 and a slightly shorter isoform called M87. M87 was detectably presented in all tissues, whereas M1 was only expressed in adult spinal cord [12]. Therefore, we introduced the p.Q347P missense mutation into M1- and M87-spastin expression HA-tag vectors and overexpressed them in HEK 293 T cell (Fig. 3a). Immunoblotting of HA showed that spastin level of p.Q347P was found to be comparable to that of WT (Additional file 2: Figure S2). To further study its influence on stability of spastin, we performed

cycloheximide (CHX, 40 μg/ml) chase assay to inhibit de-novo protein synthesis and reassessed the protein expression levels after different treatment durations. The treatment of CHX resulted in rapid degradation of p.Q347P protein (Fig. 3b and c; Additional file 2: Figure S2), indicating that the missense mutation affected protein half-life of spastin. In addition, we also validated the effect of splicing mutation c.1245 + 1_c.1245 + 2insT on patient's leukocytes derived mRNA. A different product in size from the RT-PCR of *SPAST* cDNA from the patient was detected (Fig. 3d), indicating the presence of an aberrant splice event (Fig. 3e). The sequencing of amplification products confirmed that alternative splicing result in the skipping of exon 9 in mutant transcript (Fig. 3f).

Mutations in ATL1, KIAA0196, KIF1A and ZFYVE27 gene cause ADHSP

Mutations in *KIAA0196* (SPG8), *KIF1A* (SPG30) and *ZFYVE27* (SPG33) gene of our cohort ADHSP patients were firstly presented in China. Three missense mutations and one frameshift mutation of these genes (p.T845A in *KIAA0196*, p.I37T in *KIF1A*, p. N88Rfs*7 and p.A290T in *ZFYVE27*) were detected in four ADHSP families

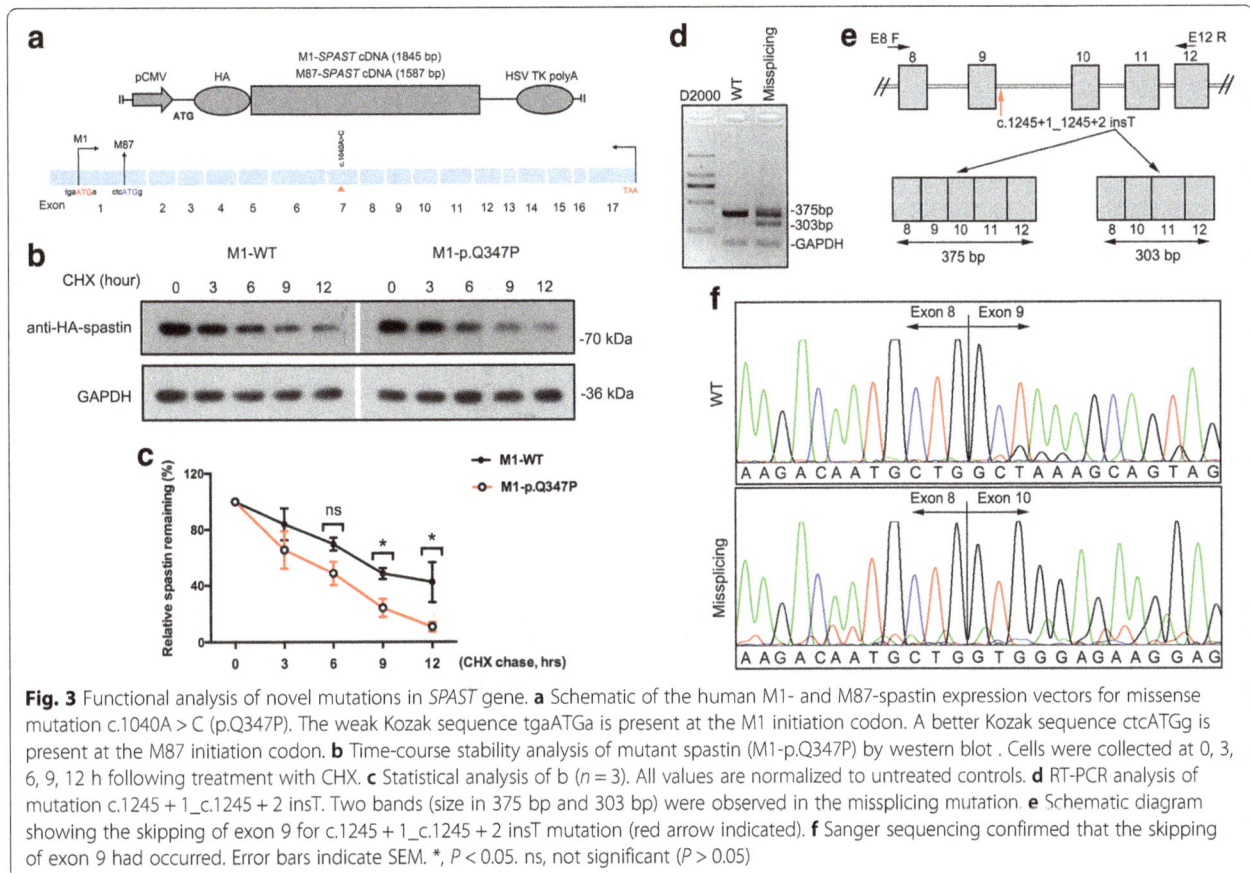

Fig. 3 Functional analysis of novel mutations in *SPAST* gene. **a** Schematic of the human M1- and M87-spastin expression vectors for missense mutation c.1040A > C (p.Q347P). The weak Kozak sequence tgaATGa is present at the M1 initiation codon. A better Kozak sequence ctcATGg is present at the M87 initiation codon. **b** Time-course stability analysis of mutant spastin (M1-p.Q347P) by western blot . Cells were collected at 0, 3, 6, 9, 12 h following treatment with CHX. **c** Statistical analysis of b (*n* = 3). All values are normalized to untreated controls. **d** RT-PCR analysis of mutation c.1245 + 1_c.1245 + 2 insT. Two bands (size in 375 bp and 303 bp) were observed in the missplicing mutation. **e** Schematic diagram showing the skipping of exon 9 for c.1245 + 1_c.1245 + 2 insT mutation (red arrow indicated). **f** Sanger sequencing confirmed that the skipping of exon 9 had occurred. Error bars indicate SEM. *, *P* < 0.05. ns, not significant (*P* > 0.05)

(Additional file 2: Figure S3). Patients carrying p.T845A in *KIAA0196* and p.A290T in *ZFYVE27*, were classified as complicated HSP, whereas others presented as pure form. Structural magnetic resonance images (MRI) of the complicated patient carrying p.A290T revealed agenesis of corpus callosum and leukoencephalopathy. In addition, we also identified two missense mutations (p.A350S and p.R416C) of *ATL1* (SPG3A) in one family with pure form and another family with complicated form, respectively (Additional file 2: Figure S3). Both probands with *ATL1* mutations had a very young AAO. Intriguingly, the mother of the proband carrying the reported mutation p.R416C, remained asymptomatic presently.

The clinical features and mutational spectrum in Chinese ARHSP

Mutations in SPG11 gene cause ARHSP

SPG11 is caused by mutations in *SPG11* gene [18]. The clinical characterization of Chinese SPG11 patients were summarized in Additional file 1: Table S6. In general, SPG11 patients had early AAO (12.71 ± 4.48 years, mean ± SD), ranging from 4 to 20 years old. The mean ± SD disease duration was 12.46 ± 8.43 years. The majority of patients (78.5%) initially presented with gait

disturbance. Except for the typical manifestation of HSP, most cases combined with cognitive deficit (78.9%), dysarthria (73.1%), mental retardation (53.9%) and peripheral neuropathy (61.6%). Notably, 92.3% of SPG11 patients presented a typical sign of thin corpus callosum on MRI.

A total of 31 subtle mutations have been detected in Chinese SPG11 patients so far (Fig. 4a). In our cohort, we identified five LOF mutations (p.M245Vfs*2, p.I415*, p.M1272Ifs*6, p.R2031* and p.W2234*) of *SPG11* gene in 4 SPG11 families (Fig. 4b). Sanger sequencing of these mutations in other family members showed a co-segregation of genotype with the disease phenotype. However, we did not find obvious clustering of these 36 mutations on the functional domain of spatacsin protein, encoded by *SPG11* gene (Fig. 4a).

Mutations in CYP7B1 gene cause ARHSP

SPG5 is caused by mutations in *CYP7B1* gene [19]. The mean ± SD AAO in Chinese SPG5 patients was 16.88 ± 10.39 years, ranging from 3 to 44 years old, with a peak in the first two decades. The mean ± SD disease duration was 9.93 ± 7.17 years. More than half of the patients (57.1%) presented as complicated forms. Interestingly,

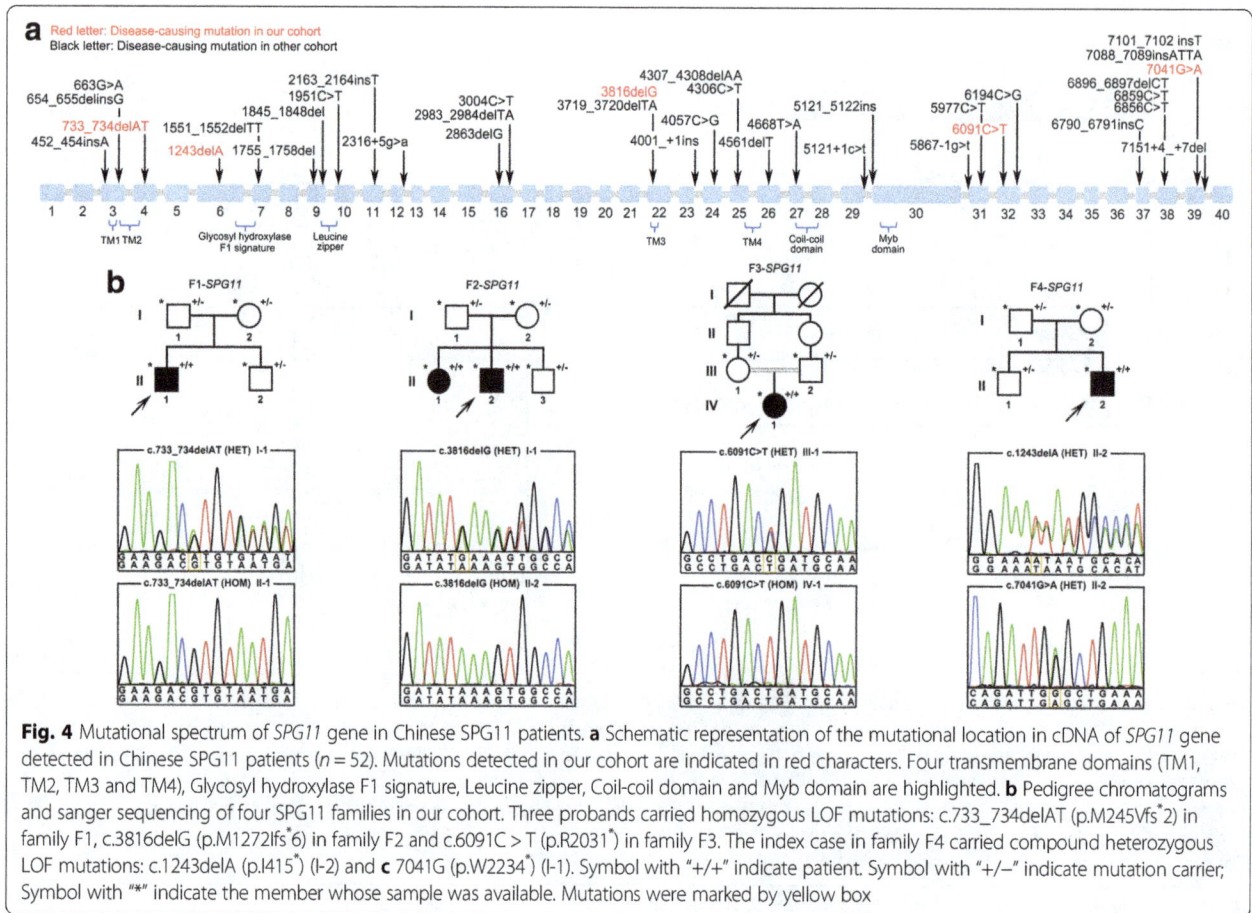

Fig. 4 Mutational spectrum of *SPG11* gene in Chinese SPG11 patients. **a** Schematic representation of the mutational location in cDNA of *SPG11* gene detected in Chinese SPG11 patients (*n* = 52). Mutations detected in our cohort are indicated in red characters. Four transmembrane domains (TM1, TM2, TM3 and TM4), Glycosyl hydroxylase F1 signature, Leucine zipper, Coil-coil domain and Myb domain are highlighted. **b** Pedigree chromatograms and sanger sequencing of four SPG11 families in our cohort. Three probands carried homozygous LOF mutations: c.733_734delAT (p.M245Vfs*2) in family F1, c.3816delG (p.M1272lfs*6) in family F2 and c.6091C > T (p.R2031*) in family F3. The index case in family F4 carried compound heterozygous LOF mutations: c.1243delA (p.I415*) (I-2) and **c** 7041G (p.W2234*) (I-1). Symbol with "+/+" indicate patient. Symbol with "+/−" indicate mutation carrier; Symbol with "*" indicate the member whose sample was available. Mutations were marked by yellow box

white matter lesions were observed in 50% of complicated SPG5 patients (Additional file 1: Table S7).

In our cohort, mutations in *CYP7B1* gene was identified in 16 SPG5 kindred (Additional file 2: Figure S4). Among these, 14 families carried the known nonsense mutation c.334 C > T (p.R112*) [20], which was homozygous in 13 families, accounting for up to 92.9%. Haplotype analysis was further performed on members of the 16 unrelated families, and revealed that cases with the mutation c.334C > T (p.R112*) shared the same unique haplotype in the 1.5-Mb interval between tagSNP rs9298109 and rs4367588 (Additional file 1: Table S8). This result implied that all the specific SPG5 patients carrying the homozygous mutation c.334C > T (p.R112*), originated from the common ancestor, which is termed as 'founder effect' (Additional file 1: Table S8). Besides that, we also identified another four novel mutations (p.L145Cfs*13, p.Y181*, p.R370C and p.P397L) of *CYP7B1* in another 3 remaining families.

Mutations in *DDHD1*, *FA2H*, *C19orf12*, *GBA2*, and *DDHD2* gene cause ARHSP

Mutations in *DDHD1* (SPG28), *C19orf12* (SPG43) and *DDHD2* (SPG54) gene of our ARHSP patients

were firstly presented in China. One previously mutation (p.G58R in *C19orf12*) and three novel mutations (p.R740* in *DDHD1*, p.Y99* and p.R112Q in *DDHD2*) were identified in three ARHSP families (Additional file 2: Figure S5). All these three families mainly presented with weakness and spasticity restricted to the lower limbs, thus they were considered as a pure form of HSP. In addition, we have also confirmed four novel mutations (p.P148L and p.L131Sfs*14 in *FA2H* (SPG35), p.W475* and p.R879W in *GBA2* (SPG46)) in two ARHSP families (Additional file 2: Figure S5). Both of them showed additional complicated features including dysarthria, cognition impairment, even skin peeling.

Functional characterization of mutant spastin and spatacsin in the patients derived fibroblast cells

SPG4 and SPG11 are the most common subtypes of ADHSP and ARHSP in China, respectively. The two groups account for up to 68.5% of all patients. To elucidate their pathogenic mechanism, we further study the function of spastin and spatacsin protein in patients derived fibroblasts.

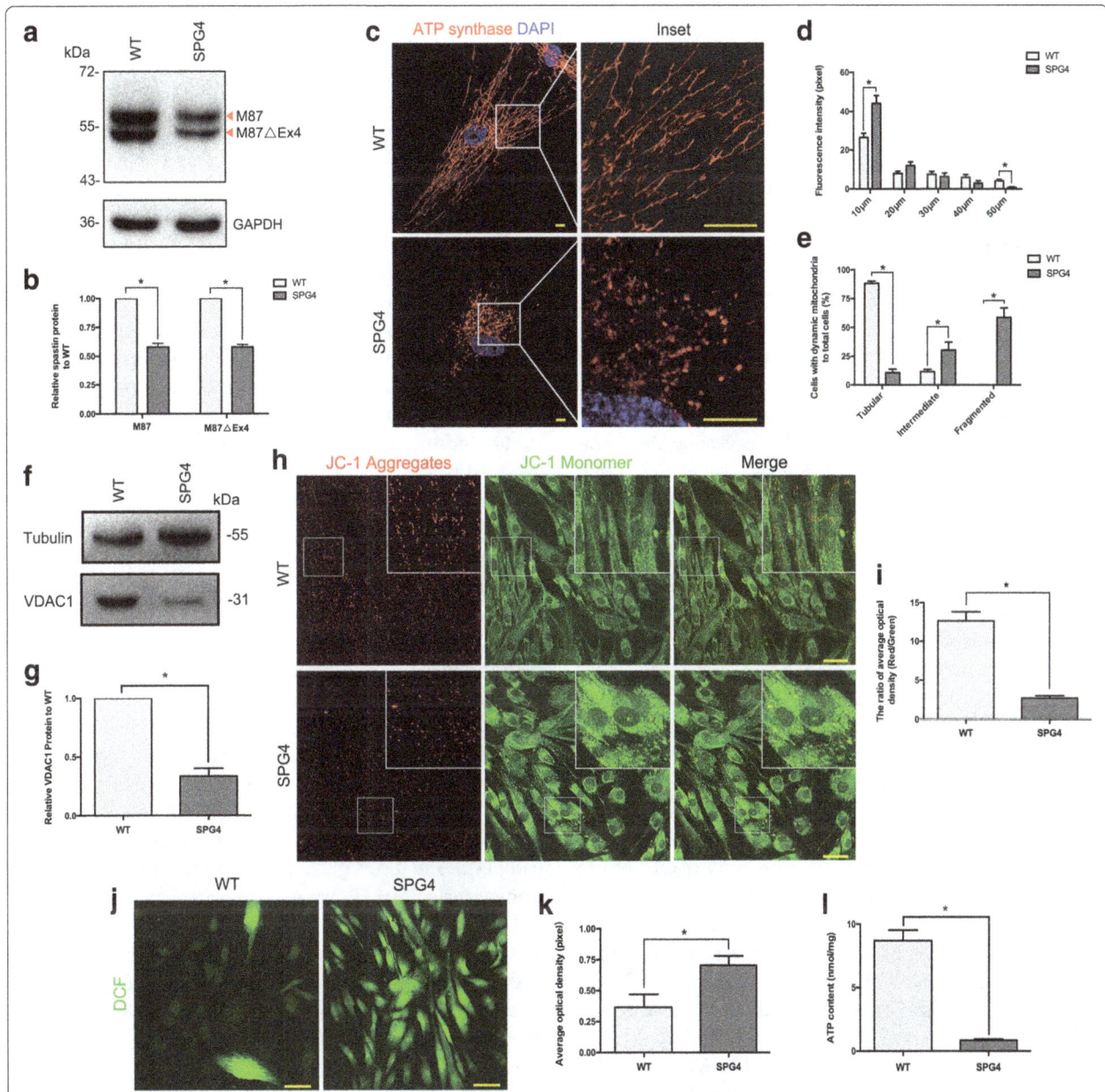

Fig. 5 Mitochondrial dynamics and oxidative metabolism were altered in the SPG4 patient derived fibroblasts. **a, b** Western blot analysis showed a significant difference in spastin isoforms (M87 and M87△Ex4) expression levels between the SPG4 patient and WT. **c** ICH of mitochondria maker (ATP synthase, red) and DAPI (blue) in fibroblasts from the WT (upper panel) and the SPG4 patient (lower panel). Insets in the images are enlarged (original magnification, ×8.0) to the right. Scale bar, 10 μm. **d** Quantification of mitochondria distribution measured from the center of the cells ($n = 3$, > 10 cells per experiment). The data showed that the number of mitochondria were significantly reduced along the branch in the SPG4 patient derived fibroblasts. **e** Quantification of cells with different mitochondrial morphology (tubular, intermediate and fragmented patterns) to total cell ($n = 3$, > 30 cells per experiment). **f, g** Western blot analysis showed a significant difference in VDAC1 protein expression levels between the SPG4 patient and WT. **h** JC-1 staining was used to measure MMP (Δψm) in fibroblasts from the WT (upper panel) and the SPG4 patient (lower panel). Boxed areas are enlarged in the insets. Scale bar, 50 μm. **i** Statistical analysis of h ($n = 3$). **j** Intracellular ROS visualization using DCFH-DA staining in WT (upper panel) and SPG4 (lower panel). Scale bar, 50 μm. **k** Statistical analysis of (**j**) ($n = 3$). **l** ATP bioluminometers analysis revealed a significant decrease of ATP content in the SPG4 patient. Error bars indicate SEM. *, $P < 0.05$

Loss of spastin results in abnormal mitochondrial dynamics and oxidative metabolism

In fact, there are two additional spastin isoforms, M1△Ex4 and M87△Ex4, that result from skipping of exon 4. We observed that the M87 and M87△Ex4 isoforms were both present in both WT and SPG4 fibroblasts, but not with M1 or M1 △Ex4 isoforms (Fig. 5a). The level of both two predominant isoforms were significantly reduced by 43% in SPG4 ($P < 0.001$, Fig. 5b). The premature termination codon within the AAA cassette domain of spastin is expected to induce nonsense mediated mRNA decay [21]. Consistent with this, we did not find the truncated isoforms (~ 50 kDa) in the SPG4 fibroblasts (Fig. 5a).

The spastin expression levels are the limiting factor in microtubule severing to maintain microtubule network. Mitochondrial motility and regional distribution have been reported to closely interact with cytoskeletal tracks, such as microtubules and actin filaments [22]. To evaluate the mitochondrial distribution pattern in SPG4, mitochondria were visualized using antibody against ATP synthase. That we observed a more pronounced concentration of mitochondria around the perinuclear region in patient derived fibroblasts ($P < 0.001$, Fig. 5c and d), suggesting the intracellular trafficking alteration. Intriguingly, we further found more fragmented and unbranched, but fewer tubular mitochondria in SPG4 fibroblasts ($P < 0.001$, Fig. 5c and e), which implied the impaired patterns of mitochondrial fission and fusion. Mitochondrial network fragmentation was further assessed by immunoblot analysis of the voltage-dependent anion channel 1(VDAC1), an outer mitochondrial membrane protein, acts as a gatekeeper for the transport of mitochondrial metabolites [23, 24]. Likewise decreased expression of the VDAC1 protein was observed in SPG4 fibroblasts ($\sim 70\%$ reduction, $P < 0.001$, Fig. 6f and g). We further sought to determine whether the mitochondrial function was altered. Fluorescence indicator, JC-1, was used to validate the level of MMP ($\Delta\psi$m). We observed the ratio of average optical density (AOD, red to green) was significantly reduced by 80% in SPG4 ($P < 0.001$, Fig. 6h and i). The loss of $\Delta\psi$m could induce the increase in intracellular ROS [25], which was strongly confirmed by DCFH-DA staining. We found that the ROS level was dramatically increased in SPG4 fibroblasts (~ 2 folds increase on average, $P < 0.001$, Fig. 6j and k). We further investigated the effect on ATP content. ATP bioluminometers analysis revealed that the relative ATP content was apparently decreased in the SPG4 fibroblasts (mean ± SEM, WT:8.70 ± 0.83 nmol/mg, SPG4: 0.85 ± 0.09 nmol/mg, $P < 0.001$, Fig. 6l). Thus, the lack of spastin in SPG4 would cause abnormal mitochondrial dynamics and oxidative metabolism.

Loss of spatacsin results in enlarged LAMP1-positive organelles and accumulation of autolysosomes

QPCR and ICH results showed that spatacsin expression level was significantly decreased by 80% in SPG11 fibroblasts ($P < 0.001$, Fig. 6a and b). Spatacsin has been reported to play a pivotal role in autophagic lysosome reformation, a pathway that generates new lysosomes [26]. With inducing autophagy by starvation of fibroblasts, we found SPG11 fibroblast cells exhibited

prominently enlarged organelles immunostained with LAMP1 (~ 2.5 folds increase on average, $P < 0.001$), a marker of late endosomes and lysosomes (Fig. 6c and d). Moreover, the number of cells with enlarged LAMP1-positive organelles (LPOs) was also significantly increased in SPG11 (~ 8 folds increase on average, $P < 0.001$, Fig. 6e), although this had no significant effect on total LAMP1 protein level ($P = 0.235$, Fig. 6f and g). Thus, we speculated that depletion of spatacsin would result in the enlarged volume of LPOs, but not in their change of total amount.

Autophagosomes fuse with lysosomes to generate autolysosomes, which is essential for autophay-dependent intracellular clearance. The accumulation of enlarged LPOs reminds us to study any dysfunction in autophagosomes status. Indeed, SPG11 fibroblasts present significantly aggregated mature autophagosomes labeled by p62 ($P < 0.001$, Fig. 6h and i), and with enhanced p62 protein level (~ 2.0 folds increase on average, $P < 0.001$, Fig. 6j and k). During autophagy, cytosolic LC3 (LC3-I) is continually modified to form a LC3-phosphatidylethanolamine conjugate (LC3-II), which can be recruited to autophagosomal membranes. The ratio of LC3-II to LC3-I is recognized as a marker for monitoring autophagosomes formation [27]. To further validate above finding, we performed immunoblot on LC3 and confirmed a significant increase in the amount of autophagosomes in SPG11 fibroblasts (~ 3.0 folds increase on average, $P < 0.001$, Fig. 6l and m). To investigate the spatial relationship between enlarged LPOs and accumulated autophagosomes, fibroblasts were coimmunostained with LC3 and LAMP1. We found that most autophagosomes labeled by LC3 were also positive with the enlarged LPOs labeled by LAMP1 in both groups ($P = 0.858$, Fig. 6n and o), indicating that normal fusion of autophagosomes with lysosomes had occurred in spatacsin-deficiency fibroblasts. Overall, the lack of spatacsin in SPG11 would lead to aberrant accumulation of the autolysosomes.

Discussion

Herein, we have analyzed and summarized 430 of ADHSP patients and 101 of ARHSP patients in China, respectively. In total, 18 SPG subtypes and more than 150 mutations have been uncovered. To the best of our knowledge, this study included the largest HSP cohort in China and presented a comprehensive overview of the clinical spectrum and genetic landscape for HSP.

As in previous studies, AD forms of HSP are mainly pure forms [28]. The AAO had a wide range from infancy to late adulthood [29, 30]. Mutations in *SPAST* (SPG4), *ATL1* (SPG3A), *KIF5A* (SPG10) and *REEP1* (SPG31) are reported as being responsible for more than 50% of all cases [6]. The present study has confirmed that SPG4 is the most common subtype of Chinese

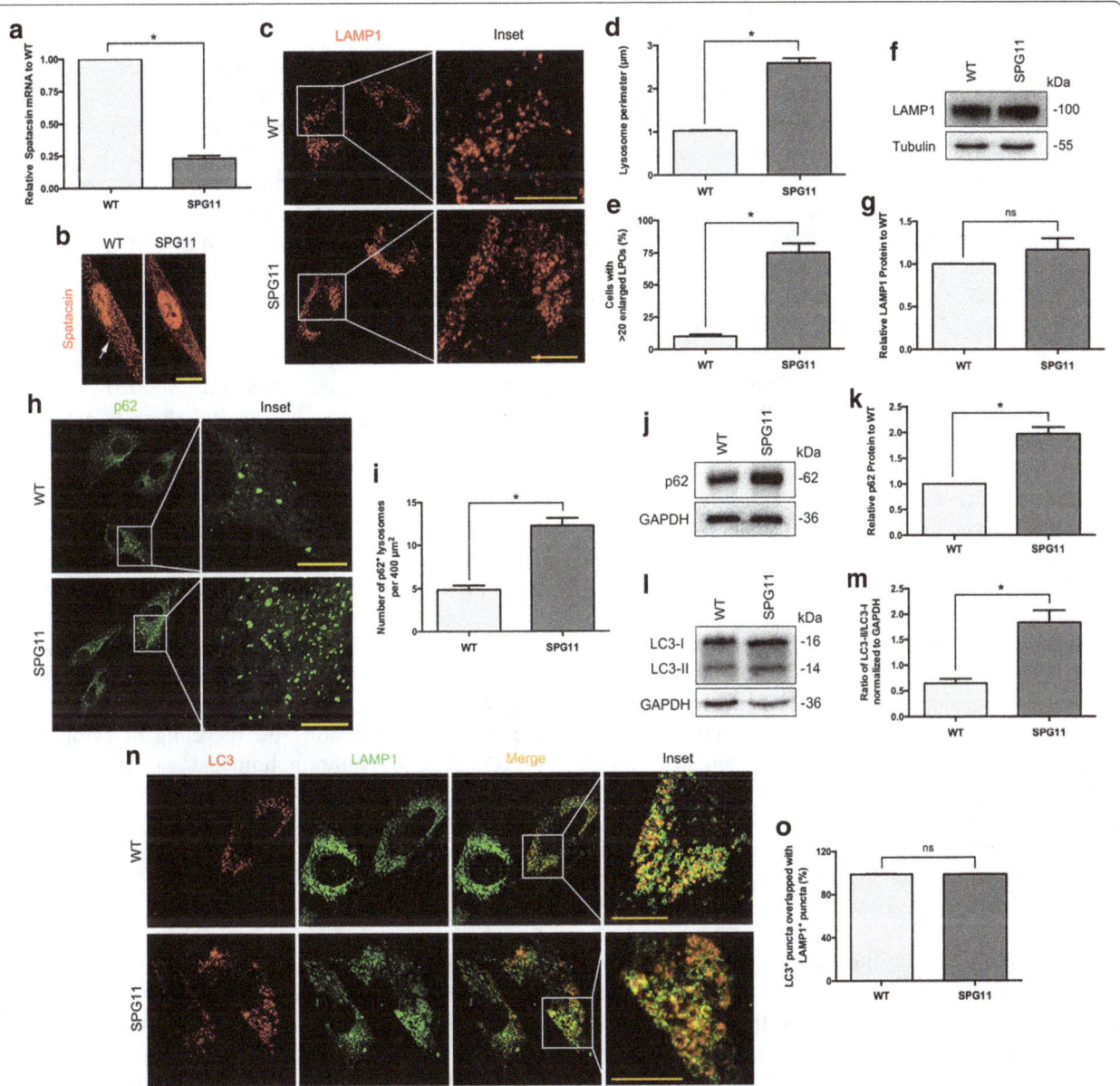

Fig. 6 Fibroblasts from the SPG11 patient exhibit enlarged LAMP1-positive organelles and accumulation of autolysosomes. **a** QPCR analysis revealed a significantly decreased expression of spatacsin mRNA in the pateint's fibroblasts. **b** ICH of spatacsin (red particles, arrow indicated) in fibroblast of WT (left panel) and the SPG4 patient (right panel). **c** ICH analysis revealed fibroblasts from the SPG11 patient exhibit prominently enlarged LPOs. Insets in the images are enlarged (original magnification, × 9.0) to the right. **d** Quantification of lysosome perimeter (20 cells, > 20 lysosomes per cell). **e** Quantification of cells with exceed 20 enlarged LPOs ($n = 3$, > 30 cells per experiment). **f**, **g** Western blot analysis showed no significant difference in LAMP1 levels between the SPG11 patient and WT. **h** ICH of p62 (green) in fibroblast of WT (upper panel) and the SPG11 patient (lower panel). Insets in the images are enlarged (original magnification, ×9.0) to the right. **i** Quantification of h (50 cells). **j**, **k** Western blot analysis revealed p62 protein was significantly accumulated in the patient derived fibroblasts. **l**, **m** Western blot analysis showed the ratio of LC3-II/LC3-I was significantly increased in autophagy induced fibroblasts from the SPG11 patient. **n**, **o** Co-immunostaining with LC3 (red) and LAMP1 (green), which showed no significant difference of their overlapping between the two groups. Insets in the images are enlarged (original magnification, ×10.5) to the right. Scale bar, 10 μm. Error bars indicate SEM. *, $P < 0.05$. ns, not significant

ADHSP patients, and followed by SPG3A, SPG6 (*NIPA1*) and SPG33 (*ZFYVE27*). Clinically, 94% of these patients were of pure HSP. However, no mutations were identified in SPG10, which appeared to be a common cause of ADHSP in previous series of other populations [31, 32]. Moreover, SPG8 (*KIAA0196*), SPG30 (*KIF1A*), SPG31and SPG42 (*SLC33A1*) seemed to be quite rare subtypes of Chinese ADHSP patients.

About 10–40% of HSP patients harbored subtle mutations and exonic rearrangements in the *SPAST* gene [3, 33]. Subtle mutations were confirmed to be the most common genetic cause for Chinese SPG4 patients, and most of them located in AAA casseete domain of Spastin protein. Spastin, a well-known AAA ATPase, is widely expressed in vertebrate cells that sever microtubules [34]. M87 is the much more abundant and effective severing isoform of spastin than M1 [35]. M1 is exclusively presented in adult spinal cord, the location of corticospinal tract axons that degenerate during HSP [21, 35]. The dynamic microtubule is functionally important for the intracellular organelles trafficking [14, 36]. Within neurons, only the short microtubules, but not the long ones, are critical for efficient axonal transport [37, 38]. In our cohort, all novel *SPAST* mutations have been shown to downregulate the expression or stability of M1- and M87-spastin protein. Based on SPG4 patient derived fibroblasts, we observed only reduced M87 and M87$^\triangle$Ex4 isoforms, and that mitochondrial dynamics and network were both altered. Of note, we further found the decreased MMP ($\Delta\psi$m), increased ROS and reduced ATP content in SPG4 fibroblasts, which have been implicated in cellular injury [39]. The neurite swelling and imbalanced axonal transport have been reported in the SPG4 stem cells derived neurons [21, 40, 41]. Indeed, in postmortem SPG4 patient brain samples, abnormal mitochondria readily accumulated in the cytosol of affected neurons [42]. On these basis, we speculate that the mitochondrial-mediated pathway plays a key role in neuron degeneration in the pathogenesis of SPG4.

In contrary to ADHSP, the AR forms of HSP appear to be more complex in clinical terms, with an early onset of symptoms [6, 43]. SPG11 was the most common cause of ARHSP [44]. In this study, 78% of Chinese ARHSP patients were suggestive of complicated HSP. Mutations in *SPG11* (SPG11) are responsioble for around 53% of ARHSP cases, and followed by *CYP7B1* (SPG5), *FA2H* (SPG35) and *GBA2* (SPG46). However, no mutations were identified in *SPG7* (SPG7) and *ZFYVE26* (SPG15) gene, which appeared to be a common cause of ARHSP in previous series of other populations [2, 6, 9, 10, 45, 46]. Indeed, subtypes for SPG14, SPG18, SPG28, SPG43, SPG54 and SPG77 of Chinses ARHSP patients are apparently orphan, affecting single family members.

In the present study, the AAO of SPG11 was generally early. The cognitive deficit, dysarthria, mental retardation, thin corpus callosum and axonal peripheral neuropathy were highly suggestive of SPG11. In previous reports, mutations in *CYP7B1* were found in both pure and complicated forms of SPG5 [47]. Cerebellar ataxia

has been the most common SPG5-related complicated phenotype [48]. Of note, white matter lesions and spastic ataxia seemed to be the two major features in Chinese SPG5 cases, accounting for approximately 50%. It was of interest to note that 82.1% of these SPG5 patients carried the unique nonsense mutation c.334C > T (p.R112*). Haplotype analysis revealed that the hotspot mutation is correlated with the founder effect.

Point mutations and rearrangements in *SPG11* have been show to make up 20% of ARHSP [49]. In our cohort, all five mutations of *SPG11* were stopgain mutation, with predicting to be LOF. Emerging studies implicated that spastic paraplegia proteins, spatacsin (SPG11) and spastizin (SPG15), were the essential components for the initiation of lysosomal tubulation [26, 50, 51]. Dysfunction of spatacsin leads to impaired axonal maintenance and cargo trafficking in the SPG11 stem cells derived neurons [52, 53]. Based on SPG11 patient derived fibroblasts, we observed that lack of spatacsin indeed induced the enlargement of LPOs and accumulation of autophagosomes. More importantly, the essence of these abnormally accumulated vesicles was shown to be autolysosomes, whose quantity and quality are crucial for autophagy. Autophagy is an intracellular activity for degradation and recycling of cytoplasmic components to maintain homeostasis [54]. The perturbed autophagy has been linked to several neurodegeneration diseases [55]. Collectively, our findings implied that the presence of autophagic dysfunction is tightly linked to SPG11.

Conclusions

In summary, our results indicated that subtypes for SPG4, SPG3A, SPG6 and SPG33 were the most frequently found in Chinese ADHSP patients, and were mainly pure forms with wide range AAO. Meanwhile, SPG11 SPG5, SPG35 and SPG46 subtypes were the most frequently found in Chinese ARHSP patients, and were more complex in clinical terms with early AAO. Moreover, we further determined that the high frequency of mutations in *CYP7B1* gene resulted from the founder effect. These studies provide the important implications on genetic counseling for suspected HSP cases. All of included patients presented with a wide range of features from asymptom to multi-system involvement, which confirming the marked heterogeneity of HSP. Stressing the mitochondrial and autophagic dysfunction hold promise as a potential therapeutic target to halt the progression of neurodegeneration in HSP. Even though, further study of a large cohort of patients should ascertain the specific correlation of genotype-phenotype in each subtype of HSP.

Additional files

Additional file 1: Summary information for mutational spectrum, targeted sequencing genes, amplification primers, antibodies, clinical features and haplotype analysis. **Table S1**. A reanalysis of the mutational spectrum in 41 reported studies exhibiting HSP in China. **Table S2**. HSP related genes included in the targeted sequencing panel. **Table S3**. Primers for amplification in the experimental procedures. **Table S4**. List of antibodies, related to immunocytochemistry (ICH) and western blotting (WB) in the experimental procedures. **Table S5**. Summary of clinical features of SPG4 patients in China (*n*=273). **Table S6**. Summary of clinical features of SPG11 patients in China (*n*=52). **Table S7**. Summary of clinical features of SPG5 patients in China (*n*=28). **Table S8**. Haplotypes of tagSNPs linkage to *CYP7B1* gene in the 16 unrelated SPG5 families.

Additional file 2: Pedigrees, sequencing chromatograms of disease-causing gene related to HSP families in our cohort. **Figure S1**. Pedigree, sequencing chromatograms of *SPAST* gene detected in 16 SPG4 families in our cohort. **Figure S2**. Western blot analysis of novel mutations of *SPAST* gene in HEK 293T cells. **Figure S3**. Pedigree, sequencing chromatograms of 6 ADHSP families in our cohort. **Figure S4**. Pedigree, sequencing chromatograms of *CYP7B1* gene detected in 16 unrelated SPG5 families in our cohort. **Figure S5**. Pedigree, sequencing chromatograms of 5 ARHSP families in our cohort.

Abbreviations

AAA: ATPases associated with diverse cellular activities; AAO: Age at onset; AD: Autosomal dominant; ADHSP: Autosomal dominant hereditary spastic paraplegia; AR: Autosomal recessive; ARHSP: Autosomal recessive hereditary spastic paraplegia; DCFH-DA: Dichlorofluorescein diacetate; DMEM: Dulbecco's modified Eagle's medium; ExAC: Exome Aggregation Consortium database; FBS: Fetal bovine serum; HSP: Hereditary spastic paraplegias; ICH: Immunocytochemistry; LOF: Loss-of-function; LPOs: LAMP1-positive organelles; MIT: Microtubule interacting and trafficking; MLPA: Multiplex ligation-dependent probe amplification; MMP: Mitochondrial membrane potential; MRI: Magnetic resonance images; MTBD: Microtubule-binding domain; NGS: Next generation sequencing; PCR: Polymerase chain reaction; qPCR: Quantification PCR; ROS: Reactive oxygen species; RT-PCR: Reverse transcription polymerase chain reaction; SPG: Spastic paraplegia; TM: Transmembrane; VDAC: Voltage-dependent anion channel

Acknowledgements

We sincerely thank the patients and their relatives for participation.

Funding

This work was supported by the grant 81322017, 81771230 and U1505222 from the National Natural Science Foundation of China, grant NCET-13-0736 from Program for New Century Excellent Talents in University, grant 2017XQ1072 from Startup Fund for scientific research of Fujian Medical University, National Key Clinical Specialty Discipline Construction Program and Key Clinical Specialty Discipline Construction Program of Fujian.

Authors' contributions

XL and WJC designed this study. ELD, CW and SW wrote the initial manuscript and constructed the figures. XL, WJC and NW contributed to the editing of the manuscript, figures and tables. ELD and CW performed the Data Analysis. SW, XHL, YQL and HZS performed the sample and history collection. XL, ELD, MZ, JH and LXM performed the mutation functional study in vitro. All authors read and approved the final manuscript.

Competing interests

The authors declare that they have no competing interests.

Author details

[1]Department of Neurology and Institute of Neurology, The First Affiliated Hospital of Fujian Medical University, Fuzhou 350005, China. [2]Department of Anatomy, Histology and Embryology, Shanghai Medical College, Fudan University, Shanghai 200032, China. [3]Fujian Key Laboratory of Molecular Neurology, Fujian Medical University, Fuzhou 350005, China.

References

1. Morais S, Raymond L, Mairey M, Coutinho P, Brandão E, Ribeiro P, Loureiro JL, Sequeiros J, Brice A, Alonso I, et al. Massive sequencing of 70 genes reveals a myriad of missing genes or mechanisms to be uncovered in hereditary spastic paraplegias. Eur J Hum Genet. 2017;25:1217–28.
2. Ruano L, Melo C, Silva MC, Coutinho P. The global epidemiology of hereditary ataxia and spastic paraplegia: a systematic review of prevalence studies. Neuroepidemiology. 2014;42:174–83.
3. Lo Giudice T, Lombardi F, Santorelli FM, Kawarai T, Orlacchio A. Hereditary spastic paraplegia: clinical-genetic characteristics and evolving molecular mechanisms. Exp Neurol. 2014;261:518–39.
4. Salinas S, Proukakis C, Crosby A, Warner TT. Hereditary spastic paraplegia: clinical features and pathogenetic mechanisms. Lancet Neurol. 2008;7:1127–38.
5. de Souza PV, de Rezende Pinto WB, de Rezende Batistella GN, Bortholin T, Oliveira AS. Hereditary spastic paraplegia: clinical and genetic hallmarks. Cerebellum. 2017;16:525–51.
6. Tesson C, Koht J, Stevanin G. Delving into the complexity of hereditary spastic paraplegias: how unexpected phenotypes and inheritance modes are revolutionizing their nosology. Hum Genet. 2015;134:511–38.
7. Estrada-Cuzcano A, Martin S, Chamova T, Synofzik M, Timmann D, Holemans T, Andreeva A, Reichbauer J, De Rycke R, Chang DI, et al. Loss-of-function mutations in the ATP13A2/PARK9 gene cause complicated hereditary spastic paraplegia (SPG78). Brain. 2017;140:287–305.
8. Loureiro JL, Miller-Fleming L, Thieleke-Matos C, Magalhaes P, Cruz VT, Coutinho P, Sequeiros J, Silveira I. Novel SPG3A and SPG4 mutations in dominant spastic paraplegia families. Acta Neurol Scand. 2009;119:113–8.
9. Schüle R, Wiethoff S, Martus P, Karle KN, Otto S, Klebe S, Klimpe S, Gallenmüller C, Kurzwelly D, Henkel D, et al. Hereditary spastic paraplegia: Clinicogenetic lessons from 608 patients. Ann Neurol. 2016;79:646–58.
10. Kara E, Tucci A, Manzoni C, Lynch DS, Elpidorou M, Bettencourt C, Chelban V, Manole A, Hamed SA, Haridy NA, et al. Genetic and phenotypic characterization of complex hereditary spastic paraplegia. Brain. 2016;139:1904–18.
11. Fink JK. Hereditary spastic paraplegia: clinico-pathologic features and emerging molecular mechanisms. Acta Neuropathol. 2013;126:307–28.
12. Solowska JM, Baas PW. Hereditary spastic paraplegia SPG4: what is known and not known about the disease. Brain. 2015;138:2471–84.
13. Harding AE. Classification of the hereditary ataxias and paraplegias. Lancet. 1983;1:1151–5.
14. McDermott CJ, Grierson AJ, Wood JD, Bingley M, Wharton SB, Bushby KM, Shaw PJ. Hereditary spastic paraparesis. Disrupted intracellular transport associated with spastin mutation. Ann Neurol. 2003;54:748–59.
15. Hazan J, Fonknechten N, Mavel D, Paternotte C, Samson D, Artiguenave F, Davoine CS, Cruaud C, Durr A, Wincker P, et al. Spastin, a new AAA protein, is altered in the most frequent form of autosomal dominant spastic paraplegia. Nat Genet. 1999;23:296–303.
16. Shoukier M, Neesen J, Sauter SM, Argyriou L, Doerwald N, Pantakani DV, Mannan AU. Expansion of mutation spectrum, determination of mutation cluster regions and predictivestructural classification of SPAST mutations in hereditary spastic paraplegia. Eur J Hum Genet. 2009;17:187–94.
17. Richards S, Aziz N, Bale S, Bick D, Das S, Gastier-Foster J, Grody WW, Hegde M, Lyon E, Spector E, et al. Standards and guidelines for the interpretation

of sequence variants: a joint consensus recommendation of the American College of Medical Genetics and Genomics and theAssociation for molecular pathology. Genet Med. 2015;17:405–24.

18. Stevanin G, Santorelli FM, Azzedine H, Coutinho P, Chomilier J, Denora PS, Martin E, Ouvrard-Hernandez AM, Tessa A, Bouslam N, et al. Mutations in SPG11, encoding spatacsin, are a major cause of spastic paraplegia with thin corpus callosum. Nat Genet. 2007;39:366–72.

19. Tsaousidou MK, Ouahchi K, Warner TT, Yang Y, Simpson MA, Laing NG, Wilkinson PA, Madrid RE, Patel H, Hentati F, et al. Sequence Alterations within CYP7B1 Implicate Defective Cholesterol Homeostasis in Motor-Neuron Degeneration. Am J Hum Genet. 2008;82:510–5.

20. Ueki I, Kimura A, Nishiyori A, Chen HL, Takei H, Nittono H, Kurosawa T. Neonatal cholestatic liver disease in an Asian patient with a homozygous mutation in the oxysterol 7alpha-hydroxylase gene. J Pediatr Gastroenterol Nutr. 2008;46:465–9.

21. Havlicek S, Kohl Z, Mishra HK, Prots I, Eberhardt E, Denguir N, Wend H, Plötz S, Boyer L, Marchetto MC, et al. Gene dosage-dependent rescue of HSP neurite defects in SPG4 patients' neurons. Hum Mol Genet. 2014;23:2527–41.

22. Okamoto K, Shaw JM. Mitochondrial morphology and dynamics in yeast and multicellular eukaryotes. Annu Rev Genet. 2005;39:503–36.

23. Shoshan-Barmatz V, Krelin Y, Chen Q. VDAC1 as a player in mitochondria-mediated apoptosis and target for modulating apoptosis. Curr Med Chem. 2017;24:4435–46.

24. Arif T, Krelin Y, Shoshan-Barmatz V. Reducing VDAC1 expression induces a non-apoptotic role for pro-apoptotic proteins in cancer cell differentiation. Biochim Biophys Acta. 1857;2016:1228–42.

25. Connolly NMC, Theurey P, Adam-Vizi V, Bazan NG, Bernardi P, Bolaños JP, Culmsee C, Dawson VL, Deshmukh M, Duchen MR, et al. Guidelines on experimental methods to assess mitochondrial dysfunction in cellular models of neurodegenerative diseases. Cell Death Differ. 2018;25:542–72.

26. Chang J, Lee S, Blackstone C. Spastic paraplegia proteins spastizin and spatacsin mediate autophagic lysosome reformation. J Clin Invest. 2014; 124:5249–62.

27. Klionsky DJ, Abdelmohsen K, Abe A, Abedin MJ, Abeliovich H, Acevedo Arozena A, Adachi H, Adams CM, Adams PD, Adeli K, et al. Guidelines for the use and interpretation of assays for monitoring autophagy (3rd edition). Autophagy. 2016;12:1–222.

28. Meijer IA, Hand CK, Cossette P, Figlewicz DA, Rouleau GA. Spectrum of SPG4 mutations in a large collection of north American families with hereditary spastic paraplegia. Arch Neurol. 2002;59:281–6.

29. Blair MA, Riddle ME, Wells JF, Breviu BA, Hedera P. Infantile onset of hereditary spastic paraplegia poorly predicts the genotype. Pediatr Neurol. 2007;36:382–6.

30. Orlacchio A, Montieri P, Babalini C, Gaudiello F, Bernardi G, Kawarai T. Late-onset hereditary spastic paraplegia with thin corpus callosum caused by a new SPG3A mutation. J Neurol. 2011;258:1361–3.

31. Goizet C, Boukhris A, Mundwiller E, Tallaksen C, Forlani S, Toutain A, Carriere N, Paquis V, Depienne C, Durr A, et al. Complicated forms of autosomal dominant hereditary spastic paraplegia are frequent in SPG10. Hum Mutat. 2009;30:E376–85.

32. Muglia M, Citrigno L, D'Errico E, Magariello A, Distaso E, Gasparro AA, Scarafino A, Patitucci A, Conforti FL, Mazzei R, et al. A novel KIF5A mutation in an Italian family marked by spastic paraparesis and congenital deafness. J Neurol Sci. 2014;343:218–20.

33. Beetz C, Nygren AO, Schickel J, Auer-Grumbach M, Burk K, Heide G, Kassubek J, Klimpe S, Klopstock T, Kreuz F, et al. High frequency of partial SPAST deletions in autosomal dominant hereditary spastic paraplegia. Neurology. 2006;67:1926–30.

34. Svenson IK, Ashley-Koch AE, Gaskell PC, Riney TJ, Cumming WJ, Kingston HM, Hogan EL, Boustany RM, Vance JM, Nance MA, et al. Identification and expression analysis of spastin gene mutations in hereditary spastic paraplegia. Am J Hum Genet. 2001;68:1077–85.

35. Solowska JM, Morfini G, Falnikar A, Himes BT, Brady ST, Huang D, Baas PW. Quantitative and functional analyses of spastin in the nervous system: implications for hereditary spastic paraplegia. J Neurosci. 2008; 28:2147–57.

36. Tortosa E, Adolfs Y, Fukata M, Pasterkamp RJ, Kapitein LC, Hoogenraad CC. Dynamic Palmitoylation targets MAP6 to the axon to promote microtubule stabilization during neuronal polarization. Neuron. 2017;94(4):809–25.

37. Baas PW, Karabay A, Qiang L. Microtubules cut and run. Trends Cell Biol. 2005;15:518–24.

38. Ahmad FJ, He Y, Myers KA, Hasaka TP, Francis F, Black MM, Baas PW. Effects of dynactin disruption and dynein depletion on axonal microtubules. Traffic. 2006;7:524–37.

39. Fang C, Bourdette D, Banker G. Oxidative stress inhibits axonal transport: implications for neurodegenerative diseases. Mol Neurodegener. 2012;7:29.

40. Abrahamsen G, Fan Y, Matigian N, Wali G, Bellette B, Sutharsan R, Raju J, Wood SA, Veivers D, Sue CM, et al. A patient-derived stem cell model of hereditary spastic paraplegia with SPASTmutations. Dis Model Mech. 2013;6:489–502.

41. Denton KR, Lei L, Grenier J, Rodionov V, Blackstone C, Li XJ. Loss of spastin function results in disease-specific axonal defects in human pluripotent stem cell-based models of hereditary spastic paraplegia. Stem Cells. 2014;32:414–23.

42. Wharton SB, McDermott CJ, Grierson AJ, Wood JD, Gelsthorpe C, Ince PG, Shaw PJ. The cellular and molecular pathology of the motor system in hereditary spastic paraparesis due to mutation of the spastin gene. J Neuropathol Exp Neurol. 2003;62:1166–77.

43. Paisan-Ruiz C, Nath P, Wood NW, Singleton A, Houlden H. Clinical heterogeneity and genotype-phenotype correlations in hereditary spastic paraplegia because of Spatacsin mutations (SPG11). Eur J Neurol. 2008;15:1065–70.

44. Samaranch L, Riverol M, Masdeu JC, Lorenzo E, Vidal-Taboada JM, Irigoyen J, Pastor MA, de Castro P, Pastor P. SPG11 compound mutations in spastic paraparesis with thin corpus callosum. Neurology. 2008;71(5):332–6.

45. Choquet K, Tetreault M, Yang S, La Piana R, Dicaire MJ, Vanstone MR, Mathieu J, Bouchard JP, Rioux MF, Rouleau GA, et al. SPG7 mutations explain a significant proportion of French Canadian spastic ataxia cases. Eur J Hum Genet. 2016;24:1016–21.

46. Klebe S, Depienne C, Gerber S, Challe G, Anheim M, Charles P, Fedirko E, Lejeune E, Cottineau J, Brusco A, et al. Spastic paraplegia gene 7 in patients with spasticity and/or optic neuropathy. Brain. 2012;135:2980–93.

47. Goizet C, Boukhris A, Durr A, Beetz C, Truchetto J, Tesson C, Tsaousidou M, Forlani S, Guyant-Maréchal L, Fontaine B, et al. CYP7B1 mutations in pure and complex forms of hereditary spastic paraplegia type 5. Brain. 2009;132: 1589–600.

48. R S, Brandt E, Karle KN, Tsaousidou M, Klebe S, Klimpe S, Auer-Grumbach M, Crosby AH, Hübner CA, Schöls L, et al. Analysis of CYP7B1 in non-consanguineous cases of hereditary spastic paraplegia. Neurogenetics. 2009; 10:97–104.

49. Stevanin G, Azzedine H, Denora P, Boukhris A, Tazir M, Lossos A, Rosa AL, Lerer I, Hamri A, Alegria P, et al. Mutations in SPG11 are frequent in autosomal recessive spastic paraplegia with thin corpus callosum, cognitive decline and lower motor neuron degeneration. Brain. 2008;131:772–84.

50. Renvoise B, Chang J, Singh R, Yonekawa S, FitzGibbon EJ, Mankodi A, Vanderver A, Schindler A, Toro C, Gahl WA, et al. Lysosomal abnormalities in hereditary spastic paraplegia types SPG15 and SPG11. Ann Clin Transl Neurol. 2014;1:379–89.

51. Vantaggiato C, Crimella C, Airoldi G, Polishchuk R, Bonato S, Brighina E, Scarlato M, Musumeci O, Toscano A, Martinuzzi A, et al. Defective autophagy in spastizin mutated patients with hereditary spastic paraparesis type 15. Brain. 2013;136:3119–39.

52. Mishra HK, Prots I, Havlicek S, Kohl Z, Perez-Branguli F, Boerstler T, Anneser L, Minakaki G, Wend H, Hampl M, et al. GSK3ß-dependent dysregulation of neurodevelopment in SPG11-patient iPSC model. Ann Neurol. 2016; https://doi.org/10.1002/ ana.24633.

53. Pérez-Branguli F, Mishra HK, Prots I, Havlicek S, Kohl Z, Saul D, Rummel C, Dorca-Arevalo J, Regensburger M, Graef D, et al. Dysfunction of spatacsin leads to axonal pathology in SPG11-linked hereditary spastic paraplegia. Hum Mol Genet. 2014;23:4859–74.

54. Varga RE, Khundadze M, Damme M, Nietzsche S, Hoffmann B, Stauber T, Koch N, Hennings JC, Franzka P, Huebner AK, et al. In vivo evidence for lysosome depletion and impaired Autophagic clearance in hereditary spastic paraplegia type SPG11. PLoS Genet. 2015;11:e1005454.

55. Walker C, El-Khamisy SF. Perturbed autophagy and DNA repair converge to promote neurodegeneration in amyotrophic lateral sclerosis and dementia. Brain. 2018; https://doi.org/10.1093/brain/awy076.

9

Blood-brain barrier-associated pericytes internalize and clear aggregated amyloid-β42 by LRP1-dependent apolipoprotein E isoform-specific mechanism

Qingyi Ma[1,2†], Zhen Zhao[1†], Abhay P Sagare[1†], Yingxi Wu[1], Min Wang[1], Nelly Chuqui Owens[1], Philip B Verghese[3], Joachim Herz[4,5,6], David M Holtzman[7] and Berislav V Zlokovic[1*]

Abstract

Background: Clearance at the blood-brain barrier (BBB) plays an important role in removal of Alzheimer's amyloid-β (Aβ) toxin from brain both in humans and animal models. Apolipoprotein E (apoE), the major genetic risk factor for AD, disrupts Aβ clearance at the BBB. The cellular and molecular mechanisms, however, still remain unclear, particularly whether the BBB-associated brain capillary pericytes can contribute to removal of aggregated Aβ from brain capillaries, and whether removal of Aβ aggregates by pericytes requires apoE, and if so, is Aβ clearance on pericytes apoE isoform-specific.

Methods: We performed immunostaining for Aβ and pericyte biomarkers on brain capillaries (< 6 μm in diameter) on tissue sections derived from AD patients and age-matched controls, and $APP^{Sw/0}$ mice and littermate controls. Human Cy3-Aβ42 uptake by pericytes was studied on freshly isolated brain slices from control mice, pericyte LRP1-deficient mice ($Lrp^{lox/lox}$; $Cspg4$-Cre) and littermate controls. Clearance of aggregated Aβ42 by mouse pericytes was studied on multi-spot glass slides under different experimental conditions including pharmacologic and/or genetic inhibition of the low density lipoprotein receptor related protein 1 (LRP1), an apoE receptor, and/or silencing mouse endogenous $Apoe$ in the presence and absence of human astrocyte-derived lipidated apoE3 or apoE4. Student's t-test and one-way ANOVA followed by Bonferroni's post-hoc test were used for statistical analysis.

Results: First, we found that 35% and 60% of brain capillary pericytes accumulate Aβ in AD patients and 8.5-month-old $APP^{Sw/0}$ mice, respectively, compared to negligible uptake in controls. Cy3-Aβ42 species were abundantly taken up by pericytes on cultured mouse brain slices via LRP1, as shown by both pharmacologic and genetic inhibition of LRP1 in pericytes. Mouse pericytes vigorously cleared aggregated Cy3-Aβ42 from multi-spot glass slides via LRP1, which was inhibited by pharmacologic and/or genetic knockdown of mouse endogenous apoE. Human astrocyte-derived lipidated apoE3, but not apoE4, normalized Aβ42 clearance by mouse pericytes with silenced mouse apoE.

Conclusions: Our data suggest that BBB-associated pericytes clear Aβ aggregates via an LRP1/apoE isoform-specific mechanism. These data support the role of LRP1/apoE interactions on pericytes as a potential therapeutic target for controlling Aβ clearance in AD.

Keywords: Pericyte, Blood-brain barrier (BBB), Amyloid-β clearance, Low-density lipoprotein receptor-related protein 1 (LRP1), Apolipoprotein E

* Correspondence: zlokovic@usc.edu
†Qingyi Ma, Zhen Zhao and Abhay P Sagare contributed equally to this work.
[1]Center for Neurodegeneration and Regeneration, Zilkha Neurogenetic Institute and Department of Physiology and Neuroscience, Keck School of Medicine, University of Southern California, Los Angeles, California 90033, USA
Full list of author information is available at the end of the article

Background

Alzheimer's disease (AD) is a progressive neurodegenerative disorder associated with cognitive impairment, early neurovascular changes, accumulation of amyloid-β (Aβ) and tau pathology, and neuron loss [1, 2]. According to the amyloid hypothesis, the build-up of Aβ in the brain parenchyma [3–5] and blood vessels [6–9] is the key event leading to other AD-related pathologies and disease symptoms. In the brain, Aβ is produced by neurons and other cell types, and is constantly removed by several clearance mechanisms. This includes receptor-mediated transport across the blood-brain barrier (BBB) into the peripheral circulation [10], enzyme-mediated Aβ proteolytic degradation [11], removal by glial cells [12], and diffusive transport across the interstitial fluid (ISF) along the perivascular spaces [13–15] leading to drainage by the meningeal lymphatic system [16, 17]. The imbalances between Aβ production and clearance result in Aβ deposition in the brain [18]. Kinetic studies in patients diagnosed with sporadic AD indicate that faulty Aβ clearance, rather than Aβ overproduction, is critical for accumulation of Aβ in the brain [19]. Moreover, recent transport studies in humans have shown that up to 50% of the Aβ in the brain is transported across the BBB to blood [20], confirming prior findings in animal models [21, 22].

The endothelial cells of the BBB, and the BBB-associated mural cells - pericytes and vascular smooth muscle cells (VSMCs), and glial cells clear Aβ, which can lead to Aβ transport across the BBB to blood, and/or Aβ degradation by mural cells, astrocytes and/or microglia [10, 18]. The low-density lipoprotein receptor-related protein 1 (LRP1), an apolipoprotein E (apoE) receptor [23, 24], mediates internalization of soluble Aβ at the abluminal side of the BBB [22, 25, 26]. This is followed by Aβ transcytosis across the BBB that is regulated by PICALM (Phosphatidylinositol Binding Clathrin Assembly Protein) and Rab5 and Rab11 small GTPases, ultimately leading to Aβ exocytosis across the luminal side of the BBB and clearance into the blood [27]. Consequently, endothelial-specific deletion of *Lrp1* gene [28] or deletion of *Picalm* gene from the endothelium [27] lead to accelerated Aβ pathology in Aβ-precursor protein (*APP*) overexpressing mice. VSMCs within the small cerebral arteries also clear Aβ via LRP1 [29, 30]. Similarly, astrocytes clear deposited Aβ via LRP1, which requires mouse endogenous apoE [31].

Brain capillary pericytes are centrally positioned between brain endothelial cells, astrocytes and neurons [32]. Besides roles in regulating BBB permeability [33, 34] and cerebral blood flow [35], pericytes show strong phagocytic activity associated with clearance of toxic foreign molecules [32], and endogenous proteins [36] including Alzheimer's Aβ, which can influence development of Aβ pathology as shown in *APP* mouse models [37, 38]. Prior studies have

demonstrated that apoE disrupts Aβ clearance across the mouse BBB [39], specifically, apoE4, which carries major genetic risk for AD [40–42], had greater disruptive effect than apoE3, which carries lower risk. However, the contribution of BBB-associated pericytes compared to endothelial trans-vascular transport to Aβ clearance at the BBB still remains elusive, particularly, whether pericytes can contribute to removal of aggregated Aβ from brain capillaries, which develop cerebral amyloid angiopathy (CAA) in AD [8], and whether removal of Aβ aggregates by pericytes requires apoE, and if so, is Aβ clearance on pericytes apoE isoform-specific? Here we show that Aβ accumulates in abundance in brain pericytes in AD and *APP*^{Sw/0} mice, suggesting their active role in Aβ removal at the BBB. Moreover, we show that pericytes internalize and clear Aβ aggregates by an LRP1/apoE isoform-specific mechanism implying that targeting LRP1/apoE pathway in pericytes has potential to control Aβ clearance in AD.

Methods

Animals

Mice were housed in plastic cages on a 12 h light cycle with ad libitum access to water and a standard laboratory diet. All procedures were approved by the Institutional Animal Care and Use Committee at the University of Southern California with National Institutes of Health guidelines. We studied *APP*^{Sw/0} mice expressing human APP transgene with the K670 M/N671 L (Swedish) double-mutation under control of the hamster prion promoter [43]. *Lrp*^{lox/lox} mice [44, 45] were crossed with *Cspg4-Cre* mice [46] to generate *Lrp*^{lox/lox};*Cspg4-Cre* mice with deletions of *Lrp1* gene from pericytes and oligodendrocyte progenitor cells. To minimize confounding effects of background heterogeneity all experiments were performed using age-matched littermates. Both, male and female mice were used in the study. All animals were randomized for their genotype information. All experiments were blinded; the operators responsible for experimental procedure and data analysis were blinded and unaware of group allocation throughout the experiments.

Human tissue immunofluorescence analysis

Written consent was obtained and approved by the University of Rochester Medical Center for all studied human subjects prior to death. The postmortem interval ranged between 4 and 16 h. Postmortem brain tissue samples including frontal cortex (Brodmann area 9/10) were obtained from subjects with a definite diagnosis of AD confirmed by neuropathological analysis including Braak stages ≥ III; CERAD (Consortium to Establish a Registry for Alzheimer's Disease) frequent, and neurologically intact controls with no AD pathology (Braak stages ≤ III; CERAD – negative). Six controls and six AD samples were used for the current study. Their demographic and clinical features were as we reported previously [47], and shown in Additional file 1: Table S1. Vascular risk factors such as atherosclerosis, hypertension and/or myocardial infarction were present in 4 out 6 AD patients and 6 out of 6 controls. The cause of death in all AD and control patients was either respiratory failure or cardiac failure. All tissues were paraformaldehyde (PFA)-fixed, paraffin-embedded and cut to 10 μm thick slices. Sections were deparaffinized with xylene and rehydrated to distilled water after serial ethanol washes. Subsequently, heat-induced antigen retrieval (HIAR) was performed following Dako's protocol. The tissue sections were then blocked in 5% donkey serum (Jackson ImmunoResearch, West Grove, PA, USA) containing 0.3% Triton X-100 (Sigma-Aldrich, St. Louis, MO, USA), and then incubated with the following primary antibodies overnight at 4 °C: goat anti-human PDGFRβ (1:100, R&D Systems, Minneapolis, MN, USA), mouse anti-human aminopeptidase N (CD13) (1:100, R&D Systems), rabbit anti-human Aβ (1:100, Cell signaling, Boston, MA, USA). Blood vessels were stained by DyLight 488 Labeled *Lycopersicon esculentum* (Tomato) Lectin (1:100, Vector Laboratories, Burlingame, CA, USA, # DL-1174) for 1 h at room temperature. Species-specific fluorochrome-conjugated secondary antibodies were incubated for 1 h at room temperature, including Alexa 568-conjugated donkey anti-goat (1:200, Invitrogen), Alexa 568-conjugated donkey anti-mouse (1:200, Invitrogen) and Alexa 647-conjugated donkey anti-rabbit (1:200, Invitrogen). Tissue sections were mounted and coverslipped using fluorescent mounting media (Dako, Carpinteria, CA, USA). All slices were scanned using Zeiss 510 confocal microscopy with Zeiss Apochromat water immersion objectives (Carl Zeiss MicroImaging Inc., Thornwood, NY, USA). All slices were scanned using Zeiss 510 confocal microscopy with Zeiss Apochromat water immersion objectives (Carl Zeiss MicroImaging Inc., Thornwood, NY, USA), with lasers and band-pass filter settings as the following: a 488-nm argon laser to excite Alexa Fluor and Dylight 488, and the emission was collected through a 500–550-nm bp filter; a 543 HeNe laser to excite Alexa Fluor 568 and Cy3 and the emission was collected through a 560–615-nm bp filter; a 633 HeNe laser to excite Alexa fluor 647 and the emission was collected through a 650–700-nm bp filter.

Aβ uptake on freshly isolated mouse brain cortical slices

Brain slices were prepared from 2-month old C57BL6 mice or $Lrp^{lox/lox}$;*Cspg4-Cre* mice. Following the urethane anesthesia, brains were quickly removed from the cranial cavity and sectioned with McIlwain tissue chopper (Ted Pella, Inc., Redding, CA, USA) into 200 μm thick slices containing cortex and hippocampus, as previously described [48]. Slices were recovered for 30 min in a submersion chamber filled with the per-warmed (at 37 °C)

artificial cerebrospinal fluid (aCSF; 126 mM NaCl, 2.5 mM KCl, 1.25 mM Na_2PO_4, 26 mM $NaHCO_3$, 1 mM $MgCl_2$, 2 mM $CaCl_2$, 0.5 mM ascorbic acid, 2 mM sodium pyruate, and 10 mM glucose, saturated with 95% O_2 and 5% CO_2). Prior to incubation with aCSF containing 5 μg/ml Cy3-Aβ42 for 30 min, slices were pre-incubated with either non-immune IgG (NI-IgG) or LRP1-specific blocking antibody [22, 29] (anti-LRP1 N20, 50 μg/ml; Santa Cruz Biotech., Santa Cruz, CA, USA) for 20 min at 37 °C. At the end of the experiment, brain slices were washed with phosphate buffer saline (PBS) and fixed with 4% PFA for 30 min. The same immunostaining procedure as for human brain tissue without antigen retrieval was performed on mouse brain slices. Primary antibodies included goat anti-mouse aminopeptidase N (CD13) (1:100, R&D Systems), and goat anti-mouse PDGFRβ (1:100, R&D Systems). Secondary antibodies were: Alexa 488-conjugated donkey anti-goat (1:200, Invitrogen). Images were obtained with Zeiss 510 confocal microscopy (Carl Zeiss MicroImaging Inc.) with lasers and band-pass filter settings as described above. The distribution of Cy3-Aβ42 in pericytes and capillary endothelium was analyzed with the NIH Image J software [49].

Pericyte isolation from the mouse brain, culture and transfection

Brain capillaries were isolated from mouse cortices pooled from 3 to 4 mouse brains for each biological replicate. In experiments in Figs. 4 and 5, we used 3–4 independent biological replicates (cultures), as indicated in the legends to these respective figures. Capillaries were isolated as we have described previously [49, 50]. In brief, mouse cortices were macroscopically dissected, and all visible white matter was discarded in ice-cold PBS containing 2% fetal bovine serum (FBS). The brain was homogenized in PBS containing 2% FBS and centrifuged at 6,000 g for 15 min after addition of Dextran (70 kDa, Sigma). The capillary pellet was collected and sequentially filtered through a 45 μm cell strainer (BD Falcon). The remaining pellet on top of the 45 μm cell strainer was collected in PBS and digested for 12 h at 37 °C with collagenase A (Roche, 10103586001), as we previously described. The cells were washed with PBS and then plated in complete medium containing DMEM, 10% FBS, 1% non-essential amino acids, 1% vitamins and 1% antibiotic/antimycotic on plastic (non-coated) tissue culture plates. After 6 to 12 h the non-adherent cells were washed away and fresh medium was replaced every 2–3 days. Cultures were confirmed to be morphological consistent with pericyte cultures and PDGFRβ-positive, SMA-positive, Desmin-positive, GFAP-negative, AQP4-negative, MAP2-negative, NeuN-negative, VWF-negative, and Iba1-negative, as previously described [37, 49]. Transfections were performed with Neon transfection system (Invitrogen, Grand Island, NY, USA) following the manufacturer's protocol. After optimization, the transfection efficiency with pEGFP plasmid was > 80%. For siRNA transfection, 15 pmol of siRNA in 1 µl was electroporated into 1×10^5 cells in a total volume of 10 µl.

Clearance of aggregated Cy3-Aβ42 by primary mouse brain pericytes

The multi-spot glass slides (Thermo Scientific, 9991090, Waltham, MA, USA) were coated with Cy3- Aβ42 [29, 51] at 1 µg per spot without cells or with brain capillary pericytes treated with non-immune IgG (NI-IgG) or LRP1-specific blocking antibody [22, 29] (anti-LRP1; 50 µg/ml) or) or apoE-specific blocking antibody (anti-apoE, HJ6.3, 50 µg/ml), scrambled siRNA (si.Control) or LRP1 siRNA (si.Lrp1) (Dharmacon, E-040764-00-0010) or apoE siRNA (si.Apoe) (Dharmacon, E-040885-00-0005), and 500 nM receptor-associated protein (RAP) [52] (EMD Bioscience), lipidated apoE3 (40 nM) or apoE4 (40 nM) [49]. Cells (5,000 per spot) were incubated for 5 days in DMEM containing 10% heat inactivated FBS, penicillin and streptomycin (Invitrogen). Cells were labeled with Cell Tracker Green CMFDA (Invitrogen C7025), and then fixed with 4% paraformaldehyde. Slides were scanned using Zeiss 510 confocal microscopy (Carl Zeiss MicroImaging Inc.). The Cy3-Aβ42 relative intensity was analyzed with the NIH Image J software.

Purification of apoE from immortalized astrocytes

Lipidated apoE isoform particles were purified from culture media of human apoE3 or apoE4 overexpressing immortalized astrocytes using an affinity column, as we described previously [53]. Briefly, astrocytes were cultured in advanced DMEM (Invitrogen) with 10% FBS. After 90–95% confluency, cells were washed by PBS and further incubated in advanced DMEM with N-2 Supplement (Invitrogen) and 3 mM 25-hydroxycholesterol (Sigma) for 3 days. Collected culture media were applied onto mouse monoclonal antibody against a human apoE (WU E-4) column. Lipidated apoE particles were eluted from the column with 3 M sodium thiocyanate, concentrated using Apollo centrifugal quantitative concentrators (QMWL: 150 kDa, Orbital Biosciences), and dialyzed against PBS.

Immunoblotting

Cell samples transfected with scrambled siRNA or LRP1 siRNA were washed in cold PBS and lysed with RIPA buffer. Proteins were quantified with BCA protein assay kit (Pierce). An equal amount of protein sample was loaded for SDS-PAGE. We used the following primary antibodies: rabbit anti-mouse LRP1 (1: 20,000, Abcam, Cambridge, MA, USA), β-actin (1:10,000, Sigma), and Aβ antibody (6E10, 1:1000, Covance). Images were scanned using ChemiDoc™ MP imager with LEDs and quantified using Image Lab™ software (Bio-Rad, Hercules, CA, USA).

Terminal deoxynucleotidyl transferase UTP nick end labeling (TUNEL)

Paraformaldehyde-fixed, paraffin embedded brain tissue sections from $APP^{Sw/0}$ mice were sectioned at a thickness of 10 µm. Immunofluorescent detection of pericytes (CD13-positive), Aβ and endothelial-specific lectin fluorescence was conducted as described above. The Dead-End Fluorometric TUNEL system (Promega) was then completed as described by the manufacturer.

Statistical analysis

All quantified data represent as mean ± s.e.m. Student's t-test or one-way analysis of variance (ANOVA) followed by Bonferroni post-hoc test was used to determine statistically significant differences. A P value < 0.05 was considered statistically significant.

Results

Aβ accumulation in pericytes from AD patients and $APP^{Sw/0}$ mice

Using 3-channel confocal microscopy, here we show that Aβ accumulates in > 30% of CD13+ and/or PDGFRβ+ pericytes on lectin+ brain endothelial capillary profiles (< 6 µm in diameter) in brain cortical sections from AD patients compared to barely detectable Aβ accumulation in pericytes in age-matched controls (see demographic Additional file 1: Table S1; Fig. 1a-f). To confirm this observation, we immunostained cortical sections of 8.5-month-old $APP^{Sw/0}$ mice for human Aβ, at a disease stage when these mice begin depositing Aβ [21]. We found that nearly 60% of CD13+ pericytes were positive for human Aβ (Fig. 1g-h). Collectively, these findings indicate that pericytes in AD and $APP^{Sw/0}$ mouse brains both accumulate Aβ. Additionally, we found that Aβ also accumulates in brain endothelium of AD patients (Additional file 1: Figure S1A, B), and in lectin+ brain endothelial cells of 8.5-month-old $APP^{Sw/0}$ mice (Additional file 1:Figure S1C).

Aβ accumulation is associated with pericyte cell death

Cultured mouse pericytes [37] and human brain pericytes [54] die when treated with excess Aβ. To verify this result in $APP^{Sw/0}$ mice in vivo, we performed quadruple TUNEL, CD13, lectin and human Aβ staining, which revealed a significant increase in TUNEL+ CD13+ pericytes in 8.5-month old, but not 3-month old, $APP^{Sw/0}$ mice compared to 8.5-month old littermate controls (Fig. 1i-j), consistent with findings that 3-month old $APP^{Sw/0}$ mice show barely detectable Aβ deposition in the brain compared to 8.5-month old mice, which begin depositing Aβ at that stage [55].

LRP1-dependent Aβ uptake by pericytes on mouse brain slices

To confirm Aβ uptake by pericytes, we next conducted Aβ uptake experiments on freshly isolated acute cortical slice

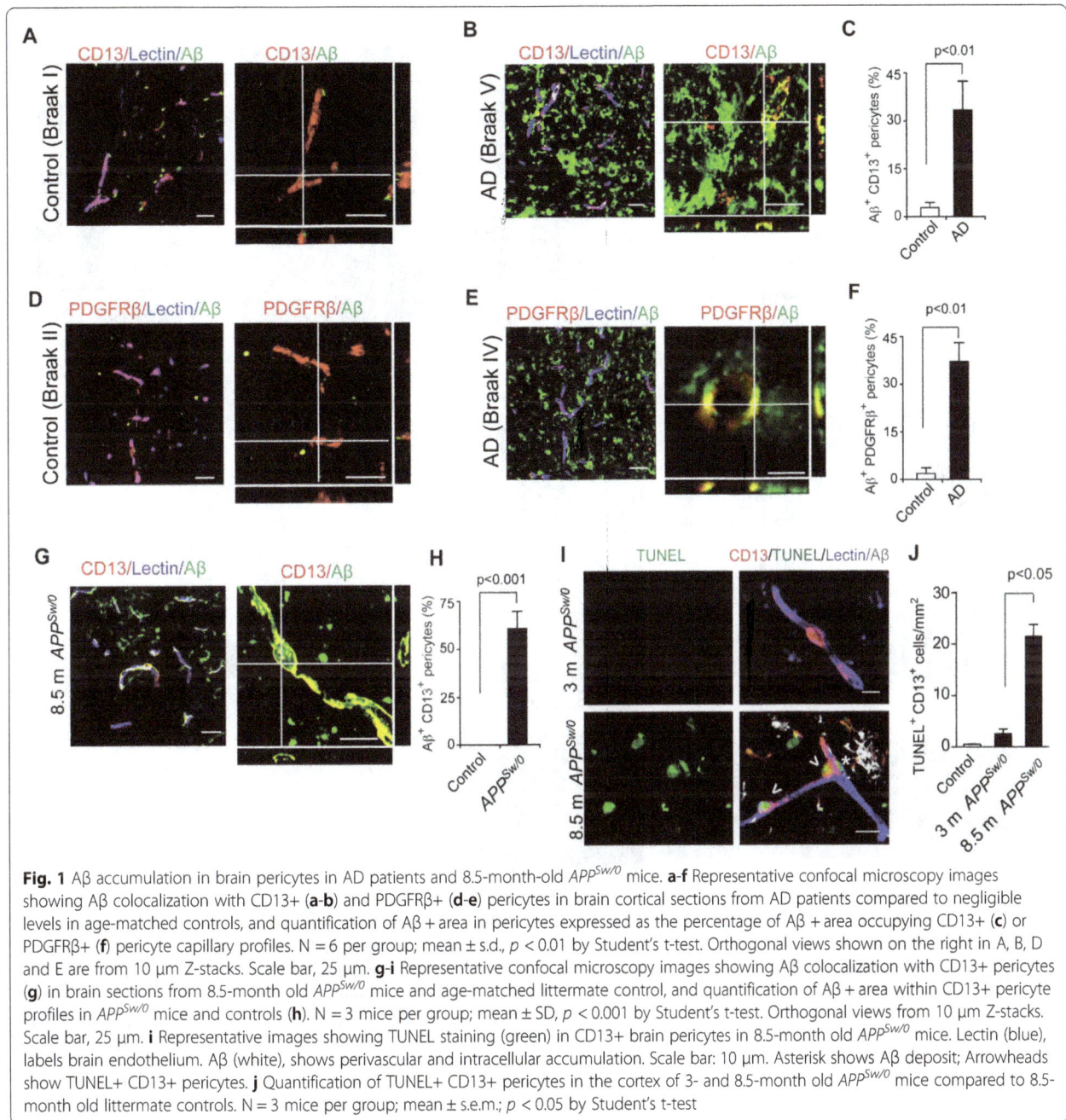

Fig. 1 Aβ accumulation in brain pericytes in AD patients and 8.5-month-old $APP^{Sw/0}$ mice. **a-f** Representative confocal microscopy images showing Aβ colocalization with CD13+ (**a-b**) and PDGFRβ+ (**d-e**) pericytes in brain cortical sections from AD patients compared to negligible levels in age-matched controls, and quantification of Aβ + area in pericytes expressed as the percentage of Aβ + area occupying CD13+ (**c**) or PDGFRβ+ (**f**) pericyte capillary profiles. N = 6 per group; mean ± s.d., $p < 0.01$ by Student's t-test. Orthogonal views shown on the right in A, B, D and E are from 10 µm Z-stacks. Scale bar, 25 µm. **g-i** Representative confocal microscopy images showing Aβ colocalization with CD13+ pericytes (**g**) in brain sections from 8.5-month old $APP^{Sw/0}$ mice and age-matched littermate control, and quantification of Aβ + area within CD13+ pericyte profiles in $APP^{Sw/0}$ mice and controls (**h**). N = 3 mice per group; mean ± SD, $p < 0.001$ by Student's t-test. Orthogonal views from 10 µm Z-stacks. Scale bar, 25 µm. **i** Representative images showing TUNEL staining (green) in CD13+ brain pericytes in 8.5-month old $APP^{Sw/0}$ mice. Lectin (blue), labels brain endothelium. Aβ (white), shows perivascular and intracellular accumulation. Scale bar: 10 µm. Asterisk shows Aβ deposit; Arrowheads show TUNEL+ CD13+ pericytes. **j** Quantification of TUNEL+ CD13+ pericytes in the cortex of 3- and 8.5-month old $APP^{Sw/0}$ mice compared to 8.5-month old littermate controls. N = 3 mice per group; mean ± s.e.m.; $p < 0.05$ by Student's t-test

cultures, as previously reported [48]. In this experiment, the mouse brains slices were left to equilibrate in aCSF for 20 min at 37 °C with aeration, that was followed by incubation with Cy3-Aβ42 (1 µM) for 30 min or 2 h. Confocal microscopy was performed to analyze Aβ internalization by pericytes (Fig. 2a). We found that uptake of Cy3-Aβ42 by pericytes was rapid and time-dependent. Compared to 30 min, at 2 h the amount of internalized Cy3-Aβ42 in CD13+ pericytes was further significantly increased (Fig. 2b-c). In these studies, Aβ42 preparation contained a mixture of Aβ42 monomers, dimers, trimers, tetramers, and small molecular weight oligomers

(Additional file 1: Figure S2). Both low (Fig. 2b) and high (Fig. 2d) magnification imaging analysis showed strong Cy3-Aβ42 fluorescence signal in CD13+ pericytes and/or PDGFRβ+ pericytes (Additional file 1: Figure S3A-B). In addition to pericytes, Cy3-Aβ42 uptake was observed by endothelial cells, astrocytes and microglia (Additional file 1: Figure S3C-E). The intracellular Cy3-Aβ42 levels in pericytes were significantly reduced in the presence of an anti-LRP1-specific antibody [22, 29] and the receptor associated protein (RAP) [52], an LRP1 antagonist which inhibits ligand binding to LRP1 (Fig. 2d), as shown by 17.1% and 21.7% of the Cy3-Aβ42+ area occupying CD13+

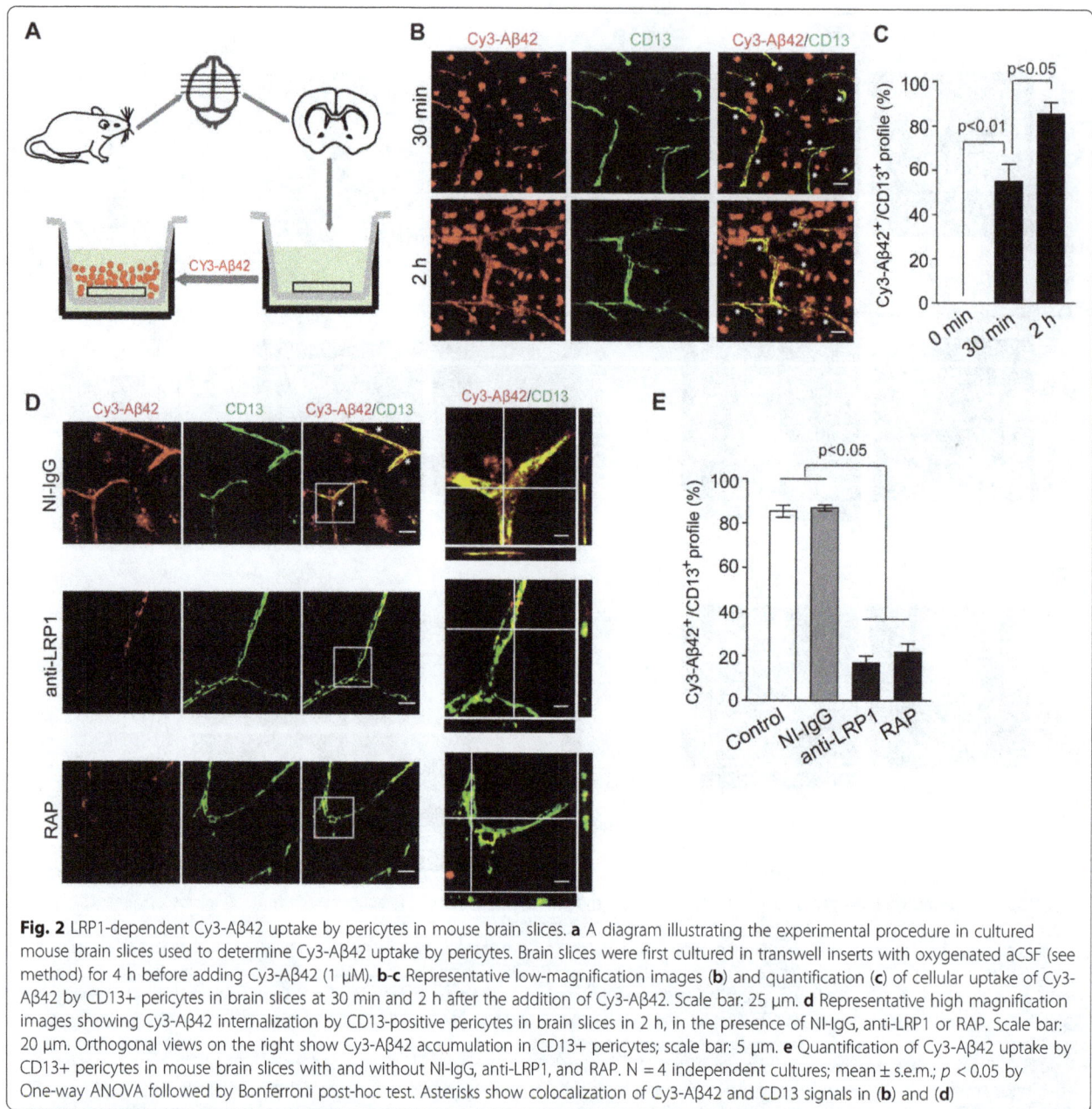

Fig. 2 LRP1-dependent Cy3-Aβ42 uptake by pericytes in mouse brain slices. **a** A diagram illustrating the experimental procedure in cultured mouse brain slices used to determine Cy3-Aβ42 uptake by pericytes. Brain slices were first cultured in transwell inserts with oxygenated aCSF (see method) for 4 h before adding Cy3-Aβ42 (1 μM). **b-c** Representative low-magnification images (**b**) and quantification (**c**) of cellular uptake of Cy3-Aβ42 by CD13+ pericytes in brain slices at 30 min and 2 h after the addition of Cy3-Aβ42. Scale bar: 25 μm. **d** Representative high magnification images showing Cy3-Aβ42 internalization by CD13-positive pericytes in brain slices in 2 h, in the presence of NI-IgG, anti-LRP1 or RAP. Scale bar: 20 μm. Orthogonal views on the right show Cy3-Aβ42 accumulation in CD13+ pericytes; scale bar: 5 μm. **e** Quantification of Cy3-Aβ42 uptake by CD13+ pericytes in mouse brain slices with and without NI-IgG, anti-LRP1, and RAP. N = 4 independent cultures; mean ± s.e.m.; $p < 0.05$ by One-way ANOVA followed by Bonferroni post-hoc test. Asterisks show colocalization of Cy3-Aβ42 and CD13 signals in (**b**) and (**d**)

pericyte profiles, respectively, compared to > 80% in control slices treated with vehicle or non-immune immunoglobulin G (IgG) (Fig. 2d-e).

To further investigate the role of LRP1 in Cy3-Aβ42 uptake by pericytes, we generated conditional knockout mice with LRP1 deficiency in pericytes (*Lrp1$^{lox/lox}$; Cspg4-Cre*) by crossing *Lrp1$^{lox/lox}$* mice [44, 45] with *Cspg4-Cre* mice [46] (Fig. 3a). As expected, CD13+ pericytes on isolated brain microvessels from *Lrp1$^{lox/lox}$; Cspg4-Cre* mice did not show a detectable LRP1 immunoreactivity in contrast to pericytes from control *Lrp1$^{lox/lox}$* mice, whereas LRP1 remained expressed in lectin+ endothelium in both *Lrp1$^{lox/lox}$; Cspg4-Cre* and

Lrp1$^{lox/lox}$ microvessels (Fig. 3b), confirming selective deletion of LRP1 from brain capillary pericytes. Both, *Lrp1$^{lox/lox}$* and *Lrp1$^{lox/lox}$; Cspg4-Cre* mice had comparable CD13+ pericyte coverage (Additional file 1: Figure S4). Next, we studied Cy3-Aβ42 uptake on brain slices from these mice, as described above. Two hours after incubation, Cy3-Aβ42 uptake by CD13+ pericytes was reduced by > 80% in *Lrp1$^{lox/lox}$; Cspg4-Cre* mice compared to control *Lrp1$^{lox/lox}$* mice (Fig. 3c-e). As expected, Aβ uptake by other cell types shown collectively as CD13- cells was not affected in this *Lrp1* conditional knockout model (Fig. 3f). In summary, these data demonstrate LRP1-depedent uptake of Aβ42 species by pericytes.

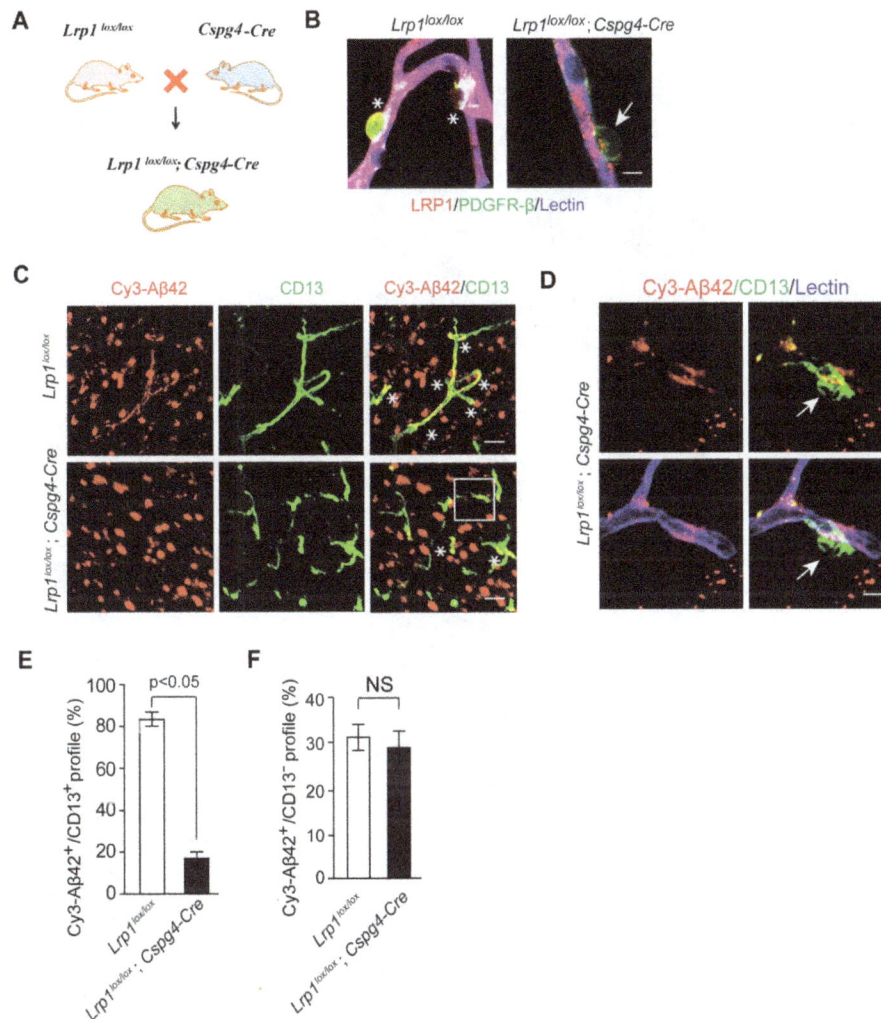

Fig. 3 LRP1 genetic deletion from pericytes inhibits Cy3-Aβ42 uptake by pericytes in mouse brain slices. **a** Diagram illustrating generation of *Lrp1*$^{lox/lox}$; *Cspg4-Cre* mice by crossing *Lrp1*$^{lox/lox}$ mice with *Cspg4-Cre* mice. **b** Representative high magnification images showing LRP1 expression in CD13+ pericytes on isolated murine brain capillaries from control *Lrp1*$^{lox/lox}$ mice, but not *Lrp1*$^{lox/lox}$; *Cspg4-Cre* mice with LRP1 deletion from pericytes. Asterisks show LRP1 immunostaining in CD13+ pericytes in control *Lrp1*$^{lox/lox}$ mice; arrow shows loss of LRP1 immunoreactivity in *Lrp1*$^{lox/lox}$; *Cspg4-Cre* mice. Scale bar: 5 μm. **c** Representative images showing Cy3-Aβ42 internalization by CD13+ pericytes in brain slices from control *Lrp1*$^{lox/lox}$ mice, and a substantial loss of Cy3-Aβ42 uptake by pericytes in *Lrp1*$^{lox/lox}$; *Cspg4-Cre* mice. Asterisks show colocalization between Cy3-Aβ42 and CD13 signals. Scale bar: 25 μm. **d** High magnification images showing greatly reduced Cy3-Aβ42 internalization by a CD13+ pericyte on brain slices from *Lrp1*$^{lox/lox}$; *Cspg4-Cre* mice, in contrast to Aβ uptake by lectin-positive endothelial cells. Arrow points to pericyte lacking Cy3-Aβ42 signal. Scale bar: 5 μm. **e, f** Quantification of Cy3-Aβ42 cellular uptake by CD13+ pericytes (**e**) compared to all other CD13- (negative) brain cells (**f**) in brain slices from control *Lrp1*$^{lox/lox}$ and *Lrp1*$^{lox/lox}$; *Cspg4-Cre* mice. N = 3 mice per group; mean ± s.e.m.; NS, not significant, p < 0.05 by Student's t-test

LRP1/apoE-dependent clearance of aggregated Cy3-Aβ42 by mouse brain capillary pericytes

To determine whether pericytes can clear aggregated Aβ, we used a slightly modified Aβ clearance model with pericytes seeded on multi-spot glass slides pre-coated with aggregated Cy3-Aβ42, as we reported previously in studies with primary VSMCs [29] (Fig. 4a). Five days after culture, the majority of Aβ42 aggregates (> 70%) were removed from the multi-spot surface by pericytes in the presence of vehicle, control non-immune IgG or scrambled short interfering si.*Control* (Fig. 4b-c), when compared to cell-free control (Fig. 4a). In contrast, only 22.8%, 27.3% and 12.9% of Cy3-Aβ42 was cleared in the presence of anti-LRP1 [22, 29], RAP [52] and si.*Lrp1* (Fig. 4c), respectively. In silencing experiment, si.*Lrp1* efficiently downregulated LRP1 in pericytes by ~ 90% when compared to si.*Control* (Additional file 1: Figure S5A). We also found a time-dependent increase in cell death of pericytes cultured on Aβ pre-coated slides, from 8.2% at 3 DIV to 18.7% at 5 DIV, whereas inhibiting LRP1 by an anti-LRP1 antibody or LRP1 silencing (si.*Lrp1*), not only significantly reduced Aβ uptake, but

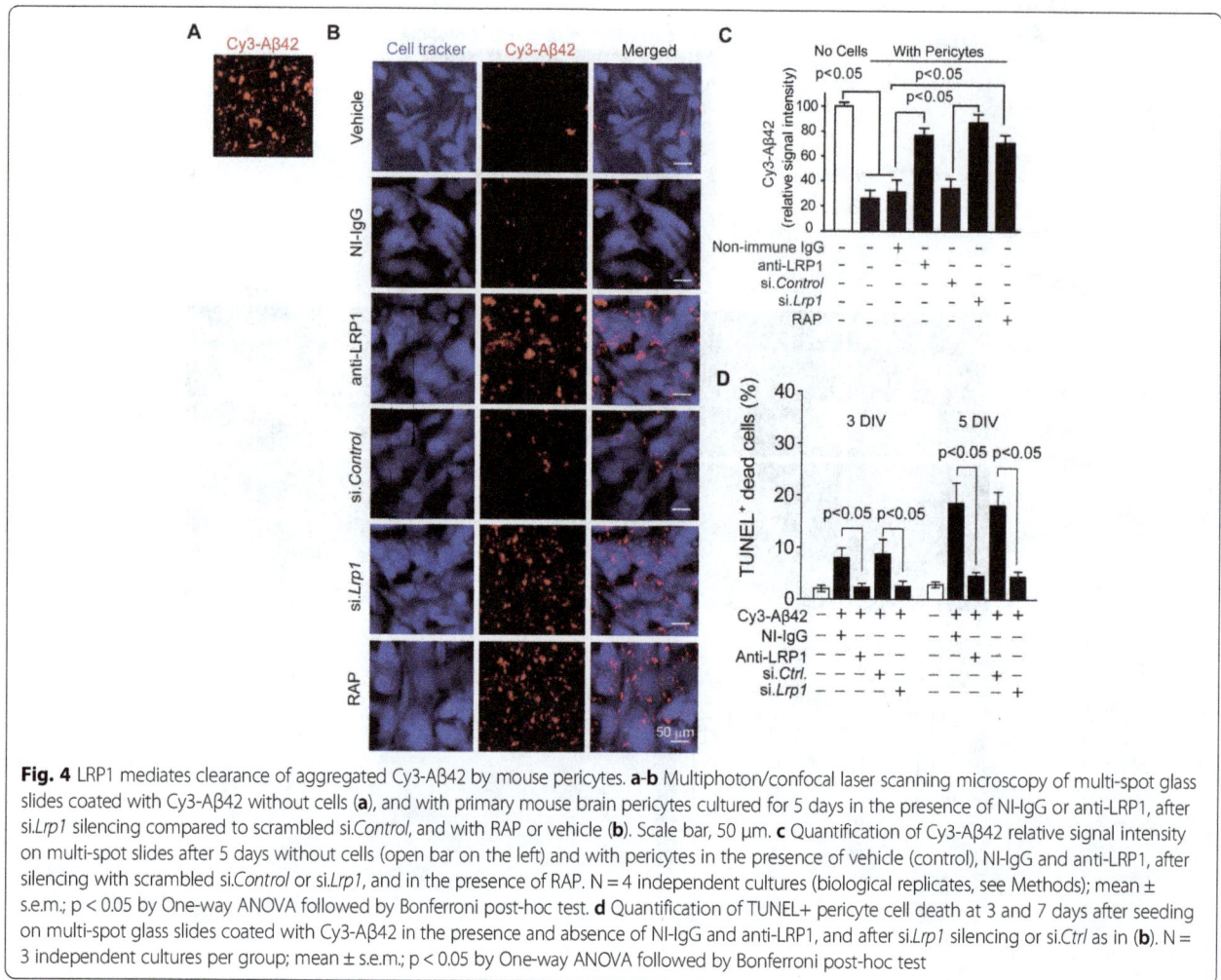

Fig. 4 LRP1 mediates clearance of aggregated Cy3-Aβ42 by mouse pericytes. **a-b** Multiphoton/confocal laser scanning microscopy of multi-spot glass slides coated with Cy3-Aβ42 without cells (**a**), and with primary mouse brain pericytes cultured for 5 days in the presence of NI-IgG or anti-LRP1, after si.Lrp1 silencing compared to scrambled si.Control, and with RAP or vehicle (**b**). Scale bar, 50 μm. **c** Quantification of Cy3-Aβ42 relative signal intensity on multi-spot slides after 5 days without cells (open bar on the left) and with pericytes in the presence of vehicle (control), NI-IgG and anti-LRP1, after silencing with scrambled si.Control or si.Lrp1, and in the presence of RAP. N = 4 independent cultures (biological replicates, see Methods); mean ± s.e.m.; p < 0.05 by One-way ANOVA followed by Bonferroni post-hoc test. **d** Quantification of TUNEL+ pericyte cell death at 3 and 7 days after seeding on multi-spot glass slides coated with Cy3-Aβ42 in the presence and absence of NI-IgG and anti-LRP1, and after si.Lrp1 silencing or si.Ctrl as in (**b**). N = 3 independent cultures per group; mean ± s.e.m.; p < 0.05 by One-way ANOVA followed by Bonferroni post-hoc test

also diminished pericyte cell death by approximately 3 and 4-fold at 3 and 5 DIV, respectively (Fig. 4d), suggesting that reducing Aβ uptake decreases Aβ toxicity consistent with previous studies with soluble Aβ [37] or Dutch Aβ peptides [54].

To check whether apoE is required for LRP1-mediated clearance of Aβ aggregates, we studied clearance by pericytes in the presence of an apoE specific blocking antibody compared to non-immune IgG, and after silencing mouse apoE (si.Apoe) compared to scrambled si.Control (Additional file 1: Figure S5B; Fig. 5a). After 5 days, we found substantially reduced Aβ clearance with either pharmacologic or genetic inhibition of murine apoE in pericytes as illustrated by representative confocal microscopy images (Fig. 5a), quantification of time-dependent Cy3-Aβ42 clearance by mouse pericytes cultured for 1, 3 and 5 days after silencing mouse endogenous apoE (si.Apoe) compared to si.Control (Fig. 5b), and quantification analysis of Cy3-Aβ42 relative signal intensity on multi-spot slides after 5 days of culture with pericytes under different experimental conditions (Fig. 5c). These data suggest that pericyte-derived apoE is

required for clearance of Aβ aggregates by cultured pericytes, which we show is mediated by LRP1, an apoE receptor (see Fig. 2d-e; Fig. 3c-e and Fig. 4b-c). Besides the self-autonomous effect of apoE in regulating clearance of Aβ aggregates by pericytes (Fig. 5a-c), to mimic in vivo situation we next studied the non-autonomous effects of astrocyte-derived apoE by adding lipidated human apoE3 or apoE4 particles prepared from immortalized astrocytes, as previously described [53]. Previous work has shown that astrocyte-derived apoE provides a major source of apoE in the brain in vivo and signals pericytes via LRP1, but not LRP2, very low density lipoprotein receptor (VLDLR), low density lipoprotein receptor (LDLR) or apoER2 [49]. The effects of apoE3 and apoE4 on Aβ clearance by pericytes was studied after silencing mouse apoE (si.Apoe). ApoE3, but not apoE4, almost completely reversed Aβ clearance by pericytes with inhibited mouse apoE (Fig. 5a-c), suggesting that astrocyte-derived apoE exerts a non-autonomous isoform-specific effect on Aβ clearance by pericytes. To additionally confirm that apoE3 effect on pericytes requires LRP1 as previously shown [49], we performed the same

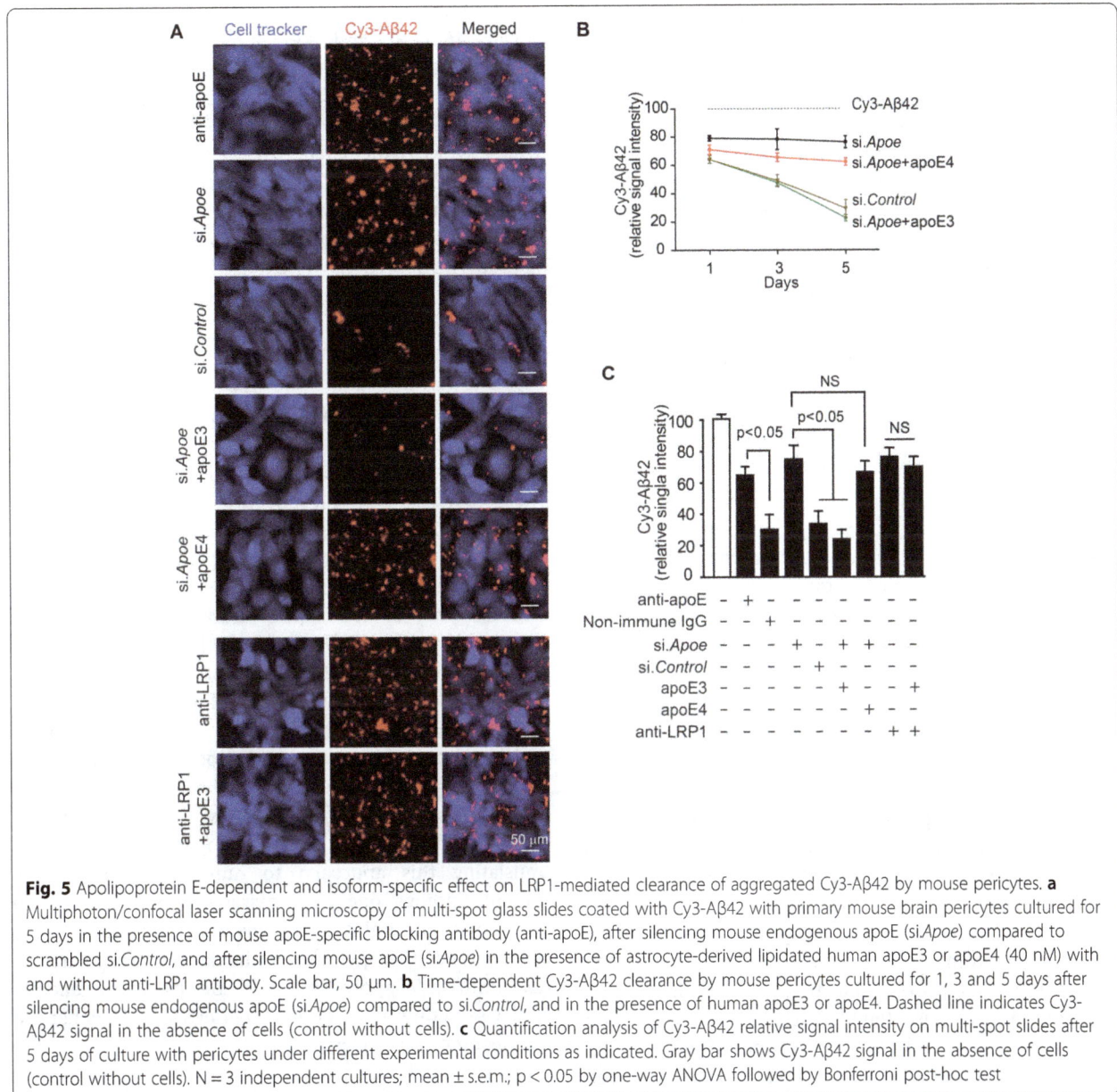

Fig. 5 Apolipoprotein E-dependent and isoform-specific effect on LRP1-mediated clearance of aggregated Cy3-Aβ42 by mouse pericytes. **a** Multiphoton/confocal laser scanning microscopy of multi-spot glass slides coated with Cy3-Aβ42 with primary mouse brain pericytes cultured for 5 days in the presence of mouse apoE-specific blocking antibody (anti-apoE), after silencing mouse endogenous apoE (si.Apoe) compared to scrambled si.Control, and after silencing mouse apoE (si.Apoe) in the presence of astrocyte-derived lipidated human apoE3 or apoE4 (40 nM) with and without anti-LRP1 antibody. Scale bar, 50 μm. **b** Time-dependent Cy3-Aβ42 clearance by mouse pericytes cultured for 1, 3 and 5 days after silencing mouse endogenous apoE (si.Apoe) compared to si.Control, and in the presence of human apoE3 or apoE4. Dashed line indicates Cy3-Aβ42 signal in the absence of cells (control without cells). **c** Quantification analysis of Cy3-Aβ42 relative signal intensity on multi-spot slides after 5 days of culture with pericytes under different experimental conditions as indicated. Gray bar shows Cy3-Aβ42 signal in the absence of cells (control without cells). N = 3 independent cultures; mean ± s.e.m.; p < 0.05 by one-way ANOVA followed by Bonferroni post-hoc test

experiment in the presence of an anti-LRP1 antibody. As expected, this experiment showed that anti-LRP1 inhibits apoE3's ability to reverse the Aβ clearing capability of mouse pericytes with silenced mouse apoE (si.Apoe) (Fig. 5a, c).

Discussion

Our data show that BBB-associated pericytes accumulate an abundance of Aβ on brain capillaries in AD patients and $APP^{Sw/0}$ mice. We also show that pericytes play a major role in clearance of different Aβ42 species including a mixture of monomers and small molecular weight oligomers, which is mediated via LRP1, similar as previously shown for Aβ40 [37]. This has been demonstrated by pharmacologic inhibition of LRP1 by an anti-LRP1

antibody [22, 29] and RAP [52], genetic $Lrp1$ knockdown with short interfering RNA (si.$Lrp1$) and deletion of LRP1 from pericytes in $Lrp^{lox/lox}$;$Cspg4$-Cre mice compared to $Lrp^{lox/lox}$ controls. Moreover, we show that pericytes efficiently clear Aβ42 aggregates by an LRP1/apoE isoform-specific mechanism. This has been demonstrated by silencing mouse $Apoe$ (si.$Apoe$) in pericytes in the absence and presence of human astrocyte-derived lipidated apoE3 or apoE4, which revealed that apoE3, but not apoE4, mediates LRP1-dependent clearance of Cy3-Aβ42 aggregates. Overall, these data point to Aβ clearance on pericytes as a possible contributory factor in the pathogenesis of AD and accumulation of Aβ in the brain and around brain capillaries causing capillary CAA as seen in

AD [8]. The data also suggest that LRP1/apoE interaction on pericytes should be explored further as a potential therapeutic approach for controlling Aβ clearance in AD.

Accumulation of Aβ in pericytes in AD and *APP* mouse brain capillaries likely reflects Aβ overload that exceeds pericytes clearance capability resulting in intracellular trapping of Aβ. This in turn may set a stage for the formation of amyloid deposits around brain capillaries and within the basement membrane between pericytes and endothelial cells, as shown in AD [7, 8] and *APP* models [21]. Consistent with these findings we also observed accumulation of Aβ in the brain endothelium in both AD and *APP^Sw/0* mice likely reflecting excess Aβ that has not been cleared via transport across the BBB [27]. Collectively, these data suggest that not only previously shown faulty clearance of Aβ on VSMCs contributes to CAA and Aβ pathology [29, 30], but also impaired clearance on pericytes may contribute to development of capillary CAA [8, 21] and retention of Aβ in the brain. This might be particularly important at disease stages when other clearance mechanisms including Aβ drainage by the perivascular route and/or the meningeal lymphatics become deficient, as recently shown in *APP* mouse models [16, 17].

Pericyte degeneration and loss have been reported in AD patients [47, 56–59] and *APP* mice [37, 60]. Consistent with previous findings demonstrating that excess Aβ in pericytes can trigger cell death in human [54] and mouse [37] pericytes, we also found that pericytes in *APP^Sw/0* mice die at the time of Aβ deposition in the brain and its accumulation in pericytes. Pericyte cell death, in turn, can exacerbate progression of AD pathology, as shown in *APP^Sw/0*; *Pdgfrb^+/−* mice with accelerated pericyte loss [37]. Similar as shown in human pericytes [54], we also found that LRP1 mediates both Aβ internalization and cell death of mouse pericytes, as illustrated by diminished Aβ uptake and reduced cell death in the presence of LRP1 inhibition by either an anti-LRP1 antibody and/or *Lrp1* silencing. Consistent with the present findings, previous studies by Verbeek and colleagues [54, 61–63] suggested that Aβ effects on pericytes are modulated by apoE isoforms. In brief, they showed that human pericytes from apoE4 carriers compared to apoE3 carriers secrete less apoE in the culture media resulting in increased accumulation of Dutch Aβ peptide on the cell surface and greater rate of cell death induced by Aβ [63].

Interestingly, loss of pericytes in human AD is significantly higher in apoE4 carriers compared to apoE3 carriers, which is associated with greater degree of BBB breakdown [56, 64], and increased risk for CAA, as shown both in human apoE4 compared to apoE3 carriers [65–69], and *APP* mouse models on apoE4 compared to apoE3 background [66, 70]. These findings are consistent with the present data showing that human astrocyte-derived apoE4, in contrast to apoE3, cannot reverse LRP-1-mediated Aβ clearance by mouse pericytes with silenced mouse endogenous apoE, and previous findings demonstrating that apoE4 compared to apoE3 poorly binds to LRP1, which leads from on one hand to BBB breakdown by activating BBB-degrading cyclophilin-A-matrix metallopropteinase-9 pathway in pericytes [49], and from the other, diminished clearance of Aβ across the BBB [39].

Finally, the present findings showing that pericytes actively contribute to Aβ removal at the BBB via LRP1-mediated apoE isoform-dependent clearance on brain capillaries should encourage future studies directed at exploring possible therapeutic potential of this pathway to control CAA and Aβ pathology in AD. For example, pharmacologic or genetic strategies that can increase activity of LRP1/apoE clearance system in pericytes and at the BBB might diminish CAA and Aβ accumulation in apoE3 carriers, but may not work as well in apoE4 carriers. On the other hand, recent cell therapy studies have shown that mouse mesodermal pericytes can improve cerebral blood flow and reduce Aβ pathology when injected into the brain of *APP* mice [38]. Based on the present findings, this therapeutic effect likely depends on mouse endogenous apoE. When translating this approach to humans, based on the present findings one can envisage using iPSC-derived pericytes from apoE3 carriers as a straight Aβ lowering cell clearance therapy, whereas in case of apoE4 carriers, CRISPER/Cas9 approach could be used to generate apoE3-secreting iPSC-derived pericytes with enhanced Aβ clearance properties.

Conclusions

In conclusion, our findings show that BBB-associated pericytes clear Aβ aggregates via an LRP1-dependent apoE isoform-specific mechanism with apoE4 disrupting Aβ clearance compared to apoE3. Overall, the present data support that the LRP1/apoE pathway in pericytes has a potential to be explored as a therapeutic target for controlling Aβ clearance and levels in AD.

Abbreviations

aCSF: Artificial cerebrospinal fluid; AD: Alzheimer's disease; apoE: Apolipoprotein E; *APP*: Aβ-precursor protein; Aβ: Amyloid-β;

BBB: Blood-brain barrier; CAA: Cerebral amyloid angiopathy; CD13: Cluster of differentiation 13; CERAD: Consortium to establish a registry for Alzheimer's disease; Cspg4: Chondroitin sulfate proteoglycan 4; Cy3: Cyanine 3; FBS: Fetal bovine serum; ISF: Interstitial fluid; LRP1: Low density lipoprotein receptor related protein 1; PFA: Paraformaldehyde; PICALM: Phosphatidylinositol binding clathrin assembly protein; RAP: Receptor-associated protein; TUNEL: Terminal deoxynucleotidyl transferase UTP nick end labeling; VSMCs: Vascular smooth muscle cells

Acknowledgements
We thank Dr. Le Ma for technical assistance on experiments using mouse brain slices.

Funding
The was supported by the National Institutes of Health grants R01NS034467, R01AG023084, R01AG039452, and the Foundation Leducq Transatlantic Network of Excellence for the Study of Perivascular Spaces in Small Vessel Disease reference no. 16 CVD 05 to BVZ, and the Cure for Alzheimer's Fund to BVZ and ZZ.

Authors' contributions
QM and ZZ designed and performed experiments and analyzed data and contributed to writing the manuscript. APS, YW, MW and NCO performed experiments. PBV, JH and DMH provided key reagent or animal model, and contributed to writing the manuscript. BVZ designed all experiments, analyzed data and wrote the paper. All authors read and approved the final manuscript.

Competing interests
DMH is an inventor on a patent filed by Washington University on the topic of anti-apoE antibodies that was licensed by Denali. DMH co-founded and is on the scientific advisory board of C2N Diagnostics. DMH consults for Genentech, AbbVie, Eli Lilly, Proclara, and Denali. Washington University receives research grants to the lab of DMH from C2N Diagnostics, AbbVie, and Denali. PBV, is a full-time employee of C2N Diagnostics, receiving stock and/or stock options.

Author details
[1]Center for Neurodegeneration and Regeneration, Zilkha Neurogenetic Institute and Department of Physiology and Neuroscience, Keck School of Medicine, University of Southern California, Los Angeles, California 90033, USA. [2]Lawrence D. Longo, MD Center for Neonatal Biology, Division of Pharmacology, Department of Basic Sciences, Loma Linda University School of Medicine, Loma Linda, CA 92350, USA. [3]C2N Diagnostics, LLC, Saint Louis, MO 63110, USA. [4]Department of Molecular Genetics, University of Texas Southwestern Medical Center, Dallas, TX, USA. [5]Department of Neuroscience, University of Texas Southwestern Medical Center, Dallas, TX, USA. [6]Department of Neurology and Neurotherapeutics and Center for Translational Neurodegeneration Research, University of Texas Southwestern Medical Center, Dallas, TX, USA. [7]Department of Neurology, Hope Center for Neurological Disorders, Knight Alzheimer's Disease Research Center, Washington University School of Medicine, Saint Louis, MO 63110, USA.

References
1. Sweeney MD, Sagare AP, Zlokovic BV. Blood-brain barrier breakdown in Alzheimer disease and other neurodegenerative disorders. Nat Rev Neurol. 2018;14:133–50.
2. Jack CR Jr, Bennett DA, Blennow K, Carrillo MC, Dunn B, Haeberlein SB, Holtzman DM, Jagust W, Jessen F, Karlawish J, et al. NIA-AA research framework: toward a biological definition of Alzheimer's disease. Alzheimers Dement. 2018;14:535–62.
3. Hardy J, Selkoe DJ. The amyloid hypothesis of Alzheimer's disease: progress and problems on the road to therapeutics. Science. 2002;297:353–6.
4. Selkoe DJ, Hardy J. The amyloid hypothesis of Alzheimer's disease at 25 years. EMBO Mol Med. 2016;8:595–608.
5. Choi SH, Kim YH, Hebisch M, Sliwinski C, Lee S, D'Avanzo C, Chen H, Hooli B, Asselin C, Muffat J, et al. A three-dimensional human neural cell culture model of Alzheimer's disease. Nature. 2014;515:274–8.
6. Zlokovic BV. Cerebrovascular effects of apolipoprotein E: implications for Alzheimer disease. JAMA Neurol. 2013;70:440–4.
7. Snyder HM, Corriveau RA, Craft S, Faber JE, Greenberg SM, Knopman D, Lamb BT, Montine TJ, Nedergaard M, Schaffer CB, et al. Vascular contributions to cognitive impairment and dementia including Alzheimer's disease. Alzheimers Dement. 2015;11:710–7.
8. Hecht M, Kramer LM, von Arnim CAF, Otto M, Thal DR. Capillary cerebral amyloid angiopathy in Alzheimer's disease: association with allocortical/hippocampal microinfarcts and cognitive decline. Acta Neuropathol. 2018; 135:681–94.
9. Wermer MJH, Greenberg SM. The growing clinical spectrum of cerebral amyloid angiopathy. Curr Opin Neurol. 2018;31:28–35.
10. Zhao Z, Nelson AR, Betsholtz C, Zlokovic BV. Establishment and dysfunction of the blood-brain barrier. Cell. 2015;163:1064–78.
11. Leissring MA. Abeta-degrading proteases: therapeutic potential in Alzheimer disease. CNS Drugs. 2016;30:667–75.
12. Tarasoff-Conway JM, Carare RO, Osorio RS, Glodzik L, Butler T, Fieremans E, Axel L, Rusinek H, Nicholson C, Zlokovic BV, et al. Clearance systems in the brain-implications for Alzheimer disease. Nat Rev Neurol. 2015;11:457–70.
13. Bakker EN, Bacskai BJ, Arbel-Ornath M, Aldea R, Bedussi B, Morris AW, Weller RO, Carare RO. Lymphatic clearance of the brain: perivascular, paravascular and significance for neurodegenerative diseases. Cell Mol Neurobiol. 2016; 36:181–94.
14. Engelhardt B, Carare RO, Bechmann I, Flugel A, Laman JD, Weller RO. Vascular, glial, and lymphatic immune gateways of the central nervous system. Acta Neuropathol. 2016;132:317–38.
15. Engelhardt B. Cluster: barriers of the central nervous system. Acta Neuropathol. 2018;135:307–10.
16. Sweeney MD, Zlokovic BV. A lymphatic waste-disposal system implicated in Alzheimer's disease. Nature. 2018;560:172–4.
17. Da Mesquita S, Louveau A, Vaccari A, Smirnov I, Cornelison RC, Kingsmore KM, Contarino C, Onengut-Gumuscu S, Farber E, Raper D, et al. Functional aspects of meningeal lymphatics in ageing and Alzheimer's disease. Nature. 2018;560:185–91.
18. Zlokovic BV. Neurovascular pathways to neurodegeneration in Alzheimer's disease and other disorders. Nat Rev Neurosci. 2011;12:723–38.
19. Mawuenyega KG, Sigurdson W, Ovod V, Munsell L, Kasten T, Morris JC, Yarasheski KE, Bateman RJ. Decreased clearance of CNS beta-amyloid in Alzheimer's disease. Science. 2010;330:1774.
20. Roberts KF, Elbert DL, Kasten TP, Patterson BW, Sigurdson WC, Connors RE, Ovod V, Munsell LY, Mawuenyega KG, Miller-Thomas MM, et al. Amyloid-beta efflux from the central nervous system into the plasma. Ann Neurol. 2014;76:837–44.
21. Montagne A, Zhao Z, Zlokovic BV. Alzheimer's disease: a matter of blood-brain barrier dysfunction? J Exp Med. 2017;214:3151–69.
22. Bell RD, Sagare AP, Friedman AE, Bedi GS, Holtzman DM, Deane R, Zlokovic BV. Transport pathways for clearance of human Alzheimer's amyloid beta-peptide and apolipoproteins E and J in the mouse central nervous system. J Cereb Blood Flow Metab. 2007;27:909–18.
23. Holtzman DM, Herz J, Bu G. Apolipoprotein E and apolipoprotein E receptors: normal biology and roles in Alzheimer disease. Cold Spring Harb Perspect Med. 2012;2:a006312.
24. Kanekiyo T, Xu H, Bu G. ApoE and Abeta in Alzheimer's disease: accidental encounters or partners? Neuron. 2014;81:740–54.
25. Shibata M, Yamada S, Kumar SR, Calero M, Bading J, Frangione B, Holtzman DM, Miller CA, Strickland DK, Ghiso J, Zlokovic BV. Clearance of Alzheimer's amyloid-ss(1-40) peptide from brain by LDL receptor-related protein-1 at the blood-brain barrier. J Clin Invest. 2000;106:1489–99.
26. Deane R, Wu Z, Sagare A, Davis J, Du Yan S, Hamm K, Xu F, Parisi M, LaRue B, Hu HW, et al. LRP/amyloid beta-peptide interaction mediates differential brain efflux of Abeta isoforms. Neuron. 2004;43:333–44.
27. Zhao Z, Sagare AP, Ma Q, Halliday MR, Kong P, Kisler K, Winkler EA, Ramanathan A, Kanekiyo T, Bu G, et al. Central role for PICALM in amyloid-beta blood-brain barrier transcytosis and clearance. Nat Neurosci. 2015;18:978–87.

28. Storck SE, Meister S, Nahrath J, Meissner JN, Schubert N, Di Spiezio A, Baches S, Vandenbroucke RE, Bouter Y, Prikulis I, et al. Endothelial LRP1 transports amyloid-beta(1-42) across the blood-brain barrier. J Clin Invest. 2016;126:123–36.

29. Bell RD, Deane R, Chow N, Long X, Sagare A, Singh I, Streb JW, Guo H, Rubio A, Van Nostrand W, et al. SRF and myocardin regulate LRP-mediated amyloid-beta clearance in brain vascular cells. Nat Cell Biol. 2009;11:143–53.

30. Kanekiyo T, Liu CC, Shinohara M, Li J, Bu G. LRP1 in brain vascular smooth muscle cells mediates local clearance of Alzheimer's amyloid-beta. J Neurosci. 2012;32:16458–65.

31. Koistinaho M, Lin S, Wu X, Esterman M, Koger D, Hanson J, Higgs R, Liu F, Malkani S, Bales KR, Paul SM. Apolipoprotein E promotes astrocyte colocalization and degradation of deposited amyloid-beta peptides. Nat Med. 2004;10:719–26.

32. Sweeney MD, Ayyadurai S, Zlokovic BV. Pericytes of the neurovascular unit: key functions and signaling pathways. Nat Neurosci. 2016;19:771–83.

33. Armulik A, Genove G, Mae M, Nisancioglu MH, Wallgard E, Niaudet C, He L, Norlin J, Lindblom P, Strittmatter K, et al. Pericytes regulate the blood-brain barrier. Nature. 2010;468:557–61.

34. Bell RD, Winkler EA, Sagare AP, Singh I, LaRue B, Deane R, Zlokovic BV. Pericytes control key neurovascular functions and neuronal phenotype in the adult brain and during brain aging. Neuron. 2010;68:409–27.

35. Kisler K, Nelson AR, Rege SV, Ramanathan A, Wang Y, Ahuja A, Lazic D, Tsai PS, Zhao Z, Zhou Y, et al. Pericyte degeneration leads to neurovascular uncoupling and limits oxygen supply to brain. Nat Neurosci. 2017;20:406–16.

36. Montagne A, Nikolakopoulou AM, Zhao Z, Sagare AP, Si G, Lazic D, Barnes SR, Daianu M, Ramanathan A, Go A, et al. Pericyte degeneration causes white matter dysfunction in the mouse central nervous system. Nat Med. 2018;24:326–37.

37. Sagare AP, Bell RD, Zhao Z, Ma Q, Winkler EA, Ramanathan A, Zlokovic BV. Pericyte loss influences Alzheimer-like neurodegeneration in mice. Nat Commun. 2013;4:2932.

38. Tachibana M, Yamazaki Y, Liu CC, Bu G, Kanekiyo T. Pericyte implantation in the brain enhances cerebral blood flow and reduces amyloid-beta pathology in amyloid model mice. Exp Neurol. 2018;300:13–21.

39. Deane R, Sagare A, Hamm K, Parisi M, Lane S, Finn MB, Holtzman DM, Zlokovic BV. apoE isoform-specific disruption of amyloid beta peptide clearance from mouse brain. J Clin Invest. 2008;118:4002–13.

40. Verghese PB, Castellano JM, Holtzman DM. Apolipoprotein E in Alzheimer's disease and other neurological disorders. Lancet Neurol. 2011;10:241–52.

41. Liao F, Yoon H, Kim J. Apolipoprotein E metabolism and functions in brain and its role in Alzheimer's disease. Curr Opin Lipidol. 2017;28:60–7.

42. Liu CC, Liu CC, Kanekiyo T, Xu H, Bu G. Apolipoprotein E and Alzheimer disease: risk, mechanisms and therapy. Nat Rev Neurol. 2013;9:106–18.

43. Hsiao K, Chapman P, Nilsen S, Eckman C, Harigaya Y, Younkin S, Yang F, Cole G. Correlative memory deficits, Abeta elevation, and amyloid plaques in transgenic mice. Science. 1996;274:99–102.

44. Boucher P, Gotthardt M, Li WP, Anderson RG, Herz J. LRP: role in vascular wall integrity and protection from atherosclerosis. Science. 2003;300:329–32.

45. Rohlmann A, Gotthardt M, Hammer RE, Herz J. Inducible inactivation of hepatic LRP gene by cre-mediated recombination confirms role of LRP in clearance of chylomicron remnants. J Clin Invest. 1998;101:689–95.

46. Zhu X, Bergles DE, Nishiyama A. NG2 cells generate both oligodendrocytes and gray matter astrocytes. Development. 2008;135:145–57.

47. Sengillo JD, Winkler EA, Walker CT, Sullivan JS, Johnson M, Zlokovic BV. Deficiency in mural vascular cells coincides with blood-brain barrier disruption in Alzheimer's disease. Brain Pathol. 2013;23:303–10.

48. Kandimalla KK, Scott OG, Fulzele S, Davidson MW, Poduslo JF. Mechanism of neuronal versus endothelial cell uptake of Alzheimer's disease amyloid beta protein. PLoS One. 2009;4:e4627.

49. Bell RD, Winkler EA, Singh I, Sagare AP, Deane R, Wu Z, Holtzman DM, Betsholtz C, Armulik A, Sallstrom J, et al. Apolipoprotein E controls cerebrovascular integrity via cyclophilin A. Nature. 2012;485:512–6.

50. Wu Z, Hofman FM, Zlokovic BV. A simple method for isolation and characterization of mouse brain microvascular endothelial cells. J Neurosci Methods. 2003;130:53–63.

51. Wyss-Coray T, Loike JD, Brionne TC, Lu E, Anankov R, Yan F, Silverstein SC, Husemann J. Adult mouse astrocytes degrade amyloid-beta in vitro and in situ. Nat Med. 2003;9:453–7.

52. Herz J, Goldstein JL, Strickland DK, Ho YK, Brown MS. 39-kDa protein modulates binding of ligands to low density lipoprotein receptor-related protein/alpha 2-macroglobulin receptor. J Biol Chem. 1991;266:21232–8.

53. Morikawa M, Fryer JD, Sullivan PM, Christopher EA, Wahrle SE, DeMattos RB, O'Dell MA, Fagan AM, Lashuel HA, Walz T, et al. Production and characterization of astrocyte-derived human apolipoprotein E isoforms from immortalized astrocytes and their interactions with amyloid-beta. Neurobiol Dis. 2005;19:66–76.

54. Wilhelmus MM, Otte-Holler I, van Triel JJ, Veerhuis R, Maat-Schieman ML, Bu G, de Waal RM, Verbeek MM. Lipoprotein receptor-related protein-1 mediates amyloid-beta-mediated cell death of cerebrovascular cells. Am J Pathol. 2007;171:1989–99.

55. Webster CI, Burrell M, Olsson LL, Fowler SB, Digby S, Sandercock A, Snijder A, Tebbe J, Haupts U, Grudzinska J, et al. Engineering neprilysin activity and specificity to create a novel therapeutic for Alzheimer's disease. PLoS One. 2014;9:e104001.

56. Halliday MR, Rege SV, Ma Q, Zhao Z, Miller CA, Winkler EA, Zlokovic BV. Accelerated pericyte degeneration and blood-brain barrier breakdown in apolipoprotein E4 carriers with Alzheimer's disease. J Cereb Blood Flow Metab. 2016;36:216–27.

57. Farkas E, Luiten PG. Cerebral microvascular pathology in aging and Alzheimer's disease. Prog Neurobiol. 2001;64:575–611.

58. Baloyannis SJ, Baloyannis IS. The vascular factor in Alzheimer's disease: a study in Golgi technique and electron microscopy. J Neurol Sci. 2012;322:117–21.

59. Miners JS, Schulz I, Love S. Differing associations between Abeta accumulation, hypoperfusion, blood-brain barrier dysfunction and loss of PDGFRB pericyte marker in the precuneus and parietal white matter in Alzheimer's disease. J Cereb Blood Flow Metab. 2018;38:103–15.

60. Park L, Zhou J, Zhou P, Pistick R, El Jamal S, Younkin L, Pierce J, Arreguin A, Anrather J, Younkin SG, et al. Innate immunity receptor CD36 promotes cerebral amyloid angiopathy. Proc Natl Acad Sci U S A. 2013;110:3089–94.

61. Verbeek MM, Van Nostrand WE, Otte-Holler I, Wesseling P, De Waal RM. Amyloid-beta-induced degeneration of human brain pericytes is dependent on the apolipoprotein E genotype. Ann N Y Acad Sci. 2000;903:187–99.

62. Wilhelmus MM, Otte-Holler I, Davis J, Van Nostrand WE, de Waal RM, Verbeek MM. Apolipoprotein E genotype regulates amyloid-beta cytotoxicity. J Neurosci. 2005;25:3621–7.

63. Bruinsma IB, Wilhelmus MM, Kox M, Veerhuis R, de Waal RM, Verbeek MM. Apolipoprotein E protects cultured pericytes and astrocytes from D-Abeta(1-40)-mediated cell death. Brain Res. 2010;1315:169–80.

64. Hultman K, Strickland S, Norris EH. The APOE varepsilon4/varepsilon4 genotype potentiates vascular fibrin(ogen) deposition in amyloid-laden vessels in the brains of Alzheimer's disease patients. J Cereb Blood Flow Metab. 2013;33:1251–8.

65. Zonneveld HI, Goos JD, Wattjes MP, Prins ND, Scheltens P, van der Flier WM, Kuijer JP, Muller M, Barkhof F. Prevalence of cortical superficial siderosis in a memory clinic population. Neurology. 2014;82:698–704.

66. Cacciottolo M, Christensen A, Moser A, Liu J, Pike CJ, Smith C, LaDu MJ, Sullivan PM, Morgan TE, Dolzhenko E, et al. The APOE4 allele shows opposite sex bias in microbleeds and Alzheimer's disease of humans and mice. Neurobiol Aging. 2016;37:47–57.

67. Esiri MM, Joachim C, Sloan C, Christie S, Agacinski G, Bridges LR, Wilcock GK, Smith AD. Cerebral subcortical small vessel disease in subjects with pathologically confirmed Alzheimer disease: a clinicopathologic study in the Oxford project to investigate memory and ageing (OPTIMA). Alzheimer Dis Assoc Disord. 2014;28:30–5.

68. Rannikmae K, Kalaria RN, Greenberg SM, Chui HC, Schmitt FA, Samarasekera N, Al-Shahi Salman R, Sudlow CL. APOE associations with severe CAA-associated vasculopathic changes: collaborative meta-analysis. J Neurol Neurosurg Psychiatry. 2014;85:300–5.

69. Shinohara M, Murray ME, Frank RD, Shinohara M, DeTure M, Yamazaki Y, Tachibana M, Atagi Y, Davis MD, Liu CC, et al. Impact of sex and APOE4 on cerebral amyloid angiopathy in Alzheimer's disease. Acta Neuropathol. 2016; 132:225–34.

70. Fryer JD, Simmons K, Parsadanian M, Bales KR, Paul SM, Sullivan PM, Holtzman DM. Human apolipoprotein E4 alters the amyloid-beta 40:42 ratio and promotes the formation of cerebral amyloid angiopathy in an amyloid precursor protein transgenic model. J Neurosci. 2005;25:2803–10.

10

Transcriptional profiling and biomarker identification reveal tissue specific effects of expanded ataxin-3 in a spinocerebellar ataxia type 3 mouse model

Lodewijk J. A. Toonen[1] (iD), Maurice Overzier[1], Melvin M. Evers[2], Leticia G. Leon[3], Sander A. J. van der Zeeuw[4], Hailiang Mei[4], Szymon M. Kielbasa[5], Jelle J. Goeman[5], Kristina M. Hettne[1], Olafur Th. Magnusson[6], Marion Poirel[7], Alexandre Seyer[7], Peter A. C. 't Hoen[1,8] and Willeke M. C. van Roon-Mom[1*]

Abstract

Background: Spinocerebellar ataxia type 3 (SCA3) is a progressive neurodegenerative disorder caused by expansion of the polyglutamine repeat in the ataxin-3 protein. Expression of mutant ataxin-3 is known to result in transcriptional dysregulation, which can contribute to the cellular toxicity and neurodegeneration. Since the exact causative mechanisms underlying this process have not been fully elucidated, gene expression analyses in brains of transgenic SCA3 mouse models may provide useful insights.

Methods: Here we characterised the MJD84.2 SCA3 mouse model expressing the mutant human ataxin-3 gene using a multi-omics approach on brain and blood. Gene expression changes in brainstem, cerebellum, striatum and cortex were used to study pathological changes in brain, while blood gene expression and metabolites/lipids levels were examined as potential biomarkers for disease.

Results: Despite normal motor performance at 17.5 months of age, transcriptional changes in brain tissue of the SCA3 mice were observed. Most transcriptional changes occurred in brainstem and striatum, whilst cerebellum and cortex were only modestly affected. The most significantly altered genes in SCA3 mouse brain were *Tmc3*, *Zfp488*, *Car2*, and *Chdh*. Based on the transcriptional changes, α-adrenergic and CREB pathways were most consistently altered for combined analysis of the four brain regions. When examining individual brain regions, axon guidance and synaptic transmission pathways were most strongly altered in striatum, whilst brainstem presented with strongest alterations in the pi-3 k cascade and cholesterol biosynthesis pathways. Similar to other neurodegenerative diseases, reduced levels of tryptophan and increased levels of ceramides, di- and triglycerides were observed in SCA3 mouse blood.

Conclusions: The observed transcriptional changes in SCA3 mouse brain reveal parallels with previous reported neuropathology in patients, but also shows brain region specific effects as well as involvement of adrenergic signalling and CREB pathway changes in SCA3. Importantly, the transcriptional changes occur prior to onset of motor- and coordination deficits.

Keywords: Spinocerebellar ataxia type 3, Mouse model, RNA sequencing, Metabolomics

* Correspondence: w.vanroon@lumc.nl
[1]Department of Human Genetics, Leiden University Medical Center, 2300 RC Leiden, The Netherlands
Full list of author information is available at the end of the article

Background

Spinocerebellar ataxia type 3 (SCA3), also known as Machado Joseph Disease (MJD), is a progressive neurodegenerative disorder, with symptoms usually presenting around midlife. SCA3 is the most common of the dominantly inherited ataxias and is caused by a CAG repeat expansion in the *ATXN3* gene [1]. The CAG repeat is translated into a polyglutamine (polyQ) stretch in the ataxin-3 protein, which upon mutational expansion to 56–84 glutamines results in a gain of toxic protein function [2]. This protein toxicity mostly shows its effects in the brain, and neuronal loss in SCA3 has been reported predominantly in the brainstem, cerebellum (spinocerebellar pathways and dentate nucleus), striatum, thalamus, substantia nigra and pontine nuclei [3]. Over time, the neuronal loss causes clinical symptoms in SCA3 patients such as progressive ataxia, dystonia, spasticity, and various other symptoms (reviewed in [1]).

The molecular mechanisms of mutant ataxin-3 toxicity have been the subject of extensive research, and a range of cellular changes have been suggested to contribute to toxicity. These include aggregation and nuclear localisation of expanded ataxin-3 protein [4, 5], impaired protein degradation [6], mitochondrial dysfunction [7] and transcriptional deregulation [8]. Transcriptional deregulation may arise due to sequestration of transcription factors such as TATA-box binding protein [9] and CREB binding protein (CBP) [10] into the polyQ aggregates, thereby interfering with their function. Previous gene expression studies have identified altered inflammatory processes, cell signalling and cell surface associated genes in cell and conditional animal models of SCA3 [8, 11, 12]. Despite these recent advances in SCA3 pathogenicity, it is currently still not fully elucidated which molecular mechanisms are altered in response to mutant ataxin-3. For this reason, it is useful to examine genetic mouse models of SCA3 for transcriptional changes that occur in different regions of the brain to infer causative disease mechanisms [13].

Apart from gaining insight into disease mechanisms, transcriptional changes may also be potentially useful as biomarkers to track disease progression in SCA3. Since it is not possible to study longitudinal gene expression changes in human brain tissue, it is useful to establish potential transcriptional changes in peripheral tissues such as blood. In addition, metabolite and lipid changes in blood can also be used as easily obtainable biomarkers, and can potentially be used to track disease progression [14]. Previous research by our group has shown that there are common gene expression signatures in blood and brain of patients with Huntington disease [15]. Since patient material is not readily available, genetic SCA3 mouse models are a good starting point to identify such potential disease biomarkers.

In this study, we set out to identify the molecular mechanisms involved in SCA3 pathology. Current next-generation sequencing techniques provide an attractive means to objectively study the transcriptome and allow for very sensitive and accurate assessment of changes in gene expression. As such, we performed RNA sequencing of brain and blood from the hemizygous MJD84.2 mouse model of SCA3, which ubiquitously expresses the full human *ATXN3* gene with 76–77 CAGs [16] and gene expression analysis was performed in 4 different regions of the brain. Additionally, blood samples from the mice were subjected to RNA sequencing and serum was used for metabolomic and lipidomic analysis to identify potential biomarkers capable of tracking disease progression.

We found that the MJD84.2 mice presented with reduced bodyweight compared to wild-type, but did not develop motor symptoms even at 17.5 months of age. Gene expression changes in blood were also not pronounced, with pathway analysis suggesting respiratory electron transport and mitochondrial function to be affected. In parallel to other neurodegenerative disorders, further metabolomic and lipidomic analyses of blood revealed decreased tryptophan and increased levels of a di- and triglycerides and ceramides in SCA3 mice. In contrast to blood, transcriptional changes were readily detected in brain, with the highest number of differentially expressed genes in brainstem and striatum. Somewhat surprisingly, the cerebellum was affected to a smaller extent compared to these two brain regions. The main deregulated pathways in brain were cellular signalling pathways (α-adrenergic and CREB signalling) and pathways related to synaptic transmission. This study hence provides additional evidence for affected CREB signalling in SCA3 and suggests affected neurotransmission pathways, particularly in striatum.

Methods

SCA3 mice and tissue sampling

MJD84.2 transgenic SCA3 mice [16] and wild-type C57BL/6 mice were obtained from Jackson Laboratories (Bar Harbor, Maine, USA). All animal experiments were carried out in accordance with European Communities Council Directive 2010/63/EU and were approved by the Leiden University animal ethical committee. Breeding was performed by crossing hemizygous SCA3 mice with wild-types. ATXN3 CAG repeat lengths were verified for each mouse through gene fragment analysis, using human specific primers (Additional file 1: Table S1) flanking the CAG repeat similar to described previously [17]. Human *ATXN3* repeat lengths were 76 or 77 for all transgenic mice. Only male mice were used, and a total of 8 transgenic and 8 wild-type mice were included in the experiment (Table 1), though 2 transgenic mice did not survive to the end of the study. Mice were group

Table 1 RNA sequencing and metabolomic/lipidomic sample overview

Analysis	Tissue	Wild-type mice	SCA3 mice
RNA-seq	brainstem	8	6
RNA-seq	cerebellum	7	6
RNA-seq	cortex	7	6
RNA-seq	striatum	8	5
RNA-seq	blood (9 and 17.5 months)	6	5
Metabolomics	plasma (4 and 16 months)	4	4
Lipidomics	plasma (4 and 16 months)	4	4 (4 months), 3 (16 months)

housed in individually ventilated cages with food and drinking water available ad libitum. Blood samples for metabolomic analyses were obtained at 4, 12 and 16 months of age from 4 wild-type and 4 SCA3 mice. Animals were fasted 4 h prior to obtaining 200 µl blood through tail cut and collection in heparin lithium tubes. Tubes were immediately spun down at 18,000 x g and the supernatant (plasma) was stored at − 80 °C. For RNA sequencing, 200 µl of blood was obtained by tail cut at 9 months and 17.5 months of age. Blood samples for RNA sequencing were collected in RNAprotect animal blood tubes (Qiagen) following manufacturer's instructions, stored overnight at 4 °C and subsequently frozen at − 80 °C until RNA isolation. At 17.5 months of age, mice were sacrificed and brainstem, cerebellum, striatum and cortex were dissected, snap-frozen in liquid nitrogen and stored at − 80 °C.

Behavioural testing
To assess the motor phenotype and coordination of the mice, a beamwalk test was performed. The beamwalk balance test consisted of 2 boxes (20 × 20 × 20 cm) elevated at 53 cm height and connected by a plastic cylindrical bar of ø 10 mm or ø 30 mm and 80 cm long. Mice were placed in the transparent elevated box and crossed the bar to an enclosed dark box. The average latency to cross from 3 trials per testing day is reported. The beamwalk test was performed when the mice were 4, 6, 7.5, 9 and 12 months of age.

Metabolite profiling in plasma
Analysis of the plasma samples was performed by Profilomics (Gif-sur-Yvette, France). For extraction of metabolites, 15 µL plasma sample was treated with 60 µL of methanol with a mixture of internal standards. Protein was precipitated at 4 °C, centrifuged and supernatants were dried under nitrogen. Samples were then resuspended in ammonium carbonate 10 mM pH 10.5/AcN 40:60 (v/v). Chromatography settings for LC-HRMS

were followed as outlined by Boudah et al... [18]. Plasma extracts were separated on a HTC PAL-system (CTC Analytics AG, Zwingen, Switzerland) coupled with a Transcend 1250 liquid chromatographic system (ThermoFisher Scientific, Les Ulis, France) using an aSequant ZICpHILIC 5 µm, 2.1 × 150 mm at 15 °C (Merck, Darmstadt, Germany). After injecting 10 µL of sample, the column effluent was directly introduced into the heated Electrospray (HESI) source of a Q-Exactive mass spectrometer (Thermo Scientific, San Jose, CA) and analysis was performed in both ionization modes. Identification of molecules was performed using TraceFinder3.1 software (ThermoFisher Scientific, Les Ulis, France). The dataset was filtered and cleaned based on quality control samples as described by Dunn et al [19].

Lipid profiling in plasma
Analysis of lipids in plasma was performed on identical samples as described for the metabolite analysis. Lipid analyses were performed at Profilomics (Gif-sur-Yvette, France), in accordance with previously described methods [20]. In brief, 50 µL of plasma was added to 245 µL of CHCl3/MeOH 1:1 (v/v) and 5 µL of internal standard mixture. Extraction was performed after 2 h at 4 °C and centrifugation at 15,000×g for 10 min at 4 °C. The upper phase (aqueous phase), containing ganglioside species and several lysophospholipids, was transferred and dried under a stream of nitrogen. The protein interphase was discarded and the lower rich-lipid phase (organic phase) was pooled with the dried upper phase. Samples were then reconstituted in 50 µl CHCl3/MeOH 1:1, vortexed for 30 s, sonicated for 60 s and diluted 100 times in MeOH/IPA/H2O 65:35:5 (v/v/v) before injection. Similar to metabolite detection, plasma total lipid extracts were separated on HTC PAL-system (CTC Analytics AG) coupled with a Transcend 1250 liquid chromatographic system (ThermoFisher Scientific) using a kinetex C8 2.6 µm 2.1 × 150 mm column (Phenomenex, Sydney, NSW, Australia). Mass spectrometry was performed similar as for the metabolites and data processing was done as previously described [20].

RNA isolation
After thawing, filled blood tubes were incubated for 4 h at 25 °C to ensure proper cell lysis. Isolation of RNA was subsequently performed using the RNeasy protect animal blood kit (Qiagen, Hilden, Germany) according to manufacturer's instructions for total RNA isolation including DNAse treatment, resulting in isolation of RNA molecules longer than approximately 200 nucleotides. Reduction of alpha and beta globin mRNA was performed on RNA samples using the GLOBINclear magnetic bead kit for mouse/rat (Qiagen) following manufacturer's instructions.

For isolation of RNA from brain tissue, approximately 30 mg of tissue was transferred to next advance pink bead tubes (Next Advance, Averill Park, US) containing 500 µl Trizol (Ambion, Thermo Fisher scientific, Waltham, MA, USA). Tissue was homogenised in a bullet blender BBX24 (Next Advance) for 3 min on setting 8. A total of 100 µl chloroform was added and samples were spun down at 10,000 x g for 15 min. The aqueous phase containing the RNA was removed and an equal volume of 70% ethanol was added. RNA purification was then performed using the PureLink RNA mini kit (Thermo Fisher scientific) in accordance with the manufacturer's protocol using provided RNA columns and a 15 min DNase step. RNA was eluted in 80 µl nuclease free water. Concentration and purity of RNA was measured using Nanodrop spectrophotometry and RNA was stored at – 80 °C.

RNA sequencing

Library preparation and RNA sequencing was performed at deCode Genetics (Reykjavik, Iceland). The quality of RNA was assessed with the LabChip GX using the 96-well RNA kit (Perkin Elmer). Approximately 1 µg of total RNA was used as starting material, and the average RIN values were 7.7 (SD ± 0.5) for brain tissue and 6.8 (SD ± 0.9) for blood. Non strand-specific sample preparation was performed using the TruSeq Poly-A v2 kit (Illumina, San Diego, USA) following manufacturer's instructions. In brief, mRNA was captured using magnetic poly-T oligo-attached magnetic beads, RNA molecules were fragmented, and cDNA synthesis was performed using SuperScript II (Invitrogen, Carlsbad CA, USA) with random hexamer primers. Subsequently, 2nd strand cDNA synthesis was performed in conjunction with RNAse-H treatment. End repair was performed to generate blunt ends and 3′ adenylation was performed, followed by ligation of indexing adapters to the ds-cDNA. PCR was performed to amplify the fragments. Quality of sequencing libraries was determined through pool sequencing on a MiSeq instrument (Illumina) to assess insert size, sample diversity and optimize cluster densities. Pooled samples (4 samples/pool) were clustered on paired-end (PE) flowcells (1 pool per lane) using a cBot instrument (Illumina). The sequencing was performed using a HiSeq 2500 with v4 SBS sequencing kits (read lengths 2 × 125 cycles). Primary processing and base calling was performed with Illumina's HCS and RTA. Demultiplexing and generation of FASTQ files was done with Illumina scripts (bcl2fastq v1.8). The FASTQ files for the mouse brain RNA can be found in the GEO repository, accession GSE107958 and blood samples are listed under accession GSE108069.

Sequencing data processing

Analysis of sequencing data was performed using the BIOPET Gentrap in-house pipeline (http://biopet--docs.readthedocs.io/en/v0.7.0/pipelines/gentrap/) The fastqc toolkit (v0.11.2) was used to evaluate sequencing quality (http://www.bioinformatics.babraham.ac.uk/projects/fastqc/). Sickle (v1.33 with default settings) and Cutadapt (v1.10, with default settings except for "-m 20") were used to clean up reads. Cleaned reads were aligned to the mouse reference genome build 10 (GRCm38/mm10) using STAR aligner version 2.3.0e [21]. The non-default settings used by STAR are "–outFilterMultimapNmax 1 –outFilterMismatchNmax 10 –outSJfilterReads Unique". Average number of reads was 84 million (SD ± 18 million). On average, 66% of reads were aligned to known genes. Gene raw read counts are generated using *HTSeq* (v0.6.1) with the Refseq gene annotation extracted from UCSC on 11–09-2015. The non-default settings used by *HTSeq are* "–format bam –stranded no". Gene expression analysis was performed using edgeR (v 3.14.0) [22]. The normalization was performed using the trimmed mean of M-values (TMM) normalization method [23].

Differential gene expression and statistical analysis

Analysis of gene expression was performed on genes exceeding an average 4 counts per million (CPM) across all samples. Principle component analysis (PCA) was performed to confirm sample consistency (i.e. clustering per brain region). Additionally, correlation between genotype and GC percentage or 5′ - 3′ ratios was assessed for potential confounding effects. Differential gene expression was performed using the generalized linear model (GLM) likelihood ratio test functionality of edgeR [22]. Analyses were performed for the 4 brain regions separately, but also as a combined dataset, which is termed "brain data combined" data throughout the manuscript. For this combined analysis of all brain regions, we modelled the effect of strain and tissue (brain region) and the interaction between them to allow detection of strain effects that were either present in all brain regions or tissue-specific. For this, a design matrix was created with the function model.matrix(~ Tissue * Strain) and dispersion was estimated accounting for this design. A general linear model was fit using the glmFit function, and likelihood ratio test then performed with glmLRT on the combination of coefficients for Strain and the interaction term Tissue*Strain. The null hypothesis is that the gene shows no differential expression in any brain region. This analysis is powerful for finding genes with weak effects in several brain regions, but does not allow inference of differential expression in any specific brain regions. For differential gene expression analysis between SCA3 and wildtype mice within individual brain regions, one coefficient was assigned to each group using model.matrix(~ 0 + group). Likelihood ratiotest was then performed using glmLRT function with contrast argument to allow pairwise genotype comparison for each brain region. Analysis of differential gene expression for blood was performed similar to brain, but due to observation of a confounding influence, GC-content correction was first performed using the conditional quantile normalization (CQN) package as previously described [24]. The GC-content correction offset obtained from CQN was then included when estimating dispersion in edgeR. The two time points (9 and 17.5 months) were included as contrasts for the likelihood ratiotest. Genes with a false discovery rate (FDR, Benjamini-Hochberg) below 0.05 were considered significant. Plots were generated using ggplot2 package [25] or graphpad Prism 7. Analysis of the metabolites and lipids in blood was performed using a Welch's t-test without multiple testing correction (due to 4 vs 4 sample size), and nominal p-values < 0.05 were considered significant.

Functional annotation of gene sets and pathway analysis

For identification of functional processes, sets of genes with a FDR of < 0.05 were used, for each individual brain region and also for all brain regions combined. This led to inclusion of 585 genes from all brain regions combined, 195 genes for brainstem and 824 genes from striatum. Cerebellum and cortex did not present with enough differentially expressed genes to perform pathway analysis. Pathway analysis and exploration of metabolite-phenotype links was performed using Ingenuity Pathway Analysis (IPA) and the Euretos Knowledge Platform (EKP) [26]. Euretos allows for semantic search for biologically interesting connections between genes, proteins, metabolites and drugs based on an underlying database of 176 integrated data sources (January 2017) [27]. Pathway analysis was performed by the use of the Fisher exact test for gene set enrichment. Overlapping significantly altered pathways between the Euretos and Ingenuity analysis were considered as the most reliable signal, and are hence listed as top overrepresented pathways.

Validation with RT-qPCR

RNA sequencing results were validated on the same RNA samples using qPCR. cDNA synthesis was performed using oligo-dT primers for brain and random hexamer primers for blood RNA, with the Transcriptor First Strand cDNA Synthesis Kit (Roche, Mannheim, Germany) similar to described previously [28], but using an incubation step of 60 min at 50 °C. qPCR was performed with SensiMix SYBR & Fluorescein Kit (Bioline, Taunton, USA) similar to previously described [28], using 3 μl of 5× diluted cDNA for brain samples and

3 μl of 15× diluted cDNA for blood. Mouse reference genes used were β-actin (*Actb*), Hypoxanthine-guanine phosophoribosyltransferase (*Hprt*), and Ribosomal Protein L22 (*Rpl22*) for brain tissue and *Actb*, vinculin (*Vcl*) and *Hprt* for blood (Additional file 1: Table S1). Primers were designed with Primer3 software [29] and PCR efficiencies and expression values (N0) were determined using LinRegPCR 2014.0 [19]. Transcript level expression was then divided by the geometric mean of the 3 reference genes expression [30]. Statistical tests were performed in graphpad (7.0) using the two-stage linear step-up multiple testing procedure of Benjamini, Krieger and Yekutieli, with Q = 5% and without assuming a consistent SD.

Western blotting

Protein isolation and western blotting of mouse brain tissue was performed following standard protocols. In brief, brain tissue was homogenized in RIPA buffer using a bullet blender BBX24 (Next Advance, Averill Park, US). Protein concentration was determined using the bicinchoninic acid kit (Thermo Fisher Scientific). A total of 30 μg protein was boiled for 5 min with 4× Laemmli sample buffer and separated on 10% Tris-glycine precast gel (Biorad, Veenendaal, the Netherlands) and transferred to a nitrocellulose membrane. Membranes were blocked in 5% low fat milk and incubated overnight at 4 °C with primary antibodies: rabbit anti-carbonic anhydrase 2 (car2) 1:2000 (Novus Biologicals, Littleton, CO, USA), rabbit anti-psat1 1:1000 (Novus Biologicals) and as loading control mouse anti-β-actin 1:5000 (Abcam, Cambridge, UK). Detection was performed using secondary antibodies IRDye 680RD and 800CW (LI-COR Biosciences, Lincoln, USA) 1:5000, and membranes were imaged using Odyssey infrared imaging system (LI-COR). Quantification was performed with Odyssey software version 3.0 (Licor) using the integrated intensity method. Intensity of car2 and psat1 protein bands were divided by the β-actin intensity to correct for protein loading.

Results

SCA3 mice do not present with overt motor symptoms at 17 months of age

The MJD84.2 mouse model ubiquitously expresses full-length mutant human ataxin-3 with 76–77 glutamines, under control of the human ataxin-3 promoter. During a 17.5 month period, the behavioural phenotype of the mice was assessed using motor tests, and blood was collected for assessment of biomarkers at transcript and metabolite/lipid level. To this end, blood RNA for sequencing was collected at two time points and blood plasma for mass-spec was collected at three time points (for experimental overview, see Fig. 1a). During the

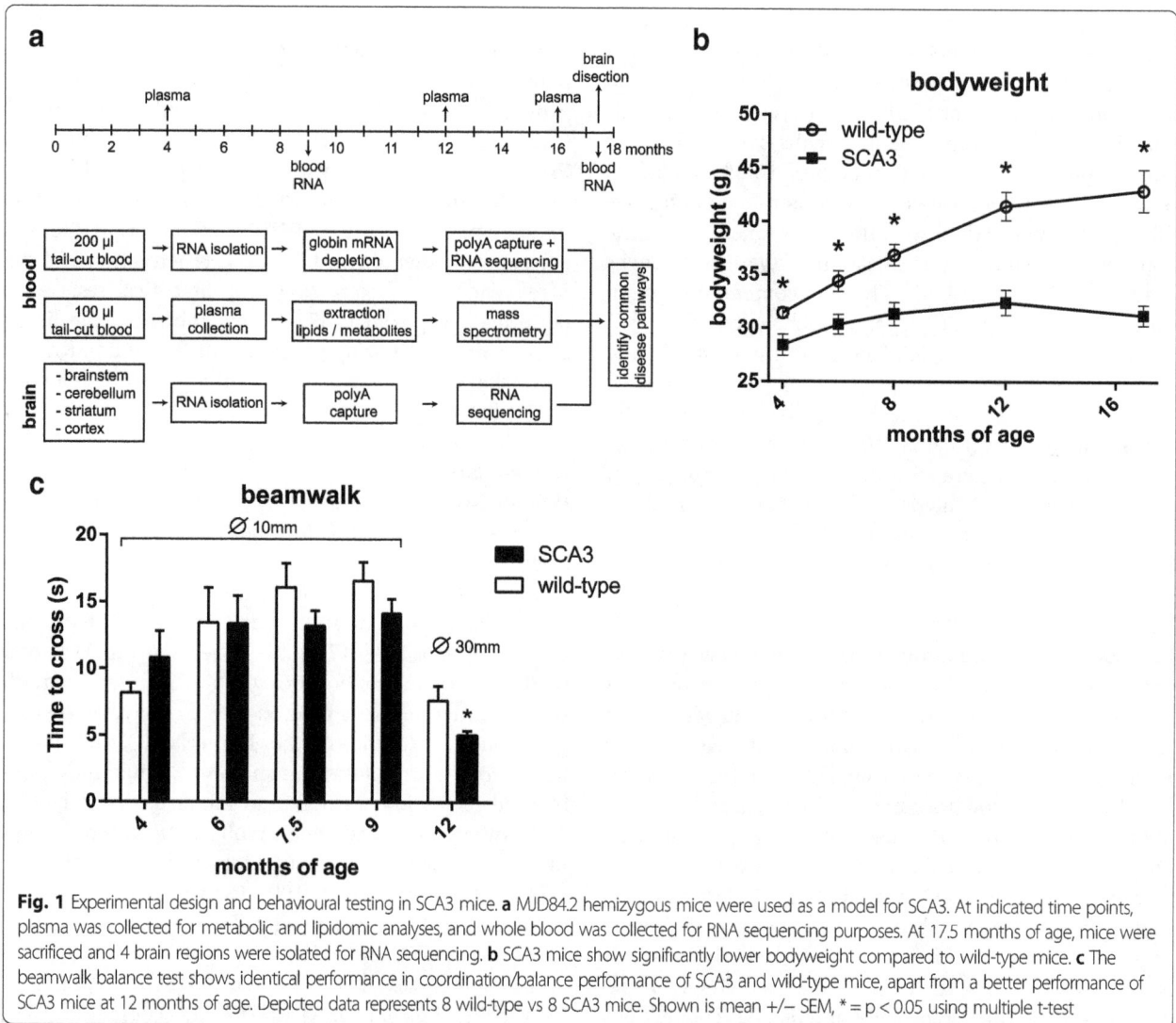

Fig. 1 Experimental design and behavioural testing in SCA3 mice. **a** MJD84.2 hemizygous mice were used as a model for SCA3. At indicated time points, plasma was collected for metabolic and lipidomic analyses, and whole blood was collected for RNA sequencing purposes. At 17.5 months of age, mice were sacrificed and 4 brain regions were isolated for RNA sequencing. **b** SCA3 mice show significantly lower bodyweight compared to wild-type mice. **c** The beamwalk balance test shows identical performance in coordination/balance performance of SCA3 and wild-type mice, apart from a better performance of SCA3 mice at 12 months of age. Depicted data represents 8 wild-type vs 8 SCA3 mice. Shown is mean +/− SEM, * = p < 0.05 using multiple t-test

testing period, the MJD84.2 mice had a significantly lower body weight compared to control mice (Fig. 1b). Assessment of an ataxic phenotype using the beamwalk balance tests at 5 time points revealed only one significant difference. This difference was a faster performance of SCA3 mice on the balance beam at 12 months of age (Fig. 1c), likely attributable to the lower bodyweight. The motor and balance performance of the SCA3 mice was identical to the wild-type mice at all other time points tested.

Individual brain regions are differently affected by mutant ataxin-3

To establish differential gene expression changes between wild-type and SCA3 mice, RNA sequencing of brain and blood tissue was performed (Table 1). After exclusion of RNA samples with low concentration (< 200 ng), a total of 53 samples were successfully sequenced. The average number of reads per

sample was 84 million (SD ± 18 million) and on average 66% of sequencing reads were aligned to exons of known genes (Additional file 2: Figure S1). Genes with average expression below 4 CPM were excluded, resulting in a total of 12,372 genes to be included for differential expression analysis. The brain RNA sequencing data can be accessed at GEO repository GSE107958. PCA plots showed good separation of samples based on brain region (Additional file 3: Figure S2) and using an FDR of < 0.05, a total of 585 genes were found significantly altered in the SCA3 brain regions combined analysis. The top 25 genes from the analysis of brain regions combined are listed in Table 2, with corresponding log2 fold change per brain region. When examining each brain region individually, the extent of differential gene expression in SCA3 mice differed greatly per brain region (Fig. 2a), with 238 genes differentially expressed in brainstem, 8 in cerebellum, 19 in cortex and 933

Table 2 Top 25 differentially expressed genes in SCA3 mice brains (regions combined)

Gene symbol	Name	FDR	Brainstem log2 fold change	Cerebellum log2 fold change	Striatum log2 fold change	Cortex log2 fold change	Protein function (GO term mol function or biological process)
Tmc3	transmembrane channel-like gene family 3	1.30E-61	1.16[a]	0.42	1.47[a]	1.16[a]	ion transport
Zfp488	zinc finger protein 488	1.05E-56	1.79[a]	1.25[a]	1.29[a]	1.45[a]	transcription, oligodendrocyte specific
Car2	carbonic anhydrase 2	3.63E-44	−1.26[a]	−0.64[a]	−1.26[a]	−0.72[a]	carbonate dehydratase activity
Chdh	choline dehydrogenase	3.26E-40	1.04[a]	0.66[a]	0.85[a]	0.87[a]	choline dehydrogenase activity
Prob1	proline rich basic protein 1	9.30E-38	1[a]	0.62[a]	0.68[a]	0.59[a]	unknown
Il33	interleukin 33	9.98E-35	−1.3[a]	−0.98[a]	−1.2[a]	−0.87[a]	cytokine activity
Fbxw15	F-box and WD-40 domain protein 15	5.97E-27	−1.8[a]	−0.84	−1.44[a]	−0.79	unknown
Rnf43	ring finger protein 43	5.64E-21	1.06[a]	0.74[a]	0.65[a]	0.88[a]	ubiquitin-protein transferase activity
Polr2a	RNA polymerase II subunit A	2.00E-20	0.74[a]	0.16	0.47[a]	0.35	DNA-directed RNA polymerase activity
Ppl	periplakin	1.50E-19	2.14[a]	0.73	0.9[a]	0.62	cadherin binding involved in cell-cell adhesion
Arsb	arylsulfatase B	2.48E-16	0.53[a]	0.2	0.32[a]	0.18	sulphate hydrolysis
Kcnk13	potassium two pore domain channel subfamily k member 13	3.04E-16	−0.97[a]	−0.73[a]	−0.81[a]	−0.44	voltage-gated ion channel
Chil1	chitinase-3-like protein 1	7.24E-16	−0.75[a]	−0.28	−0.69[a]	−0.56[a]	carbohydrate metabolic process
Serpinb1a	serpin Family B Member 1	1.16E-15	−1.34[a]	−0.86	−1.21[a]	−0.81	negative regulation of endopeptidase activity
Tspan2	tetraspanin 2	5.27E-15	−0.87[a]	−0.3	−0.99[a]	−0.41	astrocyte and microglia development
Hist1h2be	Histone H2B type 1-C/E/G	2.39E-14	0.78[a]	0.18	0.77[a]	0.66[a]	antibacterial humoral response
Acot1	Acyl-coenzyme A thioesterase 1	1.90E-13	0.74[a]	0.35	0.28	0.29	acyl-CoA metabolic process
Erbb2ip	erbin	1.86E-12	−0.89[a]	−0.44	−0.54[a]	−0.30	cellular response to tumor necrosis factor
Glul	Glutamine synthetase	1.12E-11	−0.63[a]	−0.25	−0.45[a]	−0.21	glutamine biosynthetic process
Cbs	Cystathionine beta-synthase	1.68E-11	−0.41[a]	−0.06	−0.40[a]	−0.14	catalyzes first step of the transsulfuration pathway
Qdpr	Dihydropteridine reductase	2.10E-11	−0.64[a]	−0.39	−0.70[a]	−0.36	6,7-dihydropteridine reductase activity
Sox8	Transcription factor SOX-8	6.57E-11	0.58[a]	0.37	0.42[a]	0.38	enteric nervous system development
Psat1	Phosphoserine aminotransferase	6.63E-11	0.48[a]	0.39	0.40[a]	0.46[a]	L-serine biosynthetic process
Enpp6	Ectonucleotide pyrophosphatase/phosphodiesterase family member 6	2.01E-10	0.20[a]	0.58	0.76[a]	1.25[a]	choline metabolic process
Ttyh1	Protein tweety homolog 1	1.37E-09	−0.44[a]	−0.12	−0.04	−0.14	chloride transport

Noted with [a] are genes that are also differentially expressed in individual brain regions

in striatum (FDR < 0.05) compared to wild-type mice. This observation is consistent with smaller fold-changes observed for most genes in cerebellum and cortex. Of the differentially expressed genes, 6 (*Rnf43, Zfp488, Car2, Chdh, Prob1, Il33*) were consistently significantly altered in all 4 brain regions (Fig. 2b). For each brain region that we analysed, we ranked the genes based on *p*-value, and the majority of the genes in these 4 lists were unique to that particular brain region, thus revealing tissue specific gene expression patterns. For validation we selected 6 genes from the top 25 significant genes of the

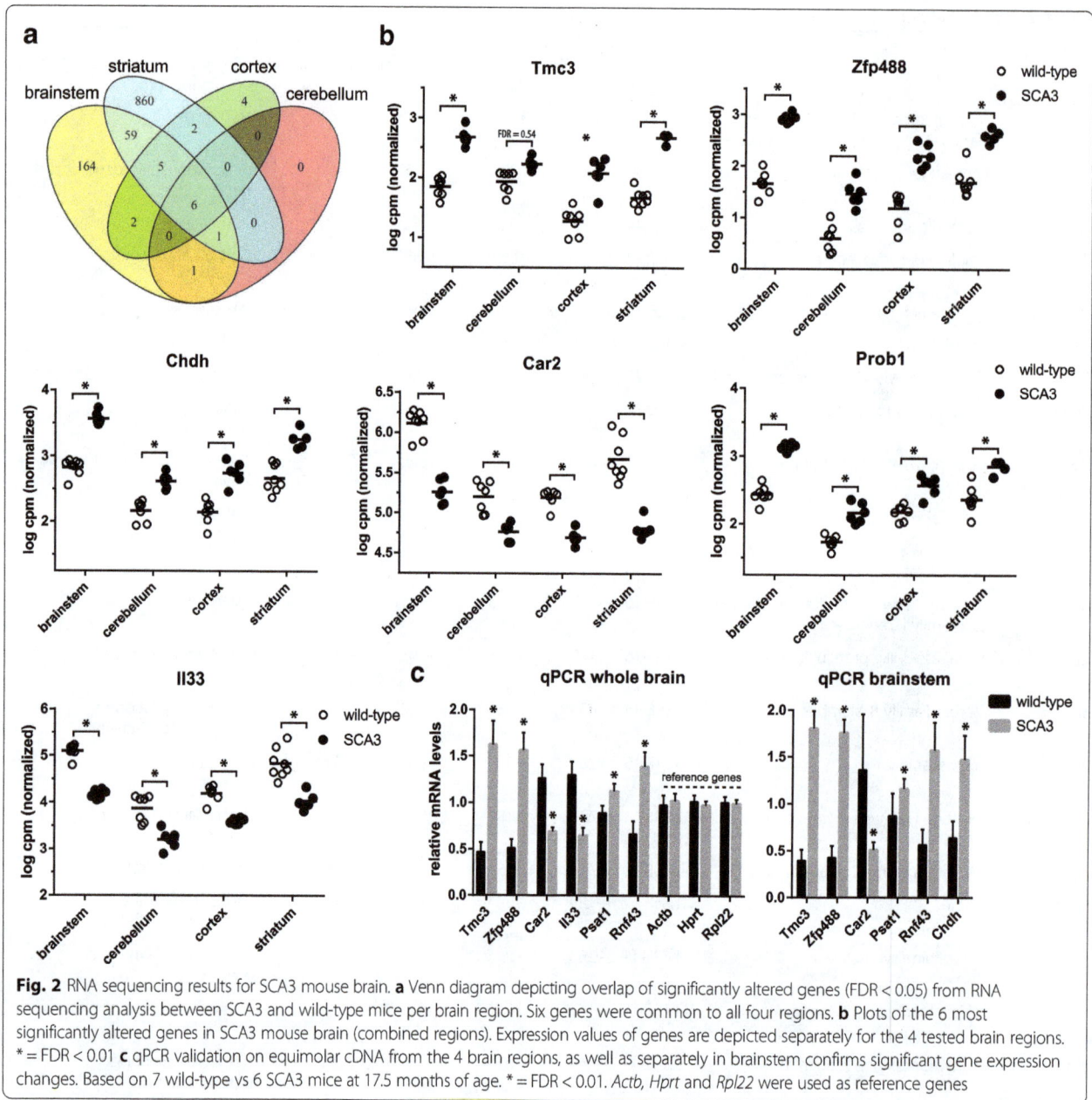

Fig. 2 RNA sequencing results for SCA3 mouse brain. **a** Venn diagram depicting overlap of significantly altered genes (FDR < 0.05) from RNA sequencing analysis between SCA3 and wild-type mice per brain region. Six genes were common to all four regions. **b** Plots of the 6 most significantly altered genes in SCA3 mouse brain (combined regions). Expression values of genes are depicted separately for the 4 tested brain regions. * = FDR < 0.01 **c** qPCR validation on equimolar cDNA from the 4 brain regions, as well as separately in brainstem confirms significant gene expression changes. Based on 7 wild-type vs 6 SCA3 mice at 17.5 months of age. * = FDR < 0.01. *Actb*, *Hprt* and *Rpl22* were used as reference genes

brain region combined analysis, based on FDR, fold change and expression level. Through qPCR on the same samples as used for RNA sequencing, we validated the significant change in expression level for all 6 genes (Fig. 2c). Finally, differential expression was confirmed at the protein level for carbonic anhydrase 2 (*Car2*) and phosphoserine aminotransferase 1 (*Psat1*), as these proteins were predicted to be differentially expressed in all 4 brain regions. Cortex and cerebellum of the SCA3 mice was available for validation of protein levels, and both brain regions showed a similar direction of protein change as was found on mRNA level and reached

significance for *Car2* in both brain regions and for *Psat1* in cerebellum (Fig. 3 and Additional file 4: Figure S3).

Cellular signalling pathways are altered in SCA3 mouse brain
To establish gene expression changes in SCA3 mice at the gene function level, the Euretos knowledge platform and Ingenuity pathway analysis (IPA) tools were used to assess pathway enrichment. Both tools showed good overlap in the top significant pathways for brain region combined analysis. The top pathways associated with the 585 differentially expressed genes in SCA3 mouse brain (4 regions combined) are listed in Table 3. The top

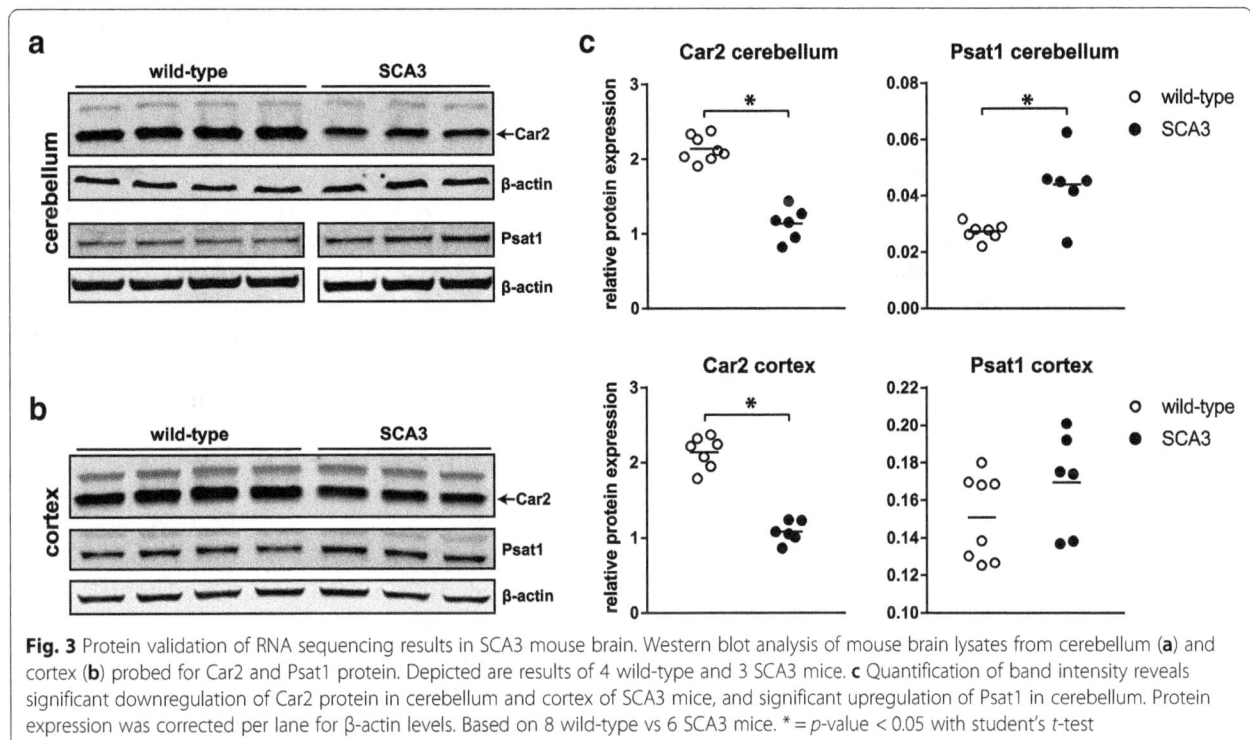

Fig. 3 Protein validation of RNA sequencing results in SCA3 mouse brain. Western blot analysis of mouse brain lysates from cerebellum (**a**) and cortex (**b**) probed for Car2 and Psat1 protein. Depicted are results of 4 wild-type and 3 SCA3 mice. **c** Quantification of band intensity reveals significant downregulation of Car2 protein in cerebellum and cortex of SCA3 mice, and significant upregulation of Psat1 in cerebellum. Protein expression was corrected per lane for β-actin levels. Based on 8 wild-type vs 6 SCA3 mice. * = p-value < 0.05 with student's t-test

pathways are sorted on ingenuity p-value, the complete list of pathway analysis can be found in (Additional file 5: Canonical pathways ingenuity). The combined region pathways signify alterations in pathways which are most consistent for the 4 brain regions, though effect size can differ per individual region. From this combined analysis, cellular signalling pathways were the most significantly enriched pathways, namely: α-adrenergic, CREB and protein kinase A (PKA) signalling, which are all predicted to be downregulated. CREB proteins can be activated by

Table 3 Top overrepresented pathways for genes differentially expressed in SCA3 mouse brain

Pathway	Number of genes	p-value	Pathway database
Brain regions combined analysis (585 genes)			
α-adrenergic signalling	11	1.23E-05	IPA
CREB signalling in neurons	25	1.95E-05	IPA
Protein kinase A signalling	25	2.57E-05	IPA
Axon guidance	24	3.63E-05	IPA + Euretos
Transmission across chemical synapses	13	5.50E-05	IPA + Euretos
Superpathway of cholesterol biosynthesis (srebp)	6	6.03E-05	IPA + Euretos
Myelination (cellular process)	24	8.02E-06	IPA + Euretos
Brainstem (195 genes)			
pi-3 k cascade	6	1.20E-04	IPA + Euretos
amino acid metabolism	9	1.31E-04	Euretos
Superpathway of Cholesterol Biosynthesis	5	1.74E-04	IPA + Euretos
Striatum (824 genes)			
axon guidance	38	2.19E-07	IPA + Euretos
neurotransmitter receptor binding and downstream transmission in the postsynaptic cell	19	9.72E-06	Euretos
synaptic transmission/long term potentiation	23	3.02E-05	IPA + Euretos

Overrepresented pathways based on Ingenuity (IPA) and Euretos pathway analyses. Where applicable, Ingenuity obtained p-values are preferentially reported. The three top pathways in brainstem were also significantly altered in striatum phosphorylation by kinases, including PKA [31], and can thus be involved in the same signalling cascade. Indeed, both CREB and PKA signalling have been implicated in Huntington disease [32, 33] and other neurodegenerative disorders [34], and CREB signalling is known to be required for long-term synaptic plasticity and axonal outgrowth [35], which was also found as one of the most significantly altered pathways. Similar to Huntington disease, sterol regulatory element binding proteins (SREBPs) and cholesterol biosynthesis [36, 37] were also among the top significantly altered pathways in the current SCA3 study. Finally, a total of 24 significantly altered genes were associated with the cellular process of myelination (go:0042552), suggesting a defect in myelin homeostasis in SCA3 brain as was also reported for Huntington disease [38].

Since ataxin-3 is ubiquitously expressed in brain, and in SCA3 patients there is no clear correlation between the affected brain regions and level of ataxin-3 expression [39], region specific pathological mechanisms are likely at play. Indeed, different pathways were observed when performing brain region combined analysis compared to brainstem and striatum individually (Table 3 and Fig. 4a). In striatum, the predominant effects were observed in axon guidance and synaptic transmission pathways (Fig. 4b) in addition to neurotransmitter receptor induced postsynaptic events. These pathways were however not apparently affected in brainstem (Fig. 4c). Of note, the affected neurotransmitter receptor pathway is most likely glutamate dependent based on involved genes (Grind2d and Grik1). Transcriptional analysis of SCA1 [40, 41] as well as SCA7 [42] mouse models have previously established a potential involvement of glutamate signalling, suggesting that this may be a signalling pathway that is more broadly affected in the polyQ cerebellar ataxias. Brainstem showed the most significant alterations in amino acid metabolism, cholesterol biosynthesis and the pi-3 k cascade, though these pathways were also significantly altered in striatum. Due to the small number of differentially expressed genes, pathway analysis was not possible for cerebellum and cortex.

Differential gene expression in blood

Blood samples were collected at 9 and 17.5 months of age, RNA was isolated and sequenced after depletion of globin transcripts. Average number of reads was 57.5 million (SD ± 10.7 million), and on average 53% were aligned to known genes (Additional file 6: Figure S4A). The blood RNA sequencing data can be found under GEO accession GSE108069. A total of 9800 genes were used for gene expression analysis. Globin transcripts were successfully reduced (Additional file 6: Figure S4B), and were < 4 CPM. However, both average GC percentage and 5′-3′ bias were significantly lower in the

samples from SCA3 mice (Additional file 6: Figure S4C and D). The GC content can have a confounding effect on differential gene expression in RNA sequencing analysis, because it may arise during PCR amplification before sequencing, and it is difficult to separate from a true signal [43]. For this reason, GC-content correction was performed prior to analysis [24]. At 9 months of age, only Uba52 was significantly downregulated in blood of SCA3 mice, while at 17.5 months of age a total of 142 genes were found differentially expressed compared to wild-type mice. The top 10 differentially expressed genes at 17.5 months are listed in Table 4 and corresponding plots of the top 5 genes are shown in (Fig. 5a). Of the significantly altered genes in SCA3 mouse blood, Tnfsf14 (Tumor Necrosis Factor (Ligand) Superfamily, Member 14) has previously been reported to be upregulated in blood of SCA3 patients [44]. Tnfsf14 showed a log fold change of 0.8 in SCA3 mouse blood, with a FDR of 0.048. Through qPCR validation we were able to verify the expression changes in SCA3 mouse blood for protein scribble homolog (Scrib, log fold change – 0.4, FDR 0.02) and cation-transporting ATPase 13A2 (Atp13a2, log fold change – 0.4, FDR 0.037), and were able to confirm a trend for 4 other genes tested (Fig. 5b). Pathway analysis of the significantly altered genes revealed an effect on respiratory electron transport and mitochondria associated genes.

Metabolic and lipid changes in blood of SCA3 mice

Plasma samples from 4 wild-type and 4 transgenic mice were collected at 4, 12 and 16 months of age and used for LC-MS detection of metabolites (Profilomics, Gif-sur-Yvette, France). A total of 195 variables were detected in both ionization modes, where 114 could be matched at a level 1 annotation (retention time, relative isotopic ratio and MS/MS spectra) and 81 with a level 2 annotation (no MS/MS data) to an in-house database of metabolites. Combining positive and negative ion modes led to detection of 148 unique metabolites. The corresponding chemical classes of the detected metabolites are depicted in (Additional file 7: Figure S5).

Alterations in metabolite levels were assessed between wild-type and SCA3 mice at individual time points using the Welch's unequal variances t-test procedure by comparing the area under the curve (AUC) using log10 areas. Due to the low sample number, there was no correction for multiple testing and nominal p-values are reported. A total of 32 metabolites were found to be significantly different (p < 0.05) between SCA3 and wild-type mice. The 10 most significantly altered metabolites, irrespective of testing time point, are listed in Table 5. At 4 months of age, DL-Dihydroorotic-acid was most significantly altered, whilst L-Threonic-acid was

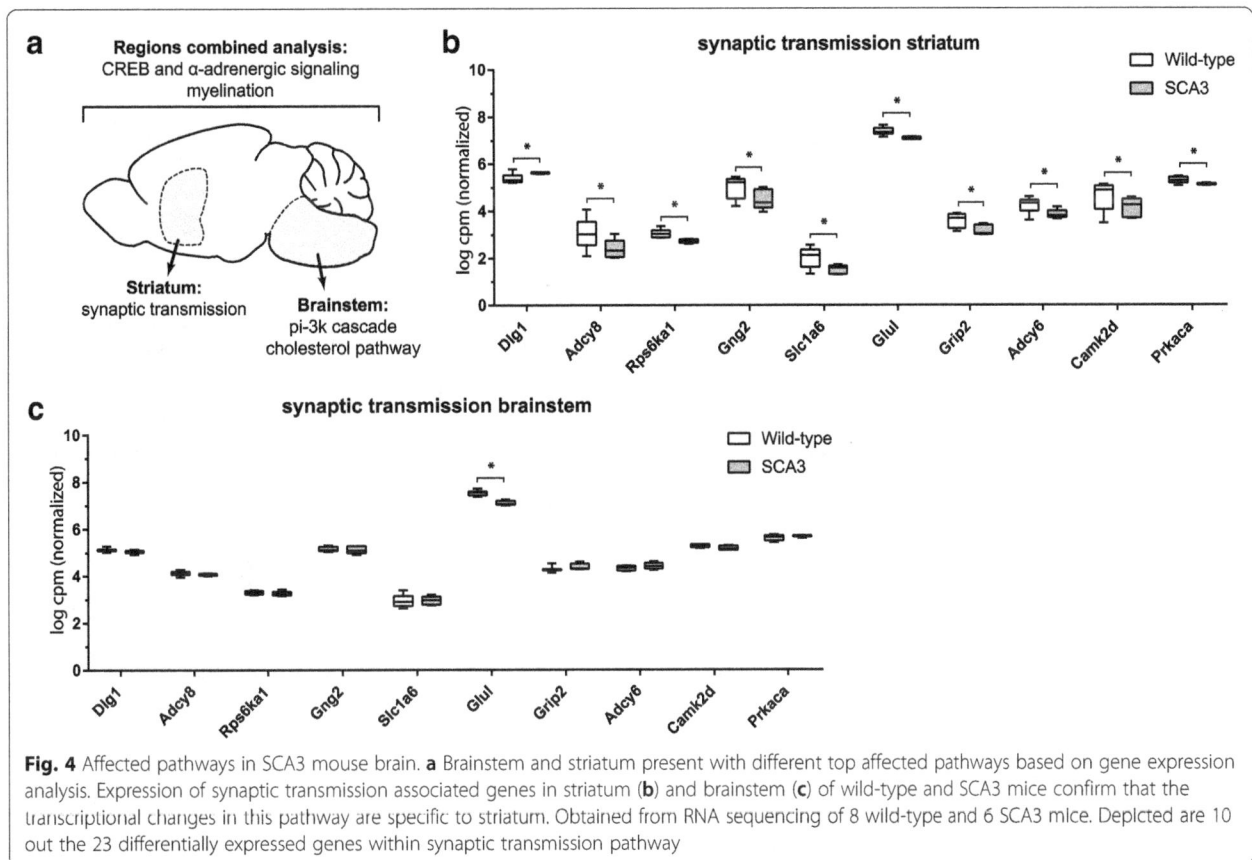

Fig. 4 Affected pathways in SCA3 mouse brain. **a** Brainstem and striatum present with different top affected pathways based on gene expression analysis. Expression of synaptic transmission associated genes in striatum (**b**) and brainstem (**c**) of wild-type and SCA3 mice confirm that the transcriptional changes in this pathway are specific to striatum. Obtained from RNA sequencing of 8 wild-type and 6 SCA3 mice. Depicted are 10 out the 23 differentially expressed genes within synaptic transmission pathway

most significantly altered at 12 months of age, and DL-tryptophan at 16 months Fig. 6a).

To assess alterations of the metabolome in SCA3 mice over time, a PCA was performed (Additional file 8: Figure S6). Age was weakly but significantly correlated with the first principal component (PC), which explains 57% of variance ($\rho = -0.586$, $p < 0.05$). Genotype also weakly but significantly correlated with PC3, explaining 7% of variance (Additional file 8: Figure S6B) ($\rho = -0.463$, $p < 0.05$), indicating that the effect

of mutant ataxin-3 expression in the mice did not induce a strong effect on blood metabolite levels. When comparing SCA3 to wild-type mice at 4, 12 and 16 months of age, the number of significantly altered metabolites in blood were 14, 20 and 4 respectively. From these metabolites, only DL-Tryptophan was altered at two of the time points, whilst the other metabolites were only found to be altered at a single time point. The full list of measured metabolites and comparisons between genotypes can be found in (Additional file 9: Blood metabolites).

Table 4 Top 10 differentially expressed genes in SCA3 mouse blood at 17.5 months old

Gene symbol	Name	FDR	Log fold change	Protein function (GO term mol. function or biological process)
Pdia6	protein disulfide isomerase associated 6	0.002	−0.6	apoptotic cell clearance
Hs3st3b1	heparan sulfate (glucosamine) 3-O-sulfotransferase 3B1	0.002	0.9	glycosaminoglycan biosynthetic process
Klk8	kallikrein related-peptidase 8	0.004	1.0	endopeptidase activity
Il18r1	interleukin 18 receptor 1	0.007	0.7	interleukin-18-mediated signaling pathway
Runx2	runt related transcription factor 2	0.007	0.8	ATP binding
Reck	reversion-inducing-cysteine-rich protein with kazal motifs	0.007	1.1	endopeptidase inhibitor activity
Tob1	transducer of ErbB-2.1	0.007	0.8	receptor tyrosine kinase binding
Phf13	PHD finger protein 13	0.007	0.6	chromatin binding
Rhoh	ras homolog family member H	0.007	−0.5	mast cell activation
Smad7	Mothers Against Decapentaplegic Homolog 7	0.010	0.7	activin binding

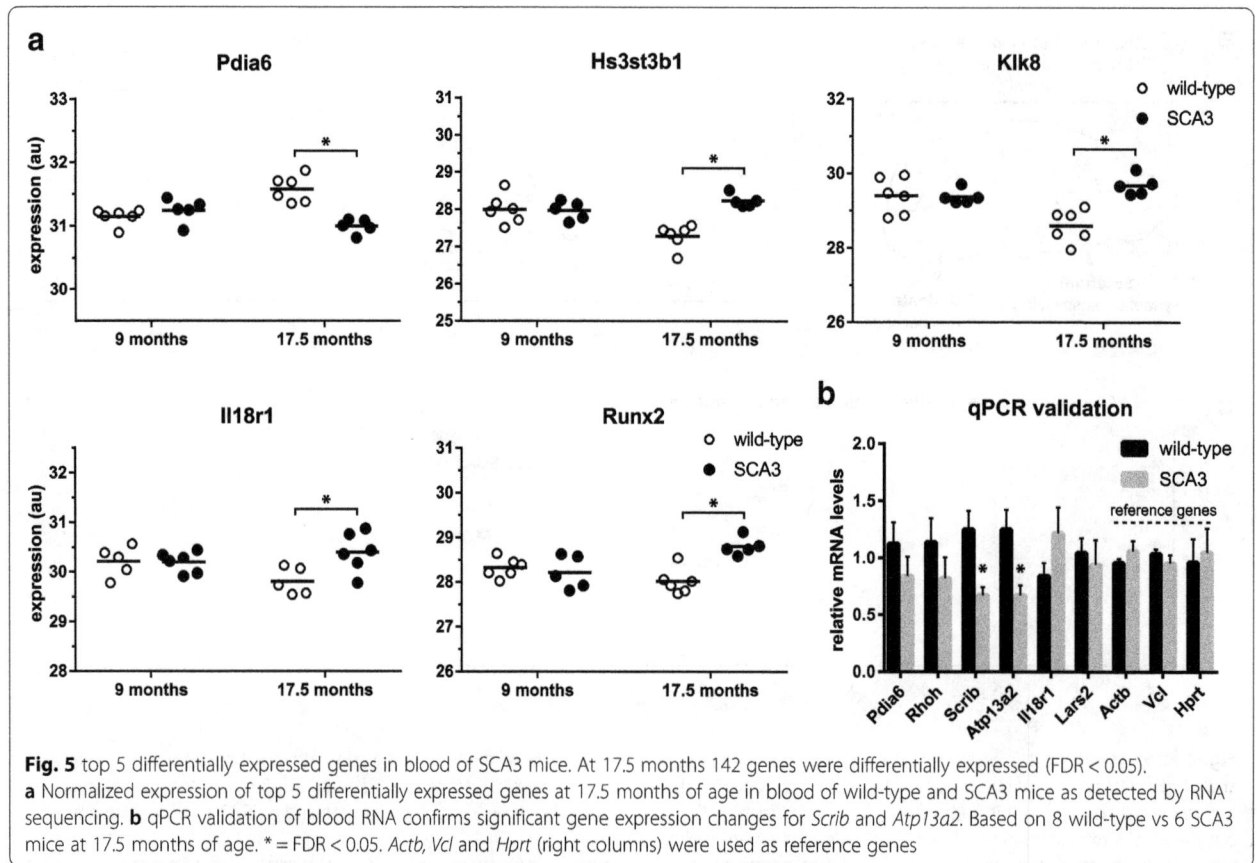

Fig. 5 top 5 differentially expressed genes in blood of SCA3 mice. At 17.5 months 142 genes were differentially expressed (FDR < 0.05). **a** Normalized expression of top 5 differentially expressed genes at 17.5 months of age in blood of wild-type and SCA3 mice as detected by RNA sequencing. **b** qPCR validation of blood RNA confirms significant gene expression changes for *Scrib* and *Atp13a2*. Based on 8 wild-type vs 6 SCA3 mice at 17.5 months of age. * = FDR < 0.05. *Actb*, *Vcl* and *Hprt* (right columns) were used as reference genes

On the same plasma samples, lipid levels were also examined. A total of 491 unique lipids were identified, divided over 26 classes (Additional file 7: Figure S5). To have an overview of the dataset, areas of all unique lipids from the same lipid class were summed. Differences in levels of the individual lipids and of the lipid classes at 4, 12 and 16 months were assessed using the Welch's unequal variance t-test without multiple testing correction (Additional file 10: Table S2). Using this method, at 4 months of age no lipid classes were found significantly

Table 5 Top altered blood metabolites in SCA3 mice at 3 time points

Compound	ChEBI ID	Fold change	*p*-value	Altered at Time points	Associated pathway
4 months					
DL-Dihydroorotic-acid	17025	1.61 ± 0.19	0.002	4 months	Pyrimidine Metabolism
N-a-acetyl-L-arginine	40521	1.95 ± 0.39	0.003	4 months	NA
3-hydroxydecanoic-acid / 10-hydroxydecanoic-acid	17409	1.51 ± 0.21	0.005	4 months	Fatty Acid
12 months					
L-Threonic-acid	15908	0.55 ± 0.08	0.001	12 months	Ascorbate and aldarate metabolism
2-Aminoisobutyric-acid / Aminobutyric-acid	27971	2.58 ± 0.69	0.002	12 months	NA
Asparagine	17196	0.68 ± 0.08	0.003	12 months	Ammonia Recycling / Aspartate Metabolism / Transcription/Translation
16 months					
Methylhistamine	29009	0.87 ± 0.06	0.019	16 months	Histidine Metabolism
DL-Tryptophan	27897	0.74 ± 0.11	0.020	12 and 16 months	NA
Threonine / D-allo-Threonine	16857	0.77 ± 0.09	0.038	16 months	Glycine and Serine Metabolism / Threonine and 2-Oxobutanoate Degradation / Transcription/Translation

Nominal p-values reported, associated pathway obtained from Profilomics database

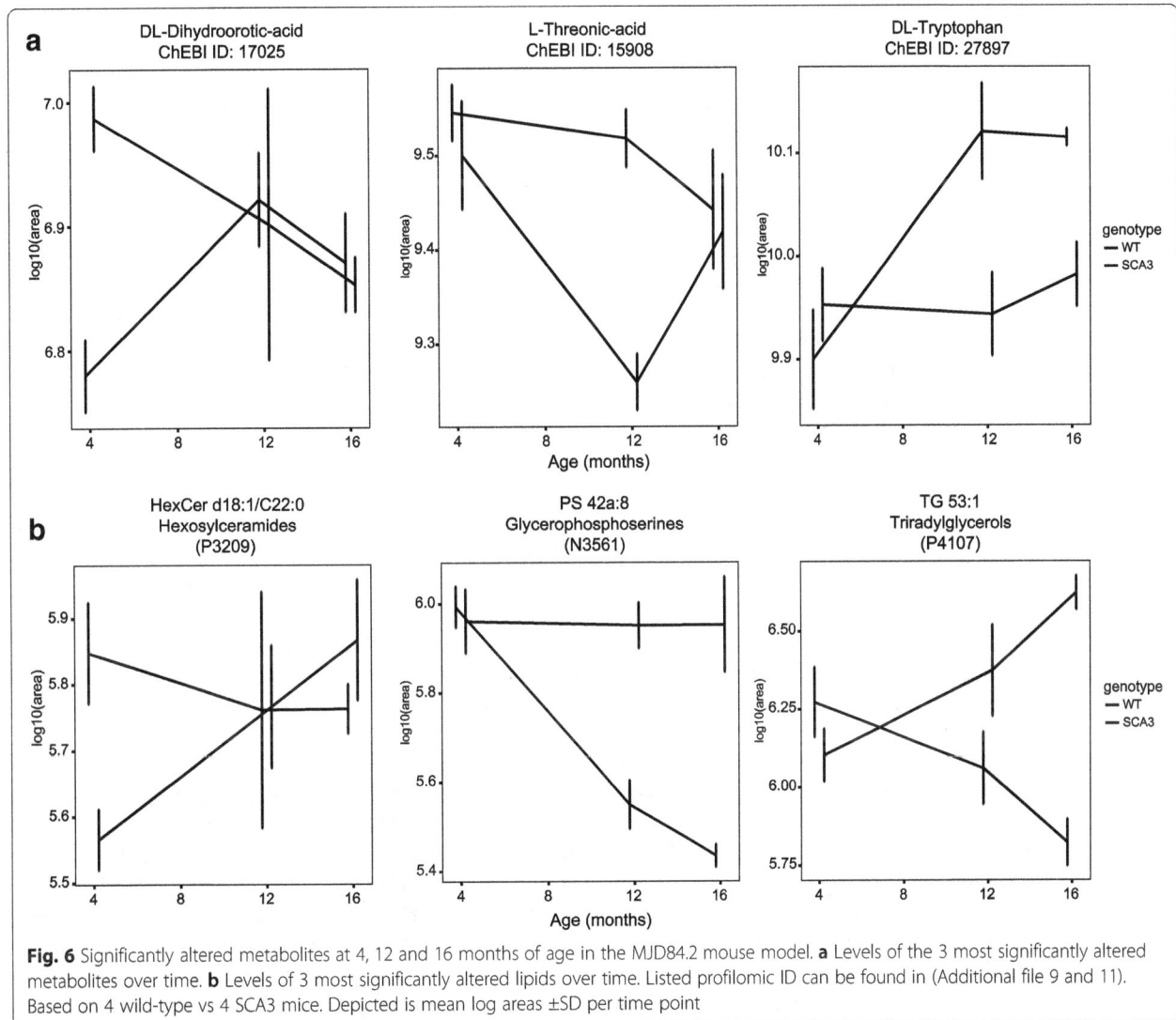

Fig. 6 Significantly altered metabolites at 4, 12 and 16 months of age in the MJD84.2 mouse model. **a** Levels of the 3 most significantly altered metabolites over time. **b** Levels of 3 most significantly altered lipids over time. Listed profilomic ID can be found in (Additional file 9 and 11). Based on 4 wild-type vs 4 SCA3 mice. Depicted is mean log areas ±SD per time point

different in plasma between SCA3 and wild-type mice. At 12 months of age, glycerophosphoserine and sulfatides were decreased significantly in the SCA3 mouse. At 16 months of age, di- and triacylglycerols and ceramides were significantly increased in plasma of SCA3 mice compared to wild-type. Both diacylglycerols and ceramides have been linked to the oxidative stress and stress signalling pathways [45, 46]. In contrast, glycerophosphoserine, lyso-phosphoinositols and sulfatide were found to be decreased in the SCA3 mice over time. Interestingly, 3 of the 4 NeuGC-GM2 gangliosides were found significantly altered at 16 months. The full list of measured lipids can be found in (Additional file 11: Blood lipids). The most significantly altered individual lipids are shown in (Fig. 5b). Due to their association with disease progression, ceramides, sulfatides, glycerophosphoserine and triradylglycerol may be of potential interest as biomarkers of disease progression in these mice.

Discussion

Here, we determined gene expression as well as metabolite and lipid changes in the SCA3 MJD84.2 mouse model [16]. Transcriptional deregulation is a known pathogenic process in SCA3 [8], but so far few studies have been performed to establish which transcriptional changes occur and how these are involved in the molecular pathogenicity in SCA3. Furthermore, there is currently a requirement for reliable (pre)clinical biomarkers capable of tracking disease progression in SCA3.

Multi-omic biomarker identification in blood of SCA3 mice

Both metabolites [47] and gene transcripts [48] may serve as biomarkers to track neurodegenerative disease progression in blood. Sequencing of whole blood RNA revealed lower levels of *Uba52* at 9 months of age, whereas 142 genes were differentially expressed at

17.5 months of age in the SCA3 mice. A total of 10 genes have been reported as transcript biomarkers in blood of SCA3 patients [44]. Of these 10 genes, only upregulation of Tumor Necrosis Factor Superfamily Member 14 (*Tnfsf14*) was also observed significantly upregulated in our dataset of the SCA3 mice. Despite the modest overlap, this observation does solidify *Tnfsf14* as a potential blood biomarker for SCA3. Pathway analysis of the 142 altered genes in our blood dataset suggested affected respiratory electron transport pathways, in line with mitochondrial abnormalities and increased oxidative damage observed in peripheral blood of Huntington patients [49] and mitochondrial DNA damage previously reported in blood and brain of SCA3 mice [50]. Interestingly, whole blood RNA sequencing of SCA2 patients also suggested affected mitochondrial function [51], suggesting a potential commonality between the different polyQ disorders.

Metabolite analysis of blood revealed a range of altered metabolites in SCA3 mouse blood at all three time points tested. However, due to the small sample size used, the results must be interpreted with caution and the most relevant alterations in metabolites are those that are represented at multiple time points and show increasing fold change over time. In this regard, DL-Tryptophan (CHEBI: 27897) was identified as the most promising biomarker. DL-tryptophan levels were found to be altered at both 12 and 16 months of age, with lower levels in SCA3 mice (fold change 0.7 +/− 0.11). Interestingly, blood tryptophan levels have been correlated with disease progression in blood of Huntington disease patients, with affected patients also showing lower levels [52, 53]. Indeed, tryptophan and its degradation products have been proposed as pathogenic factors in Huntington brain, with the tryptophan metabolite quinolinate reported to be elevated in Huntington disease brain, due to increased 3-hydroxyanthranilate oxygenase activity [54]. To our knowledge, tryptophan levels in blood of SCA3 patients have not been assessed yet, and would thus be a good starting point to establish a biomarker indicative of disease progression.

Lipidomic analyses revealed that at 16 months of age the di- and triglycerides and ceramides (CHEBI: 85812 and 85777) levels were increased considerably in the SCA3 mice (Additional file 9: Blood metabolites). Interestingly, increased triglycerides levels have been detected in blood of SCA3 patients [55], but ceramides have not yet been assessed in a clinical setting. In a mouse model for Huntington disease, increased diacylglycerol kinase (DGK) activity has been observed, and a protective effect of DGK inhibition was suggested [56]. In line with the blood transcriptional changes, ceramides have been frequently reported in relation with neurodegenerative disorders, especially in the context of oxidative stress,

inflammation and apoptosis [57–59]. For instance, in spinal cord tissue from amyotrophic lateral sclerosis spinal cord patients, increased levels of ceramides were detected and preceded the clinical phenotype in a mouse model [60]. The proposed mechanism is that the mutant protein leads to increased oxidative stress, thereby altering the sphingolipid metabolism to produce more ceramides and cholesterol esters, in turn sensitising motor neurons susceptible to excitotoxicity and oxidative stress, culminating in cell death [60]. A comparison between ceramides in blood and CNS tissue of the SCA3 mouse in future experiments may thus be useful to establish ceramides as a potential biomarker.

CREB and α-adrenergic signalling pathway transcripts are most consistently altered throughout the SCA3 mouse brain

A combined brain region differential gene expression analysis was performed in order to prioritise the most robust and consistent transcriptional alterations across all brain regions. In this manner, CREB and α-adrenergic signalling pathways were determined as most strongly affected in the SCA3 mouse brain. α-Adrenergic signalling has not yet been extensively investigated for SCA3, and further validation in other mouse models and patient brain material should thus be performed to more reliably establish this finding. However, adenosine homeostasis is reportedly changed in Huntington [61], suggestive of potential parallels between the two polyQ disorders. Additionally, an adenosine A2A receptor agonist, though pleiotropic, was shown to have beneficial effects on neurodegeneration and transcriptional dysregulation in a SCA3 transgenic mouse [62].

Downregulation of CREB signalling was the second most affected pathway based on the RNA sequencing of brain tissue in the SCA3 mice. This finding is in good agreement with previous studies where ataxin-3 was found to interact with CREB-binding protein, and inhibits transcription by this coactivator [63].This inhibition likely takes place through sequestration of CREB-binding protein by the polyglutamine, as evidenced in the polyQ disease spinal and bulbar muscular atrophy (SBMA) [64]. Furthermore, an expanded polyglutamine stretch is also known to supress phosphorylation of CREB through binding of the coactivator TAFII130, interfering with CREB-dependent transcription and subsequently contributing to polyQ pathogenicity [65]. Also, CREB deficiency enhances polyQ induced lethality in *Drosophila*, which can be partly rescued by increased CREB expression [66]. As CBP regulates CREB [67] and SREBP transcriptional activity [68], these results suggest that loss of CBP function underlies at least part of the transcriptional dysregulation in the SCA3 brain, similar to what has been suggested for Huntington disease [69]. Consistent with the synaptic transmission related gene expression changes we observed in striatum of the SCA3 mice, CREB signalling is known to be required for long-term synaptic plasticity and axonal outgrowth [35]. Together, these findings suggest that CREB dependent transcription is indeed inhibited due to presence of expanded polyQ protein, and that the resulting transcriptional dysregulation contributes to the pathogenic mechanisms in SCA3 [34].

The relation between cellular dysregulation, neuronal loss, cerebellar dysfunction and the onset of motor/coordination symptoms in SCA3 is not yet elucidated. Other reports using the MJD84.2 mouse found that changes in Purkinje cell firing are an early disease manifestation that occur prior to observable neurodegeneration, but coincide with behavioural deficits of the mice [70]. Costa et al. also reported onset of behavioural deficits in the homozygous MJD84.2 mice, with unaltered Purkinje cell counts at the same time point [71]. The 75 week time point used for transcriptional analysis in this study corresponds to the early and minor loss of Purkinje cells in the MJD84.2 mouse model reported by others [70], but there were no behavioural deficits in the current study. Other molecular hallmarks of SCA3 are however conclusively present in these mice at this time point, including increased ataxin-3 nuclear localisation and insolubility [71–73], which is considered an early stage of aberrant protein aggregation, deranged calcium signalling [72] and the increased excitability in Purkinje cells [70].

Mutant ataxin-3 affects synaptic transmission pathways more strongly in striatum

From the combined brain region transcriptional analysis, CREB and α-adrenergic signalling were found most strongly affected. However, it was clear that the contribution of each individual brain region to this list was not equal. We observed larger fold changes and more differentially expressed genes in striatum and brainstem than observed in cortex and cerebellum. As we and others have repeatedly shown similar expression of the mutant ataxin-3 transgene in the MJD84.2 mouse model in the brain regions tested here [16, 73, 74], it is unlikely that variations in expression levels can explain these differences. Since previous studies suggest that cellular *ATXN3* transcript and protein levels do not correlate well with neuronal degeneration in SCA3 [39, 75], these findings are indicative of differential effects of mutant ataxin-3 in each brain region. One of the more surprising findings in our dataset was the fact that the synaptic transmission pathways were more strongly affected in striatum compared to brainstem and cerebellum. Pathway analysis of the transcriptome in the brainstem showed that the pi-3 k cascade and cholesterol biosynthesis pathways were most significantly

altered in this brain region of the SCA3 mouse. It is not clear why different pathways are affected in brainstem compared to striatum in the SCA3 mouse. However, in a previous study we did note the strongest nuclear localisation of mutant ataxin-3 in the substantia nigra [73]. In SCA3 patients a marked reduction in dopamine transport was found in striatum [76]. Given that the dopaminergic innervation of striatum originates from substantia nigra [77, 78], pathogenic nuclear localisation of mutant ataxin-3 may interfere with this dopaminergic signalling. Indeed, in light of the requirement of CREB for dopamine dependent gene expression in the striatum [79], the observed alteration in CREB signalling in the striatum of the SCA3 mouse may reflect affected dopaminergic signalling from substantia nigra. Nonetheless, in a more severe SCA3 mouse model synaptic transmission and signal transduction pathways were found altered in cerebellum of symptomatic mice [8]. It will thus be interesting to determine whether these synaptic transmission deficiencies in cerebellum correlate with nuclear localisation or aggregation of mutant ataxin-3 and are a requirement for motor phenotype onset. The affected axon guidance pathway in striatum of SCA3 mice was also identified in a transcriptomic study with SCA2 mice, where weighted correlation network analysis of cerebellum found one module associated with axon guidance correlating to disease status [80].

Emerging role of white matter dysfunction in SCA3

In a recent study, RNAseq profiling was performed on pons of 22 week old MJD84.2 and two knock-in SCA3 models [81]. A total of 38 genes were found differentially expressed in pons of these mouse models. In our study, we were able to identify 32 of these reported genes, and indeed found significant differential expression for 23 of those genes in brainstem of the MJD84.2 mice. This overlap argues for the robustness of both studies, and since we observed altered expression for 11 genes associated with myelination (*Olig1*, *Olig 2*, *Ddx54*, *Fyn*, *Egfr*, *Cdkn1c*, *Pmp22*, *Klk6*, *Mal*, *Tspan2*, and *Aspa*), our findings further solidify white matter changes as a potential disease process in brainstem of SCA3 mice. The top downregulated protein identified in our study, Car2, accumulates on oligodendrocyte processes associated with myelinated axons and it is thought that Car2 may be involved in myelin formation in the central nervous system [82], though no major myelin abnormalities have been observed in Car2 deficient mice [83, 84]. Furthermore, *Zfp488* (zinc finger protein 488) was significantly upregulated in SCA3 mice, and plays a role in the differentiation of neural progenitor cells to mature oligodendrocytes, thereby assisting in remyelination after injury [85]. Together, these gene expression studies warrant further investigation of these white matter related processes in SCA3 pathogenicity.

Conclusions

Taken together, we report here *Tnfs14* transcript, DL-tryptophan levels and spingolipids ceramides as potential blood biomarkers for SCA3. Mechanistically, we found alterations in transcript levels for CREB and α-adrenergic pathways most consistently affected throughout all brain regions of the MJD84.2 mice. In striatum, synaptic transmission pathways were most strongly affected, whilst brainstem showed largest changes in the pi-3 k cascade.

Additional files

Additional file 1: Table S1. Primers used for qPCR validation of RNA sequencing results.

Additional file 2: Figure S1. Brain alignment summary

Additional file 3: Figure S2. Brain PCA.

Additional file 4: Figure S3. Protein validation of RNA sequencing results in SCA3 mouse brain. Western blot analysis of mouse brain lysates from cerebellum (**a**) and cortex (**b**) probed for Car2 and Psat1 proteins. Uncropped blots from those shown in Fig. 3, showing all 8 wild-type and 6 SCA3 mice.

Additional file 5: Canonical pathways ingenuity.

Additional file 6: Figure S4. number of reads and quality of blood RNA sequencing. **A** Number of reads obtained for each mouse is depicted per time point. RNA sequencing reads were aligned to mouse reference genome build 10 (GRCm38/mm10) using star aligner. **B** Distribution of reads for blood RNA sequencing indicate that globin reduction was efficient (1st rank gene account for < 10% of reads) and read distribution between samples was comparable. *n* = 22. **C** Median 5'-3' bias in reads per genotype in blood at 17.5 months of age. SCA3 mice show significantly lower values (*p* < 0.05, Welch 2 sample t-test). **D** Average GC percentage of all reads per genotype in blood at 17.5 months. Significantly lower values are seen in blood of SCA3 mice (*p* < 0.05, Welch 2 sample t-test) prior to GC-content correction.

Additional file 7: Figure S5. distribution of metabolite classes and lipid families identified from mass-spec analysis of plasma samples. LC-HRMS analysis of plasma samples led to identification of 148 unique metabolites and 491 lipids.

Additional file 8: Figure S6. principal component analysis (PCA) of measured metabolites. Individual barcodes of mice are depicted, plasma was obtained for each mouse at 3 time points **A)** Age is significantly correlated with PC1 (ρ = − 0.586, p < 0.05), hence explaining most of the variation between samples. SCA3 *n* = 4, wild-type (WT) *n* = 4. **B)** The third principal component (PC) is significantly correlated with genotype (ρ = − 0.463, p < 0.05). PC3 and PC4 are shown.

Additional file 9: Blood metabolites.

Additional file 10: Table S2. Lipid classes altered at 4, 12 and 16 months in SCA3 mice. Only lipid classes with at least one significantly altered unique lipid at any time are shown.

Additional file 11: Blood lipids.

Abbreviations
Actb: β-actin; Atp13a2: Cation-transporting ATPase 13A2; ATXN3: Ataxin-3; Car2: Carbonic anhydrase 2; CBP: CREB binding protein; CHEBI: Chemical entities of biological interest; CQN: Conditional quantile normalization; CREB: cAMP response element binding; DGK: Diacylglycerol kinase; FDR: False discovery rate; Hprt: Hypoxanthine-guanine phosophoribosyltransferase; IPA: Ingenuity Pathway Analysis; MJD: Machado-Joseph disease; PC: Principal component; PCA: Principal component analysis; PKA: Protein kinase A; PolyQ: Polyglutamine; Psat1: Phosphoserine aminotransferase 1; Rpl22: Ribosomal Protein L22; SBMA: Spinal and bulbar muscular atrophy; SCA3: Spinocerebellar ataxia type 3; Scrib: Protein scribble homolog; SREBP: Sterol regulatory element binding proteins; Tnfsf14: Tumor Necrosis Factor (Ligand) Superfamily, Member 14; Vcl: Vinculin

Acknowledgements
The authors want to thank Eleni Mina and Ioannis Moustakas for assisting with the analysis of RNA sequencing data, and want to thank Merel Boogaard for assistance with the CAG repeat sizing of the mice.

Funding
This research was supported by ZonMw 40-41900-98-018, Hersenstichting/Brugling Fund BG2013-03 and European Union Seventh Framework Programme (FP7/2007–2013) under grant agreement No. 305,121 (Neuromics) (to W.M.C.vR-M) and No. 05444 (RD-Connect). Leticia G. León was supported by an iCARE fellowship co-funded by the Italian Association for Cancer Research (AIRC) and the European Union.

Availability of materials
The FASTQ files for the mouse brain RNA sequencing can be found in the GEO repository, accession GSE107958 (https://www.ncbi.nlm.nih.gov/geo/query/acc.cgi?acc=GSE107958) and blood RNA sequencing samples are listed under accession GSE108069 (https://www.ncbi.nlm.nih.gov/geo/query/acc.cgi?acc=GSE108069).

Authors' contributions
Experiments performed by: MO, LJAT and MME. RNA sequencing performed by OTM, quality control and alignment performed by SAJvdZ and HM. Analysis of RNA sequencing by PACtH, LGL, JJG, SMK and LJAT. Metabolomic/lipid analysis by MP and AS. Pathway analysis performed by KMH and MME. Design of experiments by LJAT and WvRM. Paper written by LJAT. All authors read and approved the final manuscript.

Ethics approval
All animal experiments were approved by the Leiden University animal ethical committee.

Competing interests
Kristina M. Hettne has performed paid consultancy since November 1, 2015, for Euretos b.v, a startup founded in 2012 that develops knowledge management and discovery services for the life sciences, with the Euretos Knowledge Platform as a marketed product.

Author details
[1]Department of Human Genetics, Leiden University Medical Center, 2300 RC Leiden, The Netherlands. [2]Department of Research & Development, uniQure, Amsterdam, The Netherlands. [3]Cancer Pharmacology Lab, University of Pisa, Ospedale di Cisanello, Edificio 6 via Paradisa, 2, 56124 Pisa, Italy. [4]Sequencing Analysis Support Core, Leiden University Medical Center, 2300 RC Leiden, The Netherlands. [5]Department of Biomedical Data Sciences, Leiden University Medical Center, 2300 RC Leiden, The Netherlands. [6]deCODE genetics/Amgen, Sturlugata 8, 101 Reykjavik, Iceland. [7]MedDAY Pharmaceuticals, Paris, France. [8]Centre for Molecular and Biomolecular Informatics, Radboud Institute for Molecular Life Sciences, Radboud University Medical Center, 6500 HB, Nijmegen, The Netherlands.

References

1. Riess O, Rub U, Pastore A, Bauer P, Schols L. SCA3: neurological features, pathogenesis and animal models. Cerebellum. 2008;7:125–37.

2. Evers MM, Toonen LJ, van Roon-Mom WM. Ataxin-3 protein and RNA toxicity in spinocerebellar ataxia type 3: current insights and emerging therapeutic strategies. Mol Neurobiol. 2014;49:1513–31.

3. Matos CA, de Macedo-Ribeiro S, Carvalho AL. Polyglutamine diseases: the special case of ataxin-3 and Machado-Joseph disease. Prog Neurobiol. 2011;95:26–48.

4. Bichelmeier U, Schmidt T, Hubener J, Boy J, Ruttiger L, Habig K, Poths S, Bonin M, Knipper M, Schmidt WJ, et al. Nuclear localization of ataxin-3 is required for the manifestation of symptoms in SCA3: in vivo evidence. J Neurosci. 2007;27:7418–28.

5. Paulson HL, Perez MK, Trottier Y, Trojanowski JQ, Subramony SH, Das SS, Vig P, Mandel JL, Fischbeck KH, Pittman RN. Intranuclear inclusions of expanded polyglutamine protein in spinocerebellar ataxia type 3. Neuron. 1997;19:333–44.

6. Chai Y, Koppenhafer SL, Shoesmith SJ, Perez MK, Paulson HL. Evidence for proteasome involvement in polyglutamine disease: localization to nuclear inclusions in SCA3/MJD and suppression of polyglutamine aggregation in vitro. Hum Mol Genet. 1999;8:673–82.

7. Yu YC, Kuo CL, Cheng WL, Liu CS, Hsieh M. Decreased antioxidant enzyme activity and increased mitochondrial DNA damage in cellular models of Machado-Joseph disease. J Neurosci Res. 2009;87:1884–91.

8. Chou AH, Yeh TH, Ouyang P, Chen YL, Chen SY, Wang HL. Polyglutamine-expanded ataxin-3 causes cerebellar dysfunction of SCA3 transgenic mice by inducing transcriptional dysregulation. Neurobiol Dis. 2008;31:89–101.

9. Perez MK, Paulson HL, Pendse SJ, Saionz SJ, Bonini NM, Pittman RN. Recruitment and the role of nuclear localization in polyglutamine-mediated aggregation. J Cell Biol. 1998;143:1457–70.

10. Nucifora FC Jr, Sasaki M, Peters MF, Huang H, Cooper JK, Yamada M, Takahashi H, Tsuji S, Troncoso J, Dawson VL, et al. Interference by huntingtin and atrophin-1 with cbp-mediated transcription leading to cellular toxicity. Science (New York, NY). 2001;291:2423–8.

11. Evert BO, Vogt IR, Kindermann C, Ozimek L, de Vos RA, Brunt ER, Schmitt I, Klockgether T, Wullner U. Inflammatory genes are upregulated in expanded ataxin-3-expressing cell lines and spinocerebellar ataxia type 3 brains. J Neurosci. 2001;21:5389–96.

12. Evert BO, Vogt IR, Vieira-Saecker AM, Ozimek L, de Vos RA, Brunt ER, Klockgether T, Wullner U. Gene expression profiling in ataxin-3 expressing cell lines reveals distinct effects of normal and mutant ataxin-3. J Neuropathol Exp Neurol. 2003;62:1006–18.

13. Trancikova A, Ramonet D, Moore DJ. Genetic mouse models of neurodegenerative diseases. Prog Mol Biol Transl Sci. 2011;100:419–82.

14. Mastrokolias A, Pool R, Mina E, Hettne KM, van Duijn E, van der Mast RC, van Ommen G, t Hoen PA, Prehn C, Adamski J, van Roon-Mom W. Integration of targeted metabolomics and transcriptomics identifies deregulation of phosphatidylcholine metabolism in Huntington's disease peripheral blood samples. Metabolomics. 2016;12:137.

15. Mina E, van Roon-Mom W, Hettne K, van Zwet E, Goeman J, Neri C, ACtH P, Mons B, Roos M. Common disease signatures from gene expression analysis in Huntington's disease human blood and brain. Orphanet journal of rare diseases. 2016;11:97.

16. Cemal CK, Carroll CJ, Lawrence L, Lowrie MB, Ruddle P, Al-Mahdawi S, King RH, Pook MA, Huxley C, Chamberlain S. YAC transgenic mice carrying pathological alleles of the MJD1 locus exhibit a mild and slowly progressive cerebellar deficit. Hum Mol Genet. 2002;11:1075–94.

17. Gardiner SL, van Belzen MJ, Boogaard MW, van Roon-Mom WMC, Rozing MP, van Hemert AM, Smit JH, Beekman ATF, van Grootheest G, Schoevers RA, et al. Huntingtin gene repeat size variations affect risk of lifetime depression. Transl Psychiatry. 2017;7:1277.

18. Boudah S, Olivier MF, Aros-Calt S, Oliveira L, Fenaille F, Tabet JC, Junot C. Annotation of the human serum metabolome by coupling three liquid chromatography methods to high-resolution mass spectrometry. J Chromatogr B Analyt Technol Biomed Life Sci. 2014;966:34–47.

19. Dunn WB, Broadhurst D, Begley P, Zelena E, Francis-McIntyre S, Anderson N, Brown M, Knowles JD, Halsall A, Haselden JN, et al. Procedures for large-scale metabolic profiling of serum and plasma using gas chromatography and liquid chromatography coupled to mass spectrometry. Nat Protoc. 2011;6:1060–83.

20. Seyer A, Boudah S, Broudin S, Junot C, Colsch B. Annotation of the human cerebrospinal fluid lipidome using high resolution mass spectrometry and a dedicated data processing workflow. Metabolomics. 2016;12:91.

21. Dobin A, Davis CA, Schlesinger F, Drenkow J, Zaleski C, Jha S, Batut P, Chaisson M, Gingeras TR. STAR: ultrafast universal RNA-seq aligner. Bioinformatics (Oxford, England). 2013;29:15–21.

22. Robinson MD, McCarthy DJ, Smyth GK. edgeR: a Bioconductor package for differential expression analysis of digital gene expression data. Bioinformatics (Oxford, England). 2010;26:139–40.

23. Robinson MD, Oshlack A. A scaling normalization method for differential expression analysis of RNA-seq data. Genome Biol. 2010;11:R25.

24. Hansen KD, Irizarry RA, Wu Z. Removing technical variability in RNA-seq data using conditional quantile normalization. Biostatistics (Oxford, England). 2012;13:204–16.

25. Wickham H. ggplot2: Elegant Graphics for Data Analysis. In: Book ggplot2: Elegant Graphics for Data Analysis. New York: Springer-Verlag; 2009.

26. Euretos platform. 2017. http://www.euretos.com/.

27. Euretos platform databases. 2017. http://www.euretos.com/files/EKPSources2017.pdf.

28. Toonen LJ, Schmidt I, Luijsterburg MS, van Attikum H, van Roon-Mom WM. Antisense oligonucleotide-mediated exon skipping as a strategy to reduce proteolytic cleavage of ataxin-3. Sci Rep. 2016;6:35200.

29. Rozen S, Skaletsky H. Primer3 on the WWW for general users and for biologist programmers. Methods Mol Biol. 2000;132:365–86.

30. Ruijter JM, Ramakers C, Hoogaars WM, Karlen Y, Bakker O, van den Hoff MJ, Moorman AF. Amplification efficiency: linking baseline and bias in the analysis of quantitative PCR data. Nucleic Acids Res. 2009;37:e45.

31. Shaywitz AJ, Greenberg ME. CREB: a stimulus-induced transcription factor activated by a diverse array of extracellular signals. Annu Rev Biochem. 1999;68:821–61.

32. Wyttenbach A, Swartz J, Kita H, Thykjaer T, Carmichael J, Bradley J, Brown R, Maxwell M, Schapira A, Orntoft TF, et al. Polyglutamine expansions cause decreased CRE-mediated transcription and early gene expression changes prior to cell death in an inducible cell model of Huntington's disease. Hum Mol Genet. 2001;10:1829–45.

33. Giralt A, Saavedra A, Carreton O, Xifro X, Alberch J, Perez-Navarro E. Increased PKA signaling disrupts recognition memory and spatial memory: role in Huntington's disease. Hum Mol Genet. 2011;20:4232–47.

34. Saura CA, Valero J. The role of CREB signaling in Alzheimer's disease and other cognitive disorders. Rev Neurosci. 2011;22:153–69.

35. Alberini CM. Transcription factors in long-term memory and synaptic plasticity. Physiol Rev. 2009;89:121–45.

36. Leoni V, Caccia C. The impairment of cholesterol metabolism in Huntington disease. Biochim Biophys Acta. 2015;1851:1095–105.

37. Block RC, Dorsey ER, Beck CA, Brenna JT, Shoulson I. Altered cholesterol and fatty acid metabolism in Huntington disease. J Clin Lipidol. 2010;4:17–23.

38. Bartzokis G, Lu PH, Tishler TA, Fong SM, Oluwadara B, Finn JP, Huang D, Bordelon Y, Mintz J, Perlman S. Myelin breakdown and iron changes in Huntington's disease: pathogenesis and treatment implications. Neurochem Res. 2007;32:1655–64.

39. Nishiyama K, Murayama S, Goto J, Watanabe M, Hashida H, Katayama S, Nomura Y, Nakamura S, Kanazawa I. Regional and cellular expression of the Machado-Joseph disease gene in brains of normal and affected individuals. Ann Neurol. 1996;40:776–81.

40. Ingram M, Wozniak EA, Duvick L, Yang R, Bergmann P, Carson R, O'Callaghan B, Zoghbi HY, Henzler C, Orr HT. Cerebellar transcriptome profiles of ATXN1 transgenic mice reveal SCA1 disease progression and protection pathways. Neuron. 2016;89:1194–207.

41. Serra HG, Byam CE, Lande JD, Tousey SK, Zoghbi HY, Orr HT. Gene profiling links SCA1 pathophysiology to glutamate signaling in Purkinje cells of transgenic mice. Hum Mol Genet. 2004;13:2535–43.

42. Chou AH, Chen CY, Chen SY, Chen WJ, Chen YL, Weng YS, Wang HL. Polyglutamine-expanded ataxin-7 causes cerebellar dysfunction by inducing transcriptional dysregulation. Neurochem Int. 2010;56:329–39.

43. Benjamini Y, Speed TP. Summarizing and correcting the GC content bias in high-throughput sequencing. Nucleic Acids Res. 2012;40:e72.

44. Raposo M, Bettencourt C, Maciel P, Gao F, Ramos A, Kazachkova N, Vasconcelos J, Kay T, Rodrigues AJ, Bettencourt B, et al. Novel candidate blood-based transcriptional biomarkers of Machado-Joseph disease. Move Disord. 2015;30:968–75.

45. Denis U, Lecomte M, Paget C, Ruggiero D, Wiernsperger N, Lagarde M. Advanced glycation end-products induce apoptosis of bovine retinal

pericytes in culture: involvement of diacylglycerol/ceramide production and oxidative stress induction. Free Radic Biol Med. 2002;33:236–47.

46. Ruvolo PP. Ceramide regulates cellular homeostasis via diverse stress signaling pathways. Leukemia. 2001;15:1153–60.

47. Kori M, Aydin B, Unal S, Arga KY, Kazan D. Metabolic biomarkers and neurodegeneration: a pathway enrichment analysis of Alzheimer's disease, Parkinson's disease, and amyotrophic lateral sclerosis. Omics. 2016;20:645–61.

48. Mastrokolias A, Ariyurek Y, Goeman JJ, van Duijn E, Roos RA, van der Mast RC, van Ommen GB, den Dunnen JT, t Hoen PA, van Roon-Mom WM. Huntington's disease biomarker progression profile identified by transcriptome sequencing in peripheral blood. Eur J Human Genetics. 2015;23:1349–56.

49. Chen CM, Wu YR, Cheng ML, Liu JL, Lee YM, Lee PW, Soong BW, Chiu DT. Increased oxidative damage and mitochondrial abnormalities in the peripheral blood of Huntington's disease patients. Biochem Biophys Res Commun. 2007;359:335–40.

50. Kazachkova N, Raposo M, Montiel R, Cymbron T, Bettencourt C, Silva-Fernandes A, Silva S, Maciel P, Lima M. Patterns of mitochondrial DNA damage in blood and brain tissues of a transgenic mouse model of Machado-Joseph disease. Neurodegener Dis. 2013;11:206–14.

51. Sen NE, Drost J, Gispert S, Torres-Odio S, Damrath E, Klinkenberg M, Hamzeiy H, Akdal G, Gulluoglu H, Basak AN, Auburger G. Search for SCA2 blood RNA biomarkers highlights Ataxin-2 as strong modifier of the mitochondrial factor PINK1 levels. Neurobiol Dis. 2016;96:115–26.

52. Forrest CM, Mackay GM, Stoy N, Spiden SL, Taylor R, Stone TW, Darlington LG. Blood levels of kynurenines, interleukin-23 and soluble human leucocyte antigen-G at different stages of Huntington's disease. J Neurochem. 2010;112:112–22.

53. Widner B, Leblhuber F, Walli J, Tilz GP, Demel U, Fuchs D. Degradation of tryptophan in neurodegenerative disorders. Adv Exp Med Biol. 1999;467:133–8.

54. Schwarcz R, Okuno E, White RJ, Bird ED, Whetsell WO Jr. 3-Hydroxyanthranilate oxygenase activity is increased in the brains of Huntington disease victims. Proc Natl Acad Sci U S A. 1988;85:4079–81.

55. Pacheco LS, da Silveira AF, Trott A, Houenou LJ, Algarve TD, Bello C, Lenz AF, Manica-Cattani MF, da Cruz IB. Association between Machado-Joseph disease and oxidative stress biomarkers. Mutat Res. 2013;757:99–103.

56. Zhang N, Li B, Al-Ramahi I, Cong X, Held JM, Kim E, Botas J, Gibson BW, Ellerby LM. Inhibition of lipid signaling enzyme diacylglycerol kinase epsilon attenuates mutant huntingtin toxicity. J Biol Chem. 2012;287:21204–13.

57. Adibhatla RM, Hatcher JF. Altered lipid metabolism in brain injury and disorders. Subcell Biochem. 2008;49:241–68.

58. Arboleda G, Morales LC, Benitez B, Arboleda H. Regulation of ceramide-induced neuronal death: cell metabolism meets neurodegeneration. Brain Res Rev. 2009;59:333–46.

59. Posse de Chaves EI. Sphingolipids in apoptosis, survival and regeneration in the nervous system. Biochim Biophys Acta. 2006;1758:1995–2015.

60. Cutler RG, Pedersen WA, Camandola S, Rothstein JD, Mattson MP. Evidence that accumulation of ceramides and cholesterol esters mediates oxidative stress-induced death of motor neurons in amyotrophic lateral sclerosis. Ann Neurol. 2002;52:448–57.

61. Lee CF, Chern Y. Adenosine receptors and Huntington's disease. Int Rev Neurobiol. 2014;119:195–232.

62. Chou AH, Chen YL, Chiu CC, Yuan SJ, Weng YH, Yeh TH, Lin YL, Fang JM, Wang HL. T1-11 and JMF1907 ameliorate polyglutamine-expanded ataxin-3-induced neurodegeneration, transcriptional dysregulation and ataxic symptom in the SCA3 transgenic mouse. Neuropharmacology. 2015;99:308–17.

63. Li F, Macfarlan T, Pittman RN, Chakravarti D. Ataxin-3 is a histone-binding protein with two independent transcriptional corepressor activities. J Biol Chem. 2002;277:45004–12.

64. McCampbell A, Taylor JP, Taye AA, Robitschek J, Li M, Walcott J, Merry D, Chai Y, Paulson H, Sobue G, Fischbeck KH. CREB-binding protein sequestration by expanded polyglutamine. Hum Mol Genet. 2000;9:2197–202.

65. Shimohata M, Shimohata T, Igarashi S, Naruse S, Tsuji S. Interference of CREB-dependent transcriptional activation by expanded polyglutamine stretches—augmentation of transcriptional activation as a potential therapeutic strategy for polyglutamine diseases. J Neurochem. 2005;93:654–63.

66. Iijima-Ando K, Wu P, Drier EA, Iijima K, Yin JC. cAMP-response element-binding protein and heat-shock protein 70 additively suppress polyglutamine-mediated toxicity in Drosophila. Proc Natl Acad Sci U S A. 2005;102:10261–6.

67. Kwok RP, Lundblad JR, Chrivia JC, Richards JP, Bachinger HP, Brennan RG, Roberts SG, Green MR, Goodman RH. Nuclear protein CBP is a coactivator for the transcription factor CREB. Nature. 1994;370:223–6.

68. Oliner JD, Andresen JM, Hansen SK, Zhou S, Tjian R. SREBP transcriptional activity is mediated through an interaction with the CREB-binding protein. Genes Dev. 1996;10:2903–11.

69. Steffan JS, Kazantsev A, Spasic-Boskovic O, Greenwald M, Zhu YZ, Gohler H, Wanker EE, Bates GP, Housman DE, Thompson LM. The Huntington's disease protein interacts with p53 and CREB-binding protein and represses transcription. Proc Natl Acad Sci U S A. 2000;97:6763–8.

70. Shakkottai VG, do Carmo Costa M, Dell'Orco JM, Sankaranarayanan A, Wulff H, Paulson HL. Early changes in cerebellar physiology accompany motor dysfunction in the polyglutamine disease spinocerebellar ataxia type 3. J Neurosci. 2011;31:13002–14.

71. Costa Mdo C, Luna-Cancalon K, Fischer S, Ashraf NS, Ouyang M, Dharia RM, Martin-Fishman L, Yang Y, Shakkottai VG, Davidson BL, et al. Toward RNAi therapy for the polyglutamine disease Machado-Joseph disease. Mol Therapy. 2013;21:1898–908.

72. Chen X, Tang TS, Tu H, Nelson O, Pook M, Hammer R, Nukina N, Bezprozvanny I. Deranged calcium signaling and neurodegeneration in spinocerebellar ataxia type 3. J Neurosci. 2008;28:12713–24.

73. Toonen LJA, Rigo F, van Attikum H, van Roon-Mom WMC. Antisense oligonucleotide-mediated removal of the Polyglutamine repeat in spinocerebellar Ataxia type 3 mice. Mol Ther Nucleic Acids. 2017;8:232–42.

74. Moore LJ, Nilsen TO, Jarungsriapisit J, Fjelldal PG, Stefansson SO, Taranger GL, Patel S. Triploid atlantic salmon (Salmo salar L.) post-smolts accumulate prevalence more slowly than diploid salmon following bath challenge with salmonid alphavirus subtype 3. PLoS One. 2017;12:e0175468.

75. Schmidt T, Landwehrmeyer GB, Schmitt I, Trottier Y, Auburger G, Laccone F, Klockgether T, Volpel M, Epplen JT, Schols L, Riess O. An isoform of ataxin-3 accumulates in the nucleus of neuronal cells in affected brain regions of SCA3 patients. Brain Pathol (Zurich, Switzerland). 1998;8:669–79.

76. Wullner U, Reimold M, Abele M, Burk K, Minnerop M, Dohmen BM, Machulla HJ, Bares R, Klockgether T. Dopamine transporter positron emission tomography in spinocerebellar ataxias type 1, 2, 3, and 6. Arch Neurol. 2005;62:1280–5.

77. Nicola SM, Surmeier J, Malenka RC. Dopaminergic modulation of neuronal excitability in the striatum and nucleus accumbens. Annu Rev Neurosci. 2000;23:185–215.

78. Watabe-Uchida M, Zhu L, Ogawa SK, Vamanrao A, Uchida N. Whole-brain mapping of direct inputs to midbrain dopamine neurons. Neuron. 2012;74:858–73.

79. Andersson M, Konradi C, Cenci MA. cAMP response element-binding protein is required for dopamine-dependent gene expression in the intact but not the dopamine-denervated striatum. J Neurosci. 2001;21:9930–43.

80. Pflieger LT, Dansithong W, Paul S, Scoles DR, Figueroa KP, Meera P, Otis TS, Facelli JC, Pulst SM. Gene co-expression network analysis for identifying modules and functionally enriched pathways in SCA2. Hum Mol Genet. 2017;26:3069–80.

81. Ramani B, Panwar B, Moore LR, Wang B, Huang R, Guan Y, Paulson HL. Comparison of spinocerebellar ataxia type 3 mouse models identifies early gain-of-function, cell-autonomous transcriptional changes in oligodendrocytes. Hum Mol Genet. 2017;26:3362–74.

82. Kida E, Palminiello S, Golabek AA, Walus M, Wierzba-Bobrowicz T, Rabe A, Albertini G, Wisniewski KE. Carbonic anhydrase II in the developing and adult human brain. J Neuropathol Exp Neurol. 2006;65:664–74.

83. Cammer W, Zhang H, Tansey FA. Effects of carbonic anhydrase II (CAII) deficiency on CNS structure and function in the myelin-deficient CAII-deficient double mutant mouse. J Neurosci Res. 1995;40:451–7.

84. Ghandour MS, Skoff RP, Venta PJ, Tashian RE. Oligodendrocytes express a normal phenotype in carbonic anhydrase II-deficient mice. J Neurosci Res. 1989;23:180–90.

85. Soundarapandian MM, Selvaraj V, Lo UG, Golub MS, Feldman DH, Pleasure DE, Deng W. Zfp488 promotes oligodendrocyte differentiation of neural progenitor cells in adult mice after demyelination. Sci Rep. 2011;1:2.

11

Essential roles of mitochondrial biogenesis regulator Nrf1 in retinal development and homeostasis

Takae Kiyama[1], Ching-Kang Chen[2], Steven W Wang[3], Ping Pan[1], Zhenlin Ju[4], Jing Wang[4], Shinako Takada[5,6], William H Klein[3] and Chai-An Mao[1*]

Abstract

Background: Mitochondrial dysfunction has been implicated in the pathologies of a number of retinal degenerative diseases in both the outer and inner retina. In the outer retina, photoreceptors are particularly vulnerable to mutations affecting mitochondrial function due to their high energy demand and sensitivity to oxidative stress. However, it is unclear how defective mitochondrial biogenesis affects neural development and contributes to neural degeneration. In this report, we investigated the in vivo function of nuclear respiratory factor 1 (Nrf1), a major transcriptional regulator of mitochondrial biogenesis in both proliferating retinal progenitor cells (RPCs) and postmitotic rod photoreceptor cells (PRs).

Methods: We used mouse genetic techniques to generate RPC-specific and rod PR-specific Nrf1 conditional knockout mouse models. We then applied a comprehensive set of tools, including histopathological and molecular analyses, RNA-seq, and electroretinography on these mouse lines to study Nrf1-regulated genes and Nrf1's roles in both developing retinas and differentiated rod PRs. For all comparisons between genotypes, a two-tailed two-sample student's t-test was used. Results were considered significant when $P < 0.05$.

Results: We uncovered essential roles of Nrf1 in cell proliferation in RPCs, cell migration and survival of newly specified retinal ganglion cells (RGCs), neurite outgrowth in retinal explants, reconfiguration of metabolic pathways in RPCs, and mitochondrial morphology, position, and function in rod PRs.

Conclusions: Our findings provide in vivo evidence that Nrf1 and Nrf1-mediated pathways have context-dependent and cell-state-specific functions during neural development, and disruption of Nrf1-mediated mitochondrial biogenesis in rod PRs results in impaired mitochondria and a slow, progressive degeneration of rod PRs. These results offer new insights into the roles of Nrf1 in retinal development and neuronal homeostasis and the differential sensitivities of diverse neuronal tissues and cell types of dysfunctional mitochondria. Moreover, the conditional Nrf1 allele we have generated provides the opportunity to develop novel mouse models to understand how defective mitochondrial biogenesis contributes to the pathologies and disease progression of several neurodegenerative diseases, including glaucoma, age-related macular degeneration, Parkinson's diseases, and Huntington's disease.

Keywords: Mitochondrial biogenesis, Nrf1, Retinal progenitor cell, Retinal ganglion cell, Optic atrophy, Photoreceptor degeneration

* Correspondence: Chai-An.Mao@uth.tmc.edu; chai-an.mao@uth.tmc.edu
[1]Ruiz Department of Ophthalmology and Visual Science, McGovern Medical School at The University of Texas Health Science Center at Houston (UTHealth), 6431 Fannin St., MSB 7.024, Houston, TX 77030, USA
Full list of author information is available at the end of the article

Background

Mitochondrial biogenesis is a dynamic subcellular process through which existing mitochondria continuously import and integrate new proteins and lipids, replicate mitochondrial DNA (mtDNA), and fuse and divide upon environment changes. This process is intricately regulated to maintain a healthy mitochondrial network, essential for energy homeostasis, metabolism, signaling, and apoptosis. The vast majority of the ~ 1500 proteins involved in mitochondrial structure and function are encoded by nuclear genes, which are regulated in concert with a set of transcriptional regulators, including peroxisome proliferative activated receptor gamma coactivator 1 (PGC-1) family members, nuclear respiratory factor 1 (Nrf1), and nuclear respiratory factor 2 (Nrf2/GABP) [1–4].

Nrf1 encodes an evolutionarily conserved transcription activator [5–9]. Nrf1 binds to GC-rich DNA elements in promoters of many nuclear genes required for mitochondrial biogenesis and respiratory function [9–11]. In primary cortical neurons, Nrf1 has been shown to co-regulate all cytochrome c oxidase (COX) subunits and several glutamatergic neurochemicals, implying that a Nrf1-mediated higher-order mechanism coordinately controls the expression of genes involved in neuronal activity and energy metabolism [12–15]. In muscle, Nrf1 has been shown to be a direct PGC-1 target, the master regulator of mitochondrial biogenesis, whose dysfunction has been implicated in several neurodegenerative diseases, such as Parkinson's disease [1, 4]. In addition, Nrf1 plays a significant role in cell growth and proliferation. A recent study using chromatin immunoprecipitation sequencing (ChIP-seq) analysis identified 2470 potential Nrf1 targets in human neuroblastoma cells, indicating roles for Nrf1 in regulating genes for mitochondrial biogenesis and cell growth and in the pathogenesis of neurodegenerative diseases [16]. Interestingly, several genes involved in the glycolytic pathway, such as PFKB2, PGAM1, PGKM5, and ALDOA, were also found in this list, suggesting a possible Nrf1 role in reprogramming metabolic processes. Nrf1 also interacts with several proteins involved in different cellular functions. For example, it interacts directly with poly(ADP-ribose) polymerase 1 (PARP-1), and PARP-1 modulates Nrf1's DNA-binding domain for transcriptional regulation [17]. Dynein light chain was also shown to interact with NRF-1, although the functional significance remains unknown [18].

Several in vivo studies have revealed distinct functions of *Nrf1* in different developing organisms. In zebrafish, an insertional mutation in the *Nrf1* locus caused a cell death phenotype in developing photoreceptors [7]. In Drosophila, the *Nrf1* homolog gene *erect wing* (*ewg*) has been shown to regulate Hippo pathway activity in a neuronal subtype-specific manner to determine neuronal

fate in developing retinas [19]. In mice, *Nrf1*-null embryos fail to maintain mtDNA and die between embryonic day 3.5 (E3.5) and 6.5 [20]. These studies offer insights into the understanding of Nrf1's in vivo function in different developmental systems and cellular context, but how Nrf1-regulated pathways function in retinal development and how they contribute to defective mitochondrial biogenesis to affect neural development and contribute to neural degeneration is unknown.

In this report, we studied the function of Nrf1 during mouse retinal development. We show that *Nrf1* is expressed in proliferating retinal progenitor cells (RPCs) in embryonic retinas and enriched in retinal ganglion cells (RGCs) and rod photoreceptors cells (PRs), both of which consume large amounts of energy. Using cell-type-specific *Nrf1* knockout mice, we demonstrate that *Nrf1* controls cell proliferation in RPCs and the extension of neurite processes in developing retinal neurons. Nrf1-deficient embryonic retinas exhibited affected expression of genes involved in multiple cellular processes. In differentiated rod PRs, deleting *Nrf1* caused abnormal mitochondrial morphology, deteriorated mitochondrial functions, abnormal photoreceptor inner and outer segments, and reduced electroretinography (ERG) activities. Eventually, mutant rod PRs completely degenerated. Together, these results demonstrate the crucial role of Nrf1-mediated mitochondrial biogenesis in retinal development and homeostasis and provide new insights into Nrf1 function in neurite outgrowth and metabolic reprogramming.

Methods

Gene targeting and animal breeding

A Nrf1-targeted embryonic stem (ES) clone was obtained from the knockout mouse project repository (http://www.mousephenotype.org/data/alleles/MGI:1332235/tm1a (KOMP)Wtsi). This allele contains 2 loxP sites inserted into the third and fourth introns, and a FLP recombinase target (FRT)-site flanked T2A-LacZ-T2A-neomycin fusion cassette inserted into intron 3. Exon 4 in the floxed allele can be deleted by Cre-mediated recombination. ES cells were injected into B6(GC)-Tyrc-2 J/J blastocysts, and the injected blastocysts were transferred into C57/BL6 albino females. Chimeric males obtained by blastocyst injection were bred to wildtype B6(GC)-Tyrc-2 J/J females to generate the $Nrf1^{LacZ/+}$ allele, which was subsequently bred with a 17T17T*Rosa26-FLPeR*0T17T0T17T 0T0Ttransgene to remove a *LacZ-neomycin* fusion cassette to generate a $Nrf1^{flox/+}$ allele (Fig. 1a). PCR primers used to distinguish the $Nrf1^{flox}$ allele from the wildtype allele were U5 (5'-CCAAGACTTGTATGCATTGGTCTCAG-3') and U3 (5'-GCACTTCTGGCTCCATGGTCC-3') (Fig. 1a, b). PCR primers for *Six3-Cre* were Cre1 (5'-AACGAGTGATGAGGTTCGCAAGAAC-3') and Cre2 (5'-CGCTATTTTCCATGAGTGAACGAACC-3'); and for *Rho-iCre*

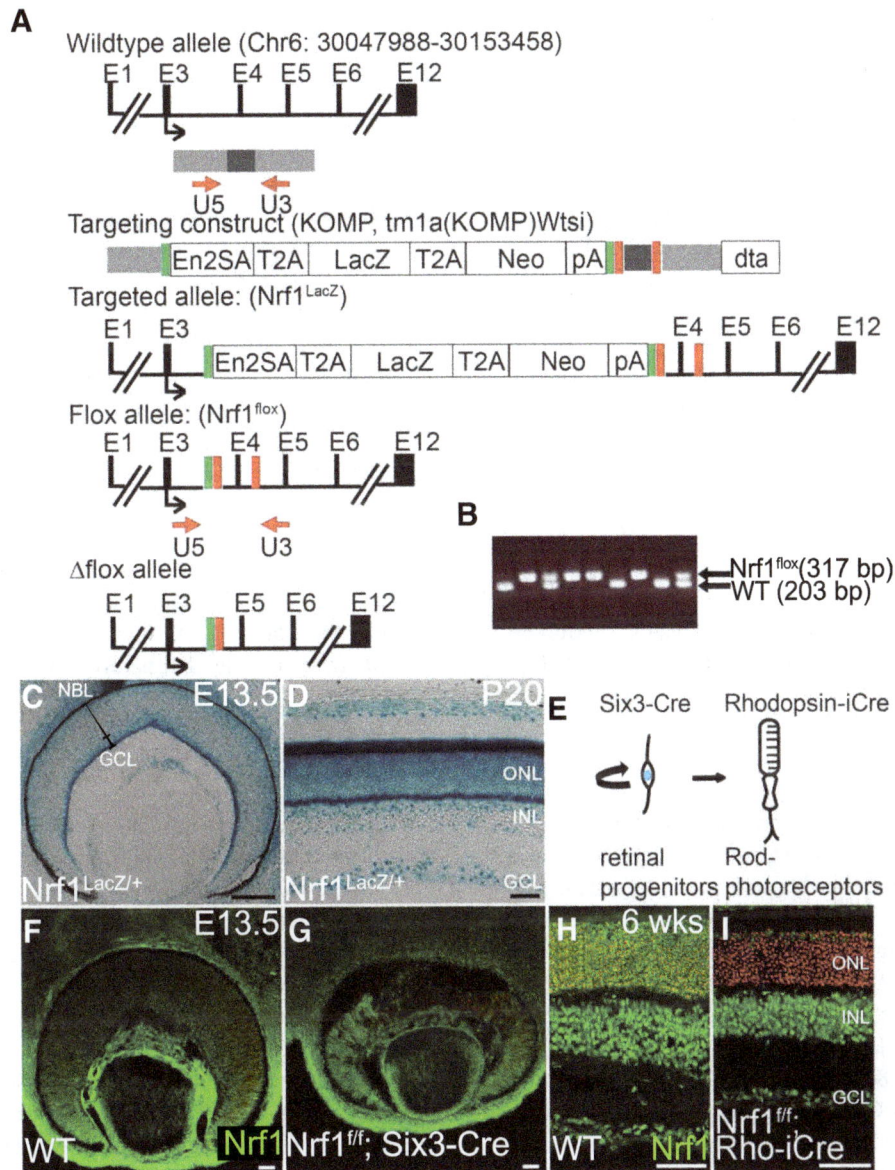

Fig. 1 Generation of Nrf1 expression and conditional *Nfr1* alleles. (**a**) Genomic structure of *Nrf1*, the targeting construct, the targeted *Nrf1^LacZ^* and *Nrf1^flox^* alleles, and the deleted allele. Exons are indicated as E1-E12. The gray and black bars indicate the regions used in the targeting construct. A black arrow indicates the translational start site for the Nrf1 protein. Red arrows indicate PCR primers used for PCR genotyping of the wildtype and floxed alleles. Red boxes indicate loxP sites, and green boxes indicate FRT sites. (**b**) PCR genotyping using U5 and U3 primers for wildtype (203 bp) and floxed (317 bp) alleles. (**c, d**) Nrf1 expression during retinogenesis revealed by LacZ expression in *Nrf1^LacZ/+^* retinas at E13.5 (**c**) and P20 (**d**). (**e**) Schematic representation of the developing retinal cells expressing Six3 and rhodopsin. Proliferative retinal progenitor cells expressing Six3 will give rise to all mature retinal cells. Rhodopsin is expressed in differentiated rod photoreceptor cells. (**f–i**) Nrf1 expression detected by immunofluorescent staining on E13.5 wildtype (**f**) and *Nrf1^f/f^;Six3-Cre* (**g**) retinal sections and on 6-week-old wildtype (**h**) and *Nrf1^f/f^;Rho-iCre* (**i**) retinal sections. Scale bars: 100 μm in C, 50 μm in **d-i**. ONL: outer nuclear layer. INL: inner nuclear layer. GCL: ganglion cell layer. WT: wildtype. NBL: neural blast layer

were iCre1 (5'-GGATGCCACCTCTGATGAAG-3') and iCre2 (5'-CACACCATTCTTTCTGACCCG-3'). Embryos were designated as E0.5 at noon on the day in which vaginal plugs were observed. Both male and female mice were used in this study, and no differences were observed according to sex.

Histology, immunohistochemistry, X-gal staining, COX activity

Embryos or eyeballs dissected from mice were fixed in 4% paraformaldehyde at 4 °C for 2 h or overnight, embedded in paraffin or optimal cutting temperature (OCT) compound, and sectioned into 7 μm thickness for histological analysis. After dewaxing and rehydration, the sections were stained with Hematoxylin and Eosin.

For immunohistochemical analysis, cryo- or paraffin-embedded embryos or eyes were sectioned into 7 μm or 30 μm thickness. Sections were heat-treated in a microwave oven at 600 W in 10 mM sodium citrate for 15 min. The sections were blocked with 2% bovine serum albumin and 5% normal serum for 2 h at room temperature. The primary antibody was applied to the sections for 1–3 days at 4°C. The primary antibodies used were mouse anti-Nrf1 (1:300, catalog #PCRP-NFR1-3D4; DSHB, The University of Iowa, Iowa City, IA), mouse anti-Isl1 (1:200, catalog# 37.3F7; DSHB), goat anti-Brn3/Pou4f2 (1:150, catalog #sc-6026; Santa Cruz Biotechnology, Dallas, TX), mouse anti-Pax6 (1:200, catalog #MAB5552; Chemicon, Burlington, MA), sheep anti-Chx10 (1:300, catalog #X1180P; Exalpha, Shirley, MA), rabbit anti-cleaved caspase-3 (1:300, catalog #9579; Cell Signaling, Danvers, MA), mouse anti-BrdU (1:10, catalog #05–633; Millipore, Burlington, MA), mouse anti-Phospho-Histone H3/PH3 (1:700, catalog #9706; Cell Signaling), rabbit anti-Cyclin D1 (1:300, catalog #MA1–39546; Thermo Fisher Scientific, Waltham, MA), mouse anti-rhodopsin (1:20, catalog #MS-1233-R7; Thermo Fisher Scientific), rabbit anti-cone arrestin (1:2000, catalog #AB16282; Millipore), and rabbit anti-Tfam (1:500, catalog #ab131607; Abcam, Cambridge, MA). Secondary antibodies conjugated with Alexa-488, 555 or 633 (Thermo Fisher Scientific) were used in 1:800 dilution. For indirect immunofluorescence, a tyramide signal amplification kit was used (PerkinElmer, Waltham, MA). HRP-conjugated secondary antibodies were from Jackson ImmunoResearch Laboratories (West Grove, PA). DAPI (2.5 μg/ml, catalog #D1306; Thermo Fisher Scientific) was used to stain nuclei. Images were captured using Olympus (Tokyo, Japan) FluoView 1000 or Zeiss (Thornwood, NY) LSM 780 confocal microscopes. SimplePCI software (Hamamatsu Corporation, Sewickley, PA) was used to analyze the number of cells.

For X-gal staining, embryos or eyes were fixed in 10% formalin for 30 min, embedded in OCT compound, and sectioned into 30 μm thickness. Sections were dried at room temperature for 3 h, washed with wash buffer (0.1 M sodium phosphate containing 2 mM MgCl₂, 0.01% deoxycholate, and 0.02% Nonidet P-40). LacZ color reaction was performed in wash buffer containing 5 mM potassium ferrocyanide, 5 mM potassium ferricyanide, and 1 mg/ml X-gal at 37°C overnight. Color reaction was terminated by incubation in 10% formalin for 10 min. Post-fixed sections were washed, dehydrated, and mounted with Cytoseal 60 (Thermo Fisher Scientific). Images were collected with a Canon EOS 10 digital camera (Melville, NY) mounted on an Olympus IX71 microscope.

Cytochrome c oxidase (COX) analysis was performed as described previously [21] with slight modifications.

E13.5 embryonic heads from wildtype and $Nrf1^{f/f}$;Six3-Cre embryos or 6 week-old adult eyeballs from wildtype and $Nrf1^{f/f}$;Rho-iCre were fixed in 10% formalin for 20 min at room temperature. Samples were washed in phosphate buffered saline (PBS) 3 times and embedded in OCT; 14 μm cryo-sections were collected. Sections were dried at 4°C for 1 hour, rehydrated, and incubated in COX reacting solution (1× DAB, 100 μM cytochrome C, and 2 μg/ml bovine catalase in 0.1 M PBS, pH 7.0) at 37°C. Color reactions were terminated by incubating in 10% formalin for 10 min. Post-fixed sections were washed, dehydrated, and mounted with Cytoseal 60. Images were collected as described for X-gal staining.

BrdU labeling and TUNEL assays
Terminal deoxynucleotidyl transferase dUTP nick end label (TUNEL) assays were performed using an in situ cell death detection kit (Roche, Pleasanton, CA). For pulse labeling with BrdU, 0.1 mg per body gram of BrdU (Sigma, St. Louis, MO) was injected intraperitoneally into pregnant females 1 h before embryo collection.

RNA sequencing analysis
Eighteen retinas from wildtype and $Nrf1^{f/f}$;Six3-Cre embryos at E13.5 of multiple littermates were pooled, and RNA was extracted using TRI reagent (Sigma) and purified with a Pure Link RNA mini kit (Thermo Fisher Scientific). RNA sequencing (RNA-seq) was performed in the Sequencing and Microarray Core Resource Facility at The University of Texas MD Anderson Cancer Center. RNAs were treated with DNase, and cDNAs were synthesized using a cDNA synthesis kit (NuGen, San Carlos, CA). One hundred nt paired-end reads were obtained using an Illumina HiSeq 3000 Next Generation Sequencing instrument (San Diego, CA). The RNA-seq experiment was duplicated, thus making statistical comparisons possible, although there is still a lack of statistical power. The RNA-seq reads were mapped to the mouse genome (mm10) via the Tophat 2.7.2 program. We performed QC and sum counts (reads) for each gene using HTseq. The differential expression analyses were performed by Cuffdiff software. Nrf1-dependent genes (fold change ≥ 1.4; adjusted P-value ≤ 0.2) were analyzed with DAVID Bioinformatics Resources 6.8 (https://david.ncifcrf.gov/home.jsp). The raw datasets and normalized count data for each gene have been deposited in NCBI (GSE101550).

Retinal explant culture
Retinal explant culture was described previously [22]. In brief, retinas were isolated from E13.5 wildtype and $Nrf1^{f/f}$;Six3-Cre embryos and cut in 4 pieces, then placed on laminin-coated coverslips and cultured in Neurobasal

media containing N2 supplement and penicillin-streptomycin (Thermo Fisher Science). Images were examined and collected using an Olympus IX-70 inverted microscope.

In situ hybridization

Embryo heads from wildtype and *Nrf1^{f/f};Six3-Cre* at E13.5 were dissected and fixed in fresh 10% neutral buffered formalin for 24 h. Samples were washed with PBS then dehydrated with serial ethanol and embedded in paraffin. Sections were cut to 7 μm or 10 μm in thickness. In situ hybridization was performed as described previously [23]. Antisense *Idh1* (957 bp) and *Ldha* (950 bp) probes were cloned by reverse transcriptase PCR using Idh1 probe F (5′-AGGTTCTGTGGTGG AGATGC-3′), Idh1 probe R (5′-GACGTCTCTTGCCC TTTCTG-3′), Ldha probe F (5′-TCCGTTACCTGATG GGAGAG-3′) and Ldha probe R (5′-ACACTTGGG TGGTTGGTTCC-3′). RNAscope in situ hybridization (ISH) was performed using the RNAscope 2.5 HD Detection Reagents-Brown kit following manufacturer's protocol (cat# 322310, Advanced Cell Diagnostics, Newark, CA). According to instructions, each mRNA molecule hybridized to a probe appears as a separate brown color dot. The probes used were mouse Cpt1a-C1 (cat# 443071) and mouse Slc16a1-C1 (cat# 423661).

Quantitative reverse transcriptase PCR (qRT-PCR)

Eight retinas from wildtype or *Nrf1^{f/f};Six3-Cre* embryos at E13.5 or one retina from wildtype or *Nrf1^{f/f}; Rho-iCre* at 6 weeks old of multiple littermates were pooled, and RNAs were extracted using TRI reagent (Sigma). First-strand cDNA was synthesized using the Superscript III First-Strand Synthesis System (Thermo Fisher Scientific). Real-time PCR was performed using CFX Connect Real-Time System (BioRad, Hercules, CA) with SsoAdvanced Universal SYBR Green Supermix (BioRad). Relative RNA levels were normalized to that of *β-actin*. Sequences of PCR primers are listed in Table 1.

Transmission electron microscopy

Eyeballs were fixed with 3% glutaraldehyde and 2% paraformaldehyde overnight at 4 °C. Retinas were washed and treated with 0.1% cacodylate-buffered tannic acid, post-fixed with 1% osmium tetroxide, stained en bloc with 1% uranyl acetate, and dehydrated with an ethanol gradient series. The samples were embedded in epon and sectioned with a JLB ultracut microtome (Leica, Wetzlar, Germany). Images were examined with a JEM 1010 REM (JEOL, Peabody, MA) and collected digitally. Fiji was used to analyze the size and circularity of inner segment (IS) and mitochondria [24].

Mitochondrial DNA quantitation

Quantification of the relative copy number of mitochondrial DNA present per nuclear genome was performed as previously described [25]. Mitochondrial DNA and genomic Pecam DNA were amplified and analyzed by quantitative PCR ($\Delta\Delta C(t)$ method). PCR primers used to amplify mitochondrial DNA were mtDNAf (5′-CCTA TCACCCTTGCCATCAT-3′) and mtDNAr (5′-GAGG CTGTTGCTTGTGTGAC-3′). PCR primers to amplify nuclear DNA were Pecamf (5′-ATGGAAAGCCTGCCATCAT G-3′) and Pecamr (5′-TCCTTGTTGTTCAGCATCAC-3′).

Electroretinography (ERG)

Mice were dark-adapted overnight and then anesthetized under infrared illumination by ketamine/xylazine/acepromazine through intraperitoneal injection (94/5/1 mg/kg), and pupils were dilated with 1% tropicamide and 2.5% phenylephrine topical eye drops (Bausch & Lomb, Tampa, FL). Body temperature was maintained at 35 °C to 37 °C by circulating 43.5 °C water through a plastic heating coil wrapped around the body. Stimulus-dependent transcorneal potential changes from both eyes were recorded simultaneously (UTAS BigShot system; LKC Technologies, Gaithersburg, MD) following the delivery of a white light flash with an intensity of 25 Candela sec m^{-2}, as described previously [26]. The inter-stimulus interval was 120 s, and responses from 3 independent measurements were averaged and analyzed. Photopic ERG recordings ensued immediately after scotopic recordings by exposing the animals to a white background light of 30 Candela m^{-2} for 10 min. Transcorneal potential changes were then elicited by flashes of 25 Candela sec m^{-2} in intensity and presented at 1 Hz for 90 s, averaged, and then analyzed. A typical recording session lasted 1 h, and 5 μl of sterile-filtered PBS was applied every 20 min to ensure good electrical contact and delay the formation of corneal clouding and cataract.

Experimental design

Six E13.5 littermate embryos of each genotype (wildtype and *Nrf1^{f/f};Six3-Cre*) were used for counting BrdU+ and PH3+ cells' RPCs. Four sections near the central retinas from each embryo were stained with BrdU or PH3. The most representative sections from each embryo were used for cell counting. Total RNAs were isolated and pooled from 9 pairs of E13.5 wildtype and *Nrf1^{f/f};Six3-Cre* retinas for RNA-seq. For RNA-seq data validation using qRT-PCR, 3 sets of 6 pairs of E13.5 wildtype and *Nrf1^{f/f};Six3-Cre* retinas were isolated and pooled, and 2 independent experiments were conducted. For each qRT-PCR experiment, total RNAs from 4 pairs of E13.5 wildtype and *Nrf1^{f/f};Six3-Cre* retinas were isolated and pooled, and 5 sets of independent experiments were

Table 1 Primer sets used for qRT-PCR

Gene	Position	5'-sequence-3'
b-actin	Forward	CAACGGCTCCGGCATGTGC
	Reverse	CTCTTGCTCTGGGCCTCG
CCND1	Forward	GCACTTTTGGTCAGCTAGCT
	Reverse	GACATGGCCCTAAACCTTCT
Gli1	Forward	ACTGGGGTGAGTTCCCTTCT
	Reverse	AGGACTACCCAGCAAATCCT
Mapt	Forward	AATGGAAGACCATGCTGGAG
	Reverse	TCCCAATCTGAGTCCCAAAG
Ret	Forward	TGGCACACCTCTGCTCTATG
	Reverse	CTGTTCCCAGGAACTGTGGT
Stmn3	Forward	CCCGAACACCATCTACCAGT
	Reverse	CTTCTGCAGCTCTTCCAAGG
Ncan	Forward	GTGGCTGCTTCTCCTAGTGG
	Reverse	AATGTCTCGCAGGGAGCTTA
Ina	Forward	TTCGGGAATACCAGGACTTG
	Reverse	GTGCTAAACCGCGTCTCTTC
Islr2	Forward	CTCTGCCTTTTCAAGGATGC
	Reverse	CGCTGAGTTGAAAGGCCTAC
Nell2	Forward	CACAGTTGACCTTTCCTGCT
	Reverse	CAGCACAAATGGCCATTCTT
Stmn2	Forward	GCAATGGCCTACAAGGAAAA
	Reverse	GGTGGCTTCAAGATCAGCTC
Gap43	Forward	GTGCTGCTAAAGCTACCACT
	Reverse	CTTCAGAGTGGAGCTGAGAA
Nrn1	Forward	CCAGGGGAATGACTTCAAGA
	Reverse	TTTCGCTTTTCTGGAGGAGA
Syt4	Forward	TGTTGTAGGTGATGGTTTCA
	Reverse	AGACCATGGTTCTTAGGTGA
Dcx	Forward	ACAGATGTCAACCGGGAAAG
	Reverse	TCGTTCGTCAAAATGTCCAA
Pou4f1	Forward	AGGCCTATTTGCCGTACAA
	Reverse	CGTCTCACACCCTCCTCAGT
Irx4	Forward	GAGACCACCAGCACACTGAA
	Reverse	AGGTGGAAACCTGTGTGAGG
Cx3cr1	Forward	AGCCCAGGGGAAGAAATAGA
	Reverse	CTCTGTTGGCTCCAGTCTCC
Capn3	Forward	GCTTCTGGAGGAAGACGATG
	Reverse	TTTGGGAACCTCGTAGATGG
Igfbp7	Forward	GGAAAATCTGGCCATTCAGA
	Reverse	TGCGTGGCACTCATACTCTC
Vit	Forward	GCGTCTACGCGTCTTACTCC
	Reverse	CCCTTTTGGGGCTTACTTTC
Nid1	Forward	ACCATCACCTTCCAGGAGTG
	Reverse	GCATAGCGCAAGATCCTCTC

Table 1 Primer sets used for qRT-PCR *(Continued)*

Gene	Position	5'-sequence-3'
Stab1	Forward	ACAAGATCTTCAGCCGCCTA
	Reverse	AGTTTGTCACGGTGGTCCTC
Spp1	Forward	TGCACCCAGATCCTATAGCC
	Reverse	CTCCATCGTCATCATCATCG
Tgfbi	Forward	GGATGTCCTGAAGGGAGACA
	Reverse	ATTGGTGGGAGCAAAAACAG
Cox4i2	Forward	AGCTGAGCCAAGCAGAGAAG
	Reverse	GCCCATCACTGTCTTCCATT
Idh1	Forward	AGGTTCTGTGGTGGAGATGC
	Reverse	GACGCCCACGTTGTATTTCT
Dna2	Forward	CGAAGTTCTGTGCATCCTGA
	Reverse	TTCTCAGACACCGAATGCTG
Gdap1	Forward	CTGTGAGGCCACTCAGATCA
	Reverse	TGAGCTCAGGATGCAAAATG
Shmt2	Forward	CTCTTTGCTTCGGACCACTC
	Reverse	TTCTCCCTCTGCAGAAGCTC
Cpt1a	Forward	CCAGGCTACAGTGGGACATT
	Reverse	AAGGAATGCAGGTCCACATC
Sardh	Forward	ACTCGGTTGTCTTCCCACAC
	Reverse	CCTGTCGCTCTTGAAACACA
Ucp2	Forward	GCCACTTCACTTCTGCCTTC
	Reverse	GAAGGCATGAACCCCTTGTA
Pmaip1	Forward	CCCAGATTGGGGACCTTAGT
	Reverse	AGTTATGTCCGGTGCACTCC
Rab32	Forward	CTCTTCTCCCAGCACTACCG
	Reverse	CAAATGCTCCAAGAGCTTCC
Ldha	Forward	AGGCTCCCCAGAACAAGATT
	Reverse	TCTCGCCCTTGAGTTTGTCT
HK1	Forward	GAAGCCAAATGGGACTGTGT
	Reverse	CACGCACAGATTGGTTATGC
Pfkp	Forward	GAAGCCAAATGGGACTGTGT
	Reverse	CACGCACAGATTGGTTATGC
Tpi1	Forward	CCTGGCCTATGAACCTGTGT
	Reverse	CAGGTTGCTCCAGTCACAGA
Pgam2	Forward	AGGAGCTGCCTACCTGTGAA
	Reverse	GGGCTGCAATAAGCACTCTC
Mfn1	Forward	GCTGTCAGAGCCCATCTTTC
	Reverse	CAGCCCACTGTTTTCCAAAT
Mfn2	Forward	GTCCTGGACGTCAAAGGGTA
	Reverse	GCAGAACTTTGTCCCAGA
Opa1	Forward	GATGACACGCTCTCCAGTGA
	Reverse	TCGGGGCTAACAGTACAACC

conducted. The ratio of $Nrf1^{f/f}$;Six3-Cre to wildtype expression was calculated for each experiment and averaged for further analysis. For counting photoreceptors, 20 littermates from each genotype (wildtype and $Nrf1^{f/f}$;Rho-iCre) were used for the study. Five littermates per genotype were sacrificed, and 4 sections from the central area of each retina were stained. One representative section from each sample was used to count the number of rows of photoreceptors at each study time point (3, 6, 7, and 8 weeks). For electron microscopy analysis, 2 pairs of wildtype and $Nrf1^{f/f}$;Rho-iCre littermates were used. Images were collected from both mouse retinas. Four images of the IS of each genotype were used to quantify the shape and size of the IS and number of mitochondria. For ERG, 3 pairs of wildtype and $Nrf1^{f/f}$;Rho-iCre littermates were used.

Statistical analysis

All data are presented as mean ± standard deviation for each genotype. For all comparisons between genotypes, a two-tailed two-sample student's t-test was used for all measurements. Results were considered significant when $P < 0.05$. Statistical tests were conducted using Excel (Microsoft, Redmond, WA).

Results

Nrf1 expression in the developing retina

To determine the expression and function of Nrf1 in the retina, we generated $Nrf1^{LacZ}$ and Nrf1^{flox} targeted mouse lines (Fig. 1a, b). The $Nrf1^{LacZ}$ knock-in allele contains a LacZ cassette, which was used to trace the spatiotemporal expression of Nrf1. We first examined the expression of Nrf1 in developing and adult retinas. In E13.5 developing retinas, strong LacZ activity was detected near the apical and basal layers of the neural retina, suggesting Nrf1 is highly expressed in developing RGCs and photoreceptor precursor cells (Fig. 1c). Notably, weaker LacZ activity could also be detected in the neuroblast layer where proliferating RPCs and postmitotic precursor cells reside (Fig. 1c). Along the developmental progression, a similar pattern of LacZ expression was observed in E16.5 and P0 retinas (data not shown). In adult retinas, robust LacZ activity was observed in the ganglion cell layer and outer nuclear layer (ONL), where the metabolic activity is high (Fig. 1d) [27], while a moderate level of LacZ activity was observed in the inner nuclear layer (INL). The dynamic expression pattern of Nrf1 in both developing and mature retinas suggests that Nrf1 may play multiple roles in proliferating RPCs in the developing retina and in the differentiated retinal neurons.

To determine the functions of Nrf1 in RPCs and differentiated retinal neurons, we performed conditional knockout of Nrf1 by breeding the $Nrf1^{flox}$ allele with either Six3-Cre to delete Nrf1 in the proliferating RPCs or with Rho-iCre to delete Nrf1 in the rod PRs, respectively (Fig. 1e). During retinal development, the Six3-Cre transgenic line begins to activate Cre expression in the central retina at E11 [28], and the Rho-iCre transgenic line starts to activate Cre activity in differentiated rod PRs at P7 [26]. By immunostaining, Nrf1 protein was detected in developing RGCs and photoreceptor precursor cells, as well as in the neuroblast layer at E13.5 (Fig. 1f) and in cells in all nuclear layers in adult retinas (Fig. 1h). Consistent with the onset of Cre expression in both lines, the expression of Nrf1 protein was completely abolished in the central $Nrf1^{f/f}$; Six3-Cre retina (compare Fig. 1f and g) and in the rod PRs of $Nrf1^{f/f}$; Rho-iCre retinas (compare Fig. 1h and g) respectively, suggesting effective conditional deletion of Nrf1 in RPCs by Six3-Cre or in rod PRs by Rho-iCre.

Deleting Nrf1 in RPCs causes RGC loss and retinal degeneration

To determine whether deleting Nrf1 in embryonic retinas affects retinal development, we first examined the histology and morphology of Six3-Cre-mediated Nrf1 mutant retinas ($Nrf1^{f/f}$;Six3-Cre) at different developmental stages. At E16.5, $Nrf1^{f/f}$; Six3-Cre retinas were substantially smaller and thinner than those of the wildtype retinas (Fig. 2a, b), causing a large sub-retinal space between the retina and the pigmented epithelium. The central regions of $Nrf1^{f/f}$;Six3-Cre retinas near the optic disc were completely disrupted and acellular (arrowheads in Fig. 2b). At P20, $Nrf1^{f/f}$;Six3-Cre retinas were relatively thinner than those of wildtype retinas. Decreased cell numbers in all cellular layers were observed with near complete abolishment of RGCs. Although the stereotypic laminar structure was retained in Nrf1-mutant retinas, the cells in each laminar layer were not properly aligned as in control retinas (Fig. 2c, d). In 7-month-old $Nrf1^{f/f}$;Six3-Cre retinas, the number of retinal cells was further reduced, and the laminar layers were completely disrupted (Fig. 2e, f). The surface of the whole retina from $Nrf1^{f/f}$;Six3-Cre was much smaller, underlying only a limited area near the optic disc in the eyeball (Fig. 2g, h). There were no visible optic nerves or optic chiasms in $Nrf1^{f/f}$;Six3-Cre mice (Fig. 2i, j). These data suggest that deleting Nrf1 in RPCs causes substantial RGC loss followed by the degeneration of the entire retina.

Delayed RGC differentiation, defective RGC migration, and apoptotic RGCs in Nrf1$^{f/f}$;Six3-Cre retinas

Because a significant loss of RGCs was seen in $Nrf1^{f/f}$;Six3-Cre retinas, we examined whether and how the RGC differentiation program was affected. RGCs are the

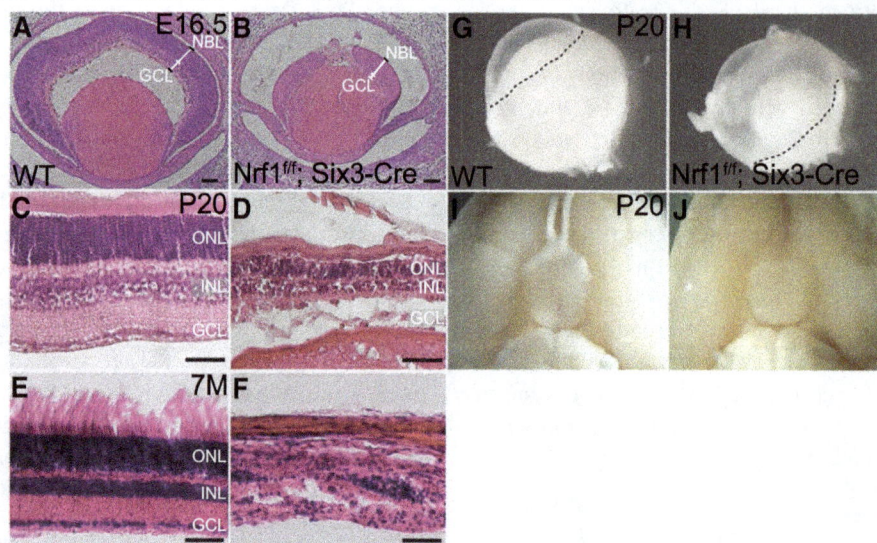

Fig. 2 Loss of retinal ganglion cells and severe retinal degeneration in Nrf1-deficient RPCs. (**a–f**) Hematoxylin and eosin staining of retinal sections from wildtype (**a**, **c** and **e**) and *Nrf1^{f/f};Six3-Cre* (**b**, **d**, and **f**) at E16.5, P20, and 7 months old. (**g**, **h**) Eyeballs from wildtype (**g**) and *Nrf1^{f/f};Six3-Cre* (**h**) animals. The peripheral rim of underlying retinas is plotted with dotted lines. (**i**, **j**) Ventral view of the brains showing the optic nerve and optic chiasm in wildtype (**i**) and *Nrf1^{f/f};Six3-Cre* (**j**) animals. Scale bars: 50 µm. ONL: outer nuclear layer. INL: inner nuclear layer. GCL: ganglion cell layer. WT: wildtype. NBL: neural blast layer

first retinal cell type to differentiate from Atoh7-expressing precursor cells during retinogenesis. RGC differentiation is marked by the onset of Pou4f2 and Isl1 expression in the central retina around E12 [29, 30]. To determine when RGCs began to differentiate in *Nrf1^{f/f};Six3-Cre* retina, we monitored Isl1 and Pou4f2 expression by immunostaining at different embryonic stages.

In E12.5 wildtype retinas, while the newly differentiated Isl1+ RGCs could be readily detected in the central retina (Fig. 3a), only a few Isl1+ cells were present in *Nrf1* mutant retinas (Fig. 3b). At E14.5, while differentiating Pou4f2+ RGCs were widespread across the neuroblast and ganglion cell layers in wildtype retinas (Fig. 3c), fewer Pou4f2+ RGCs were detected in Nrf1 mutant retinas (Fig. 3d). No clear ganglion cell layer could be seen in *Nrf1* mutant retinas. Furthermore, Pou4f2+ RGCs were distributed unevenly and formed patched clumps in the central region of the mutant retina (arrowheads in Fig. 3d). In E16.5 wildtype retinas, a distinct ganglion cell layer was formed, and newly differentiated Pou4f2+ RGCs were seen in the neuroblast layer (Fig. 3e). In contrast, a much thinner ganglion cell layer was observed in *Nrf1^{f/f};Six3-Cre* retinas, and Pou4f2+ RGCs were spread to the peripheral region (Fig. 3f). Together, these data suggest that RGC differentiation was delayed, and newly differentiated RGCs had defects in migrating toward the vitreous layer in the *Nrf1^{f/f};Six3-Cre* retinas.

To detect RPCs, wildtype and *Nrf1^{f/f};Six3-Cre* retinal sections were immunolabeled with anti-Pax6 or Chx10 antibodies (Fig. 4a–d). Pax6 and Chx10 were expressed in both wildtype and *Nrf1^{f/f};Six3-Cre* retinas. However, Pax6+ or Chx10+ RPCs were unevenly distributed in the central region of Nrf1^{f/f} retinas compared to the peripheral region (Fig. 4b, d). Interestingly, several clumps of RPCs lacking Pax6 expression were formed in Nrf1 mutant retinas, and the nuclei of these Pax6-negative cells appeared granulated, suggesting these were cells undergoing apoptosis (Fig. 4b, b', b''). Similarly, mis-patterned Chx10 expression and granular-shaped nuclei were observed in the central region of *Nrf1^{f/f};Six3-Cre* retinas (Fig. 4d, d', d''). Consistently, *Nrf1^{f/f};Six3-Cre* retinas contained significantly more apoptotic cells than wildtype retinas (Fig. 5a, b). The majority of apoptotic cells were found in the central region of *Nrf1*-mutant retinas. In addition, these apoptotic cells (marked by cleaved caspase 3 expression) were Pou4f2+ (Fig. 5c-e), indicating that ganglion cells had differentiated but could not migrate to the RGC layer and eventually died in situ.

Severe reduction of proliferation in *Nrf1^{f/f};Six3-Cre* retina

The *Nrf1^{f/f};Six3-Cre* retina was substantially smaller and thinner than the wildtype retina, suggesting that the proliferation of RPCs in the *Nrf1*-mutant retina was compromised. To examine this phenotype, wildtype and *Nrf1^{f/f};Six3-Cre* retinas were immuno-labeled with several cell cycle markers. To detect S-phase proliferating RPCs, we pulse-labeled E13.5 embryos with BrdU and then conducted immunostaining using anti-BrdU antibody on retinal sections. We counted the number of BrdU+ cells in

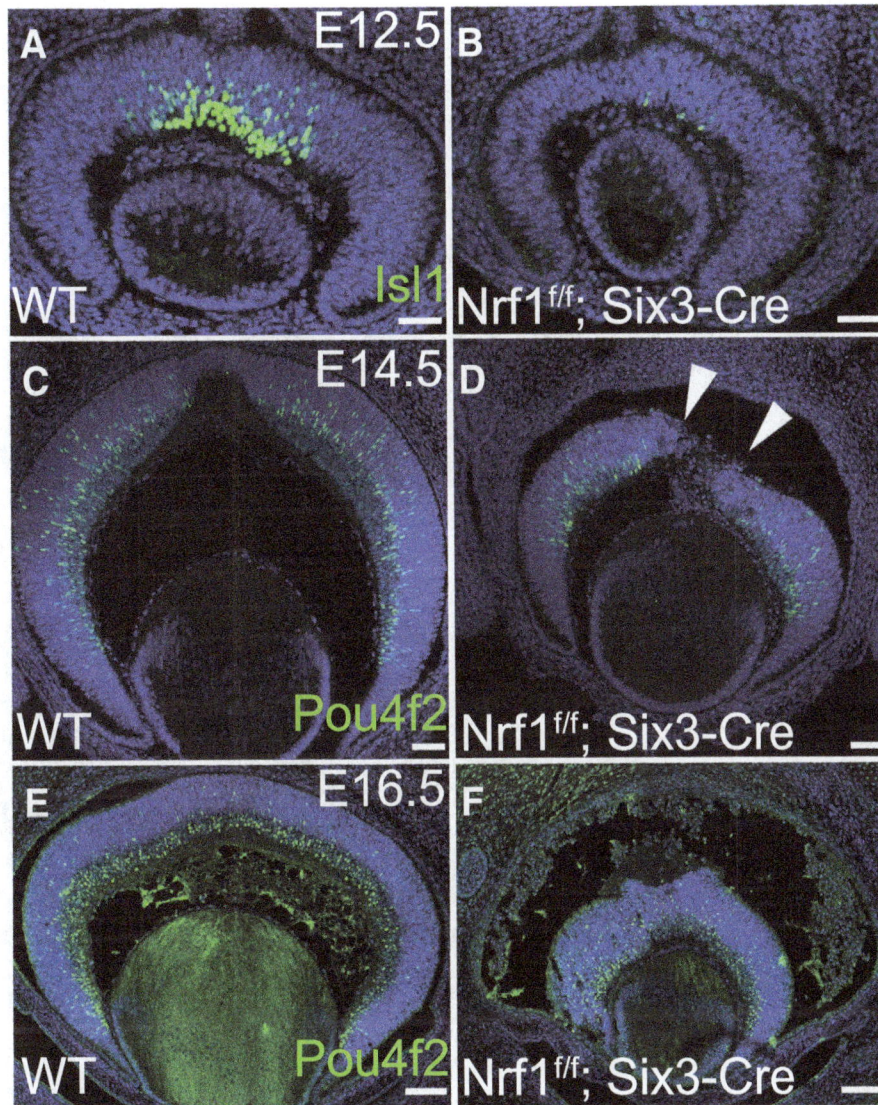

Fig. 3 Delayed onset of RGC differentiation in *Nrf1^(f/f)^;Six3-Cre* retina. (**a–f**) Immunostaining of wildtype (**a**, **c**, and **e**) and *Nrf1^(f/f)^;Six3-Cre* (**b**, **d**, and **f**) retinas. (**a**, **b**) E12.5 retinal sections labeled with anti-Isl1 antibody. (**c**, **d**) E14.5 and (**e**, **f**) E16.5 retinal sections labeled with anti-Pou4f2 antibody. Arrowheads indicate clumped Pou4f2+ cells in the central area of *Nrf1^(f/f)^;Six3-Cre* retina. Scale bars: 50 μm in **a–d**, 100 μm in **e** and **f**. WT: wildtype

sections and found that the number of BrdU+ S-phase RPCs were reduced to ∼ 50% in *Nrf1^(f/f)^;Six3-Cre* retinas compared to wildtype retinas (Fig. 6a-c, *P* = 0.0009). We then conducted immunostaining using anti-PH3 and anti-cyclin D1 (Ccnd1) antibodies on retinal sections to detect RPCs in M-phase and G1-phase, respectively. The number of PH3+ M-phase RPCs per section from *Nrf1^(f/f)^;Six3-Cre* was also reduced to ∼ 50% compared to wildtype retinas (Fig. 6d-f, *P* = 0.002), and Ccnd1+ RPCs were nearly absent in the central region of *Nrf1*-mutant retinas (Fig. 6g, h). The PH3+ RPCs in the *Nrf1*-mutants were not properly positioned at the apical side as in control retinas (Fig. 6d, e). In addition, using qRT-PCR, we found that the expression levels of *Ccnd1* were reduced to ∼ 10% in *Nrf1*-mutant

retinas compared with wildtype retina, and *Gli1*, the key downstream effector of Shh pathway in RPCs [31, 32], was reduced to ∼ 30% (Fig. 6i, *Ccnd1*: *P* = 0.001, *Gli1*: *P* = 0.006). Other Shh pathway genes, such as Shh and Ptch1, were also downregulated in *Nrf1*-mutant retinas (in GSE101550 dataset described in next section). Together, these data indicate that the RPC proliferation is reduced in *Nrf1*-mutant retinas.

Identification of Nrf1-dependent retina-expressed genes at E13.5

To further investigate how Nrf1 regulates retinal development, we performed RNA-seq analysis on E13.5

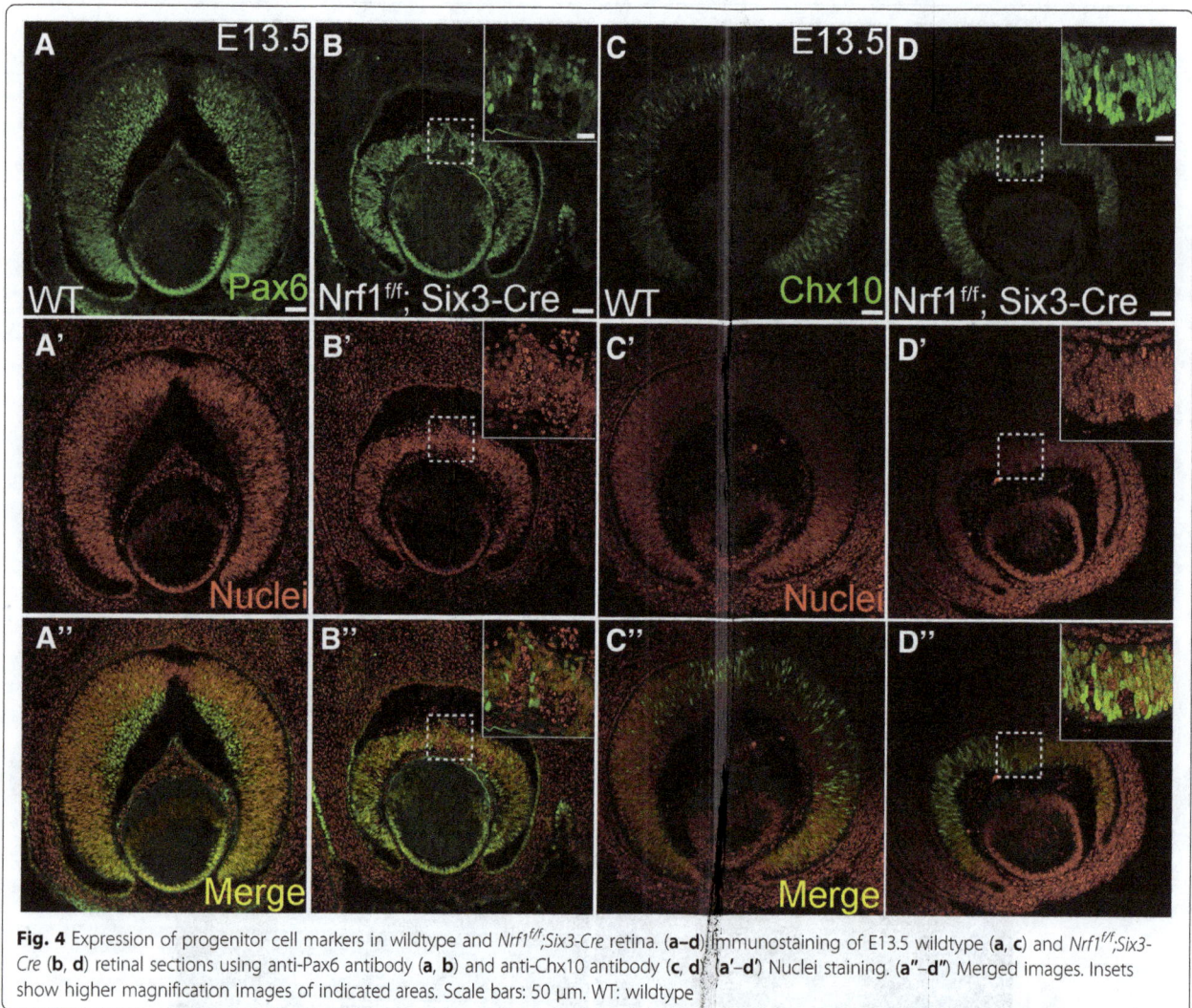

Fig. 4 Expression of progenitor cell markers in wildtype and *Nrf1^{f/f};Six3-Cre* retina. (**a–d**) Immunostaining of E13.5 wildtype (**a, c**) and *Nrf1^{f/f};Six3-Cre* (**b, d**) retinal sections using anti-Pax6 antibody (**a, b**) and anti-Chx10 antibody (**c, d**). (**a′–d′**) Nuclei staining. (**a″–d″**) Merged images. Insets show higher magnification images of indicated areas. Scale bars: 50 μm. WT: wildtype

wildtype and *Nrf1^{f/f};Six3-Cre* retinas to identify genes whose expression was affected in the *Nrf1^{f/f};Six3-Cre* retinas. The data discussed here have been deposited in NCBI's Gene Expression Omnibus [33] and are accessible through GEO Series accession number GSE101550 (https://www.ncbi.nlm.nih.gov/geo/query/acc.cgi?acc=GSE101550). The analysis revealed 488 downregulated and 595 upregulated genes in *Nrf1*-mutant retinas compared to control retinas. We first conducted qRT-PCR analysis on the 22 most affected genes (14 down- and 8 up-regulated) and found that their relative expression levels between the E13.5 control and *Nrf1*-mutant retinas are consistent with the RNA-seq output, demonstrating the reliability of the RNA-seq data (Fig. 7a). Using gene ontology for biological process analysis (GO-BP) of these gene lists, the top 5 categories of the downregulated genes are genes involved in nervous system development, neurogenesis, neuron differentiation, generation of neurons, and neuron projection development (Table 2), and the upregulated genes are involved

in cell adhesion, biological adhesion, regulation of cell projection, angiogenesis, and positive regulation of developmental process (Table 3).

Since severe RGC loss was observed in *Nrf1^{f/f};Six3-Cre* retinas, we expected that RGC gene expression would be reduced in *Nrf1*-deficient retinas. Atoh7 is a key factor essential for RGC development. RNA-seq data revealed that *Atoh7* expression was slightly reduced by ~ 19.5% in *Nrf1*-mutant retinas; however, Atoh7-expressing precursor cells can be readily detected in *Nrf1*-mutant retinas (data not shown), suggesting that the RGC loss phenotype is mainly due to a defective RGC differentiation process. Transcriptome analysis comparing Atoh7+ RPCs and Atoh7-negative cells in E13.5 has revealed 236 genes with altered expression levels [34]. We compared the 488 genes that are downregulated in *Nrf1^{f/f};Six3-Cre* retinas with the 236 genes enriched in Atoh7+ RPCs and found 121 common genes (Table 4). The majority of these genes were expressed in RGCs, including *Pou4f1*, *Pou4f2*, *Isl1*, and *Myt1*, which are known to be expressed in differentiating RGCs [35]. In addition, 41 genes

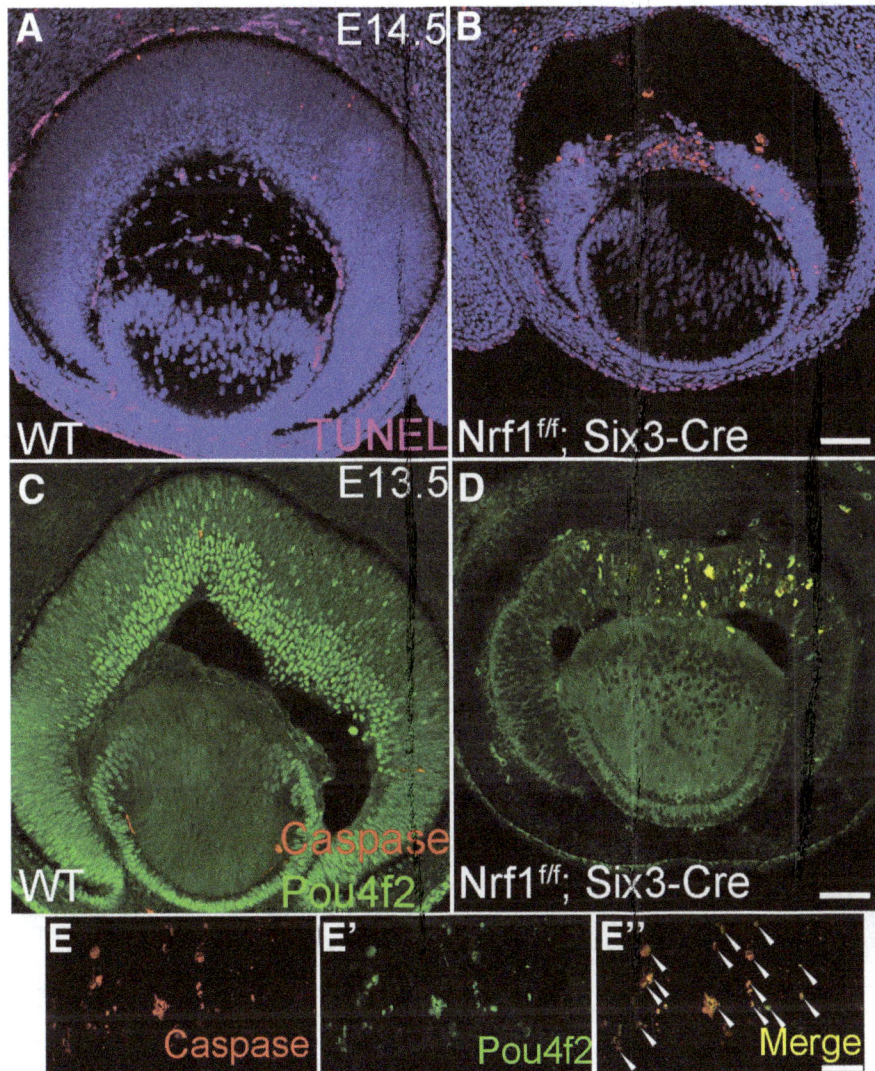

Fig. 5 Differentiated RGCs undergo apoptosis in *Nrf1^f/f^;Six3-Cre* retina. (**a**, **b**) TUNEL assay on E14.5 wildtype (**a**) and *Nrf1^f/f^;Six3-Cre* (**b**) retinal sections. (**c-e**) E13.5 wildtype (**e**) and *Nrf1^f/f^;Six3-Cre* (**d**, **e**) sections labeled with anti-Pou4f2 and anti-cleaved caspase 3 antibodies. (**e**, **e'** and **e"**) Higher magnification images of *Nrf1^f/f^;Six3-Cre* sections labeled with anti-caspase (**e**) and Pou4f2 (**e'**) antibodies. (**e"**) Merged images. Arrowheads indicate cells that are double positive for caspase and Pou4f2. Scale bars: 50 μm in **a** and **b**, 100 μm in **c** and **d**. WT: wildtype

involved in neuronal differentiation were found, such as *neurofilament light chain* (*Nefl*) and *neurofilament middle chain* (*Nefm*). We also compared the 488 downregulated genes in *Nrf1^f/f^;Six3-Cre* to the 49 significantly downregulated genes in the *Pou4f2^-/-^* retina [36] and found 18 common genes downregulated in both *Nrf1^f/f^;Six3-Cre* and *Pou4f2^-/-^* retinas (data not shown). Among them, 7 genes are enriched in Atoh7+ retinas. These results indicate *Nrf1* depletion affects RGC gene expression.

Defective axon outgrowth in *Nrf1^f/f^;Six3-Cre* retinas

To determine whether retinal neurons were defective in neurite outgrowth, we cultured retinal explants from E13.5 wildtype and *Nrf1^f/f^;Six3-Cre* embryos to examine axonal outgrowth. Consistent with the RNA-seq analysis, we found that retinal explants from *Nrf1^f/f^;Six3-Cre* embryos failed to form and extend well-bundled axons as in wildtype explants (Fig. 7b, c), indicating an important function for Nrf1 in regulating genes involved in neurite outgrowth.

Altered expression of genes associated with mitochondrial function and energy production in *Nrf1^f/f^;Six3-Cre* retinas

Because Nrf1 is a key regulator of nuclear-encoded genes involved in mitochondrial functions, we then tested whether genes involved in mitochondrial functions were altered in *Nrf1*-deficient retinas. By comparing the gene list in MitoCarta 2.0 [37, 38], we revealed a

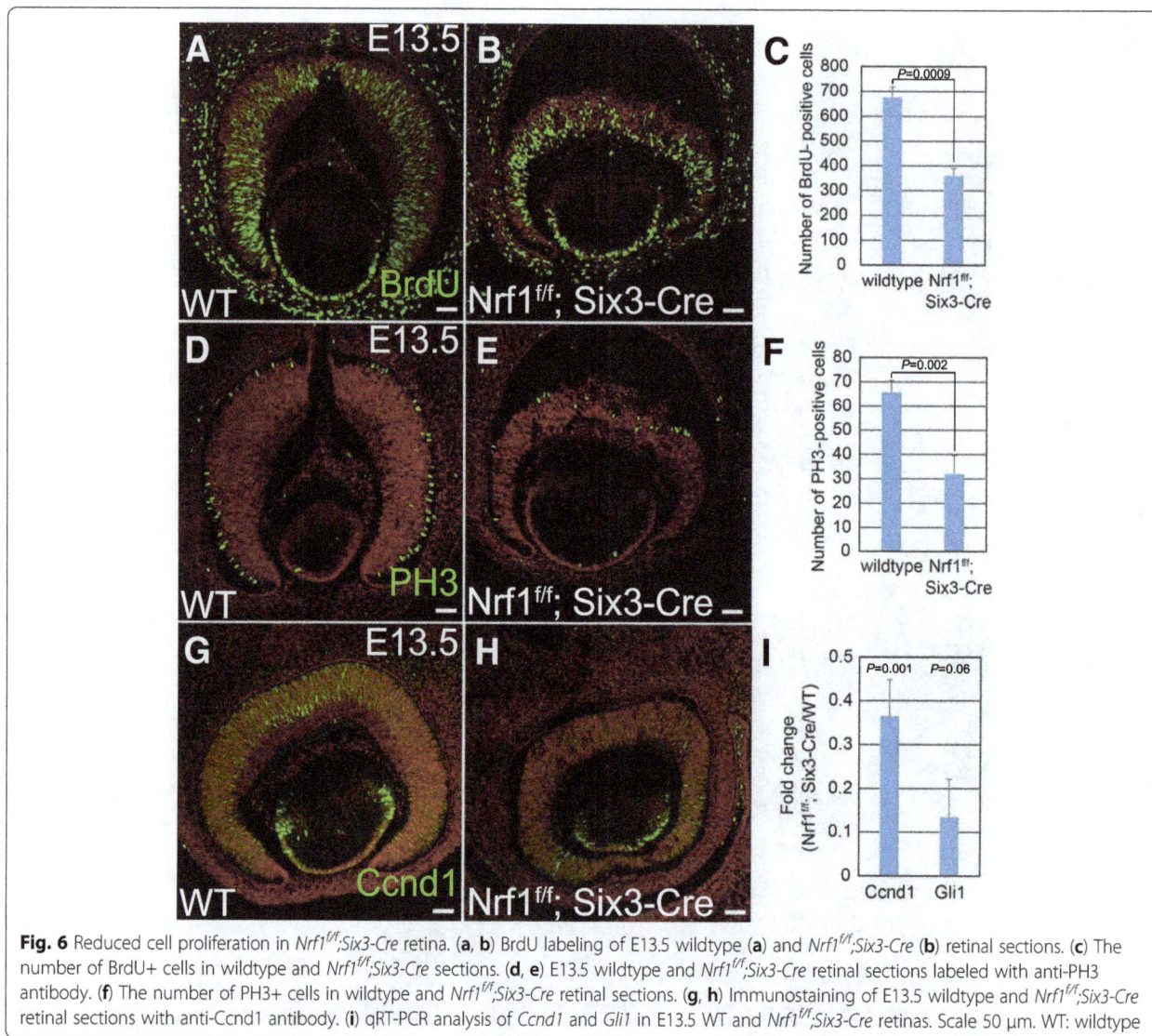

Fig. 6 Reduced cell proliferation in *Nrf1^{f/f}*;*Six3-Cre* retina. (**a, b**) BrdU labeling of E13.5 wildtype (**a**) and *Nrf1^{f/f}*;*Six3-Cre* (**b**) retinal sections. (**c**) The number of BrdU+ cells in wildtype and *Nrf1^{f/f}*;*Six3-Cre* sections. (**d, e**) E13.5 wildtype and *Nrf1^{f/f}*;*Six3-Cre* retinal sections labeled with anti-PH3 antibody. (**f**) The number of PH3+ cells in wildtype and *Nrf1^{f/f}*;*Six3-Cre* retinal sections. (**g, h**) Immunostaining of E13.5 wildtype and *Nrf1^{f/f}*;*Six3-Cre* retinal sections with anti-Ccnd1 antibody. (**i**) qRT-PCR analysis of *Ccnd1* and *Gli1* in E13.5 WT and *Nrf1^{f/f}*;*Six3-Cre* retinas. Scale 50 μm. WT: wildtype

subset of genes with altered expression levels in *Nrf1*-mutant retinas, and color-coded and mapped them to various functional subdomains in the mitochondria (Fig. 7d). In addition, 5 glycolysis genes with affected expression levels in *Nrf1*-deficient retinas were identified (Fig. 7e, q). For example, mRNA levels of *cytochrome c oxidase subunit 4i2* (*Cox4i2*) in *Nrf1*-mutant retinas were reduced to ∼44% of those in wildtype retinas. We tested mitochondrial respiratory activity in *Nrf1^{f/f}*;*Six3-Cre* retinas by examining the histochemical activity of COX. Intense COX activity was detected in RGCs (arrowhead in Fig. 7f) and the outermost area of retina where photoreceptor precursors resided (arrow in Fig. 7f). In contrast, COX activity was diminished to background levels in the *Nrf1^{f/f}*;*Six3-Cre* retina (Fig. 7g). We then performed qRT-PCR analysis on a small, selected set of these affected genes and found that the levels of expression of all of them

were consistent with the RNA-seq data (Fig. 7h, *Cox4i2*: $P = 0.038$, *Idh*: $P = 0.0001$, *Dna2*: $P = 0.003$, *Gdap1*: $P = 0.002$, *Shmt2*: $P = 0.003$, *Cpt1a*: $P = 0.0001$, *Sardh*: $P = 0.003$, *Ucp2*: $P = 0.013$, *Pmaip1*: $P = 0.048$, *Rab32*: $P = 0.014$).

Furthermore, we performed in situ hybridization (ISH) for several genes whose expression was either upregulated (*Cpt1a* and *Slc16a1*) or downregulated (*Idh1*, *Ldha*) in *Nrf1* mutants by RNA-seq analysis. *Cpt1a*, encoding carnitine palmitoyltransferase 1a, is involved in lipid transfer in mitochondria. In E13.5 wildtype retinas, *Cpt1a* was expressed at extremely low levels, barely detectable even by ultrasensitive RNAscope ISH (Fig. 7i). In *Nrf1*-mutant retinas, weak but detectable *Cpta1* transcripts were visible in the central retina (arrowheads in Fig. 7j). *Slc16a1*, encoding solute carrier family 16 (monocarboxylic acid transporters) member 1, is involved in lactate/pyruvate transport in mitochondria. *Slc16a1* was expressed in the peripheral retina in E13.5

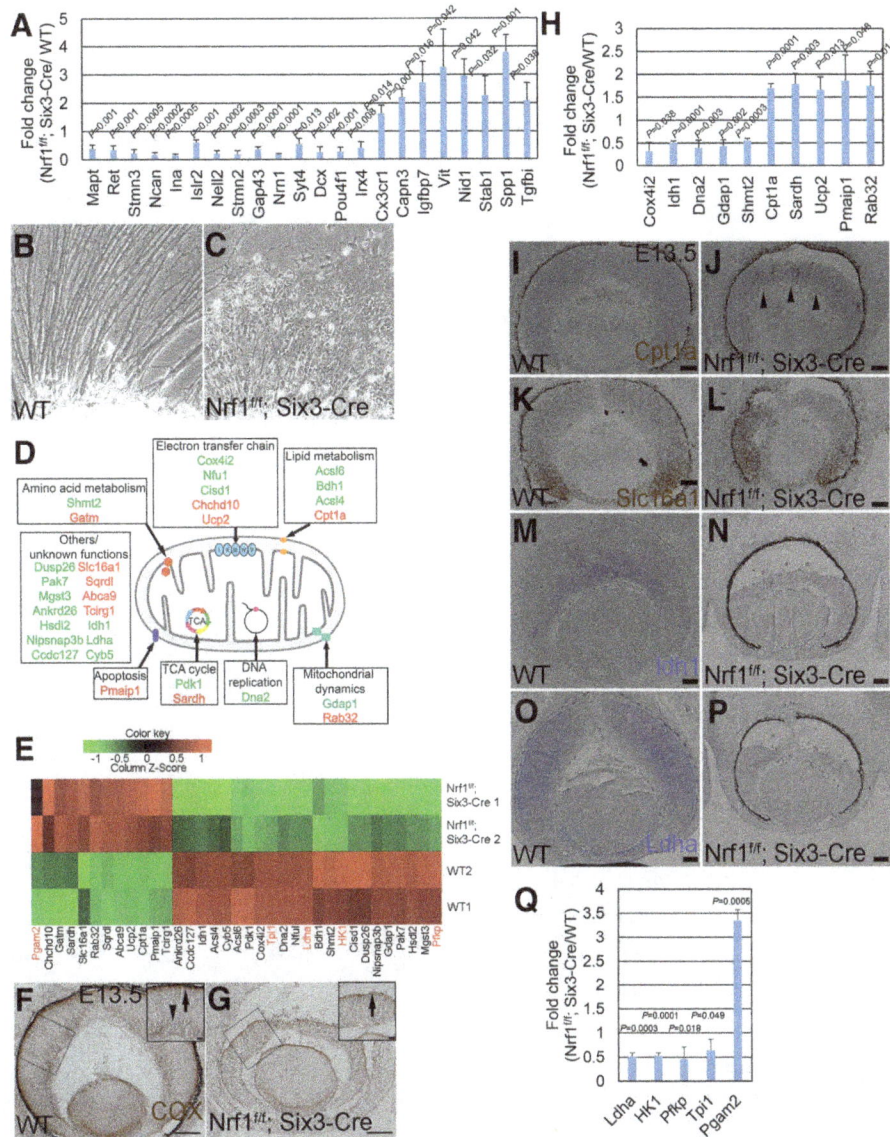

Fig. 7 RNA-seq identifies genes involved in neurite outgrowth, mitochondrial functions, and energy production in *Nrf1^{f/f};Six3-Cre* retina. (**a**) qRT-PCR analysis of the 22 top affected genes identified in *Nrf1^{f/f};Six3-Cre* retinas, confirming changes in mRNA expression detected by RNA-seq. (**b, c**) Representative images of retinal explant cultures from E13.5 wildtype (**b**) and *Nrf1^{f/f};Six3-Cre* (**c**) embryos. (**d**) Schematic mapping of mitochondrial and functional annotation of upregulated (red) and downregulated (green) genes in *Nrf1^{f/f};Six3-Cre* retinas detected by RNA-seq. (**e**) Heatmap from *Nrf1^{f/f}; Six3-Cre* RNA-seq showing 30 mitochondrial and 5 glycolytic genes whose expression changed. Mitochondrial genes are labeled in black, and glycolytic genes are labeled in red. (**f, g**) COX activity in E13.5 wildtype (**f**) and *Nrf1^{f/f};Six3-Cre* (**g**) retinas. Insets show higher magnification images of the indicated areas. Arrows indicate COX activities in the future photoreceptor layer; arrowheads indicate COX activities in ganglion cell layer. (**h**) qRT-PCR analysis of a subset of affected mitochondria genes between wildtype and *Nrf1^{f/f};Six3-Cre* retinas confirming changes of mRNA expression detected by RNA-seq. (**i–p**) In situ hybridization of mitochondrion-associated genes on E13.5 wildtype (**i, k, m**, and **o**) and *Nrf1^{f/f};Six3-Cre* (**j, l, n**, and **p**) retinal sections. Arrowheads indicate increased expression of *Cpt1a* in the central area of *Nrf1^{f/f};Six3-Cre* retina. (**q**) qRT-PCR analysis of glycolytic genes of wildtype and *Nrf1^{f/f};Six3-Cre* retinas. Scale bars: 100 μm in **f** and **g**, 20 μm in insets and 50 μm in **i–j**. WT: wildtype

wildtype retinas and upregulated in the central area of *Nrf1^{f/f};Six3-Cre* retinas (Fig. 7k, l). *Idh1*, encoding isocitrate dehydrogenase 1, was highly expressed in RGCs in wildtype retinas, whereas its expression was drastically reduced in *Nrf1^{f/f};Six3-Cre* retinas (Fig. 7m, n). *Ldha*, encoding lactate dehydrogenase A, which catalyzes the conversion of lactate to pyruvate in the glycolysis pathway, was highly expressed in RPCs in wildtype retinas but downregulated in *Nrf1^{f/f};Six3-Cre* retinas (Fig. 7o, p). To confirm the effect of *Nrf1* deletion on the 5 genes involved in the glycolysis pathway, we performed qRT-PCR analysis for these 5 glycolysis-associated genes (Fig. 7q, *Ldha: P* = 0.0003, *HK1:*

Table 2 Top 10 GO terms relevant to 488 downregulated genes in E13.5 *Nrf1^{f/f}; Six3-Cre* retinas

Rank	GO Category	GO ID	GO Term	Number of Focused Genes	P Value	FDR
1	GOTERM_BP_FAT	GO:0030182	nervous system development	156	1.70E-39	6.96E-36
2	GOTERM_BP_FAT	GO:0048666	neurogenesis	126	1.80E-35	3.80E-32
3	GOTERM_BP_FAT	GO:0031175	neuron differentiation	114	1.40E-34	2.00E-31
4	GOTERM_BP_FAT	GO:0048667	generation of neurons	119	8.00E-34	8.40E-31
5	GOTERM_BP_FAT	GO:0000904	neuron projection development	91	6.90E-33	5.80E-30
6	GOTERM_BP_FAT	GO:0048812	neuron development	99	7.00E-33	4.90E-30
7	GOTERM_BP_FAT	GO:0007409	neuron projection morphogenesis	68	5.00E-29	3.00E-26
8	GOTERM_BP_FAT	GO:0030030	cell morphogenesis involved in neuron differentiation	62	5.50E-26	2.90E-23
9	GOTERM_BP_FAT	GO:0019226	axonogenesis	55	2.70E-25	1.30E-22
10	GOTERM_BP_FAT	GO:0048858	cell projection organization	99	1.40E-24	5.90E-22
1	GOTERM_CC_FAT	GO:0030424	axon	54	4.00E-27	1.30E-24
2	GOTERM_CC_FAT	GO:0045202	synapse	57	5.30E-23	8.90E-21
3	GOTERM_CC_FAT	GO:0043025	neuronal cell body	58	1.40E-22	1.60E-20
4	GOTERM_CC_FAT	GO:0043005	neuron projection	51	5.70E-22	4.80E-20
5	GOTERM_CC_FAT	GO:0016020	membrane	243	9.40E-16	6.00E-14
6	GOTERM_CC_FAT	GO:0030425	dendrite	46	1.90E-15	1.10E-13
7	GOTERM_CC_FAT	GO:0010469	postsynaptic density	31	1.10E-14	1.70E-12
8	GOTERM_CC_FAT	GO:0030054	cell junction	53	1.80E-13	7.50E-12
9	GOTERM_CC_FAT	GO:0043195	terminal bouton	21	1.10E-12	4.10E-11
10	GOTERM_CC_FAT	GO:0030426	growth cone	24	1.80E-12	6.10E-11
1	GOTERM_MF_FAT	GO:0008092	cytoskeletal protein binding	52	2.40E-10	2.40E-07
2	GOTERM_MF_FAT	GO:0022836	gated channel activity	26	6.10E-08	2.70E-05
3	GOTERM_MF_FAT	GO:0005216	ion channel activity	29	2.60E-07	7.50E-05
4	GOTERM_MF_FAT	GO:0022838	substrate-specific channel activity	29	4.90E-07	1.10E-04
5	GOTERM_MF_FAT	GO:0015631	tubulin binding	23	7.60E-07	1.30E-04
6	GOTERM_MF_FAT	GO:0005261	cation channel activity	23	1.20E-06	1.80E-04
7	GOTERM_MF_FAT	GO:0022803	passive transmembrane transporter activity	29	2.00E-06	2.50E-04
8	GOTERM_MF_FAT	GO:0015267	channel activity	29	2.00E-06	2.50E-04
9	GOTERM_MF_FAT	GO:0019905	syntaxin binding	12	7.10E-06	7.80E-04
10	GOTERM_MF_FAT	GO:0017075	syntaxin-1 binding	7	1.10E-05	1.00E-03

GO gene ontology, *FDR* false discovery rate

$P = 0.0001$, *Pfkp*: $P = 0.018$, *Tpi1*: $P = 0.049$, *Pgam2*: $P = 0.0005$) and confirmed that expression levels of these genes were indeed affected as revealed by RNA-seq analysis. These data indicate that Nrf1 is important in regulating various metabolic pathways, including lipid metabolism, glycolysis, and oxidative phosphorylation, during retinal development.

Deleting *Nrf1* in rod photoreceptors caused complete rod degeneration

To investigate the in vivo function of *Nrf1* in differentiated neurons, we choose to use rod PRs as a model system, because rod PRs are the major neuronal type in the retina, and a large number of genetic mutations causing PR degeneration have been identified [39]. We bred a *Rho-iCre*

transgenic mouse line with mice harboring *Nrf1^{flox}* allele to delete *Nrf1* in the photoreceptor cells. Prior to 6 weeks of age, *Nrf1^{f/f};Rho-iCre* retinas did not show any sign of histological phenotype compared with wildtype retinas (Fig. 8a, b). Starting from 8 weeks, the thickness of the ONLs in the *Nrf1^{f/f};Rho-iCre* retinas was notably thinner than that in the control retinas (Fig. 8c, d), and the number of PRs decreased to 50% of that in wildtype retinas (Fig. 8m, 3 weeks: $P = 0.373$, 6 weeks: $P = 0.070$, 7 weeks: $P = 0.001$, 8 weeks: $P = 0.0001$). At 5 months, the ONLs had almost disappeared (Fig. 8e, f).

To determine whether cone photoreceptors were also affected in rod-*Nrf1*-mutants, we immunolabeled wildtype and

Table 3 Top 10 GO terms relevant to 595 upregulated genes in E13.5 *Nrf1^f/f; Six3-Cre* retinas

Rank	GO Category	GO ID	GO Term	Number of Focused Genes	P Value	FDR
1	GOTERM_BP_FAT	GO:0007155	cell adhesion	70	1.40E-22	5.00E-33
2	GOTERM_BP_FAT	GO:0022610	biological adhesion	70	1.60E-22	3.90E-33
3	GOTERM_BP_FAT	GO:0042127	regulation of cell projection	57	4.80E-15	3.70E-31
4	GOTERM_BP_FAT	GO:0001525	angiogenesis	23	2.40E-10	3.30E-31
5	GOTERM_BP_FAT	GO:0051094	positive regulation of developmental process	29	9.60E-10	7.80E-31
6	GOTERM_BP_FAT	GO:0007423	sensory organ development	31	1.00E-09	9.90E-31
7	GOTERM_BP_FAT	GO:0048514	blood vessel morphogenesis	27	1.20E-09	1.10E-29
8	GOTERM_BP_FAT	GO:0001568	blood vessel development	30	2.00E-09	1.10E-29
9	GOTERM_BP_FAT	GO:0009611	response to wounding	36	2.10E-09	1.20E-28
10	GOTERM_BP_FAT	GO:0001944	vasculature development	30	9.60E-09	1.20E-28
1	GOTERM_CC_FAT	GO:0031012	extracellular matrix	77	7.30E-29	4.10E-26
2	GOTERM_CC_FAT	GO:0005578	proteinaceous extracellular matrix	62	9.90E-27	2.80E-24
3	GOTERM_CC_FAT	GO:0044421	extracellular region part	231	9.50E-24	1.80E-21
4	GOTERM_CC_FAT	GO:0031982	membrane-bounded vehicle	206	5.60E-21	7.90E-19
5	GOTERM_CC_FAT	GO:0005576	extracellular region	245	9.40E-21	1.10E-18
6	GOTERM_CC_FAT	GO:0009986	cell surface	88	1.30E-20	1.20E-18
7	GOTERM_CC_FAT	GO:0044420	extracellular matrix component	33	4.50E-19	3.70E-17
8	GOTERM_CC_FAT	GO:1903561	extracellular vesicle	168	2.70E-18	1.90E-16
9	GOTERM_CC_FAT	GO:0043230	extracellular organelle	168	3.50E-18	2.20E-16
10	GOTERM_CC_FAT	GO:0070062	extracellular exosome	166	9.20E-18	5.20E-16
1	GOTERM_MF_FAT	GO:0005212	structural constituent of eye lens	16	9.60E-18	1.10E-17
2	GOTERM_MF_FAT	GO:0005515	protein biding	196	9.70E-14	1.60E-12
3	GOTERM_MF_FAT	GO:0005178	integrin binding	22	1.20E-12	1.80E-11
4	GOTERM_MF_FAT	GO:0005518	collagen binding	16	1.10E-10	4.50E-10
5	GOTERM_MF_FAT	GO:0005509	calcium ion binding	52	2.60E-09	5.00E-09
6	GOTERM_MF_FAT	GO:0005201	extracellular matrix structural constituent	12	1.90E-08	3.20E-08
7	GOTERM_MF_FAT	GO:0008201	heparin binding	21	2.10E-08	6.10E-08
8	GOTERM_MF_FAT	GO:0050840	extracellular matrix binding	10	6.80E-08	2.70E-07
9	GOTERM_MF_FAT	GO:0004872	receptor activity	21	1.90E-07	4.00E-07
10	GOTERM_MF_FAT	GO:0004714	transmembrane receptor protein tyrosine kinase activity	12	4.10E-07	6.10E-07

GO gene ontology, *FDR* false discovery rate

Nrf1^f/f;Rho-iCre retinas with rod-specific rhodopsin and cone-specific arrestin (CAR). At 6 weeks of age, rhodopsin was enriched in the outer segments (OSs) of rod PRs. We observed slightly upregulated rhodopsin in *Nrf1^f/f;Rho-iCre* retinas compared to wildtype retinas. There was no difference in numbers of CAR+ cells between control and mutant retinas. OSs and ISs were shorter in *Nrf1^f/f;Rho-iCre* retinas than in wildtype retinas (Fig. 8g, h). In 8-week-old retinas, rhodopsin+ PRs in *Nrf1^f/f;Rho-iCre* retinas were reduced to ~ 30% of wildtype retinas, while strong rhodopsin staining was detected in ONLs of *Nrf1^f/f;Rho-iCre* retinas (Fig. 8i, j). At this stage, the number of cone photoreceptor cells was also reduced in *Nrf1^f/f;Rho-iCre* retinas compared with wildtype retinas (Fig. 8i, j). In 5-month-old

mutant retinas, no rhodopsin+ PRs were detected, while the few remaining cone photoreceptors formed a single column in the ONLs without the distinguishable normal cone-shaped morphology (Fig. 8k, l). Since rod PRs are required for cone survival [40, 41], the cone degeneration in *Nrf1^f/f;Rho-iCre* retinas was likely secondary to rod PR degeneration. These results clearly indicate that *Nrf1* is essential for the survival of photoreceptor cells.

Abnormal mitochondrial morphology and impaired mitochondrial functions in *Nrf1^f/f;Rho-iCre* inner segments

To examine how *Nrf1* deletion affected mitochondria in rod PRs, we used transmission electron microscopy to

Table 4 Genes downregulated in *Nrf1^{f/f}*; *Six3-Cre* that are enriched in Atoh7+ cells

	Gene name	FC	Spatial expression
Transcription factor	Barhl2	−1.63	RGC
	Ebf1	−2.63	RGC
	Ebf3	−3.09	RGC
	Irx2	−2.35	RGC
	Irx3	−1.97	RGC
	Irx5	−2.43	RGC
	Irx6	−2.18	RGC
	Isl1	−2.43	RGC
	Myt1	−2.14	RGC
	Onecut3	−2.15	RGC
	Pou4f1	−2.62	RGC
	Pou4f2	−1.89	RGC
	Pou6f2	−2.28	RGC
	Ptf1a	−2.02	retina
	Tub	−2.38	RGC
Neuron differentiation	Actl6b	−2.2	RGC
	Adcyap1	−1.71	RGC
	Bsn	−2.27	RGC
	Celsr3	−2.35	RGC
	Cend1	−1.89	RGC
	Cntn2	−3.09	RGC
	Dcx	−2.87	RGC
	Dner	−2.08	RGC
	Dnm3	−1.7	unknown
	Dok5	−1.52	retina
	Dscam	−2.5	retina
	Elavl3	−1.52	RGC
	Elavl4	−2.67	retina
	Gap43	−3.02	RGC
	Gprin1	−2.51	retina
	Ina	−3.56	RGC
	Insc	−1.88	unknown
	Islr2	−3.49	RGC
	Kif5a	−2.66	RGC
	Klhl1	−1.76	RGC
	L1cam	−2.65	RGC
	Mapt	−4.37	RGC
	Mmp24	−2.32	RGC
	Myo16	−1.61	RGC
	Myt1l	−2.61	RGC
	Nefl	−3.67	RGC
	Nefm	−2.46	RGC
	Nell2	−3.49	RGC
	Nptx1	−1.63	RGC
	Nrn1	−2.91	RGC
	Ret	−3.75	RGC
	Scn3b	−2.77	RGC
	Scrt1	−2.11	RGC
	Sez6l	−2.56	RGC
	Slit1	−1.81	RGC
	Snap25	−2.41	RGC
	Stmn2	−3.26	RGC
	Stmn3	−3.65	RGC
	Th	−2.45	retina
	Tnik	−1.63	unknown
	Tubb3	−2.38	RGC
	Unc13a	−2.62	RGC
Others	1810041L15Rik	−2.49	RGC
	A930011O12Rik	−2.08	unknown
	Ajap1	−1.66	RGC
	Akap6	−3.68	RGC
	Apba2	−1.93	RGC
	Arg1	−1.55	RGC
	Atp1a3	−1.7	retina
	Cacna1b	−2.28	RGC
	Calb2	−2.96	RGC
	Ccnd1	−1.83	RPC
	Cda	−1.56	RGC
	Celf3	−2.19	RGC
	Celf5	−1.89	retina
	Chga	−1.65	RGC
	Chgb	−1.72	RGC
	Chst8	−1.95	RGC
	Coro2a	−1.85	RGC
	Crmp1	−2.78	RGC
	D930028M14Rik	−1.8	RGC
	Disp2	−2.82	RGC
	Dnajc6	−1.78	RGC
	Dusp26	−2.37	RGC
	Eya2	−1.59	RGC
	Fam155a	−1.76	RGC
	Fam78b	−1.73	unknown
	Fgf15	−1.61	RPC
	Gabbr2	−1.97	unknown
	Gdap1l1	−1.91	RGC
	Grm2	−2.67	unknown

Table 4 Genes downregulated in *Nrf1^{f/f}*; *Six3-Cre* that are enriched in Atoh7+ cells (*Continued*)

Gene name	FC	Spatial expression
Hecw1	−2.5	RGC
Hspa12a	−2.21	retina adult
Igfbpl1	−2.25	RGC
Iqsec3	−1.53	RGC
Kcnq2	−2.47	unknown
Mapk11	−1.75	RGC
Mtus2	−2.7	RGC
Nacad	−2.65	RGC
Nhlh2	−2.68	RGC
Nmnat2	−2.43	RGC
Nsg2	−3.26	RGC
Pak7	−2.04	unknown
Ppp2r2b	−1.8	RGC
Ppp2r2c	−1.88	unknown
Rab3c	−2.12	RGC
Rph3a	−2.58	RGC
Rtn1	−2.59	RGC
Rundc3a	−2.27	RGC
Rusc1	−1.92	RGC
Scg3	−2.94	RGC
Scn3a	−2.4	unknown
Sez6l2	−2.56	RGC
Slc17a6	−2.88	RGC
Smpd3	−1.97	RGC
Sncg	−4.74	RGC
Spire2	−1.54	RGC
Srrm3	−2	unknown
Sst	−2.14	RGC
Stk32a	−1.83	RGC
Svop	−2.17	RGC
Thsd7b	−2.45	unknown
Trim46	−1.56	unknown
Trp53i11	−1.79	RGC
Tubb2a	−2.35	unknown
Unc79	−2.31	unknown
Vwa5b2	−1.67	RGC
Xkr7	−1.69	unknown

488 downregulated genes in *Nrf1^{f/f}*; *Six3-Cre* retinas compared with 236 genes enriched in Atoh7+ retinal cells [34] identified 121 common genes. They are listed with official gene name, RNA-seq fold difference, and spatial expression pattern. Italicized gene names indicated downregulated genes in E14.5 Pou4f2^{−/−} retinas [35]. *FC* fold change

inspect the morphology of mitochondria in 6-week-old *Nrf1^{f/f}*;*Rho-iCre* retinas, when the ISs had not yet degenerated. We collected transmission electron microscopy images of ISs from wildtype *Nrf1^{f/f}*;*Rho-iCre* photoreceptors and analyzed with Fiji for the circularity of IS, size of IS, and number of mitochondria. We found that the ISs in *Nrf1^{f/f}*;*Rho-iCre* retinas were slightly wider than the wildtype ISs (Fig. 9a-c, $P = 0.002$), resulting in a ~ 40% increase in size compared to wildtype retinas (Fig. 9d, $P = 0.008$). The number of mitochondria in a *Nrf1^{f/f}*;*Rho-iCre* IS section was 2.5 times than that of wildtype (Fig. 9e, $P = 0.003$). The mitochondria in the *Nrf1^{f/f}*;*Rho-iCre* ISs were notably smaller and displayed a more rounded shape compared to mitochondria in the control retinas and were more widely distributed within the ISs (Fig. 9a, b). A cluster of mitochondria was observed near the outer limiting membranes while no mitochondria were present in the same area in the wildtype ISs (asterisks in Fig. 9b). We also noticed that the OSs in *Nrf1^{f/f}*;*Rho-iCre* photoreceptors were shorter than that of the controls (Fig. 9f, g).

Nuclear-encoded mitochondrial transcription factor A (Tfam/mtTFA), a key regulator of mitochondrial transcription and mitochondrial genome replication, is a known downstream target of Nrf1 [42]. To examine whether Tfam was affected in Nrf1-deficient rod PRs, we inspected Tfam expression by immunostaining and found that Tfam expression was abolished in *Nrf1^{f/f}*;*Rho-iCre* ISs whereas strong expression of Tfam was observed in the wildtype ISs (Fig. 9h, i). Abnormalities in the number, morphology, and distribution of mitochondria, and the downregulation of a key mitochondrial regulator Tfam in *Nrf1^{f/f}*;*Rho-iCre* ISs prompted us to determine whether mitochondrial function was compromised. We performed a COX assay to examine the mitochondrial enzymatic activity. As expected, COX activity was weaker in *Nrf1^{f/f}*;*Rho-iCre* ISs compared with wildtype ISs (Fig. 9j, k). Furthermore, we tested whether the expression levels of genes involved in mitochondrial fusion were affected in *Nrf1^{f/f}*;*Rho-iCre* retinas. Mitofusion-1 (Mfn1), Mfn2, and Optic Atrophy 1 (Opa1) are key mitochondrial proteins mediating mitochondrial fusion [43–45]. Deletion of *Mfn1* and *Mfn2* in skeletal muscle results in reduction of mtDNA and respiratory deficiencies [25]. We performed qRT-PCR to compare mRNA expression levels of *Mfn1*, *Mfn2*, and *Opa1* in 6-week-old wildtype and *Nrf1^{f/f}*;*Rho-iCre* retinas. In *Nrf1^{f/f}*;*Rho-iCre* retinas, *Mfn1*, *Mfn2*, and *Opa1* levels decreased to ~ 50% of wildtype retinas (Fig. 9l, *Mfn1*: $P = 0.0009$, *Mfn2*: $P = 0.0002$, *Opa1*: $P = 0.0002$). In addition, the copy numbers of mtDNA in *Nrf1^{f/f}*;*Rho-iCre* retinas was ~ 38% compared to that of wildtype retinas (Fig. 9m), consistent with Tfam's role as a major regulator of mtDNA replication and mitochondrial transcription.

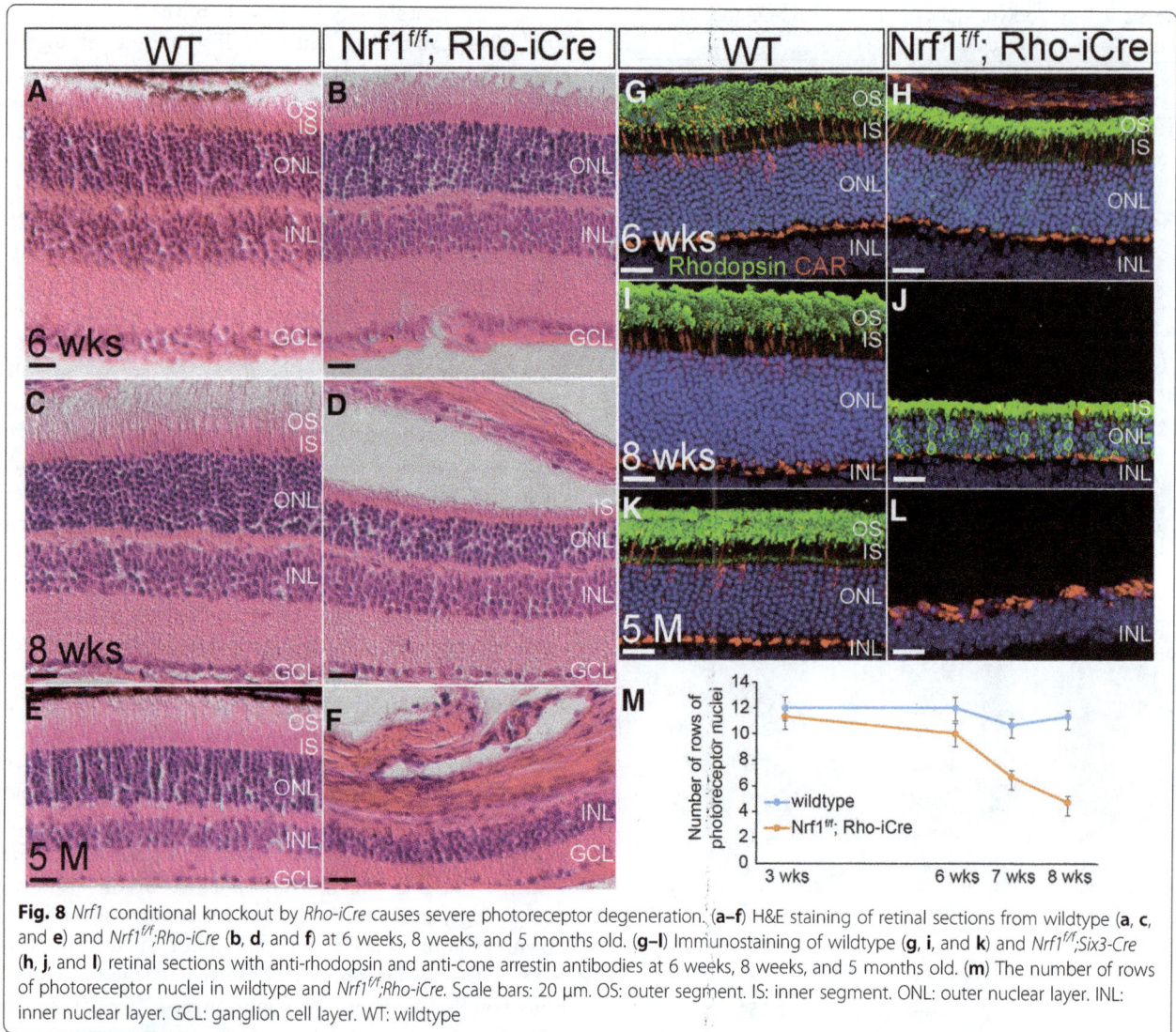

Fig. 8 *Nrf1* conditional knockout by *Rho-iCre* causes severe photoreceptor degeneration. (**a–f**) H&E staining of retinal sections from wildtype (**a**, **c**, and **e**) and *Nrf1^{f/f};Rho-iCre* (**b**, **d**, and **f**) at 6 weeks, 8 weeks, and 5 months old. (**g–l**) Immunostaining of wildtype (**g**, **i**, and **k**) and *Nrf1^{f/f};Six3-Cre* (**h**, **j**, and **l**) retinal sections with anti-rhodopsin and anti-cone arrestin antibodies at 6 weeks, 8 weeks, and 5 months old. (**m**) The number of rows of photoreceptor nuclei in wildtype and *Nrf1^{f/f};Rho-iCre*. Scale bars: 20 μm. OS: outer segment. IS: inner segment. ONL: outer nuclear layer. INL: inner nuclear layer. GCL: ganglion cell layer. WT: wildtype

Because *Nrf1^{f/f};Rho-iCre* retinas displayed severe rod degeneration followed by cone degeneration, we set out to track outer retina function using electroretinography (ERG). Dark-adapted wildtype and *Nrf1^{f/f};Rho-iCre* mice were exposed to calibrated light flashes for ERG recording. The scotopic a-wave amplitudes of *Nrf1^{f/f};Rho-iCre* mice were similar to those of wildtype before 5 weeks of age, began to decline at 6 weeks, and had completely diminished by 3 months (Fig. 9n, 4 weeks: $P = 0.3101$, 5 weeks: $P = 0.4548$. Six weeks: $P = 1.6988E-05$, 7 weeks: $P = 3.0756E-09$, 8 weeks: $P = 9.7899E-12$, 9 weeks: $P = 2.7743E-16$, 10 weeks: $P = 9.8167E-05$, 11 weeks: $P = 0.00497$). Photopic ERG b-wave amplitudes from light-adapted wildtype and *Nrf1^{f/f};Rho-iCre* mice were similar before 7 weeks of age, started to decline noticeably at 8 weeks, and were undetectable beyond 10 weeks (Fig. 9o, 5 week: $P = 0.7052$, 6 weeks: $P = 0.2420$, 7 weeks: $P = 0.4169$, 8 weeks: $P = 0.0522$, 9 weeks: $P =$

$8.0496E-05$, 10 weeks: $P = 0.0002$, 11 weeks: $P = 6.8768E-05$). These data indicate that PR functional loss precedes morphological defects and further demonstrate that deleting *Nrf1* in rod PRs causes abnormal mitochondria and impaired mitochondrial function, resulting in reduced outer retina activity and eventual complete photoreceptor loss.

Discussion

Functional mitochondrial biogenesis is essential for energy metabolism, calcium homeostasis, the biosynthesis of amino acids, cholesterol, and phospholipids, elimination of excessive reactive oxygen species, and apoptosis. Nrf1 was identified as a major transcriptional regulator that connects the regulation of nuclear-encoded genes and mitochondrial biogenesis and has been implicated in the pathology of several neurodegenerative diseases [16, 46]. However, little is known about its role in central

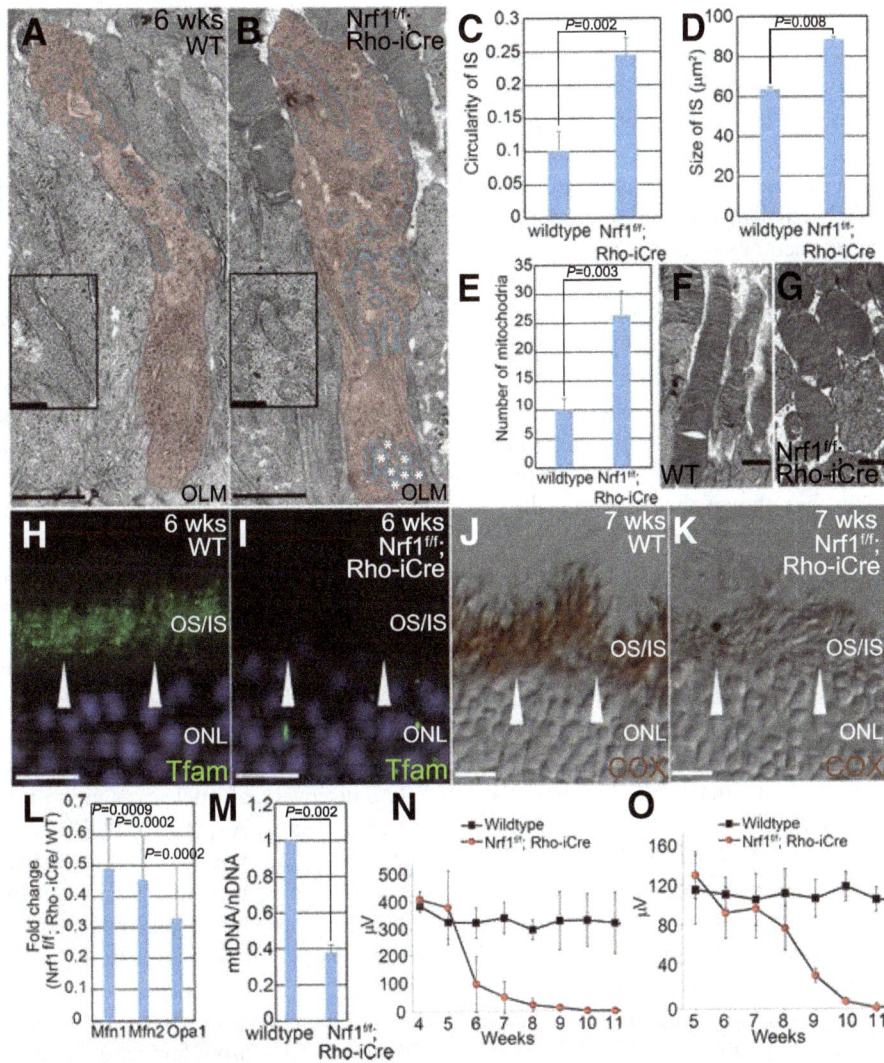

Fig. 9 Defective mitochondria and ERG response in *Nrf1^f/f^;Rho-iCre* retina. (**a**, **b**) Transmission electron microscopy (TEM) images of the inner segments of wildtype and *Nrf1^f/f^;Rho-iCre* photoreceptors. Inner segment is color-labeled in red, and mitochondria are circled in blue. Asterisks indicate clustered mitochondria near the OLM in *Nrf1^f/f^;Rho-iCre* ISs. Insets show higher magnification images of indicated areas. (**c–e**) TEM images were analyzed with Fiji for the circularity of ISs (**c**), size of ISs (**d**) and the number of mitochondria (**e**). **f**, **g** TEM images of the outer segments of wildtype (**f**) and *Nrf1^f/f^;Rho-iCre* (**g**) photoreceptors. (**h**, **i**) Immunostaining of 6-week wildtype (**h**) and *Nrf1^f/f^;Rho-iCre* (**i**) retinal sections with anti-Tfam antibody. Arrowheads indicate Tfam staining in ISs. (**j**, **k**) COX activity of 7-week wildtype (**j**) and *Nrf1^f/f^;Rho-iCre* (**k**) retinal sections. Arrowheads indicate COX activities in ISs. (**l**) qRT-PCR analysis of genes involved in mitochondria fusion of wildtype and *Nrf1^f/f^;Rho-iCre* retinas. (**m**) Mitochondria copy number of 6-week-old wildtype and *Nrf1^f/f^;Rho-iCre* retinas. (**n**, **o**) ERGs of wildtype and *Nrf1^f/f^;Rho-iCre* littermates under dark-adapted (scotopic, **n**) and light-adapted (photopic, **o**) conditions. Scale bars: 1 μm in **a**, **b**, **f** and **g**, 10 μm in **h–k**. OLM: outer limiting membrane. OS: outer segment. IS: inner segment. ONL: outer nuclear layer. WT: wildtype

nervous system development because of the lack of an appropriate animal model. To fill this gap of knowledge, we generated *Nrf1* conditional knockout mouse models and used these mouse lines to conduct the first comprehensive in vivo study to delineate various roles of Nrf1 in proliferating neural progenitor cells, newly differentiated RGCs, and terminally differentiated rod PRs.

Previous studies have provided evidence for *Nrf1*'s role in cell growth and proliferation. For example, a genome-wide ChIP-chip study has revealed that Nrf1

binds and regulates a number of E2F-targeted genes involved in DNA replication and repair, mitosis and chromosome dynamics, and metabolism [47]. A ChIP-seq study using SK-N-SH human neuroblastoma cells has revealed that Nrf1 target genes contain genes associated with cell cycle regulation [16]. Cyclin D1-dependent kinase phosphorylates Nrf1 and inhibits its transcriptional activity [48]. *Nrf1*-deleted mouse embryos die during the peri-implantation stage between embryonic days 3.5 and 6.5 in part due to reduced cell proliferation [20]. In our study, we showed that deleting *Nrf1* in the proliferating RPCs reduced cell proliferation indices in the developing retina. The few surviving RPCs that exited the cell cycle and differentiated into RGCs failed to migrate from the neuroblast layer to the ganglion cell layer. Using RNA-seq analysis, we discovered that genes involved in neurite outgrowth are significantly downregulated in *Nrf1*-deficient retinas. Consistent with the RNA-seq data, we demonstrated that neurite outgrowth activity was reduced in *Nrf1*-deleted retinal explants compared to control explants. Although we cannot exclude the possibility that the RGC migration and neurite outgrowth phenotypes seen in *Nrf1*-mutants are caused indirectly by defective mitochondria, a recent study on a RPC-specific knockout of Ronin, a key transcriptional regulator for mitochondrial gene expression and RPC proliferation, has shown that conditionally deleting Ronin in RPCs causes defective mitochondrial function and premature cell cycle exit in RPCs, leading to the generation of more RGCs [49]. Interestingly, these extra, newly differentiated RGCs survive and do not display any defects as observed in *Nrf1*-mutants, suggesting that Nrf1 directly regulates subsets of genes for RGC migration and neurite outgrowth during retinal development. Together this in vivo and ex vivo evidence supports the previous findings that *Nrf1* is essential for cell growth, proliferation, and neurite outgrowth [50].

In the developing mouse retina, the proliferating RPCs and the terminally differentiated retinal neurons adopt different metabolic pathways for energy production. In RPCs, aerobic glycolysis is a predominant way to produce ATP, whereas oxidative phosphorylation is utilized in differentiated neurons [51]. Such a transition is observed in many developmental systems, suggesting that the reconfiguration of energy metabolic pathways is likely intricately mapped onto the regulatory networks controlling cell cycle progression and differentiation. In *Nrf1*-mutant retinas, *Ldha*, which encodes the enzyme that converts pyruvate to lactate and generates the nicotinamide adenine dinucleotide (NAD+) necessary for aerobic glycolysis [52], was significantly downregulated. Additionally, several glycolytic pathway genes were also downregulated in *Nrf1*-mutant RPCs, suggesting that *Nrf1*-mutant RPCs may shift to utilize oxidative phosphorylation to produce energy. Consistent with this, pyruvate dehydrogenase kinase isoenzyme 1 (Pdk1), a metabolic checkpoint enzyme that inactivates pyruvate dehydrogenase, was also downregulated in *Nrf1* mutant RPCs. Hence the increased pyruvate dehydrogenase activity would enable pyruvate to enter the tricarboxylic acid cycle. Despite Nrf1's known function as a transcriptional activator, a subset of genes carrying out various mitochondrial functions, and *Pgam2*, encoding phosphoglycerate mutase which is involved in glycolysis, are upregulated in *Nrf1*-mutant retinas. Among

them we observed the upregulation of *Cpt1a* and *Slc16a1* in mutant RPCs. It is currently unknown whether Nrf1 functions as a repressor that directly modulates the transcriptional levels of these genes or if deleting *Nrf1* indirectly leads to reprogramming in their transcriptional regulatory regions in RPCs. Nevertheless, these data taken together implicate Nrf1 in a regulatory role to enable RPCs to alter their metabolic program and advance to a committed neuronal fate. Although the molecular mechanism regulating the metabolic transition is currently unclear, the potential roles of metabolites in epigenetic control at several levels, including DNA methylation/demethylation and histone modifications, could influence the cellular state and fate [53]. Interestingly, a recent study showed that in vivo Nrf1 binding to its target sites is inhibited by de novo DNA methylation, and active demethylation and obstruction of de novo methylation through the binding of methylation-insensitive transcription factors could de-methylate the nearby genome, thus restoring Nrf1 binding and transcriptional activity [54]. Future research is required to uncover and compare the in vivo occupancy of Nrf1 and the methylome in proliferating RPCs and differentiated rod photoreceptors to determine whether this novel mechanism is actively utilized by Nrf1 and co-regulators in regulating metabolic transition.

The discovery of nuclear-encoded mitochondrial transcription factor A (Tfam/mtTFA) as a target of Nrf1 established the regulatory link between nuclear and mitochondrial gene expression [42]. In wildtype retinal photoreceptors, Tfam was transported to and enriched in the ISs, but its expression was undetectable in 6-week-old *Nrf1*-mutant ISs, confirming that *Tfam* is a bona fide in vivo target of Nrf1. The small, rounded mitochondrial morphology and the increased number of mitochondria seen in the ISs in *Nrf1*-deficient rods suggest that the normal mitochondrial fusion/fission processes are defective in *Nrf1*-mutant rods. Continuous mitochondrial fusion and fission are essential for maintaining a functional mitochondrial network to ensure sufficient exchange of mitochondrial contents, which might be otherwise damaged under stressed environments [55, 56]. Several key molecular regulators for mitochondrial fusion, including *Mfn1*, *Mfn2*, and *Opa1*, were downregulated in 6-week-old *Nrf1*-deficient rods. Because loss of any of these genes causes defects in mitochondrial fusion, impairs mitochondrial oxidative phosphorylation, and eventually leads to apoptosis, it is likely that defective mitochondrial fusion in *Nrf1*-null rods is a major cause of rod degeneration. Consistent with this, *ewg*, the Drosophila homolog of *Nrf1*, has been shown to play a role in regulating mitochondrial fusion and expression of the *Opa1*-like gene during muscle growth in the fly [57]. It is noteworthy that mutations in human *OPA1*, a direct target of human NRF1, are the cause of autosomal dominant optic atrophy [58], which leads to retinal ganglion cell death. Thus, it would be interesting to test whether downregulation of *Nrf1* contributes to RGC death in several glaucoma animal models.

For mammals with vascular retinas, mitochondria in the rod PRs migrate toward and localize in the outer part of the IS (the ellipsoid) for oxygen supplied from choriocapillaris [59, 60]. In *Nrf1*-null rods, however, mitochondria were often trapped near the base of the outer limiting membrane. Proper mitochondrial trafficking within a neuron is critical for clearing the older, damaged components and delivering the new materials encoded by nuclear genes [61]. It is therefore conceivable that mitochondrial trafficking defects in *Nrf1*-mutant retinas also contribute to the death of rod PRs.

Many mouse models of inherited retinal degenerative disease have been established to understand disease mechanisms and design treatment strategies for human diseases [62, 63]. In our study, we showed that *Rho-iCre* efficiently and specifically deleted *Nrf1* in rod cells as early as P10; however, the *Nrf1*-deficient rods degenerated at a relatively slow pace. By 4 weeks of age, we did not find histological differences between the controls and mutants. The first sign of degeneration in rod-Nrf1 mutants was the slight thinning of the ONLs and OSs and the reduction of the scotopic a-wave amplitudes. It took approximately 3 months for the *Nrf1*-deficient rods to completely degenerate. The reason for such resiliency is currently unknown. It is possible that the glycolysis pathway partially supports the energy demand in *Nrf1*-deficient rods. Alternatively, other transcriptional factors and epigenetic memory may transiently compensate for the loss of *Nrf1* to maintain the expression of *Nrf1*-regulated downstream genes. Nevertheless, the slow, progressive rod degeneration found in this new mouse model offers a unique opportunity to investigate how defective mitochondrial biogenesis affects different cellular processes whose defects frequently link to retinal degeneration. Furthermore, mitochondrial function declines with age and is associated with age-related disorders and cell death. It is of interest to test whether any of components in the Nrf1-regulated mitochondrial biogenesis pathway are associated with aging retinas and whether they can be used as therapeutic targets for ameliorating retinal degenerative diseases.

Conclusions

Our findings confirm some of the known functions of Nrf1 that were previously revealed mainly through in vitro studies. Additionally, we uncovered a novel role for Nrf1 in metabolic reprogramming, although the degree to which Nrf1 is involved in this process during neural development remains to be determined. Our data also

shed new light on how dysfunctional mitochondrial biogenesis may be involved in various neurodegenerative diseases. For example, we have shown that RPCs and newly differentiated RGCs are very sensitive to *Nrf1* deletion. In contrast, rod PRs, an energy demanding neuronal type, are much more tolerant of *Nrf1* deletion. We also found that the terminally differentiated RGCs are less sensitive to *Nrf1* deletion (data not shown). This difference may be in part due to the varying roles of *Nrf1* in different cell types and developmental stages; however, it also suggests that different neuronal tissues and cell lineages may have diverse sensitivities to mitochondrial defects. Future experiments using tissue- and cell-specific *Nrf1* deletions will be critical in directly addressing how dysfunctional mitochondrial biogenesis contributes to the pathology and disease progression in neurodegenerative diseases.

Abbreviations

CAR: Cone-specific arrestin; Ccnd1: Cyclin D1; ChIP-seq: Chromatin immunoprecipitation sequencing; COX: Cytochrome c oxidase; ERG: Electroretinography; ES: Embryonic stem; ewg: Erect wing; FRT: FLP recombinase target; GCL: Ganglion cell layer; INL: Inner nuclear layer; IS: Inner segment; ISH: In situ hybridization; Mfn1: Mitofusion-1; Mfn2: Mitofusion-2; mtDNA: Mitochondrial DNA; nefl: Neurofilament light chain; nefm: Neurofilament middle chain; Nrf1: Nuclear respiratory factor 1; Nrf2/GABP: Nuclear respirator factor 2; OCT: Optimal cutting temperature; OLM: Outer limiting membrane; ONL: Outer nuclear layer; Opa1: Optic atrophy 1; OS: Outer segments; PARP-1: poly(ADP-ribose) polymerase 1; PGC-1: Peroxisome proliferative activated receptor gamma coactivator 1; PR: Photoreceptor; qRT-PCR: Quantitative reverse transcriptase PCR; RGC: Retinal ganglion cell; RNA-seq: RNA sequencing; RPC: Retinal progenitor cell; TEM: Transmission electron microscopy; Tfam: Mitochondrial transcription factor A; TUNEL: Transferase dUTP nick end label; WT: Wildtype

Acknowledgements

We are grateful to Dr. Yasuhide Furuta (RIKEN) for sharing the Six3-Cre mouse strain. We acknowledge the Genetically Engineered Mouse Facility, Kenneth Dunner, Jr. of the High Resolution Electron Microscope Facility, and the Sequencing and Microarray Facility at The University of Texas MD Anderson Cancer Center for their assistance, and Dr. Kimberly Mankiewicz at UTHealth for reading and editing the manuscript.

Funding

This work was supported by grants from the National Institutes of Health-National Eye Institute to C.-A.M. (EY024376), C.-K.C (EY013811, EY022228), and W.H.K. (EY011930) and from the National Institute of Allergy and Infectious Diseases to S.T. (AI057504). This work was also supported by National Eye Institute Vision Core Grant P30EY010608 (UTHealth).

Authors' contributions

TK, C-KC, SWW, ST, WHK and C-AM designed experiments. TK, C-KC, SWW, PP, ST and C-AM performed experiments. ZJ and JW conducted bioinformatics analysis. TK, C-KC, WHK and C-AM wrote the manuscript.

Ethics approval

All animal procedures followed the US Public Health Service Policy on Humane Care and Use of Laboratory Animals and were approved by the Institutional Animal Care and Use Committee at The University of Texas MD Anderson Cancer Center, Animal Welfare Committee at The University of Texas Health Science Center at Houston, and Animal Welfare Committee at Baylor College of Medicine.

Competing interests

The authors declare that they have no competing interests.

Author details

[1]Ruiz Department of Ophthalmology and Visual Science, McGovern Medical School at The University of Texas Health Science Center at Houston (UTHealth), 6431 Fannin St., MSB 7.024, Houston, TX 77030, USA. [2]Department of Ophthalmology, Baylor College of Medicine, 1 Baylor Plaza, Houston, TX 77030, USA. [3]Department of Systems Biology, The University of Texas MD Anderson Cancer Center, 1515 Holcombe Blvd, Houston, TX 77030, USA. [4]Department of Bioinformatics and Computational Biology, The University of Texas MD Anderson Cancer Center, 1515 Holcombe Blvd, Houston, TX 77030, USA. [5]Department of Biochemistry and Molecular Biology, The University of Texas MD Anderson Cancer Center, 1515 Holcombe Blvd, Houston, TX 77030, USA. [6]Present Address: Office of Scientific Review, National Institute of General Medical Sciences, National Institutes of Health, Bethesda, MD 20892, USA.

References

1. Wu Z, Puigserver P, Andersson U, Zhang C, Adelmant G, Mootha V, Troy A, Cinti S, Lowell B, Scarpulla RC, Spiegelman BM. Mechanisms controlling mitochondrial biogenesis and respiration through the thermogenic coactivator PGC-1. Cell. 1999;98:115–24.
2. Virbasius CA, Virbasius JV, Scarpulla RC. NRF-1, an activator involved in nuclear-mitochondrial interactions, utilizes a new DNA-binding domain conserved in a family of developmental regulators. Genes Dev. 1993;7: 2431–45.
3. Hock MB, Kralli A. Transcriptional control of mitochondrial biogenesis and function. Annu Rev Physiol. 2009;71:177–203.
4. Spiegelman BM. Transcriptional control of mitochondrial energy metabolism through the PGC1 coactivators. Novartis Found Symp. 2007;287:60–3 discussion 63-69.
5. Calzone FJ, Hoog C, Teplow DB, Cutting AE, Zeller RW, Britten RJ, Davidson EH. Gene regulatory factors of the sea urchin embryo. I. Purification by affinity chromatography and cloning of P3A2, a novel DNA-binding protein. Development. 1991;112:335–50.
6. DeSimone SM, White K. The Drosophila erect wing gene, which is important for both neuronal and muscle development, encodes a protein which is similar to the sea urchin P3A2 DNA binding protein. Mol Cell Biol. 1993;13:3641–9.
7. Becker TS, Burgess SM, Amsterdam AH, Allende ML. Hopkins N: not really finished is crucial for development of the zebrafish outer retina and encodes a transcription factor highly homologous to human nuclear respiratory factor-1 and avian initiation binding repressor. Development. 1998;125:4369–78.
8. Schaefer L, Engman H, Miller JB. Coding sequence, chromosomal localization, and expression pattern of Nrf1: the mouse homolog of Drosophila erect wing. Mamm Genome. 2000;11:104–10.
9. Evans MJ, Scarpulla RC. NRF-1: a trans-activator of nuclear-encoded respiratory genes in animal cells. Genes Dev. 1990;4:1023–34.
10. Scarpulla RC. Nuclear control of respiratory chain expression in mammalian cells. J Bioenerg Biomembr. 1997;29:109–19.
11. Gleyzer N, Vercauteren K, Scarpulla RC. Control of mitochondrial transcription specificity factors (TFB1M and TFB2M) by nuclear respiratory factors (NRF-1 and NRF-2) and PGC-1 family coactivators. Mol Cell Biol. 2005; 25:1354–66.
12. Dhar SS, Ongwijitwat S, Wong-Riley MT. Nuclear respiratory factor 1 regulates all ten nuclear-encoded subunits of cytochrome c oxidase in neurons. J Biol Chem. 2008;283:3120–9.
13. Dhar SS, Liang HL, Wong-Riley MT. Transcriptional coupling of synaptic transmission and energy metabolism: role of nuclear respiratory factor 1 in co-regulating neuronal nitric oxide synthase and cytochrome c oxidase genes in neurons. Biochim Biophys Acta. 2009;1793:1604–13.
14. Dhar SS, Ongwijitwat S, Wong-Riley MT. Chromosome conformation capture of all 13 genomic loci in the transcriptional regulation of the multisubunit bigenomic cytochrome C oxidase in neurons. J Biol Chem. 2009;284:18644–50.
15. Scarpulla RC. Nucleus-encoded regulators of mitochondrial function: integration of respiratory chain expression, nutrient sensing and metabolic stress. Biochim Biophys Acta. 2012;1819:1088–97.
16. Satoh J, Kawana N, Yamamoto Y. Pathway analysis of ChIP-Seq-based NRF1 target genes suggests a logical hypothesis of their involvement in the pathogenesis of neurodegenerative diseases. Gene Regul Syst Bio. 2013;7:139–52.
17. Hossain MB, Ji P, Anish R, Jacobson RH, Takada S. Poly(ADP-ribose) polymerase 1 interacts with nuclear respiratory factor 1 (NRF-1) and plays a role in NRF-1 transcriptional regulation. J Biol Chem. 2009;284:8621–32.
18. Herzig RP, Andersson U, Scarpulla RC. Dynein light chain interacts with NRF-1 and EWG, structurally and functionally related transcription factors from humans and drosophila. J Cell Sci. 2000;113(Pt 23):4263–73.
19. Hsiao HY, Jukam D, Johnston R, Desplan C. The neuronal transcription factor erect wing regulates specification and maintenance of Drosophila R8 photoreceptor subtypes. Dev Biol. 2013;381:482–90.
20. Huo L, Scarpulla RC. Mitochondrial DNA instability and peri-implantation lethality associated with targeted disruption of nuclear respiratory factor 1 in mice. Mol Cell Biol. 2001;21:644–54.
21. Ross JM. Visualization of mitochondrial respiratory function using cytochrome c oxidase/succinate dehydrogenase (COX/SDH) double-labeling histochemistry. J Vis Exp. 2011;e3266.
22. Wang SW, Mu X, Bowers WJ, Klein WH. Retinal ganglion cell differentiation in cultured mouse retinal explants. Methods. 2002;28:448–56.
23. Mao CA, Kiyama T, Pan P, Furuta Y, Hadjantonakis AK, Klein WH. Eomesodermin, a target gene of Pou4f2, is required for retinal ganglion cell and optic nerve development in the mouse. Development. 2008; 135:271–80.
24. Schindelin J, Arganda-Carreras I, Frise E, Kaynig V, Longair M, Pietzsch T, Preibisch S, Rueden C, Saalfeld S, Schmid B, et al. Fiji: an open-source platform for biological-image analysis. Nat Methods. 2012;9:676–82.
25. Chen H, Vermulst M, Wang YE, Chomyn A, Prolla TA, McCaffery JM, Chan DC. Mitochondrial fusion is required for mtDNA stability in skeletal muscle and tolerance of mtDNA mutations. Cell. 2010;141:280–9.
26. Li S, Chen D, Sauve Y, McCandless J, Chen YJ, Chen CK. Rhodopsin-iCre transgenic mouse line for Cre-mediated rod-specific gene targeting. Genesis. 2005;41:73–80.
27. Wong-Riley MT. Energy metabolism of the visual system. Eye Brain. 2010;2:99–116.
28. Furuta Y, Lagutin O, Hogan BL, Oliver GC. Retina- and ventral forebrain-specific Cre recombinase activity in transgenic mice. Genesis. 2000;26:130–2.
29. Wu F, Kaczynski TJ, Sethuramanujam S, Li R, Jain V, Slaughter M, Mu X. Two transcription factors, Pou4f2 and Isl1, are sufficient to specify the retinal ganglion cell fate. Proc Natl Acad Sci U S A. 2015;112:E1559–68.
30. Pan L, Deng M, Xie X, Gan L. ISL1 and BRN3B co-regulate the differentiation of murine retinal ganglion cells. Development. 2008;135:1981–90.
31. Zhang XM, Yang XJ. Regulation of retinal ganglion cell production by sonic hedgehog. Development. 2001;128:943–57.
32. Dakubo GD, Wang YP, Mazerolle C, Campsall K, McMahon AP, Wallace VA. Retinal ganglion cell-derived sonic hedgehog signaling is required for optic disc and stalk neuroepithelial cell development. Development. 2003;130:2967–80.

33. Edgar R, Domrachev M, Lash AE. Gene expression omnibus: NCBI gene expression and hybridization array data repository. Nucleic Acids Res. 2002; 30:207–10.

34. Gao Z, Mao CA, Pan P, Mu X, Klein WH. Transcriptome of Atoh7 retinal progenitor cells identifies new Atoh7-dependent regulatory genes for retinal ganglion cell formation. Dev Neurobiol. 2014;74:1123–40.

35. Mu X, Fu X, Beremand PD, Thomas TL, Klein WH. Gene regulation logic in retinal ganglion cell development: Isl1 defines a critical branch distinct from but overlapping with Pou4f2. Proc Natl Acad Sci U S A. 2008;105:6942–7.

36. Mu X, Beremand PD, Zhao S, Pershad R, Sun H, Scarpa A, Liang S, Thomas TL, Klein WH. Discrete gene sets depend on POU domain transcription factor Brn3b/Brn-3.2/POU4f2 for their expression in the mouse embryonic retina. Development. 2004;131:1197–210.

37. Pagliarini DJ, Calvo SE, Chang B, Sheth SA, Vafai SB, Ong SE, Walford GA, Sugiana C, Boneh A, Chen WK, et al. A mitochondrial protein compendium elucidates complex I disease biology. Cell. 2008;134:112–23.

38. Calvo SE, Clauser KR, Mootha VK. MitoCarta2.0: an updated inventory of mammalian mitochondrial proteins. Nucleic Acids Res. 2016;44:D1251–7.

39. Wright AF, Chakarova CF, Abd El-Aziz MM, Bhattacharya SS. Photoreceptor degeneration: genetic and mechanistic dissection of a complex trait. Nat Rev Genet. 2010;11:273–84.

40. Ait-Ali N, Fridlich R, Millet-Puel G, Clerin E, Delalande F, Jaillard C, Blond F, Perrocheau L, Reichman S, Byrne LC, et al. Rod-derived cone viability factor promotes cone survival by stimulating aerobic glycolysis. Cell. 2015;161:817–32.

41. Cronin T, Raffelsberger W, Lee-Rivera I, Jaillard C, Niepon ML, Kinzel B, Clerin E, Petrosian A, Picaud S, Poch O, et al. The disruption of the rod-derived cone viability gene leads to photoreceptor dysfunction and susceptibility to oxidative stress. Cell Death Differ. 2010;17:1199–210.

42. Virbasius JV, Scarpulla RC. Activation of the human mitochondrial transcription factor a gene by nuclear respiratory factors: a potential regulatory link between nuclear and mitochondrial gene expression in organelle biogenesis. Proc Natl Acad Sci U S A. 1994;91:1309–13.

43. Koshiba T, Detmer SA, Kaiser JI, Chen H, McCaffery JM, Chan DC. Structural basis of mitochondrial tethering by mitofusin complexes. Science. 2004;305:858–62.

44. Meeusen S, McCaffery JM, Nunnari J. Mitochondrial fusion intermediates revealed in vitro. Science. 2004;305:1747–52.

45. Meeusen S, DeVay R, Block J, Cassidy-Stone A, Wayson S, McCaffery JM, Nunnari J. Mitochondrial inner-membrane fusion and crista maintenance requires the dynamin-related GTPase Mgm1. Cell. 2006;127:383–95.

46. Taherzadeh-Fard E, Saft C, Akkad DA, Wieczorek S, Haghikia A, Chan A, Epplen JT, Arning L. PGC-1alpha downstream transcription factors NRF-1 and TFAM are genetic modifiers of Huntington disease. Mol Neurodegener. 2011;6:32.

47. Cam H, Balciunaite E, Blais A, Spektor A, Scarpulla RC, Young R, Kluger Y, Dynlacht BD. A common set of gene regulatory networks links metabolism and growth inhibition. Mol Cell. 2004;16:399–411.

48. Wang C, Li Z, Lu Y, Du R, Katiyar S, Yang J, Fu M, Leader JE, Quong A, Novikoff PM, Pestell RG. Cyclin D1 repression of nuclear respiratory factor 1 integrates nuclear DNA synthesis and mitochondrial function. Proc Natl Acad Sci U S A. 2006;103:11567–72.

49. Poche RA, Zhang M, Rueda EM, Tong X, McElwee ML, Wong L, Hsu CW, Dejosez M, Burns AR, Fox DA, et al. RONIN is an essential transcriptional regulator of genes required for mitochondrial function in the developing retina. Cell Rep. 2016;14:1684–97.

50. Wang JL, Tong CW, Chang WT, Huang AM. Novel genes FAM134C, C3orf10 and ENOX1 are regulated by NRF-1 and differentially regulate neurite outgrowth in neuroblastoma cells and hippocampal neurons. Gene. 2013; 529:7–15.

51. Agathocleous M, Love NK, Randlett O, Harris JJ, Liu J, Murray AJ, Harris WA. Metabolic differentiation in the embryonic retina. Nat Cell Biol. 2012;14:859–64.

52. Lunt SY, Vander Heiden MG. Aerobic glycolysis: meeting the metabolic requirements of cell proliferation. Annu Rev Cell Dev Biol. 2011;27:441–64.

53. Mathieu J, Ruohola-Baker H. Metabolic remodeling during the loss and acquisition of pluripotency. Development. 2017;144:541–51.

54. Domcke S, Bardet AF, Adrian Ginno P, Hartl D, Burger L, Schubeler D. Competition between DNA methylation and transcription factors determines binding of NRF1. Nature. 2015;528:575–9.

55. Westermann B. Mitochondrial fusion and fission in cell life and death. Nat Rev Mol Cell Biol. 2010;11:872–84.

56. Chen H, Chan DC. Emerging functions of mammalian mitochondrial fusion and fission. Hum Mol Genet. 2005;14 Spec No. 2:R283–9.

57. Rai M, Katti P, Nongthomba U. Drosophila Erect wing (Ewg) controls mitochondrial fusion during muscle growth and maintenance by regulation of the Opa1-like gene. J Cell Sci. 2014;127:191–203.

58. Alexander C, Votruba M, Pesch UE, Thiselton DL, Mayer S, Moore A, Rodriguez M, Kellner U, Leo-Kottler B, Auburger G, et al. OPA1, encoding a dynamin-related GTPase, is mutated in autosomal dominant optic atrophy linked to chromosome 3q28. Nat Genet. 2000;26:211–5.

59. Stone J, van Driel D, Valter K, Rees S, Provis J. The locations of mitochondria in mammalian photoreceptors: relation to retinal vasculature. Brain Res. 2008;1189:58–69.

60. Bentmann A, Schmidt M, Reuss S, Wolfrum U, Hankeln T, Burmester T. Divergent distribution in vascular and avascular mammalian retinae links neuroglobin to cellular respiration. J Biol Chem. 2005;280:20660–5.

61. Lovas JR, Wang X. The meaning of mitochondrial movement to a neuron's life. Biochim Biophys Acta. 2013;1833:184–94.

62. Chang B, Hawes NL, Hurd RE, Davisson MT, Nusinowitz S, Heckenlively JR. Retinal degeneration mutants in the mouse. Vis Res. 2002;42:517–25.

63. Veleri S, Lazar CH, Chang B, Sieving PA, Banin E, Swaroop A. Biology and therapy of inherited retinal degenerative disease: insights from mouse models. Dis Model Mech. 2015;8:109–29.

12

The *Trem2* R47H variant confers loss-of-function-like phenotypes in Alzheimer's disease

Paul J. Cheng-Hathaway[1,2,3†], Erin G. Reed-Geaghan[1†], Taylor R. Jay[1†], Brad T. Casali[1,2,3], Shane M. Bemiller[3,4], Shweta S. Puntambekar[3,4], Victoria E. von Saucken[2,3], Roxanne Y. Williams[2,3], J. Colleen Karlo[1], Miguel Moutinho[2,3], Guixiang Xu[3,4], Richard M. Ransohoff[5,6], Bruce T. Lamb[1,3,4,5] and Gary E. Landreth[1,2,3*]

Abstract

Background: The R47H variant of Triggering Receptor Expressed on Myeloid cells 2 (TREM2) confers greatly increased risk for Alzheimer's disease (AD), reflective of a central role for myeloid cells in neurodegeneration. Understanding how this variant confers AD risk promises to provide important insights into how myeloid cells contribute to AD pathogenesis and progression.

Methods: In order to investigate this mechanism, CRISPR/Cas9 was used to generate a mouse model of AD harboring one copy of the single nucleotide polymorphism (SNP) encoding the R47H variant in murine *Trem2*. TREM2 expression, myeloid cell responses to amyloid deposition, plaque burden, and neuritic dystrophy were assessed at 4 months of age.

Results: AD mice heterozygous for the *Trem2* R47H allele exhibited reduced total *Trem2* mRNA expression, reduced TREM2 expression around plaques, and reduced association of myeloid cells with plaques. These results were comparable to AD mice lacking one copy of *Trem2*. AD mice heterozygous for the *Trem2* R47H allele also showed reduced myeloid cell responses to amyloid deposition, including a reduction in proliferation and a reduction in CD45 expression around plaques. Expression of the *Trem2* R47H variant also reduced dense core plaque number but increased plaque-associated neuritic dystrophy.

Conclusions: These data suggest that the AD-associated TREM2 R47H variant increases risk for AD by conferring a loss of TREM2 function and enhancing neuritic dystrophy around plaques.

Keywords: TREM2, Neuroinflammation, Innate immunity, CRISPR/Cas9, Single nucleotide polymorphism, Alzheimer's disease

Background

Alzheimer's disease (AD) is accompanied by a robust inflammatory response [1]. However, until recently, it has been unclear whether myeloid cells (including brain-resident microglia and possibly infiltrating monocytes) actively contribute to AD pathogenesis and progression. Recent Genome Wide Association Studies have linked single nucleotide polymorphisms (SNPs) in inflammation-related genes to increased AD risk [2], including a SNP encoding the R47H variant in Triggering Receptor Expressed on Myeloid cells 2 (*TREM2*). The *TREM2* R47H variant not only constitutes one of the strongest single allele genetic risk factors for AD [3, 4], but also confers elevated risk for Parkinson's disease, amyotrophic lateral sclerosis, and frontotemporal dementia [5]. Furthermore, homozygous *TREM2* variants cause Nasu-Hakola disease, which is characterized by extensive white matter loss and frontotemporal-like dementia [6]. These genetic studies definitively demonstrate that myeloid cell perturbations can contribute to neurodegenerative disease. However, it remains unclear how the *TREM2*

* Correspondence: glandret@iu.edu
†Paul J. Cheng-Hathaway, Erin G. Reed-Geaghan and Taylor R. Jay contributed equally to this work.
[1]Department of Neurosciences, Case Western Reserve University, School of Medicine, Cleveland, OH 44106, USA
[2]Department of Anatomy and Cell Biology, Indiana University, School of Medicine, Indianapolis, IN 46202, USA
Full list of author information is available at the end of the article

R47H variant alters myeloid cell function to enhance disease risk.

In the brain, TREM2 is expressed exclusively by myeloid cells [7, 8] and has been implicated in a diverse range of myeloid cell functions [5]. A number of studies have investigated the role of TREM2 in AD pathogenesis using *Trem2* deficient mice. Myeloid cells accumulate around amyloid plaques in the AD brain, but the abundance of these plaque-associated myeloid cells is substantially diminished in AD mice lacking *Trem2*, consistent with its known roles in myeloid cell survival and proliferation. Yuan et al. postulate that the loss of plaque-associated myeloid cells promotes plaque expansion and damage to surrounding neurites in *Trem2* deficient mice [9]. In support of this hypothesis, *Trem2* deficient AD mice exhibit enhanced amyloid pathology at late stages in disease [10, 11] accompanied by increased plaque-associated neuritic dystrophy [9, 11, 12]. However, at early stages of disease progression, *Trem2* deficiency reduces amyloid burden [10, 13].

While these studies have elucidated some important aspects of TREM2 function in the context of AD, how these studies relate to disease-associated TREM2 variants has only recently begun to be investigated. In vitro studies have demonstrated that the TREM2 R47H variant reduces affinity for TREM2 ligand binding [9, 11, 14–18], and alters glycosylation [19, 20], leading to speculation that the TREM2 R47H variant may result in a loss of TREM2 function. The function of the R47H variant was recently assessed for the first time in vivo. Song et al. expressed the human *TREM2* R47H variant using a bacterial artificial chromosome (BAC) transgenic and found that the R47H variant could not rescue aspects of TREM2 function in AD mice lacking endogenous *Trem2* expression [21]. This study is in agreement with the in vitro data suggesting the *TREM2* R47H variant results in a loss of TREM2 function. However, because of the approach used in this study, it is unclear whether the loss of function phenotypes observed could be attributed to impairments in association of human TREM2 with mouse signaling pathways. In addition, these mice expressed eight copies of the *TREM2* gene and, because TREM2 overexpression has previously been associated with changes in microglial function and pathology [22], it is difficult to determine which phenotypes observed in this study were due to the TREM2 R47H variant or overexpression of the TREM2 protein. In the current study, we use a complementary approach that maintains endogenous regulation of *Trem2* expression. We address the critical question of how the R47H *Trem2* variant alters TREM2 function in vivo, including AD-associated myeloid cell responses, using AD mouse models in which CRISPR/Cas9 was used to knock the R47H variant into the endogenous mouse *Trem2* gene.

Using this model, we demonstrate that the *Trem2* R47H variant dramatically reduces TREM2 expression, compromising myeloid cell responses to AD-like amyloid pathology. Furthermore, we are the first to demonstrate that these myeloid cell changes with the R47H *Trem2* variant alter plaque structure to enhance neuritic dystrophy.

Methods

Contact for reagent and resource sharing
Further information and requests for resources and reagents should be directed to corresponding authors Gary Landreth (glandret@iu.edu) or Bruce Lamb (btlamb@iu.edu).

Experimental model
CRISPR/Cas9-mediated insertion of the SNP encoding the TREM2 R47H variant into the mouse *Trem2* gene was performed by injecting embryos with Cas9, short-guide RNA (sgRNA) and replacement oligo. The sequences are as follows: *Trem2* targeted region 3'-CGCAAGGCCTGGTG TCGGCAGCTGGGTGAG, sgRNA (antisense) 5'-CCAC AGCCGTCGACCCACTC, and replacement oligo 3'-CACA AGGCTTGGTGTCGGCAGCTGGGTGAG. The first codon in the replacement oligo corresponds to the SNP encoding the R47H variant, while the third codon corresponds to a silent mutation that ablates the protospacer adjacent motif (PAM) site, necessary for initial binding of CRISPR/Cas9. Using Sanger sequencing, mice from six different founder lines were identified to carry the SNP encoding the TREM2 R47H mutation in either heterozygosity or homozygosity. SNP-based genotyping (Thermo Fisher) was used to identify carriers in subsequent crosses using the following: forward primer: 5'-ATGTACTTATGACGCCTTG AAGCA, reverse primer: 5'-ACCCAGCTGCCGACAC, SNP reporter 1: 5'-CCTTGCGTCTCCC, SNP reporter 2: 5'-CCTTGTGTCTCCC.

In order to determine whether off-target mutations occurred with CRISPR/Cas9-targeting, genomic DNA was extracted using the DNeasy Blood and Tissue Kit (Qiagen, 69504) from F1 mice from four independently generated *Trem2* R47H founder lines (R104, R202, R506, and R1019) and independently maintained APPPS1-21; *Trem2*$^{+/+}$ or *Trem2*$^{+/+}$ mice. HiSeqX Sequencing was conducted with at least 30× coverage, 75% of bases above Q30 at 2×150 bp (Garvan Institute of Medical Research). Following alignment to the mouse reference genome (MM9), the presence of insertion and deletion mutations were assessed using the variant calling tools GATK-HC and Samtools Mpileup. Sequences are available via http://www.ncbi.nlm.nih.gov under BioProject accession PRJNA471261. CRISPR off-target prediction software (http://www.crispor.tefor.net) was used to determine potential off-target genes in exonic regions of chromosome 17 [23]. Mutations are shown for the only predicted off-target gene *Rab11fip3* and the CRISPR/ Cas-9 target (Additional file 1: Table S1). Additionally, in order to address dysregulation of *Trem*-like genes within 5 kb of the *Trem2* locus that may affect myeloid cell function [24], mutations were also assessed in *Treml1, Treml2,* and *Treml6.* Mutations were detected in lines R202 and R506 and these lines were therefore not used for the current study. However, no off-target mutations were identified in R104 or R1019 lines, consistent with the low rate of expected off-target mutations due to CRISPR/Cas9 targeting [25]. These two founder lines were maintained independently and mice from generations F1-F3 were used in the analyses presented here.

Trem2 deficient mice (*Trem2*^tm1(KOMP)Vlcg) with replacement of exons 2, 3, and part of 4 with *LacZ* were used to generate *Trem2*^+/+ *and Trem2*^+/− controls. WT *Trem2* was genotyped using the following primers: forward 5'-TGGTGAGCACACACGGT, reverse 5'-TGCTCCCAT TCCGCTTCTT and *LacZ* was genotyped using the following primers: forward 5'-ATCACGACGCGCGCTGTATC, reverse: 5'-ACATCGGGCAAATAATATC. *Trem2*^R47H and *Trem2*^tm1(KOMP)Vlcg mice were crossed into the APPPS1– 21 AD mouse model (kindly provided by Mathias Jucker) which expresses the Swedish APP mutation (KM670/ 671NL) and the L166P mutation in PSEN1 driven under the *Thy-1* promoter [26]. All mice used in this study were maintained on a C57BL6/J background. Both male and female mice were used in this study.

Method details

Tissue isolation

Following deep anesthetization with ketamine/xylazine, mice were perfused with ice-cold PBS, and brains removed. For immunohistochemistry, one hemisphere was drop-fixed in 4% PFA in PBS for 24–48 h, transferred and stored at 4 °C in 30% sucrose in PBS. After embedding in OCT Compound (VWR), 30 μm thick sections were obtained on a Leica CM 1950 cryostat and stored in cryoprotection buffer containing 30% sucrose, 1% PVP-40, and 30% ethylene glycol in 0.1 M phosphate buffer at − 20 °C until use.

For qPCR and ELISA studies, cortical and hippocampal regions from the other hemisphere were microdissected, snap frozen in liquid nitrogen, and stored at − 80 °C until proceeding to extraction. Tissue was homogenized in buffer containing 1% NP-40, 0.5% sodium deoxycholate, 0.1% SDS, 1:100 protease inhibitor cocktail (Sigma Aldrich, P8340). For Aβ extractions, brain homogenates were stored at − 80 °C. For qPCR, samples were stored in an equal volume of RNA-Bee (Amsbio, CS-104B) at − 80 °C until proceeding to RNA extraction.

Quantitative RT-PCR

RNA was isolated using phenol-chloroform extraction and a Purelink RNA Mini Kit (Life Technologies) with an on-column DNAse Purelink Kit (Life Technologies). RNA-to-cDNA conversion was conducted on 500 ng RNA with QuantiTech Reverse Transcription Kit (Qiagen) and qPCR was conducted using a StepOne Real Time PCR System with Taqman Assays (Life Technologies). Gene expression was normalized to *Gapdh* and *18s.* Relative gene expression is graphed as fold change, and ΔCT values were used for statistical analysis. The following genes were assessed: *Arg1* (Mm00475977_m1), *Fizz1* (Mm00445109_m1), *Ym1* (Mm00657889_mH), *Il-1b* (Mm00434228_m1), *Il-6* (Mm00446191_m1), *iNos* (Mm00440502_m1), *Tlr4* (Mm445273_m1), *Tnfa* (Mm443258_m1), and *Trem2* (Mm04209424_g1).

Immunohistochemistry

Sections were permeabilized with PBS containing 0.1% Triton X-100. Antigen retrieval was conducted using 10 mM sodium citrate, pH 6.0, with 0.5% Tween-20, except for TREM2 and CD45 for which Reveal Decloaker (Biocare Medical, RV1000) was used. Sections were exposed to antigen retrieval for 10 min at 95 °C, cooled for 20 min, and incubated in blocking buffer containing 5% normal goat serum, 0.3% Triton X-100, in PBS. Sections were incubated in primary antibodies diluted in blocking buffer overnight at 4 °C, washed, and incubated in the appropriate Alexa-Fluor-conjugated secondary antibodies at 1:1000 in blocking buffer for 1 h at room temperature (RT). To detect TREM2, sections were incubated in primary antibody for 48 h at 4 °C and secondary antibody for 6 h at RT. Nuclei were counterstained with DAPI, and slices were mounted and coverslipped with Prolong Gold (Thermo Fisher, P36930). Mouse on Mouse Blocking Reagent (Vector Laboratories, MKB-2213) was used for primary antibodies generated in mouse or rat at 1:1000. TREM2 (R&D Systems, AF1729), 6E10 (Bio Legend 9153– 005), IBA1 (Wako, 019–19741), Ki67 (Cell Signaling Technology, RM9106–50), CD45 (ABD Serotec, MCA1388), and n-APP (EMD Milliopore, MAB348) were used at 1:500, and ubiquitin (Thermo Fisher PA1–10023) was used at 1:2000. For dense core plaque staining, sections were washed with PBS, mounted, and stained with 1% *w/v* Thioflavin S.

Aβ₁₋₄₀ and Aβ₁₋₄₂ ELISAs

Extraction of Aβ species was conducted as described previously [27]. Briefly, cortical tissue-enriched homogenates were combined in equal volume with 0.4% diethylamine (DEA), subjected to ultracentrifugation, and supernatant containing the soluble protein fraction was neutralized with 0.5 M Tris-HCl. The pellet was dissolved in ice-cold 95% formic acid (FA), subjected to ultracentrifugation, and supernatant containing the insoluble protein fraction was neutralized in buffer containing 0.5 M Tris base, 0.5 M Na_2HPO_4, and 0.05% NaN_3. Fractions were stored at -80 °C until use.

For ELISA detection of $A\beta_{1-40}$ and $A\beta_{1-42}$, F8 Maxisorp Nunc-Immuno Module (Thermo Fisher) wells were coated with 6E10 ascites antibody (Bio Legend, SIG-39300) at 1:1000 diluted in 100 mM carbonate buffer, pH 9.6, overnight at 4 °C. Wells were washed with PBS containing 0.025% Tween-20 and blocked with 1% nonfat milk in PBS for 1 h at 37 °C. DEA fractions, FA fractions, and recombinant $A\beta_{1-40}$ (Bachem, 4014442) and $A\beta_{1-42}$ (Bachem, 4061966) protein standards were diluted in PBS containing 0.025% Tween-20 and 0.5% BSA and incubated overnight at 4 °C. Following incubation with anti-$A\beta_{1-40}$-conjugated HRP (Biolegend, 805407) at 1:2500 or anti-$A\beta_{1-42}$-conjugated HRP (Biolegend, 805507) at 1:1250 for 1 h at RT, $A\beta_{1-40}$ and $A\beta_{1-42}$ were detected using the Pierce TMB Substrate Kit (Thermo Fisher, 34021) and a BioTek Synergy HTX plate reader at 450 nm. Total levels of $A\beta$ were normalized to total protein levels in each fraction using the Pierce BCA Protein Assay Kit (Thermo Fisher, 23225) and values are represented as fold change to APPPS1; $Trem2^{+/+}$ animals.

Image acquisition
Epifluorescent images for percent area and plaque burden were acquired on a CTR5000 upright epifluorescent microscope (Leica). Confocal images for IBA1-positive cell number were obtained on a LSM 510 META microscope (Zeiss).

Quantification and statistical analysis
Quantification of all immunohistochemistry experiments was conducted by observers blinded to $Trem2$ genotype. Values within one image were averaged together and then averaged for each biological replicate. Data are graphed as the mean ± SEM.

Plaque-associated percent area
Plaque-associated percent area of TREM2 and CD45 were assessed using one medial and one lateral matched section per animal. Images were acquired from three cortical regions (motor, somatosensory, and visual cortex) and three hippocampal regions at 20× magnification. A circular ROI centered on 6E10-positive plaques was used to define regions for quantification. Images were manually thresholded and quantified using the Multi-measure ROI function in Image J (NIH).

Plaque-associated myeloid cell number
IBA1-positive cell number per plaque was assessed by acquiring confocal Z stacks 0.25 um apart in one medial and one lateral matched section per animal from three cortical regions (motor, somatosensory, and visual cortex) at 20× magnification. Stacks were collapsed into a single image and the number of IBA1-positive cell soma within the ROI centered around 6E10-positive plaques was scored using Image J.

Proliferating myeloid cell number
The total number of Ki67, IBA1-double positive cells within one medial and one lateral matched section per animal was manually scored.

Plaque burden
For plaque burden, every 12th sagittal section (10–12 sections per animal) was stained with Thioflavin S or 6E10. Images were acquired from three cortical regions (motor, somatosensory, and visual cortex) at 10× magnification and the dorsal hippocampus at 5× magnification per section. 6E10 and Thioflavin S-positive plaque number and area were quantified using the Particle Analysis function in Image J following manual thresholding.

Dystrophic Neurite Area & Plaque Size
For the analyses relating plaque size to dystrophic neurite area, images were acquired from three cortical regions (motor, somatosensory, and visual cortex) and three hippocampal regions at 20× magnification from one medial and one lateral matched section per animal. ROIs centered on 6E10-positive plaques were drawn individually for each plaque to include the total area of plaque-associated dystrophic neurites (ubiquitin and n-APP). Following manual thresholding, 6E10 immunoreactive plaque size and dystrophic neurite immunoreactive area for each respective ROI was quantified using the Particle Analysis function in Image J. Dystrophic neurite area was divided by 6E10 plaque size for each plaque. These values were averaged within each image and then across images for each animal to yield the results for dystrophic neurite area / plaque size.

Statistical analysis
Prism (Graphpad) was used for all statistical analyses. Grubb's test with a cutoff of $\alpha = 0.05$ was used to determine statistical outliers. Statistical significance was determined using a one-way or two-way ANOVA with Bonferroni post hoc analysis, with p-values less than 0.05 considered as significant. Each n represents a single biological replicate. Data shown are representative of three independent experiments.

Supplemental material
Additional file 2: Figure S1 details the experimental model, main findings in the manuscript across $Trem2$ R47H founder lines, $Trem2$ expression in non-AD transgene expressing animals, and $Trem2$ expression by sex. Additional file 3: Figure S2 details IBA1+ plaque number according to plaque size and the expression of a panel of inflammation-related genes. Additional file 4: Figure S3

shows changes in expression of genes related to Aβ production and Aβ species using ELISA. Additional file 1: Table S1 provides the variant calls for mutations in the off-target predicted gene *Rab11fip3*, *Trem2*, and *Trem--like* genes in mice derived from the first cross from *Trem2* R47H founders.

Results

To assess whether the *Trem2* R47H variant affects TREM2 expression, myeloid cell function and pathology in AD, we used CRISPR/Cas9 targeting to introduce the G→A single nucleotide polymorphism (SNP) encoding the variant in the endogenous mouse *Trem2* gene. Successful knock in of *Trem2* R47H was validated using Sanger sequencing (Additional file 2: Figure S1A) and whole genome sequencing did not identify any off-target mutations (Additional file 1: Table S1). Founder lines positive for the SNP were crossed to the APPPS1–21 AD mouse model [26], generating APPPS1–21;*Trem2*$^{+/R47H}$ mice. Mice from two founder lines were maintained independently and generations F1-F3 from both lines were used throughout this study. While working with early generations of these mice does increase the chance that off-target mutations are present, we observed no significant differences in phenotype between the two independent lines (Additional file 2: Figure S1B). These

mice were compared to APPPS1–21;*Trem2*$^{+/+}$ and APPPS1–21;*Trem2*$^{+/-}$ at 4 months of age.

Trem2 R47H impairs the myeloid cell response to amyloid pathology

To determine whether the *Trem2* R47H variant affects *Trem2* expression, we evaluated *Trem2* RNA levels in the brains of *Trem2*$^{+/+}$, and *Trem2*$^{+/R47H}$ mice and found a significant 42% decrease in *Trem2* RNA in *Trem2*$^{+/R47H}$ mice compared to *Trem2*$^{+/+}$ mice (Additional file 2: Figure S1C). This suggests that the *Trem2* R47H variant impairs TREM2 expression when endogenous regulation of its expression is maintained, an important consideration when interpreting previous in vitro studies in which *Trem2* R47H expression is induced at WT levels. A significant reduction was observed in *Trem2* expression in APPPS1–21;*Trem2*$^{+/R47H}$ mice compared to APPPS1–21;*Trem2*$^{+/+}$ mice (64% in the hippocampus), similar to the levels observed in APPPS1–21;*Trem2*$^{+/-}$ mice (Fig. 1b, Additional file 2: Figure S1D). This reduction in *Trem2* expression in the context of AD suggests that, in addition to reducing baseline *Trem2* expression, the *Trem2* R47H variant may also impair upregulation of *Trem2* expression in response to AD pathology.

As TREM2 protein expression in the AD brain is primarily upregulated on plaque-associated myeloid cells [9, 13], we

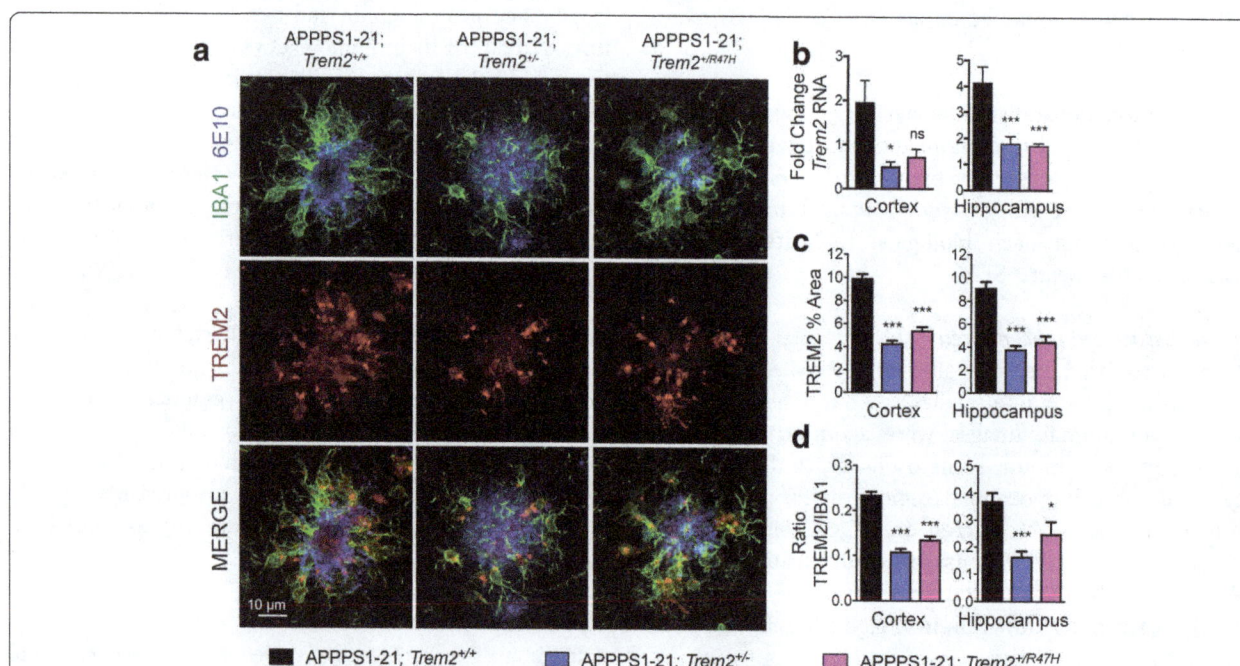

Fig. 1 TREM2 expression is significantly reduced in AD mice expressing the *Trem2* R47H variant. **a** Immunohistochemistry was used to identify myeloid cells (IBA1, green), plaques (6E10, blue), and TREM2 (red). **b** *Trem2* RNA levels were assessed in cortical and hippocampal lysates from APPPS1–21;*Trem2*$^{+/+}$ (*n* = 14), APPPS1–21;*Trem2*$^{+/-}$ (*n* = 13), and APPPS1–21;*Trem2*$^{+/R47H}$ (*n* = 10) mice. Data are presented as fold change normalized gene expression relative to *Trem2*$^{+/+}$ mice (*n* = 9). **c** Images were quantified to assess TREM2-immunoreactive area and (**d**) the ratio of TREM2 to IBA1 immunoreactive area around plaques (n = 10–13 mice / genotype). Data are presented as mean ± SEM. *$p < 0.05$; ***$p < 0.001$; ns - not significant. Representative images are from the cortex

next evaluated how TREM2 expression was affected in this cell population. Similar to the observed reductions in *Trem2* RNA, the *Trem2* R47H variant resulted in a significant reduction in plaque-associated TREM2 protein expression in APPPS1–21; *Trem2*$^{+/R47H}$ mice compared to APPPS1–21; *Trem2*$^{+/+}$ mice (45% reduction in the cortex and 51% reduction in the hippocampus), similar to the levels observed in APPPS1–21; *Trem2*$^{+/-}$ mice (Fig. 1a and c). This reduction in plaque-associated TREM2 protein expression could be due to a reduction in cellular TREM2 expression or due to a reduction in the number of plaque-associated myeloid cells. We found that altered TREM2 expression was not solely due to changes in the presence of myeloid cells around plaques, as TREM2 percent area was still significantly reduced when normalized to the myeloid cell marker IBA1 (Fig. 1d). Together, these data suggest that the *Trem2* R47H variant reduces TREM2 expression in the context of AD.

It has been consistently reported that *Trem2* deficiency leads to a specific reduction in accumulation of myeloid cells around plaques, while not significantly affecting non-plaque-associated myeloid cell number [9–13, 28, 29]. To assess whether the *Trem2* R47H variant confers a similar phenotype, we examined the number of IBA1 positive cells around plaques. We found a significant reduction in the number of plaque-associated myeloid cells in APPPS1–21; *Trem2*$^{+/R47H}$ mice compared to APPPS1–21; *Trem2*$^{+/+}$ mice (37% reduction in the cortex and 39% in the hippocampus), at levels comparable to APPPS1–21; *Trem2*$^{+/-}$ mice (Fig. 2a), which was consistent across plaque size (Additional file 3: Figure S2A). Thus, AD mice expressing the *Trem2* R47H variant exhibit an impairment in myeloid cell accumulation around plaques consistent with a loss of TREM2 function.

We previously reported that *Trem2* deficiency results in preferential loss of CD45^{hi}-expressing myeloid cells around plaques [10, 13]. Canonically, CD45^{hi} has been used to identify peripherally derived myeloid cells [30], though we cannot exclude the possibility that these cells represent a phenotypically distinct subset of reactive microglia. Regardless of their provenance, TREM2 has been shown to be required for accumulation of this cell population in the AD brain. We found a significant reduction in the area of high CD45 immunoreactivity around plaques in APPPS1–21; *Trem2*$^{+/R47H}$ mice relative to APPPS1–21; *Trem2*$^{+/+}$ mice (33% reduction in cortex, 21% in hippocampus), comparable to the reduction observed in APPPS1–21; *Trem2*$^{+/-}$ mice (Fig. 2b). Similar to what has been observed with *Trem2* deficiency, our findings suggest the *Trem2* R47H variant preferentially reduces accumulation of myeloid cells expressing high levels of CD45 around plaques.

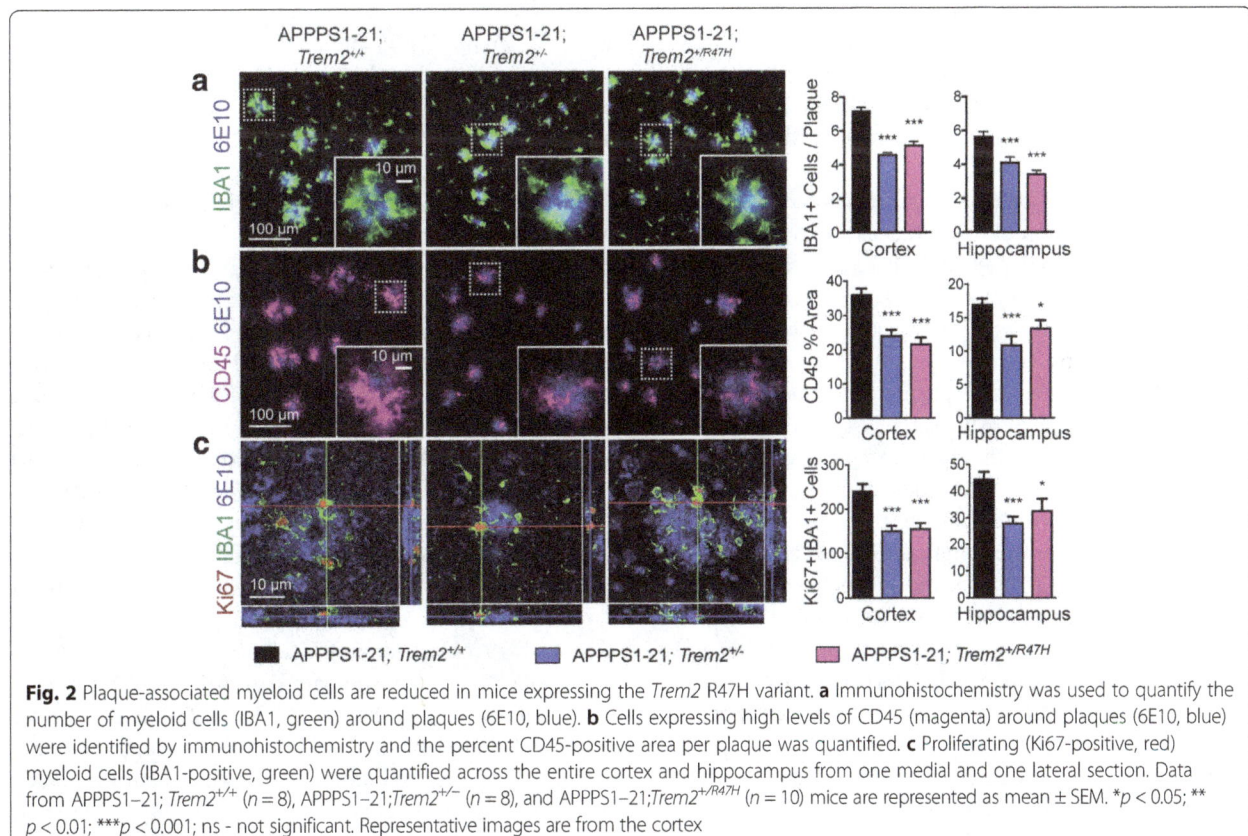

Fig. 2 Plaque-associated myeloid cells are reduced in mice expressing the *Trem2* R47H variant. **a** Immunohistochemistry was used to quantify the number of myeloid cells (IBA1, green) around plaques (6E10, blue). **b** Cells expressing high levels of CD45 (magenta) around plaques (6E10, blue) were identified by immunohistochemistry and the percent CD45-positive area per plaque was quantified. **c** Proliferating (Ki67-positive, red) myeloid cells (IBA1-positive, green) were quantified across the entire cortex and hippocampus from one medial and one lateral section. Data from APPPS1–21; *Trem2*$^{+/+}$ ($n = 8$), APPPS1–21;*Trem2*$^{+/-}$ ($n = 8$), and APPPS1–21;*Trem2*$^{+/R47H}$ ($n = 10$) mice are represented as mean ± SEM. *$p < 0.05$; ** $p < 0.01$; ***$p < 0.001$; ns - not significant. Representative images are from the cortex

The *Trem2* R47H variant could also contribute to reduced myeloid cell number around plaques by increasing myeloid cell death or decreasing myeloid cell proliferation [10, 12]. We only rarely observed cleaved caspase-3 positive myeloid cells across genotypes, so we were unable to assess how the *Trem2* R47H variant affected myeloid cell death. However, proliferation of myeloid cells, assessed using immunohistochemistry to identify Ki67+ IBA1+ cells, was reduced in APPPS1–21; *Trem2*$^{+/R47H}$ mice compared to APPPS1–21; *Trem2*$^{+/+}$ mice (35% reduction in cortex, 27% in hippocampus), similar to APPPS1–21; *Trem2*$^{+/-}$ mice (Fig. 2c). These findings suggest the *Trem2* R47H variant reduces plaque associated myeloid cells, at least in part, through reducing myeloid cell proliferation.

Recent work suggests that TREM2 is required for the myeloid cell-mediated inflammatory response in AD [28, 31]. Therefore, we wanted to assess whether the *Trem2* R47H variant would also impair the inflammatory response to AD pathology. Relative to controls, we detected a significant increase in the RNA levels of *Arg1*, *Ym1*, and *Fizz1*, similar to our previous observations in *Trem2* deficient AD mice (Additional file 3: Figure S2B) [13]. Interestingly, we also observed a significant increase in *IL-6* in mice with the *Trem2* R47H variant. None of these cortical gene expression changes were evident in APPPS1–21; *Trem2*$^{+/-}$ mice. There were also significant increases in *Fizz1* and *IL-6* in hippocampal lysates from APPPS1–21; *Trem2*$^{+/R47H}$ and APPPS1–21; *Trem2*$^{+/-}$ mice relative to APPPS1–21; *Trem2*$^{+/+}$ controls (Additional file 3: Figure S2C). A more detailed analysis will be required to fully address the role of *Trem2* R47H on inflammatory responses in AD.

Trem2 R47H reduces compact plaque number

Reduced accumulation of myeloid cells around plaques due to loss of TREM2 has previously been shown to result in changes in plaque deposition [10, 11, 13]. *Trem2* deficiency alters plaque burden in a disease progression-dependent manner, increasing plaque accumulation at advanced disease stages, but reducing plaque accumulation early in disease [10]. Consistent with earlier plaque deposition in the cortex relative to the hippocampus in APPPS1–21 mice, at 4 months of age, previous studies found a reduction in amyloid accumulation in the hippocampus with *Trem2* deficiency, but no significant differences in the cortex [13]. These changes occurred independent of changes in AD transgene expression, which we also found were unaltered in mice expressing the *Trem2* R47H variant [10] (Additional file 4: Figure S3A). In order to assess whether the *Trem2* R47H variant modifies total plaque burden, we measured the number and percent area of 6E10 positive plaques. While a modest increase in total cortical plaque number and percent area were noted in APPPS1–21; *Trem2*$^{+/-}$ mice compared to APPPS1–21; *Trem2*$^{+/+}$ mice,

no difference in 6E10 positive plaque number or percent area was observed in APPPS1–21; *Trem2*$^{+/R47H}$ mice (Fig. 3a). Previous studies have demonstrated that *Trem2* deficient mice exhibit a shift in plaque structure, from compact, fibrillar plaques to diffuse plaques [9]. To determine whether the *Trem2* R47H variant affected the relative abundance of these different plaque types, we quantified the number and percent area of fibrillar, thioflavin S positive plaques. A significant reduction in thioflavin S positive plaque number (31%) and percent area (36%) were observed in the hippocampus of APPPS1–21; *Trem2*$^{+/R47H}$ mice compared to APPPS1–21; *Trem2*$^{+/+}$ mice (Fig. 3b).

To assess whether this shift in plaque morphology was due to alterations in the presence of different Aβ species, we used ELISAs to assess soluble and insoluble Aβ$_{1–40}$ and Aβ$_{1–42}$. We observed a significant decrease in soluble Aβ$_{1–40}$ in the cortex of APPPS1–21; *Trem2*$^{+/R47H}$ mice compared to APPPS1–21; *Trem2*$^{+/+}$ mice (Additional file 4: Figure S3B), and thus an increased ratio of Aβ42/40 (Additional file 4: Figure S3C) in APPPS1–21; *Trem2*$^{+/R47H}$ mice relative to APPPS1–21; *Trem2*$^{+/+}$ controls. We also observed a significant increase in soluble Aβ$_{1–40}$ in the hippocampus of APPPS1–21; *Trem2*$^{+/-}$ mice compared to APPPS1–21; *Trem2*$^{+/+}$ mice but no significant changes in other Aβ species in mice expressing the *Trem2* R47H variant. Together, these data suggest that changes in the relative abundance of these species are not the primary contributor to changes in plaque structure in mice with the *Trem2* R47H variant. However, fibrillar plaques are specifically reduced in mice bearing the *Trem2* R47H variant, consistent with results from *Trem2* deficient mice and human carriers of *TREM2* R47H [9].

Trem2 R47H significantly increases plaque-associated neuritic dystrophy

Damage to axons and dendrites in the vicinity of plaques, termed neuritic dystrophy, is thought to contribute to cognitive impairment in AD [32] and is reported to be enhanced in AD mice lacking *Trem2* and humans carrying an R47H allele [9, 12]. To determine whether the changes in plaque structure observed in AD mice with the *Trem2* R47H variant similarly affected neuritic dystrophy, we next analyzed plaque-associated N-terminal APP (n-APP), which is elevated in dystrophic neurites due to impaired anterograde transport, and ubiquitin, which is increased in response to cellular stress and protein dyshomeostasis. A significant 33% increase in ubiquitin percent area around plaques was observed in the hippocampus of APPPS1–21; *Trem2*$^{+/R47H}$ mice compared to APPPS1–21; *Trem2*$^{+/+}$ mice, similar to levels in APPPS1–21; *Trem2*$^{+/-}$ mice (Fig. 4a). Comparable trends in neuritic dystrophy were observed using the additional dystrophic neurite marker n-APP, though the changes with *Trem2* genotype were only significant in the cortex of APPPS1–21; *Trem2*$^{+/-}$ mice

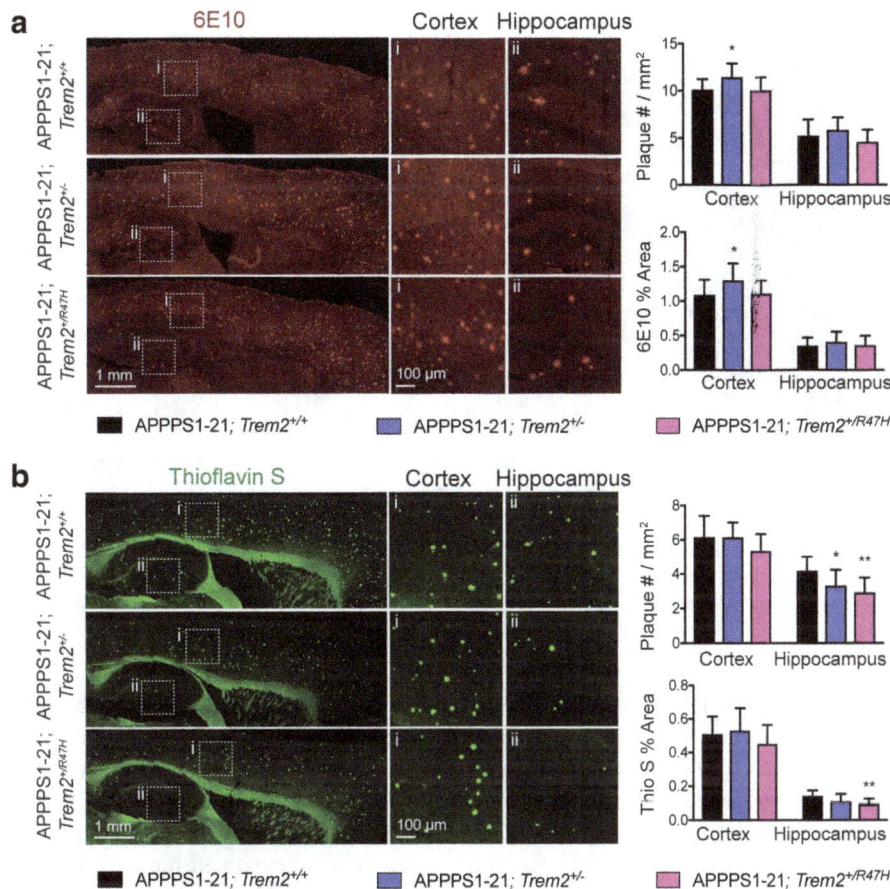

Fig. 3 Compact plaque number is specifically reduced in mice expressing the *Trem2* R47H variant. Quantification of plaque burden was performed in APPPS1–21;*Trem2$^{+/+}$* ($n = 15$), APPPS1–21;*Trem2$^{+/-}$* ($n = 13$), and APPPS1–21;*Trem2$^{+/R47H}$* ($n = 10$) mice by (**a**) measuring 6E10 (red) and (**b**) Thioflavin S (green) positive plaque number and percent area across three cortical and one hippocampal region from 10 to 12 sagittal sections. Higher magnification of cortical (i) and hippocampal (ii) regions are shown. Data are presented as mean ± SEM. *$p < 0.05$; **$p < 0.01$

relative to APPPS1–21;*Trem2$^{+/+}$* mice (Fig. 4b). The ratio of ubiquitin area to plaque size was significantly increased in APPPS1–21;*Trem2$^{+/R47H}$* mice compared to APPPS1–21;*Trem2$^{+/+}$* mice (Fig. 4c). Interestingly, the correlation between plaque size and ubiquitin positive area was preserved across genotypes (Fig. 4d and e) and there was a trend toward an increase in the slope of the best fit line between ubiquitin positive area and plaque size in mice with the *Trem2* R47H variant (Fig. 4f). This indicates that larger plaques may be even more strongly affected by the loss of TREM2 function. Together, our data demonstrate overall enhanced neuritic dystrophy with the *Trem2* R47H variant, when normalized to plaque size, suggesting a possible mechanism by which the variant could increase synaptic loss and neuronal dysfunction, and ultimately confer AD risk.

Discussion

In order to investigate how the *Trem2* R47H variant affects TREM2 function and AD pathology, we developed a CRISPR/Cas9 knock-in of the R47H variant into the mouse

Trem2 gene. Because this approach maintains endogenous regulation of TREM2 expression, we were able to determine that expression of one copy of the R47H variant reduces *Trem2* expression in a wild-type background and further impairs upregulation of *Trem2* expression in an AD mouse model. This finding differs from a previous study that found no changes in TREM2 expression in postmortem tissue from human AD patients heterozygous for the *TREM2* R47H variant [33]. While many factors could contribute to this discrepancy, *Trem2* levels are known to change throughout disease progression [13], and our study evaluates *Trem2* changes at a relatively early stage in pathology in the APPPS1–21 model, while the postmortem samples are from humans at a late stage in disease. It will be interesting to assess in future studies whether *Trem2* levels are differentially affected by the R47H variant throughout disease progression.

Importantly, this finding also merits consideration when interpreting studies of TREM2 R47H function in vitro, which have all used systems where *Trem2* R47H

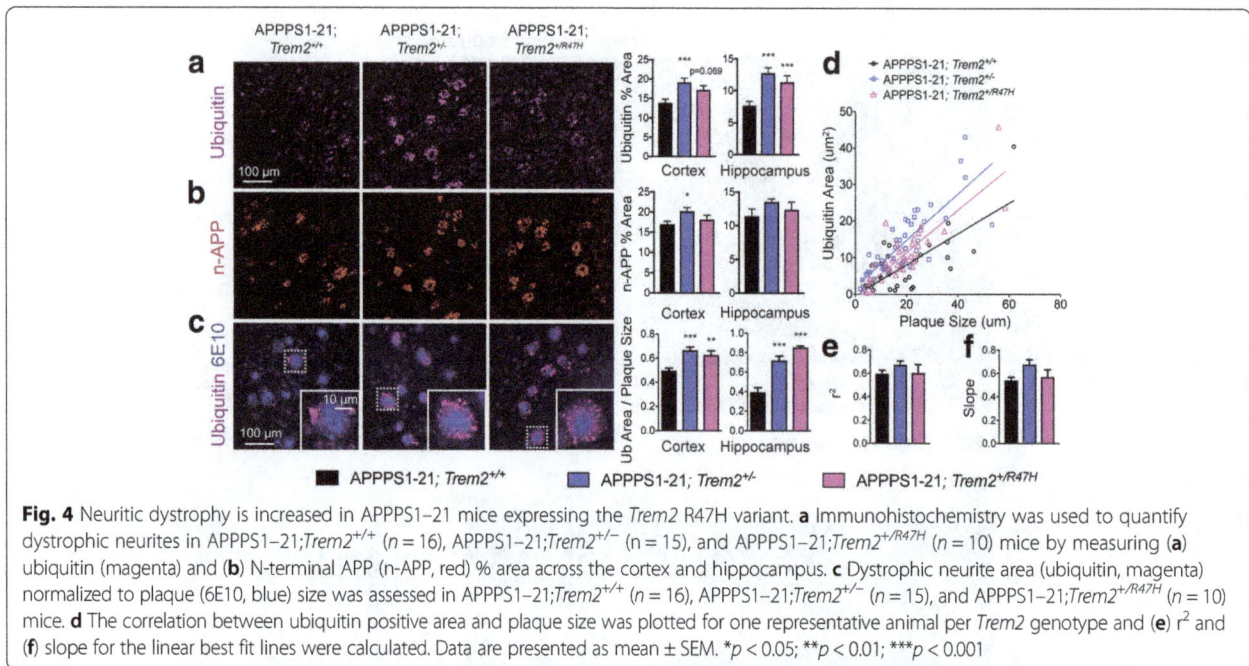

Fig. 4 Neuritic dystrophy is increased in APPPS1–21 mice expressing the *Trem2* R47H variant. **a** Immunohistochemistry was used to quantify dystrophic neurites in APPPS1–21;*Trem2*$^{+/+}$ ($n = 16$), APPPS1–21;*Trem2*$^{+/-}$ (n = 15), and APPPS1–21;*Trem2*$^{+/R47H}$ ($n = 10$) mice by measuring (**a**) ubiquitin (magenta) and (**b**) N-terminal APP (n-APP, red) % area across the cortex and hippocampus. **c** Dystrophic neurite area (ubiquitin, magenta) normalized to plaque (6E10, blue) size was assessed in APPPS1–21;*Trem2*$^{+/+}$ ($n = 16$), APPPS1–21;*Trem2*$^{+/-}$ ($n = 15$), and APPPS1–21;*Trem2*$^{+/R47H}$ ($n = 10$) mice. **d** The correlation between ubiquitin positive area and plaque size was plotted for one representative animal per *Trem2* genotype and (**e**) r^2 and (**f**) slope for the linear best fit lines were calculated. Data are presented as mean ± SEM. *$p < 0.05$; **$p < 0.01$; ***$p < 0.001$

expression is maintained at WT levels, and the recent evaluation of *Trem2* R47H variant function using BAC transgenics where *Trem2* was overexpressed. It is possible that the observed loss-of-function phenotypes may arise, at least in part, through reduced expression of TREM2. Furthermore, by knocking the R47H variant into the mouse *Trem2* gene, we maintain the appropriate interaction of mouse TREM2 with its endogenous ligands and signaling molecules. However, despite a high degree of homology between human *TREM2* and mouse *Trem2* genes, it is possible that the R47H variant affects human TREM2 differently than it affects mouse TREM2 structure and function. This caveat of our approach is addressed by complementary work using a BAC to express human TREM2 R47H in *Trem2*-deficient AD model [21]. Notably, our CRISPR/Cas9 knock-in approach and their BAC transgenic yield comparable results in myeloid cell accumulation around plaques, Together, these findings suggest that the *Trem2* R47H variant confers phenotypes consistent with loss of TREM2 function in a mouse model of AD-like amyloid deposition.

AD mice expressing the *Trem2* R47H variant exhibit reduced plaque-associated myeloid cells. We find that this is, in part, due to reduced proliferation. In addition, we demonstrate a selective reduction in plaque-associated cells expressing high levels of CD45 in mice expressing the *Trem2* R47H variant. It remains unclear whether the reduction in myeloid cell number represents impaired recruitment or survival of peripherally derived macrophages in the AD brain or diminished phenotypic conversion of resident microglia to adopt expression of this marker. Other possible mechanisms may also contribute to the

reduction of myeloid cells around plaques in mice expressing the *Trem2* R47H variant, including deficits in myeloid cell migration [34] and survival [11].

The alterations in myeloid cell accumulation are also reflected by changes in inflammation-related gene expression. While changes in hippocampal gene expression are largely similar between APPPS1–21;*Trem2*$^{+/R47H}$ mice and APPPS1–21;*Trem2*$^{+/-}$ mice, in the cortex, increases in mRNA levels of *Arg1*, *Fizz1*, *Ym1* and *IL-6* are specific to mice expressing the *Trem2* R47H variant. This demonstrates that there are some functional measures in which the R47H variant does not completely phenocopy loss of one copy of *Trem2*. These differences in cortical gene expression between APPPS1–21;*Trem2*$^{+/R47H}$ and APPPS1–21;*Trem2*$^{+/-}$ mice are not reflected in differences in the other myeloid cell phenotypes or features of pathology assessed in this manuscript. Additional experiments will be required to fully address whether these region-specific alterations in gene expression relate to other meaningful differences in myeloid cell function and pathology.

Our data show that the *Trem2* R47H variant does not alter 6E10 positive plaque burden, but does reduce compact, thioflavin S positive plaques, suggesting that the changes in myeloid cell function mediated by the *Trem2* R47H variant result in altered plaque structure. Yuan et al. suggested that this could be due to impaired accumulation of myeloid cells around plaques, which may normally limit plaque growth. However, it has also been shown that TREM2 influences the phagocytic activity of myeloid cells, which could also contribute to changes in plaque structure.

It has been previously postulated that myeloid cells form a barrier around plaques, protecting surrounding neurites from damaging Aβ species [35], leading to the prediction that impaired association of myeloid cells with plaques would increase neuritic dystrophy. Indeed, studies have previously shown enhanced neuritic dystrophy with reduced myeloid cell plaque coverage in AD mice deficient for *Trem2*, and in AD patients carrying the *TREM2* R47H variant [9, 12]. Consistent with these findings, we observed an increase in dystrophic neurites, relative to plaque size, in mice expressing the *Trem2* R47H variant. However, it has also been shown that larger plaques typically have less microglial coverage and more neuritic dystrophy. Thus, we expected that reduced myeloid cell accumulation around plaques with changes in *Trem2* genotype would preferentially increase neuritic dystrophy around small plaques, and have less impact on larger plaques, since these plaques already exhibit little myeloid cell coverage. In contrast, however, we find that dystrophic neurite area correlated just as strongly with plaque size in both APPPS1–21;*Trem2*$^{+/R47H}$ and APPPS1–21;*Trem2*$^{+/-}$ mice. Furthermore, there was a trend toward an increase in the slope between dystrophic neurite area and plaque size in APPPS1–21;*Trem2*$^{+/R47H}$ and APPPS1–21;*Trem2*$^{+/-}$ mice relative to controls, suggesting that larger plaques may be even more strongly affected by the loss of TREM2 function, and consequently reduced accumulation of plaque-associated myeloid cells. Together, these data are suggestive of additional roles for TREM2 in modulating neuritic dystrophy other than limiting access of plaque species to surrounding neurites. These findings suggest that TREM2 may be involved in other mechanisms of dystrophic neurite formation, or perhaps more likely, given its demonstrated role of phagocytosis in vitro, in the clearance of these dystrophic neurites [5]. It will be important to determine whether the enhanced neuritic dystrophy also correlates with neurodegeneration and cognitive deficits.

A central question arising from this work is how the changes observed in our study relate to the approximate three-fold elevation in AD risk in heterozygous carriers of the *TREM2* R47H variant. Our data demonstrate that the *Trem2* R47H variant impairs TREM2 function, in part by reducing TREM2 expression. This results in a reduced myeloid cell response to AD pathology, and increased neuritic dystrophy. Our results highlight the important functional roles of myeloid cells in AD pathogenesis and progression, and suggest that enhancing TREM2 signaling may be beneficial in the context of sporadic AD. In addition, because the *TREM2* R47H variant confers risk for other neurodegenerative diseases, this study also provides a basis for understanding important myeloid cells functions and provides potential avenues for therapeutic targets in other disease contexts. Collectively, understanding the mechanism by which the *Trem2* R47H variant affects myeloid cell function and pathology across multiple disease models promises to decipher common mechanisms by which myeloid cells modulate neurodegenerative disease pathology.

Conclusions

In summary, our findings indicate that the Alzheimer's disease-associated *Trem2* R47H variant confers a loss of TREM2 function, impairing myeloid cell responses to pathology. This results in a reduction in TREM2 expression, myeloid cell proliferation, reduced compact plaque burden and enhanced neuritic dystrophy in an Alzheimer's disease mouse model. These findings were comparable to AD mice lacking one copy of *Trem2*.

Additional files

Additional file 1: Table S1. Variant calling for APPPS1–21;*Trem2*$^{+/R47H}$ mice for the CRISPR predicted off target gene *Rab11fip3*, *Trem2*, and *Trem*-like genes *Treml1*, *Treml2*, and *Treml6*. "0/1" indicates a heterozygous variant and "./." indicates no variants detected. Variants detected in *Trem2* R47H lines but not APPPS1–21; *Trem2*$^{+/+}$ or *Trem2*$^{+/+}$ mice were considered to be true.

Additional file 2: Figure S1. (A) The SNP encoding for the arginine-to-histidine missense mutation was knocked into exon 2 of mouse *Trem2* using CRISPR/Cas9 targeting. The sequences for the reference genome, guide RNA (antisense), and homology directed repair (HDR) oligonucleotide containing the AD-associated R47H variant (red) and a silent mutation (blue) to ablate the protospacer adjacent motif (PAM), are indicated. Sanger sequence alignment from a representative *Trem2*$^{+/R47H}$ mouse is shown. (B) Comparison of major findings across two independently generated *Trem2* R47H founder lines are shown for APPPS1–21; *Trem2*$^{+/R47H}$ mice from line R104 ($n = 7$) and line R1019 ($n = 3$). (C) RNA levels of *Trem2* were assessed in cortical lysates from *Trem2*$^{+/+}$ ($n = 9$), and *Trem2*$^{+/R47H}$ ($n = 10$) mice. (D) RNA levels of *Trem2* were assessed in cortical and hippocampal lysates from APPPS1–21;*Trem2*$^{+/+}$ ($n = 6$ females, $n = 6$ males), APPPS1–21;*Trem2*$^{+/-}$ ($n = 5$ females, $n = 8$ males), and APPPS1–21;*Trem2*$^{+/R47H}$ ($n = 5$ females, $n = 5$ males) mice. Data are presented as fold change normalized gene expression relative to *Trem2*$^{+/+}$ mice ($n = 4$ females, $n = 4$ males) and were analyzed using a two-way ANOVA. $*p < 0.05$; $***p < 0.001$; ns - not significant.

Additional file 3: Figure S2. (A) IBA1+ cell number per plaque was assessed relative to plaque size in cortex from APPPS1–21;*Trem2*$^{+/+}$ ($n = 4$), APPPS1–21;*Trem2*$^{+/-}$ ($n = 6$), and APPPS1–21;*Trem2*$^{+/R47H}$ ($n = 4$) mice. Data are presented as mean ± SEM. (B) Inflammation-related genes were assessed in cortical and (C) hippocampal lysates from APPPS1–21;*Trem2*$^{+/+}$ ($n = 15$), APPPS1–21;*Trem2*$^{+/-}$ ($n = 12$), and APPPS1–21;*Trem2*$^{+/R47H}$ ($n = 10$) mice. Data are presented as fold change normalized gene expression,$*p < 0.05$, $**p < 0.01$, $****p < 0.0001$.

Additional file 4: Figure S3. (A) Expression of amyloid precursor protein (*App*) and related genes were assessed in cortical lysates from APPPS1–21;*Trem2*$^{+/+}$ ($n = 13$), APPPS1–21;*Trem2*$^{+/-}$ ($n = 13$), and APPPS1–21;*Trem2*$^{+/R47H}$ ($n = 8$) mice. Data are presented as fold change normalized gene expression. (B) ELISAs for Aβ$_{1–40}$ and Aβ$_{1–42}$ and (C) ratio of Aβ$_{1–42}$/Aβ$_{1–40}$ were performed on DEA (soluble) and FA (insoluble) fractions from cortex and hippocampus from APPPS1–21;*Trem2*$^{+/+}$ ($n = 17$), APPPS1–21;*Trem2*$^{+/-}$ ($n = 14$), and APPPS1–21;*Trem2*$^{+/R47H}$ ($n = 10$) mice. Data are presented as fold change normalized protein expression. $*p < 0.05$, $**p < 0.01$.

Abbreviations

AD: Alzheimer's disease; BAC: Bacterial artificial chromosome; CRISPR: Clustered regularly interspaced short palindromic repeats; IBA1: Ionized calcium-binding adapter molecule 1; PAM: Protospacer adjacent motif; SNP: Single nucleotide polymorphism; TREM2: Triggering receptor expressed on myeloid cells 2

Acknowledgements

This work was supported by grants from the Alzheimer's Association (BTL and GEL); CWRU Neurodegenerative Diseases training grant T32 NS077888

(PJC-H), Medical Scientist Training Program training grant T32 GM725039 (PJC-H); NIA National Service Research Award F30 AG055261 (PJC-H) and F31 AG048704 (TRJ); NIA R01 AG051495 (BTL and GEL) and AG050597 (GEL); NIA U54 AG054345 (BTL). In addition, this study was supported by generous donations from the Jane & Lee Seidman Fund, Chet & Jane Scholtz, and Dave & Susan Roberts. We also thank the Case Transgenic Core and Targeting Center for the generation of the *Trem2* R47H founder lines and off-target mutation prediction. We also thank the Case Western Reserve University School of Medicine Genetics Core for conducting whole genome sequencing, performing sequencing alignment and mutation analysis.

Authors' contributions

Conceptualization, PJC-H, EGR-G, TRJ, BTL and GEL; Methodology, PJC-H, EGR-G and TRJ; Formal Analysis, PJC-H, EGR-G and TRJ; Investigation, PJC-H, EGR-G, TRJ, BTC, SMB, SSP, VEV, RYW, JCK, MM, and GX; Writing – Original Draft, PJC-H, EGR-G and TRJ; Writing – Review & Editing, PJC-H, EGR-G, TRJ, BTC, RMR, BTL and GEL; Funding Acquisition, PJC-H, TRJ, BTL and GEL; Supervision, BTL and GEL. All authors read and approved the final manuscript.

Ethics approval

Animals used in this study were housed in the Association for Assessment and Accreditation of Laboratory Animal Care International accredited facility in the Cleveland Clinic Biological Resources Unit and all experimental procedures were approved by the Cleveland Clinic Foundation Institutional Animal Care and Use Committee (IACUC).

Competing interests

The authors declare that they have no competing interests.

Author details

[1]Department of Neurosciences, Case Western Reserve University, School of Medicine, Cleveland, OH 44106, USA. [2]Department of Anatomy and Cell Biology, Indiana University, School of Medicine, Indianapolis, IN 46202, USA. [3]Paul and Carole Stark Neurosciences Research Institute, Indiana University, School of Medicine, Indianapolis, IN 46202, USA. [4]Department of Medical and Molecular Genetics, Indiana University, School of Medicine, Indianapolis, IN 46202, USA. [5]Cleveland Clinic Lerner Research Institute, Cleveland, OH 44195, USA. [6]Third Rock Ventures, Boston, MA 02116, USA.

References

1. Heneka MT, Carson MJ, El Khoury J, Landreth GE, Brosseron F, Feinstein DL, Jacobs AH, Wyss-Coray T, Vitorica J, Ransohoff RM, et al. Neuroinflammation in Alzheimer's disease. Lancet Neurol. 2015;14:388–405.
2. Karch CM, Goate AM. Alzheimer's disease risk genes and mechanisms of disease pathogenesis. Biol Psychiatry. 2015;77:43–51.
3. Guerreiro R, Wojtas A, Bras J, Carrasquillo M, Rogaeva E, Majounie E, Cruchaga C, Sassi C, Kauwe JS, Younkin S, et al. TREM2 variants in Alzheimer's disease. N Engl J Med. 2013;368:117–27.
4. Jonsson T, Stefansson H, Steinberg S, Jonsdottir I, Jonsson PV, Snaedal J, Bjornsson S, Huttenlocher J, Levey AI, Lah JJ, et al. Variant of TREM2 associated with the risk of Alzheimer's disease. N Engl J Med. 2013;368:107–16.
5. Jay TR, von Saucken VE, Landreth GE. TREM2 in neurodegenerative diseases. Mol Neurodegener. 2017;12:56.
6. Paloneva J, Manninen T, Christman G, Hovanes K, Mandelin J, Adolfsson R, Bianchin M, Bird T, Miranda R, Salmaggi A, et al. Mutations in two genes encoding different subunits of a receptor signaling complex result in an identical disease phenotype. Am J Hum Genet. 2002;71:656–62.
7. Colonna M. TREMs in the immune system and beyond. Nat Rev Immunol. 2003;3:445–53.
8. Schmid CD, Sautkulis LN, Danielson PE, Cooper J, Hasel KW, Hilbush BS, Sutcliffe JG, Carson MJ. Heterogeneous expression of the triggering receptor expressed on myeloid cells-2 on adult murine microglia. J Neurochem. 2002;83:1309–20.
9. Yuan P, Condello C, Keene CD, Wang Y, Bird TD, Paul SM, Luo W, Colonna M, Baddeley D, Grutzendler J. TREM2 Haplodeficiency in mice and humans impairs the microglia barrier function leading to decreased amyloid compaction and severe axonal dystrophy. Neuron. 2016;90:724–39.
10. Jay TR, Hirsch AM, Broihier ML, Miller CM, Neilson LE, Ransohoff RM, Lamb BT, Landreth GE. Disease progression-dependent effects of TREM2 deficiency in a mouse model of Alzheimer's disease. J Neurosci. 2017;37:637–47.
11. Wang Y, Cella M, Mallinson K, Ulrich JD, Young KL, Robinette ML, Gilfillan S, Krishnan GM, Sudhakar S, Zinselmeyer BH, et al. TREM2 lipid sensing sustains the microglial response in an Alzheimer's disease model. Cell. 2015; 160:1061–71.
12. Wang Y, Ulland TK, Ulrich JD, Song W, Tzaferis JA, Hole JT, Yuan P, Mahan TE, Shi Y, Gilfillan S, et al. TREM2-mediated early microglial response limits diffusion and toxicity of amyloid plaques. J Exp Med. 2016;213:667–75.
13. Jay TR, Miller CM, Cheng PJ, Graham LC, Bemiller S, Broihier ML, Xu G, Margevicius D, Karlo JC, Sousa GL, et al. TREM2 deficiency eliminates TREM2 + inflammatory macrophages and ameliorates pathology in Alzheimer's disease mouse models. J Exp Med. 2015;212:287–95.
14. Atagi Y, Liu CC, Painter MM, Chen XF, Verbeeck C, Zheng H, Li X, Rademakers R, Kang SS, Xu H, et al. Apolipoprotein E is a ligand for triggering receptor expressed on myeloid cells 2 (TREM2). J Biol Chem. 2015;290:26043–50.
15. Bailey CC, DeVaux LB, Farzan M. The triggering receptor expressed on myeloid cells 2 binds apolipoprotein E. J Biol Chem. 2015;290:26033–42.
16. Kober DL, Alexander-Brett JM, Karch CM, Cruchaga C, Colonna M, Holtzman MJ, Brett TJ. Neurodegenerative disease mutations in TREM2 reveal a functional surface and distinct loss-of-function mechanisms. Elife. 2016;5: e20391.
17. Yeh FL, Wang Y, Tom I, Gonzalez LC, Sheng M. TREM2 binds to apolipoproteins, including APOE and CLU/APOJ, and thereby facilitates uptake of amyloid-Beta by microglia. Neuron. 2016;91:328–40.
18. Song W, Hooli B, Mullin K, Jin SC, Cella M, Ulland TK, Wang Y, Tanzi RE, Colonna M. Alzheimer's disease-associated TREM2 variants exhibit either decreased or increased ligand-dependent activation. Alzheimers Dement. 2017;13:381–7.
19. Park J-S, Ji IJ, An HJ, Kang M-J, Kang S-W, Kim D-H, Yoon S-Y. Disease-associated mutations of TREM2 Alter the processing of N-linked oligosaccharides in the Golgi apparatus. Traffic. 2015;16:510–8.
20. Park J-S, Ji IJ, Kim D-H, An HJ, Yoon S-Y. The Alzheimer's disease-associated R47H variant of TREM2 has an altered glycosylation pattern and protein stability. Front Neurosci. 2017;10:618.
21. Song WM, Joshita S, Zhou Y, Ulland TK, Gilfillan S, Colonna M. Humanized TREM2 mice reveal microglia-intrinsic and -extrinsic effects of R47H polymorphism. J Exp Med. 2018;215:745–60.
22. Jiang T, Tan L, Zhu XC, Zhang QQ, Cao L, Tan MS, Gu LZ, Wang HF, Ding ZZ, Zhang YD, Yu JT. Upregulation of TREM2 ameliorates neuropathology and rescues spatial cognitive impairment in a transgenic mouse model of Alzheimer's disease. Neuropsychopharmacology. 2014;39:2949–62.
23. Haeussler M, Schönig K, Eckert H, Eschstruth A, Mianné J, Renaud J-B, Schneider-Maunoury S, Shkumatava A, Teboul L, Kent J, et al. Evaluation of off-target and on-target scoring algorithms and integration into the guide RNA selection tool CRISPOR. Genome Biol. 2016;17:148.
24. Zheng H, Liu CC, Atagi Y, Chen XF, Jia L, Yang L, He W, Zhang X, Kang SS, Rosenberry TL, et al. Opposing roles of the triggering receptor expressed on myeloid cells 2 and triggering receptor expressed on myeloid cells-like transcript 2 in microglia activation. Neurobiol Aging. 2016;42:132–41.
25. Iyer V, Shen B, Zhang W, Hodgkins A, Keane T, Huang X, Skarnes WC. Off-target mutations are rare in Cas9-modified mice. Nat Methods. 2015;12:479.
26. Radde R, Bolmont T, Kaeser SA, Coomaraswamy J, Lindau D, Stoltze L, Calhoun ME, Jaggi F, Wolburg H, Gengler S, et al. Abeta42-driven cerebral amyloidosis in transgenic mice reveals early and robust pathology. EMBO Rep. 2006;7:940–6.
27. Casali B, Landreth G. Abeta extraction from murine brain homogenates. Bio Protoc. 2016;6:e1787.
28. Krasemann S, Madore C, Cialic R, Baufeld C, Calcagno N, El Fatimy R, Beckers L, O'Loughlin E, Xu Y, Fanek Z, et al. The TREM2-APOE pathway drives the

transcriptional phenotype of dysfunctional microglia in neurodegenerative diseases. Immunity. 2017;47:566–581.e569.

29. Ulrich JD, Finn MB, Wang Y, Shen A, Mahan TE, Jiang H, Stewart FR, Piccio L, Colonna M, Holtzman DM. Altered microglial response to Abeta plaques in APPPS1-21 mice heterozygous for TREM2. Mol Neurodegener. 2014;9:20.

30. Sedgwick JD, Schwender S, Imrich H, Dorries R, Butcher GW, ter Meulen V. Isolation and direct characterization of resident microglial cells from the normal and inflamed central nervous system. Proc Natl Acad Sci U S A. 1991;88:7438–42.

31. Keren-Shaul H, Spinrad A, Weiner A, Matcovitch-Natan O, Dvir-Szternfeld R, Ulland TK, David E, Baruch K, Lara-Astaiso D, Toth B, et al. A unique microglia type associated with restricting development of Alzheimer's disease. Cell. 2017;169:1276–1290.e1217.

32. Serrano-Pozo A, Frosch MP, Masliah E, Hyman BT. Neuropathological alterations in Alzheimer disease. Cold Spring Harb Perspect Med. 2011;1:a006189.

33. Ma L, Allen M, Sakae N, Ertekin-Taner N, Graff-Radford NR, Dickson DW, Younkin SG, Sevlever D. Expression and processing analyses of wild type and p.R47H TREM2 variant in Alzheimer's disease brains. Mol Neurodegener. 2016;11:72.

34. Mazaheri F, Snaidero N, Kleinberger G, Madore C, Daria A, Werner G, Krasemann S, Capell A, Trumbach D, Wurst W, et al. TREM2 deficiency impairs chemotaxis and microglial responses to neuronal injury. EMBO Rep. 2017;18:1186-98.

35. Condello C, Yuan P, Schain A, Grutzendler J. Microglia constitute a barrier that prevents neurotoxic protofibrillar Abeta42 hotspots around plaques. Nat Commun. 2015;6:6176.

13

AMPA-ergic regulation of amyloid-β levels in an Alzheimer's disease mouse model

Jane C. Hettinger[1], Hyo Lee[1], Guojun Bu[2], David M. Holtzman[1] and John R. Cirrito[1*] (iD)

Abstract

Background: Extracellular aggregation of the amyloid-β (Aβ) peptide into toxic multimers is a key event in Alzheimer's disease (AD) pathogenesis. Aβ aggregation is concentration-dependent, with higher concentrations of Aβ much more likely to form toxic species. The processes that regulate extracellular levels of Aβ therefore stand to directly affect AD pathology onset. Studies from our lab and others have demonstrated that synaptic activity is a critical regulator of Aβ production through both presynaptic and postsynaptic mechanisms. AMPA receptors (AMPA-Rs), as the most abundant ionotropic glutamate receptors, have the potential to greatly impact Aβ levels.

Methods: In order to study the role of AMPA-Rs in Aβ regulation, we used in vivo microdialysis in an APP/PS1 mouse model to simultaneously deliver AMPA and other treatments while collecting Aβ from the interstitial fluid (ISF). Changes in Aβ production and clearance along with inflammation were assessed using biochemical approaches. IL-6 deficient mice were utilized to test the role of IL-6 signaling in AMPA-R-mediated regulation of Aβ levels.

Results: We found that AMPA-R activation decreases in ISF Aβ levels in a dose-dependent manner. Moreover, the effect of AMPA treatment involves three distinct pathways. Steady-state activity of AMPA-Rs normally promotes higher ISF Aβ. Evoked AMPA-R activity, however, decreases Aβ levels by both stimulating glutamatergic transmission and activating downstream NMDA receptor (NMDA-R) signaling and, with extended AMPA treatment, acting independently of NMDA-Rs. Surprisingly, we found this latter, direct AMPA pathway of Aβ regulation increases Aβ clearance, while Aβ production appears to be largely unaffected. Furthermore, the AMPA-dependent decrease is not observed in IL-6 deficient mice, indicating a role for IL-6 signaling in AMPA-R-mediated Aβ clearance.

Conclusion: Though basal levels of AMPA-R activity promote higher levels of ISF Aβ, evoked AMPA-R signaling decreases Aβ through both NMDA-R-dependent and -independent pathways. We find that evoked AMPA-R signaling increases clearance of extracellular Aβ, at least in part through enhanced IL-6 signaling. These data emphasize that Aβ regulation by synaptic activity involves a number of independent pathways that together determine extracellular Aβ levels. Understanding how these pathways maintain Aβ levels prior to AD pathology may provide insights into disease pathogenesis.

Keywords: Alzheimer's disease, Amyloid-beta, AMPA, Clearance, IL-6, Microdialysis

Background

Alzheimer's disease (AD) follows a protracted course with pathology detected years, even decades before clinical symptoms manifest. The preclinical stage of AD appears to be initiated by the aggregation of the peptide amyloid-β (Aβ) into toxic oligomers and plaques within the brain extracellular space, thereby triggering a host of biochemical and cellular pathological events [1–3]. The shift from normal production of soluble Aβ to its pathogenic aggregation is heavily influenced by the concentration of Aβ. Consequently, the rate at which Aβ is produced and secreted from the neuron, as well as its clearance from the extracellular space, appears to be directly linked to the formation of toxic amyloid species [4–6].

Our lab and others have shown that an important regulator of extracellular Aβ levels is synaptic activity [7, 8]. Elevated synaptic activity drives clathrin-

---

* Correspondence: cirritoj@neuro.wustl.edu
[1]Department of Neurology, Knight Alzheimer's Disease Research Center, Hope Center for Neurological Disorders, Washington University School of Medicine, Campus Box 8111, 660 South Euclid Avenue, St. Louis, MO 63110, USA
Full list of author information is available at the end of the article

mediated endocytosis at the presynaptic membrane, thereby increasing endocytosis of the amyloid precursor protein (APP) and subsequent Aβ generation [9]. At the systems level, the regional distribution of amyloid plaque deposition in AD brains correlates with default mode network connectivity, suggesting that chronic high levels of network activity contribute to plaque formation [10, 11]. However, not all increased neuronal activity results in increased Aβ concentrations. Indeed, a number of postsynaptic receptors have been shown to decrease Aβ production. Stimulation of serotonin receptors activates the extracellular regulated kinase (ERK) signaling pathway, which enhances α-secretase activity and non-amyloidogenic APP processing [12, 13]. NMDA receptor (NMDA-R) activation regulates Aβ levels bidirectionally – low concentrations of NMDA elevate Aβ levels through increased presynaptic membrane endocytosis, while higher concentrations of NMDA decrease Aβ production through dendritic, calcium-dependent signaling and increased α-secretase activity [12]. These experiments show that the relationship between neuronal activity and Aβ production is complex, with even the same receptors in some cases having opposing effects depending on the extent of activation.

AMPA receptors (AMPA-Rs) are the predominant postsynaptic glutamate-gated ion channels and are responsible for the majority of fast excitatory transmission in the CNS, making them well positioned to impact the relationship between Aβ levels and synaptic activity. Furthermore, growing evidence suggests AMPA-Rs can act as independent activators of second messenger signaling in addition to their well-established role as the primary agents of postsynaptic depolarization [14–18]. Most of the research involving AMPA-Rs and AD has focused on the deleterious effect of pathological amyloid species on AMPA-Rs [19–21], while the inverse relationship, that of AMPA-R's effects on Aβ, has received much less attention. A notable exception is a compelling study by Hoey and colleagues, which reported increased non-amyloidogenic processing of APP following calcium-permeable AMPA-R activation in primary cortical neurons [22]. Given the AMPA-R's dominant role in synaptic transmission and its active signaling capabilities, we hypothesized that AMPA-Rs regulate Aβ metabolism.

Using in vivo microdialysis, we found that baseline AMPA-R activity maintains higher levels of Aβ, whereas evoked activation of AMPA-Rs leads to reduced Aβ levels in the interstitial fluid (ISF) of the mouse hippocampus. Interestingly, the effect of exogenous AMPA treatment resolves into two phases. Initially, AMPA-Rs decrease Aβ levels through synaptic release of glutamate and downstream activation of NMDA-Rs. After prolonged treatment with AMPA, however, Aβ levels are reduced through an NMDA-R-independent pathway that does not rely on presynaptic transmission. Surprisingly,

we found that AMPA-Rs directly influence Aβ levels by altering Aβ clearance, implicating synaptic activity with clearance mechanisms. Moreover, data collected from IL-6 deficient mice indicate a critical role for IL-6 signaling in this pathway. These findings highlight the complexity behind the overlapping pathways regulating extracellular Aβ levels.

Methods

Animals

The mice used for these studies were hemizygous *APPswe/PS1ΔE9* (APP/PS1) and bred on a wild-type C3H/B6 background, C57BL/6j-IL-6^{tm1Kopf} mice (hereafter referred to as IL-6$^{-/-}$ mice), or littermate controls (WT) [23, 24].

Original APP/PS1 transgenic breeders as well as IL-6$^{-/-}$ mice were purchased from Jackson Laboratory (Bar Harbor, Maine), and colonies were maintained at Washington University. Equal numbers of male and female mice were used in each study at 2–4 months of age. All studies were performed in accordance with the guidelines of AAALAC and the IACUC at Washington University.

Aβ microdialysis

In vivo microdialysis was performed in awake and behaving APP/PS1 mice as previously described [12, 25]. Briefly, guide cannulas (BR-style, Bioanalytical Systems, West Lafayette, IN) were stereotaxically implanted above the left hippocampus, coordinates bregma – 3.1 mm, 2.5 mm lateral to midline, and 1.2 mm below dura at a 12° angle. The cannulas were securely affixed to the head with dental cement, and microdialysis probes (BR-2, 2 mm, 38 kDa MWCO, Bioanalytical Systems) were inserted into the hippocampus through the guide cannula. In APP/PS1 mice, probes were perfused with artificial cerebrospinal fluid (aCSF; 1.3 mM CaCl$_2$, 1.2 mM MgSO$_4$, 3 mM KCl, 04 mM KH$_2$PO$_4$, 25 mM NaHCO$_3$, and 122 mM NaCl, pH 7.35) with 0.15% bovine serum albumin (BSA; Sigma-Aldrich, St. Louis, MO) at a rate of 1.0 μL/min with samples of hippocampal ISF collected every 90 min during basal collection or every 60 min during treatment. Because WT murine Aβ concentrations are lower than in amyloidogenic transgenic mice, microdialysis was run at 0.5 μL/min and samples collected every 3 h to increase concentration of each sample. Murine Aβ was also analyzed in the experiment using IL-6$^{-/-}$ mice. For this experiment, microdialysis was run at 1.0 μL/min and samples were collected every 2.5 h. Basal sampling began at least 16 h following surgery. These experiments took place under constant light conditions to diminish circadian-related fluctuation in Aβ levels. At the conclusion of the experiment, all ISF samples were analyzed for either human or murine Aβ$_{x-40}$ or Aβ$_{x-42}$ levels by sandwich ELISA.

Compounds

Reverse microdialysis was used to administer compounds directly into the hippocampus. Drugs were diluted into the perfusion buffer of artificial CSF and 0. 15% BSA, allowing the drugs to diffuse into the brain continuously for the duration of the experiment at the same time that Aβ is collected. Due to the complexity of determining the final concentration of compound delivered to the brain, only the starting concentrations of drugs in the perfusion buffer are given. We estimate approximately 10% of the drug is delivered across the probe membrane where it is further diluted in the brain CSF. AMPA (0.5, 2, 5, 7.5, and 10 μM), MK801 (100 μM), NMDA (40 μM), and thiorphan (10 μM) were purchased from Sigma. Cyclothiazide (CTZ; 300 μM), tetrodotoxin (TTX; 5 μM), NBQX (100 μM), and GM6001 (25 μM) were purchased from Tocris Bioscience (Ellisville, MO). LY411575 (Sigma-Aldrich) was diluted in corn oil and administered subcutaneously at 5 mg/kg.

Aβ sandwich ELISAs

ISF samples were analyzed for $A\beta_{x-40}$ or $A\beta_{x-42}$ concentration using methods previously described (Fisher et al., 2016). A mouse monoclonal anti-$A\beta_{40}$ capture antibody (mHJ2) or anti-$A\beta_{42}$ capture antibody (mHJ7.4) made in-house was used in conjunction with a biotinylated central domain detection antibody (mHJ5.1) and streptavidin-poly-HRP-40 (Fitzgerald Industries, Acton, MA). Super Slow ELISA TMB (Sigma-Aldrich) was then used to develop, and absorbance was read by a BioTek Epoch plate reader at 650 nm. The same assay can be used for both human and murine $A\beta_{x-40}$. Standard curves for ELISAs were generated using synthetic human $A\beta_{40}$ or $A\beta_{42}$ (American Peptide, Sunnyvale, CA). Basal levels of ISF Aβ levels were calculated by averaging the Aβ concentrations taken every 90 min for 9 h prior to drug treatment. All Aβ levels for each mouse were then normalized by calculating percent of basal for each point. Mean ± SEM per group are shown.

Western blotting

Guide cannula implantation and microdialysis were performed as described above using 2–4 month old APP/PS1 mice. 5 μM AMPA or vehicle was administered to APP/PS1 mice via reverse microdialysis for 8 or 14 h. Immediately following treatment, perfusion buffer was changed to aCSF containing 0.1% Evans Blue dye for 30 min. During this period, the area of the hippocampus directly surrounding the microdialysis probe was dyed blue, approximating the area of tissue affected by reverse microdialysis drug delivery. Following the 30-min of Evans Blue administration, the mice were sacrificed and the dyed tissue surrounding the probe was microdissected

and snap frozen on dry ice, generating approximately 5-7 mg of tissue per mouse. The collected hippocampal tissue was homogenized by sonication at a 10:1 volume: wet weight in 150 mM NaCl, 50 mM Tris, pH 7.4, 0.5% deoxycholic acid, 0.1% SDS, 1% Triton X-100, 2.5 mM EDTA, and protease inhibitors. Gel electrophoresis of 20 μg protein samples was performed under reducing conditions using 4–12% Bis-Tris NuPAGE gels (Thermo-Fisher Scientific, Waltham, MA) and then transferred to nitrocellulose membrane. Blots were probed for glial fibrillary acidic protein (GFAP; 1:500; ThermoFisher), low density lipoprotein receptor-related protein 1 (LRP1; 1: 5000; Abcam, Cambridge, MA), insulin-degrading enzyme (IDE; 1μg/mL; Abcam), neprilysin (1:1000; Millipore, Billerica, MA), matrix metalloproteinase-9 (MMP-9; 1:1000; Millipore), C-terminal fragments of APP (1:1000; Sigma-Aldrich), total soluble APP (22C11; 1:5000; Millipore), soluble APP-α (poly18268; BioLegend, San Diego, CA), soluble APP-β (poly8134; 1:1000; BioLegend), β-amyloid 1–16 (6E10; 1:500; BioLegend), glutamate receptor 2 (GluR2; 1:1000; Millipore), tubulin (1:2500; Sigma), and glyceraldehyde 3-phosphate dehydrogenase (GAPDH; 1: 10,000; Sigma). HRP-conjugated goat anti-rabbit IgG (1: 1000; Cell Signaling Technology, Danvers, MA) and HRP-conjugated Amersham ECL sheep anti-mouse IgG (1: 1000; GE Healthcare, Chicago, IL) were used as secondary antibodies. Membranes were developed using SuperSignal West Pico Substrate (ThermoFisher) or Lumigen-TMA6 (GE Healthcare) and imaged using the Kodak ImageStation 440CF (Rochester, NY). Band intensity was quantified using the Kodak 1D Image Analysis software, and normalized using tubulin or GAPDH signals as loading controls. Values shown are these normalized band intensities relative to the experimental control group. Mean ± SEM per group are shown.

Quantitative real-time PCR (qPCR)

Using the same tissue preparation as used for Western blotting (described above), APP/PS1 mice were treated with 5 μM AMPA for 8 or 14 h, followed by 30 min of 0.1% Evans Blue solution via reverse microdialysis. Dyed tissue around the probe was microdissected and frozen. Quantitative PCR was performed as described previously (Fisher et al., 2016). The RNeasy Mini Kit (Qiagen, Valencia, CA) was used to extract RNA, which was then reverse transcribed with a High Capacity cDNA Reverse Transcription kit (ThermoFisher). The Harvard Medical School Primer Bank was used to design primers [26–28]. Real-time detection of PCR product was performed using the Fast SYBR Green Master Mix (Applied Biosystems, Foster City, CA) in ABI 7900HT (Applied Biosystems) with the default thermal cycling program. *cFos* was used as a positive control due to its established role as a mark of neuronal activity [29]. *Gapdh* was used as a reference gene for relative expression calculations. Relative mRNA levels were calculated using the comparative Ct method using the formula $2^{-\Delta\Delta Ct}$. Mean ± SEM per group are shown.

Histology

2–4 month-old wild-type mice (n = 6 per group) or APP/PS1 mice (n = 3 per group) were treated with 8 h or 14 h, respectively, of AMPA or artificial CSF via reverse microdialysis then immediately transcardially perfused with ice-cold phosphate buffer saline (PBS) with 0. 3% heparin. Brains were removed, fixed in 4% paraformaldehyde for 24 h at 4 °C, then placed in 30% sucrose prior to freezing and sectioning. Coronal brain sections 50 μm wide were sliced in 300 μm intervals using a freezing sliding microtome. Sections were then immunostained to visualize astrocytes or microglia using antibodies against glial fibrillary acidic protein (GFAP; 1:500, ThermoFisher) as an astrocytic marker or against ionized calcium-binding adaptor molecule 1 (Iba1; 1:500; Wako Laboratory Chemicals, Richmond, VA) as a microglial marker. Biotinylated secondary antibody, horseradish peroxidase-conjugated streptavidin, and DAB reaction (Sigma) were used to develop. Brain sections were imaged with a Nanozoomer slide scanner (Hamamatsu Photonics, Bridgewater, NJ). Staining density was qualitatively evaluated by blinded observers and vehicle- and AMPA-treated groups were compared. Images shown are representative.

Aβ elimination half-life

Half-life of ISF Aβ was measured using methods described previously [25]. Microdialysis was performed as detailed above and basal ISF Aβ levels were collected. Reverse microdialysis was then used to treat APP/PS1 mice with either 5 μM AMPA or vehicle for 14 h, followed by co-administration with LY411575, a potent and selective γ-secretase inhibitor (Sigma-Aldrich; 5 mg/kg in corn oil, subcutaneous injection) to block Aβ production. ISF Aβ levels were measured using sandwich ELISA, and the half-life was calculated using the slope of the semi-log plot of percent change in Aβ levels versus time. The slope was calculated based only on Aβ values that were continually decreasing, excluding points at which levels plateaued. Mean ± SEM per group are shown.

MesoScale discovery (MSD) multiplex cytokine assay

Hippocampal tissue was collected from APP/PS1 mice treated with either vehicle (n = 7) or AMPA (n = 9) for 14 h via reverse microdialysis. Only tissue directly surrounding the probe was used. Tissue was homogenized following the manufacturer protocol in 500 mM NaCl, 50 mM Tris, pH 7.4, 0.5% deoxycholic acid, 0.1% SDS, 1% Triton X-100, 2 mM EDTA, and protease inhibitors (MesoScale Discovery, Rockville, MD, USA). Samples were assayed for interleukin(IL)-1β, IL-6, and tumor necrosis factor (TNF)-α using a custom MSD Proinflammatory Panel multiplex assay using the manufacturer's protocol. Samples were assayed duplicate. Data analysis was performed using MSD Workbench software.

Experimental design and statistical analysis

Littermate mice were randomly assigned into treatment groups, with equal numbers of male and females. Based on power analyses for detecting changes in ISF Aβ in microdialysis experiments, we used n = 4–8 mice per treatment group. A full description of statistical tests and the number of mice used can be found in the figure legends. Two-tailed unpaired t-tests were used to compare between two groups. One-way or two-way ANOVA was used when comparing one or two independent variables, respectively, between multiple groups. The appropriate correction for multiple comparisons was used (Sidak, Tukey, or Bonferroni; refer to figure legends). Analysis of microdialysis experiments was performed by averaging the final three data points of a specific treatment period and using one-way or two-way ANOVA with an appropriate correction for multiple comparisons. Values were accepted as significant is $p \leq 0.05$. Data in figures are presented as mean ± SEM. Prism 6.0b for Mac OS X (GraphPad, San Diego, CA) was used for all statistical analyses.

Results

Local administration of AMPA decreases ISF Aβ in a dose-dependent manner

Both synaptic activity and NMDA-Rs have distinct, established roles in regulating Aβ, but the involvement of AMPA-R signaling in Aβ regulation has been largely unexplored. To address this, we used in vivo microdialysis to measure the concentration of ISF Aβ in the hippocampus of mice [9, 25]. Crucially, this technique allows us to monitor changes in ISF Aβ levels over time in freely moving mice with functional glutamatergic synapses and intact neuronal networks. Through reverse microdialysis, we are also able to locally and continuously deliver small-molecule compounds, such as AMPA, into the hippocampus without needing to cross the blood-brain barrier.

Using microdialysis in the hippocampus of young, plaque-free (2–4 month old) *APPswe/PS1Δe9* hemizygous (APP/PS1) mice [23, 24], we collected hourly samples of ISF while infusing AMPA in increasing concentrations from 0.5 μM to 10 μM for 8 h each (Fig. 1a). AMPA delivered at 0.5 μM or 2 μM had no effect on ISF Aβ. However, beginning with the 5 μM AMPA concentration, ISF Aβ levels gradually decreased over time before stabilizing at a 32% decrease from baseline levels. An even greater decrease is seen following 10 μM AMPA treatment, with levels of Aβ stabilizing at a 75% decrease from baseline levels (Fig. 1a). In the following experiments, we used 5 μM AMPA in order to observe further increases and decreases in ISF Aβ levels after they are already lowered by AMPA treatment. In this study, we focus primarily on ISF $A\beta_{40}$ because it is produced in much higher quantities than $A\beta_{42}$ in our mouse model and therefore simpler to detect using microdialysis. To determine if AMPA treatment acts on both species of Aβ similarly, ISF samples from 5 μM AMPA-treated mice were measured for $A\beta_{42}$. We found that AMPA decreases ISF $A\beta_{42}$ similarly to $A\beta_{40}$, indicating that it acts on both species of Aβ in the same manner (Fig. 1b). Next, wild-type (WT) mice were treated with 5 μM AMPA to eliminate potential confounds due to the transgenes in APP/PS1 mice. Murine ISF Aβ levels in WT animals reacted to 5 μM AMPA treatment similarly to APP/PS1 mice with a 45% decrease from baseline levels (Fig. 1c).

AMPA-Rs rapidly desensitize following AMPA or glutamate exposure [30]. One possible explanation for the observed effect on ISF Aβ, therefore, could be reduced activity due to decreased AMPA-R signaling. To test this possibility, we treated the APP/PS1 mice with cyclothiazide (CTZ), a thiazide diuretic, which inhibits desensitization and potentiates AMPA-mediated glutamate currents [31]. The mice were pre-treated with CTZ for 4 h before and then during treatment with increasing doses of AMPA (0.5 μM–5 μM) lasting 4 h each (Fig. 1d). Potentiated AMPA-R signaling enhanced the suppression in ISF Aβ levels with AMPA treatment starting at just 0.5 μM, a dose that has no effect on ISF Aβ without CTZ. This decrease is dose-dependent, with a maximal decrease in ISF Aβ of 83% from basal levels (Fig. 1d). These data indicate that the observed decrease in ISF Aβ is due to AMPA-R activity and not desensitization.

AMPA decreases Aβ levels through multiple distinct pathways

The exogenous application of AMPA through reverse microdialysis allows us to directly and selectively target AMPA-Rs. However, infusion of AMPA does not necessarily reproduce endogenous AMPA-R signaling. To address this, we treated mice with NBQX, a competitive AMPA-R antagonist (Fig. 2a). When baseline levels of

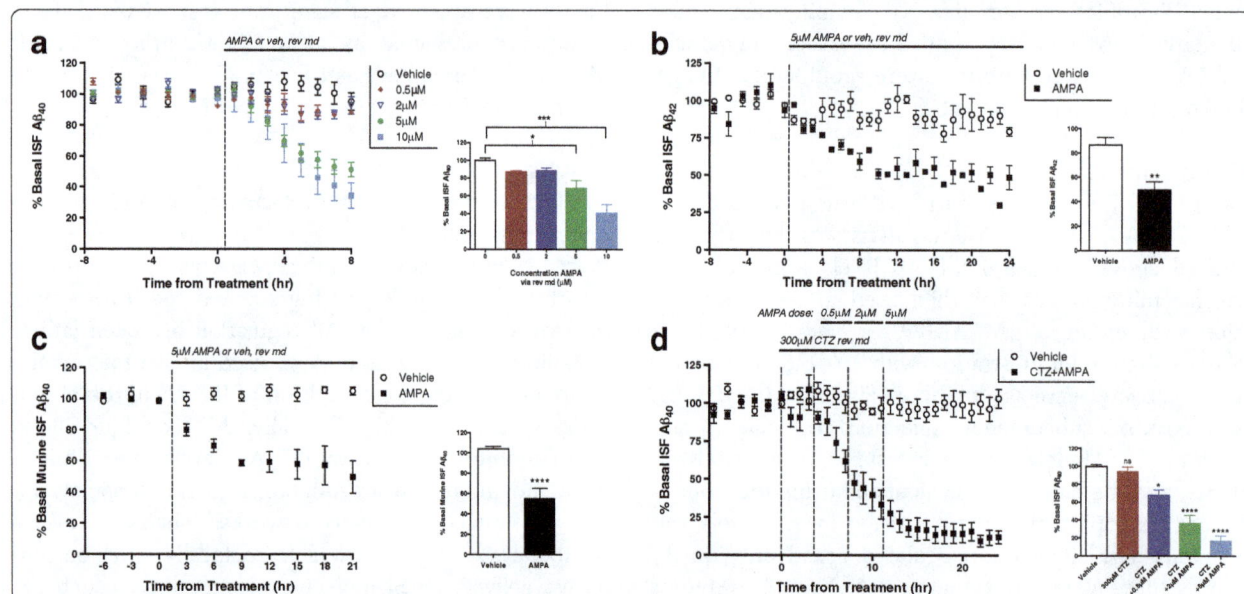

Fig. 1 AMPA treatment decreases levels of ISF Aβ levels. **a** Varying doses of AMPA or vehicle (artificial CSF) were administered to 2–4 month-old APP/PS1 mice via reverse microdialysis (rev md), and changes in interstitial fluid (ISF) $A\beta_{40}$ were measured using ELISA. AMPA has a dose-dependent effect on ISF Aβ levels. Though treatment with 0.5 μM and 2 μM AMPA did not alter ISF Aβ levels significantly ($n = 3$, $n = 5$ respectively), treatment with 5 μM AMPA decreased levels $31.7 \pm 9.5\%$ ($p = 0.015$, $n = 4$, one-way ANOVA, Dunnet's post hoc test), and 10 μM AMPA decreased levels by $73.8 \pm 12.2\%$ ($p < 0.0001$, $n = 2$, one-way ANOVA, Dunnet's post hoc test). **b** APP/PS1 mice ($n = 4$) were treated with 5 μM AMPA for 24 h and ISF $A\beta_{42}$ levels decreased by $37.0 \pm 9.4\%$ ($p < 0.0043$, two-tailed t-test). **c** Wild-type, littermate C3H/B6 mice were dosed with 5 μM AMPA using rev md and levels of murine ISF $A\beta_{40}$ levels decreased by $49.4 \pm 8.4\%$ ($p < 0.0001$, $n = 6$, two-tailed t-test). **d** APP/PS1 mice were treated with 300 μM cyclothiazide (CTZ) for 4 h ($n = 6$), after which increasing doses of AMPA (0.5, 2, and 5 μM) were added to the perfusion buffer. CTZ administered alone did not change ISF Aβ levels. Aβ levels decreased $31.9 \pm 11.1\%$ ($p = 0.030$, one-way ANOVA, Dunnet's post hoc test) by 0.5 μM AMPA, $63.6 \pm 11.1\%$ ($p < 0.0001$, one-way ANOVA, Dunnet's post hoc test) by 2 μM, and maximally decreased $83.2 \pm 11.1\%$ ($p < 0.0001$, one-way ANOVA, Dunnet's post hoc test) when treated with 5 μM AMPA. Data plotted as mean ± SEM

AMPA-R signaling were blocked, ISF Aβ levels decreased by 32%, suggesting that AMPA-R activation increases Aβ during normal activity.

Next, we treated mice with tetrodotoxin (TTX) for 16 h to prevent the production of action potentials and therefore block evoked presynaptic release of glutamate (Fig. 2b). Following 16 h of TTX treatment, we co-infused TTX with NBQX. As previously reported, treatment with TTX alone decreases ISF Aβ levels by about 40% from basal levels [8]. Blocking AMPA-Rs in addition to TTX treatment leads to a further decrease in Aβ levels of 33% despite the cessation of presynaptic activity (Fig. 2b). Thus, AMPA-Rs activated during steady-state, tonic levels of activity appear to drive higher ISF Aβ levels independently of evoked glutamatergic signaling. Interestingly, antagonizing basally active AMPA-Rs induces a full effect on ISF Aβ levels regardless if action potentials are intact or blocked with TTX, suggesting that basal AMPA-ergic regulation of Aβ is driven by spontaneous glutamate release via miniature EPSCs ("minis") as opposed to evoked activity.

We next determined the extent to which AMPA-mediated Aβ regulation relies on presynaptic activity. As before, mice were pre-treated with TTX followed by co-treatment with TTX and AMPA. During the initial 8 h of TTX and AMPA treatment, the decrease in Aβ levels caused by AMPA treatment (Fig. 2c) is abolished. However, a longer AMPA treatment of 14 h significantly decreased ISF Aβ levels by 30% of post-TTX levels (Fig. 2b). These results imply that, initially, evoked glutamatergic transmission is necessary for AMPA treatment to decrease ISF Aβ. With longer treatment, however, ISF Aβ levels are reduced through postsynaptic AMPA-R signaling alone, without the need of action potentials or further glutamatergic activity stimulation.

Given that high levels of NMDA-R activation result in decreased Aβ levels through calcium–dependent ERK signaling [32, 33], we hypothesized that AMPA treatment might reduce ISF Aβ levels through the indirect activation of NMDA-Rs expressed on downstream post-synaptic neurons. To determine the contribution of NMDA-Rs to the changes in Aβ levels following AMPA

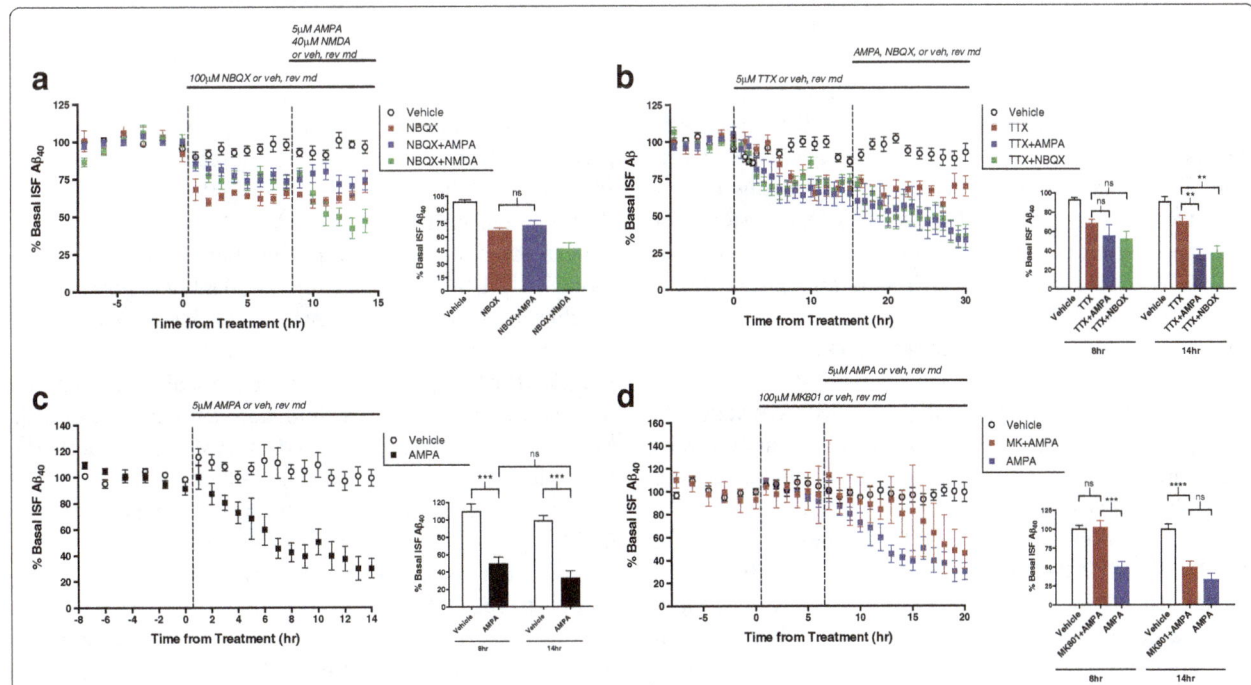

Fig. 2 AMPA treatment alters Aβ levels through multiple pathways. **a** APP/PS1 mice ($n = 6$) were treated with 100 μM NBQX, an AMPA receptor antagonist, for 8 h then co-treated with either 40 μM NMDA ($n = 6$), 5 μM AMPA ($n = 7$), or vehicle ($n = 12$). After 6 h of co-treatment with NBQX, the addition of AMPA had no effect on Aβ levels, though NMDA still reduced Aβ by 37.5 ± 3.3% ($p < 0.0001$, one-way ANOVA, Bonferroni post hoc test). **b** Animals ($n = 6$ per group) were treated with 5 μM tetrodotoxin (TTX) for 16 h then co-treated with TTX and either 5 μM AMPA, 100 μM NBQX, or vehicle for an additional 14 h. After 8 h of co-treatment, ISF Aβ levels remained unchanged in all groups. 14 h co-treatment with AMPA reduced Aβ levels by 34.6 ± 9.9% ($p = 0.0027$, two-way ANOVA, Sidak post hoc test) and co-treatment with NBQX reduced levels by 32.8 ± 9.3% ($p = 0.0027$, two-way ANOVA, Sidak post hoc test). **c** APP/PS1 mice were treated with either 5 μM AMPA ($n = 7$) or vehicle ($n = 5$) for 14 h, leading to a decrease in ISF Aβ levels of 66.3 ± 11.8% ($p = 0.0001$, two-way ANOVA, Sidak post hoc test). **d** 100 μM MK801 or vehicle was administered by reverse microdialysis for 6 h to APP/PS1 mice followed by co-administration with 5 μM AMPA or vehicle. After 8 h, mice treated with AMPA alone had significance decreases in ISF Aβ as compared to vehicle-treated mice, but mice receiving both MK801 and AMPA showed no change ($p = 0.996$, two-way ANOVA, Sidak post hoc test). After 14 h, however, AMPA treatment significantly decreased ISF Aβ levels to the same extent regardless of the presence of MK801 ($p = 0.384$, two-way ANOVA, Sidak post hoc test). Data plotted as mean ± SEM

treatment, mice were pre-treated with MK801, a NMDA-R open channel blocker, via reverse microdialysis for 6 h before co-treatment with MK801 and 5 µM AMPA (Fig. 2d). Within the first 8 h of treatment, co-application of MK801 and AMPA does not effect an AMPA-related change in Aβ levels. The ability of AMPA to alter ISF Aβ is therefore dependent on NMDA-R activation at this time point. By hour 14 of AMPA treatment, however, Aβ levels began to decline regardless of the presence of MK801 (Fig. 2d). These data imply that AMPA's effects on ISF Aβ levels are dependent on NMDA-R signaling for only a limited period. After prolonged treatment with AMPA, Aβ levels decrease through an NMDA-R-independent mechanism.

In consideration of these results, we questioned if AMPA-R signaling might be responsible for any part of NMDA-Rs' effect on Aβ levels. To test this, we first treated the mice with 100 µM NBQX, a competitive AMPA-R antagonist, through reverse microdialysis then co-treated with NMDA (Fig. 2a). As observed in previous experiments [32], 40 µM NMDA reduced ISF Aβ levels to approximately 50% of basal levels within 6 h of treatment, even in the presence of an AMPA-R antagonist (Fig. 2a). Though the effect of AMPA treatment on ISF Aβ in part relies on NMDA-R involvement, the opposite does not appear true; NMDA treatment decreases Aβ levels independently from AMPA-R activation. To ensure the specificity of AMPA treatment, animals were treated with NBQX to block AMPA-Rs prior to the addition of AMPA. As was expected, NBQX completely blocked the effect of AMPA-Rs on Aβ (Fig. 2a).

AMPA treatment results in long-lasting changes in ISF Aβ levels

Previous data show that activation of NMDA-R signaling rapidly decreases ISF Aβ levels by approximately 50% [32]. Once NMDA is no longer administered, ISF Aβ gradually returns to baseline levels within 30 h. AMPA treatment, however, results in a longer-lasting change in Aβ levels. APP/PS1 mice were perfused with 5 µM AMPA for 8 h. After this period, AMPA treatment ended and Aβ levels were monitored every 1–2 h for an additional 44 h (Fig. 3a). Levels of ISF Aβ decreased steadily during the AMPA treatment and continued to decrease for 3 h into the washout period to reach a maximal decrease of 60% from basal levels. From this lowest point, Aβ levels significantly increased from the trough to reach a level only 35% decreased from basal levels after 44 h of recovery (Fig. 3a). The washout study was terminated after a total of 60 h of ISF collection due to limitations in the reliable duration of microdialysis experiments, so it is possible that Aβ levels may completely recover from AMPA treatment with a longer washout period. A recovery in ISF Aβ suggests that

AMPA treatment does not cause major cell death and that the area surrounding the microdialysis probe continues to function normally following treatment.

APP/PS1 mice were treated with AMPA for 8 h followed by co-administration with NBQX (Fig. 3b). The decrease in Aβ levels following AMPA application did not recover to baseline levels with the addition of NBQX despite the cessation of AMPA-R activation. Because the Aβ decrease was preserved without AMPA-ergic transmission, the effect on Aβ is likely due to a long-lasting intracellular event and not a feed-forward increase in continued glutamatergic transmission. This observed long-lived change in Aβ levels was initiated by an AMPA treatment period of only 30 min, which resulted in a 30% decrease in ISF Aβ (Fig. 3c).

Transcription of APP processing-related genes and the levels of APP fragments are unchanged following AMPA treatment

We demonstrated above that extended treatment with AMPA influences ISF Aβ levels without the need for NMDA-R activation. NMDA-Rs receptors are often associated with intracellular signaling and transcriptional regulation, while AMPA-Rs are generally thought of in terms of neuronal depolarization. However, there is growing evidence to suggest that AMPA-Rs may also play an active role in cellular signaling. For example, Plant et al. (2006) found that transient calcium signaling through calcium-permeable AMPA-Rs promotes the maintenance of long-term potentiation (LTP) [34]. Additionally, AMPA-R signaling, independent of depolarization, is sufficient to activate the transcription factor CREB as well as to initiate ERK signaling [17, 18, 35]. Given these results, the AMPA-R-dependent decrease in ISF Aβ that we observe could be due to the initiation of a signaling cascade by AMPA-Rs. First, we tested if AMPA-Rs affect the transcription of genes related to APP processing or Aβ clearance (Fig. 4a, b). APP/PS1 mice were administered 5 µM AMPA for 8 or 14 h by reverse microdialysis. At the end of treatment, probes were infused with Evans Blue for 30 min to mark the surrounding tissue reached by reverse microdialysis. The dyed hippocampal tissue was lysed and used for quantitative real-time PCR (qPCR) for a selection of genes involved in Aβ metabolism. Expression of the immediate early gene, cFos, was used as a control due to its increased expression following glutamatergic transmission [29]. As expected, AMPA treatment increased the expression of cFos in both the 8- and 14-h groups. However, we found no significant changes in the expression of APP, in genes related to α-secretase (ADAM10 and ADAM17), in genes related to β-secretase (BACE1), nor in genes related to Υ-secretase (PS1, PS2, PSEN2, APH1, BSG, and NIC) following 8 or 14 h of AMPA treatment (Fig. 4a, b). Further, AMPA treatment did not change expression in ERK1 or

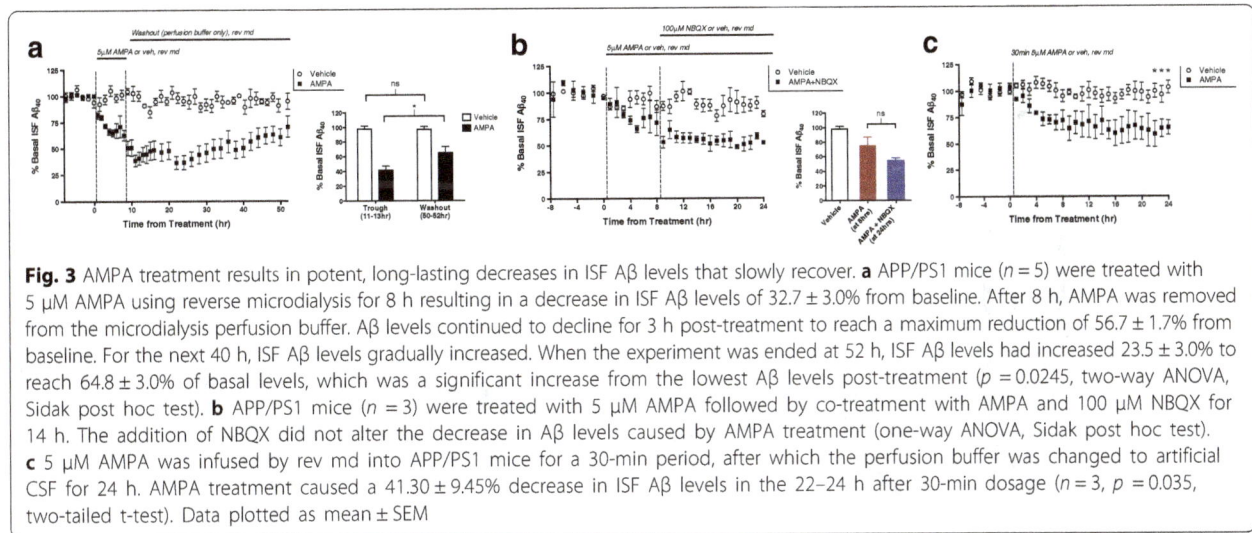

Fig. 3 AMPA treatment results in potent, long-lasting decreases in ISF Aβ levels that slowly recover. **a** APP/PS1 mice ($n = 5$) were treated with 5 μM AMPA using reverse microdialysis for 8 h resulting in a decrease in ISF Aβ levels of $32.7 \pm 3.0\%$ from baseline. After 8 h, AMPA was removed from the microdialysis perfusion buffer. Aβ levels continued to decline for 3 h post-treatment to reach a maximum reduction of $56.7 \pm 1.7\%$ from baseline. For the next 40 h, ISF Aβ levels gradually increased. When the experiment was ended at 52 h, ISF Aβ levels had increased $23.5 \pm 3.0\%$ to reach $64.8 \pm 3.0\%$ of basal levels, which was a significant increase from the lowest Aβ levels post-treatment ($p = 0.0245$, two-way ANOVA, Sidak post hoc test). **b** APP/PS1 mice ($n = 3$) were treated with 5 μM AMPA followed by co-treatment with AMPA and 100 μM NBQX for 14 h. The addition of NBQX did not alter the decrease in Aβ levels caused by AMPA treatment (one-way ANOVA, Sidak post hoc test). **c** 5 μM AMPA was infused by rev md into APP/PS1 mice for a 30-min period, after which the perfusion buffer was changed to artificial CSF for 24 h. AMPA treatment caused a $41.30 \pm 9.45\%$ decrease in ISF Aβ levels in the 22–24 h after 30-min dosage ($n = 3$, $p = 0.035$, two-tailed t-test). Data plotted as mean ± SEM

ERK2 or in genes associated with Aβ clearance (*LRP1*, *LRPR*, *AQP4*, *NEP*, *MMP2*, and *MMP9*). Finally, none of the AMPA-R subunits genes (*GRIA1–4*) were altered by AMPA treatment (Fig. 4a, b).

Extended treatment with AMPA promotes increased ISF Aβ clearance

To the best of our knowledge, all previous studies investigating the relationship between synaptic signaling and alterations in Aβ levels, including several from our laboratory, have found that synaptic signaling primarily affects Aβ production [4, 6–8, 25, 36]. However, after 14 h of AMPA administration, we found no change in full-length APP levels or in the cleavage products β-C-terminal fragment (β-CTF), soluble APP-α (sAPP-α), and sAPP-β as determined by Western blot (Fig. 5a). In combination with the lack of transcriptional changes in production-related genes (Fig. 4a, b), these data suggest that extended treatment with AMPA does not have a pronounced effect on Aβ production. It is important to note, however, that small changes in gene or protein levels, such that occur when only a subpopulation of cells is affected, can be masked when total brain lysates are analyzed. Considering the large effect that AMPA has on ISF Aβ levels, though, we hypothesized that AMPA-Rs act on ISF Aβ through a different mechanism, namely by altering its clearance.

Aβ is eliminated from the ISF through five main pathways: receptor-mediated transport across the blood brain barrier (BBB), enzymatic degradation, cellular uptake, glymphatic-mediated clearance, or passive bulk-flow clearance for (reviews see [37–39]). If any of these pathways is targeted by AMPA treatment, the rate of ISF Aβ clearance could increase. To test this possibility, we measured half-life of ISF Aβ in mice treated with either 5 μM AMPA or vehicle using reverse

microdialysis (Fig. 5b). AMPA treatment leads to a rapid decrease in Aβ that stabilizes by 6–8 h of treatment. After 14 h, mice were subcutaneously injected with LY411575, a potent γ-secretase inhibitor that rapidly inhibits Aβ production. LY411575 enters the brain and within 15 min reaches a concentration approximately 200-fold in excess of its IC_{50} for γ-secretase inhibition [25]. Once γ-secretase is inhibited, all new production of Aβ is precluded and microdialysis is used to monitor the levels of remaining ISF Aβ over time. The rate at which Aβ in the ISF is eliminated can be measured by calculating the slope of the semi-log plot of percentage baseline Aβ levels versus time. This elimination rate was determined for both groups, and the Aβ half-life calculated. Interestingly, the half-life of ISF Aβ was significantly shorter by over 30% in mice receiving AMPA treatment ($t_{1/2} = 0.93$ h) than those in the control group ($t_{1/2} = 1.38$ h), indicating that AMPA treatment increases the clearance of ISF Aβ (Fig. 5c). It is important to note that 6 of 12 AMPA-treated mice had ISF Aβ levels decrease so much that a reliable half-life could not be calculated. If this greater decrease following AMPA treatment was also due to enhanced clearance, then the observed effect of AMPA on Aβ would be even greater so, we could be underestimating the effect of AMPA on Aβ clearance. Next, we measured the levels of key proteins involved in Aβ clearance in the hippocampal tissue surrounding the microdialysis probe for mice treated with 14 h of AMPA or vehicle (Fig. 6a). Similar to the qPCR experiments (Fig. 4b), only the positive control cFos showed a significant change in protein levels with AMPA treatment (Fig. 6a). Though these data suggest that none of the Aβ clearance-related proteins selected is involved in AMPA-mediated regulation of Aβ, Western blots do not

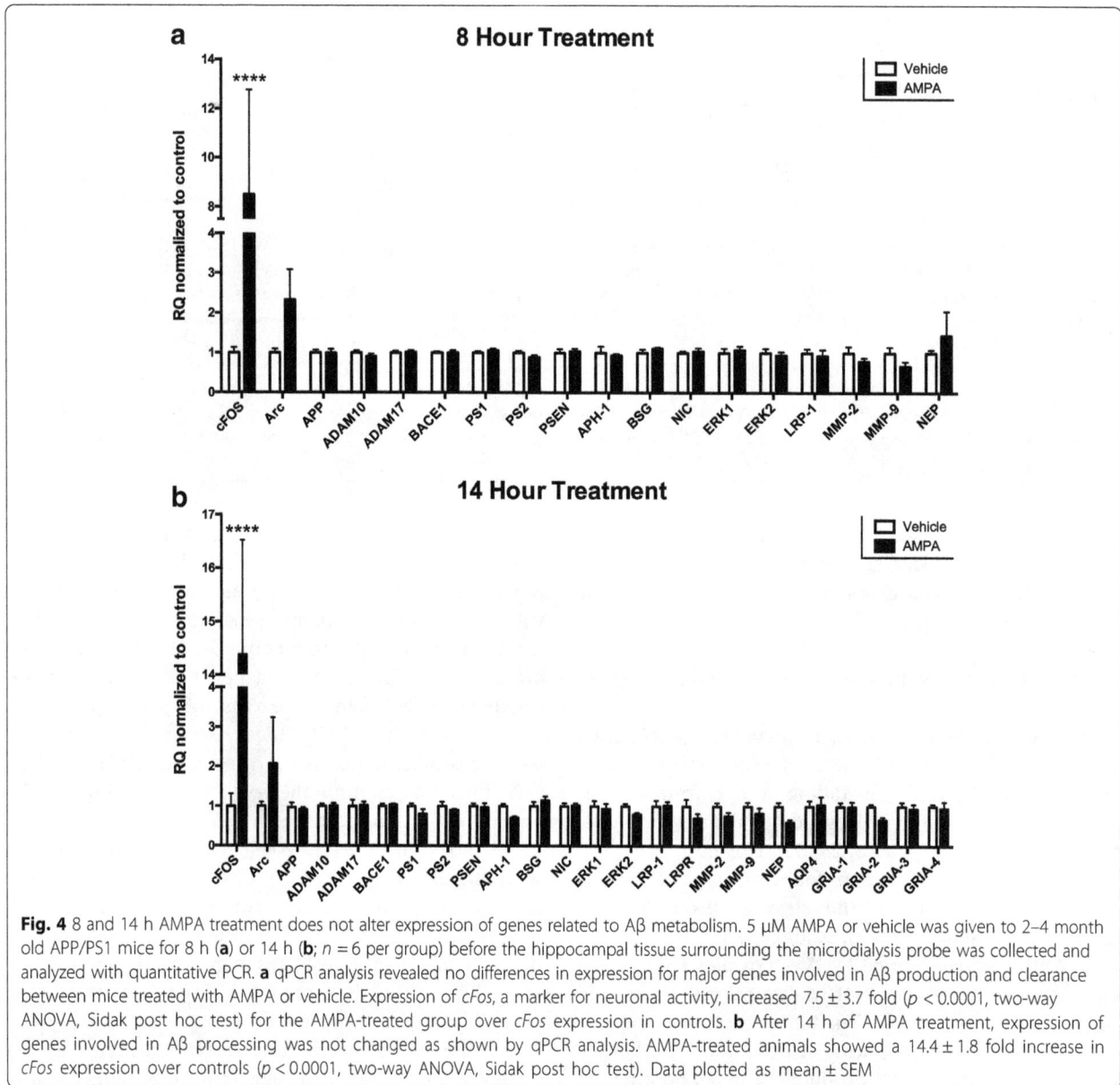

Fig. 4 8 and 14 h AMPA treatment does not alter expression of genes related to Aβ metabolism. 5 μM AMPA or vehicle was given to 2–4 month old APP/PS1 mice for 8 h (**a**) or 14 h (**b**; $n = 6$ per group) before the hippocampal tissue surrounding the microdialysis probe was collected and analyzed with quantitative PCR. **a** qPCR analysis revealed no differences in expression for major genes involved in Aβ production and clearance between mice treated with AMPA or vehicle. Expression of *cFos*, a marker for neuronal activity, increased 7.5 ± 3.7 fold ($p < 0.0001$, two-way ANOVA, Sidak post hoc test) for the AMPA-treated group over *cFos* expression in controls. **b** After 14 h of AMPA treatment, expression of genes involved in Aβ processing was not changed as shown by qPCR analysis. AMPA-treated animals showed a 14.4 ± 1.8 fold increase in *cFos* expression over controls ($p < 0.0001$, two-way ANOVA, Sidak post hoc test). Data plotted as mean ± SEM

detect cell type-specific changes in protein levels, alterations in protein function, or changes in protein localization. To test if AMPA treatment increases protease activity and thus Aβ degradation, we pre-treated APP/PS1 mice with the neprilysin inhibitor, thiorphan, or with the broad-spectrum metalloproteinase (MMP) inhibitor, GM6001, before co-treating with AMPA. Inhibition of neprilysin and all MMP family members both blocks Aβ clearance pathways and potentially inhibits α-secretase, which increases ISF Aβ levels when those agents are administered singly (Fig. 6b). Importantly, the addition of AMPA still decreased Aβ by a comparable amount as observed without the protease inhibitors, indicating

that AMPA does not affect degradation of Aβ through these proteases.

AMPA-R activation does not induce broad inflammation

A potential concern is that AMPA treatment decreases ISF Aβ by causing cellular toxicity and/or creating a lesion through increased glutamatergic activity [40]. If AMPA does cause cellular damage, an inflammatory response would involve the recruitment and activation of microglia and astrocytes [41–43]. To monitor inflammatory responses, mice were treated with 5 μM AMPA or with vehicle for 8 or 14 h before brains were collected and fixed in 4% formaldehyde. The brains were stained for Iba1, a marker of microglia [44], and GFAP, a marker

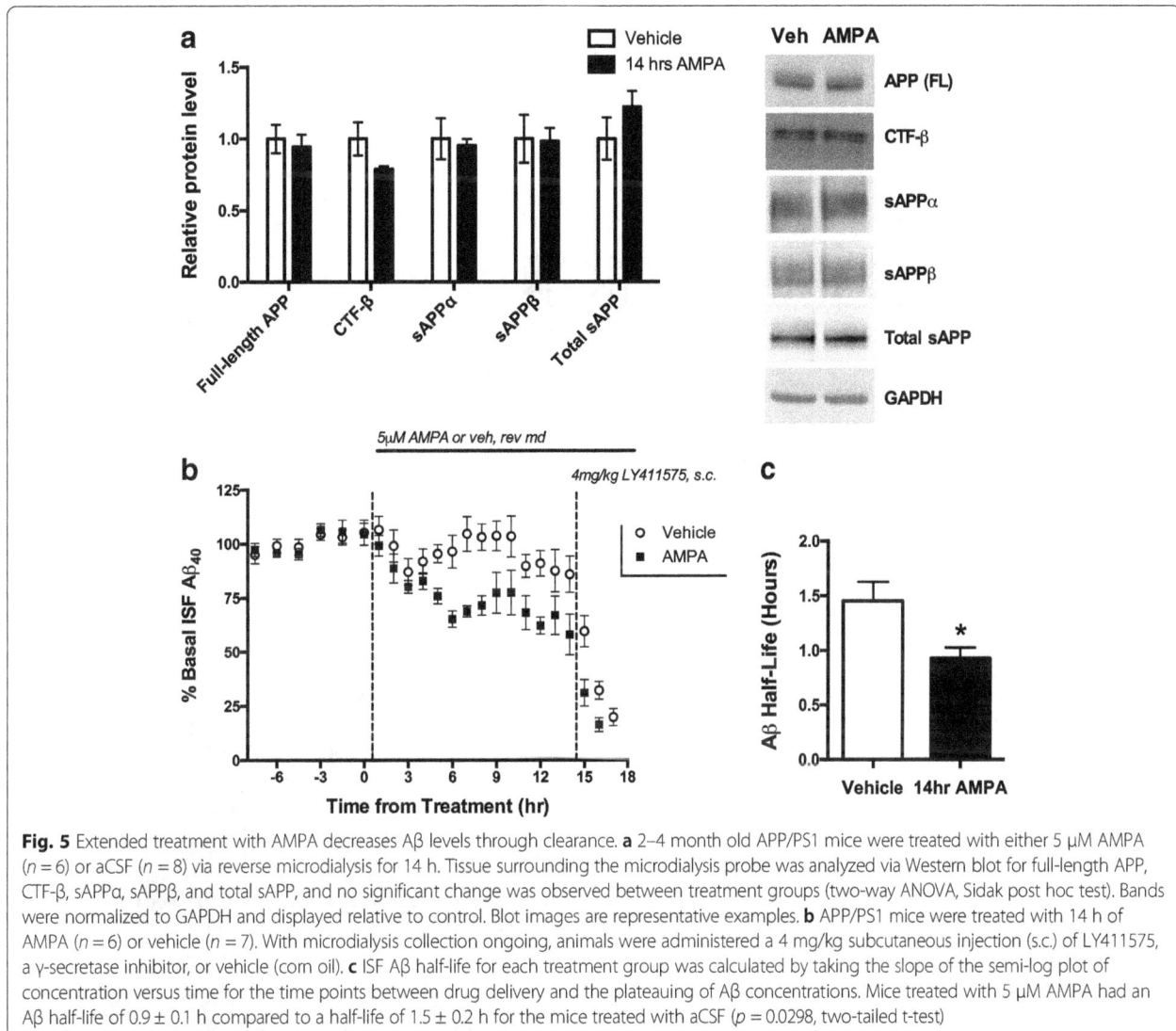

Fig. 5 Extended treatment with AMPA decreases Aβ levels through clearance. **a** 2–4 month old APP/PS1 mice were treated with either 5 μM AMPA (*n* = 6) or aCSF (*n* = 8) via reverse microdialysis for 14 h. Tissue surrounding the microdialysis probe was analyzed via Western blot for full-length APP, CTF-β, sAPPα, sAPPβ, and total sAPP, and no significant change was observed between treatment groups (two-way ANOVA, Sidak post hoc test). Bands were normalized to GAPDH and displayed relative to control. Blot images are representative examples. **b** APP/PS1 mice were treated with 14 h of AMPA (*n* = 6) or vehicle (*n* = 7). With microdialysis collection ongoing, animals were administered a 4 mg/kg subcutaneous injection (s.c.) of LY411575, a γ-secretase inhibitor, or vehicle (corn oil). **c** ISF Aβ half-life for each treatment group was calculated by taking the slope of the semi-log plot of concentration versus time for the time points between drug delivery and the plateauing of Aβ concentrations. Mice treated with 5 μM AMPA had an Aβ half-life of 0.9 ± 0.1 h compared to a half-life of 1.5 ± 0.2 h for the mice treated with aCSF (*p* = 0.0298, two-tailed t-test)

for astrocytes [42, 45]. As expected, we found increased Iba1 and GFAP staining around the microdialysis probe tract, but no change in staining density between the AMPA- and vehicle-treated tissue at either time point (Fig. 7a). For confirmation, we measured protein levels of GFAP and CD45, another microglial marker [46], using hippocampal lysates from APP/PS1 mice treated with either 5 μM AMPA or vehicle for 14 h (Fig. 7b). In agreement with the immunostaining results, AMPA treatment did not increase GFAP or CD45 protein levels, indicating a lack of glial recruitment (Fig. 7b). In addition to monitoring the glial response, we measured pro-inflammatory cytokines levels in the hippocampal lysates of mice following AMPA treatment. Though IL-1β and TNF-α levels were unchanged, the levels of IL-6 showed a dramatic increase of over 500% (Fig. 7c). IL-6 is a neuropoietic cytokine with both neuromodulatory and neuroprotective roles, known to be induced by

neuronal activity [47–49]. Without a visible increase in gliosis and with no significant increase in IL-1β or TNF-α, there does not appear to be a broad inflammatory response. These data, along with the partial recovery of ISF Aβ in the 44 h sampled following AMPA treatment (Fig. 3a), strongly suggest AMPA is not causing widespread toxicity accounting for the effects on Aβ observed in this study.

IL-6 is a neuropoietic cytokine with both neuromodulatory and neuroprotective roles, known to be induced by neuronal activity [47–49]. Intriguingly, IL-6 has previously been linked to enhanced Aβ clearance [50, 51]. Because levels of IL-6 increased greatly following AMPA treatment, we tested the possibility that enhanced IL-6 signaling is involved in the decrease in ISF Aβ levels following AMPA-R stimulation. To do this, we utilized 3-month-old IL-6-deficient mice (IL-6$^{-/-}$ mice). These mice develop normally and produce normal levels of

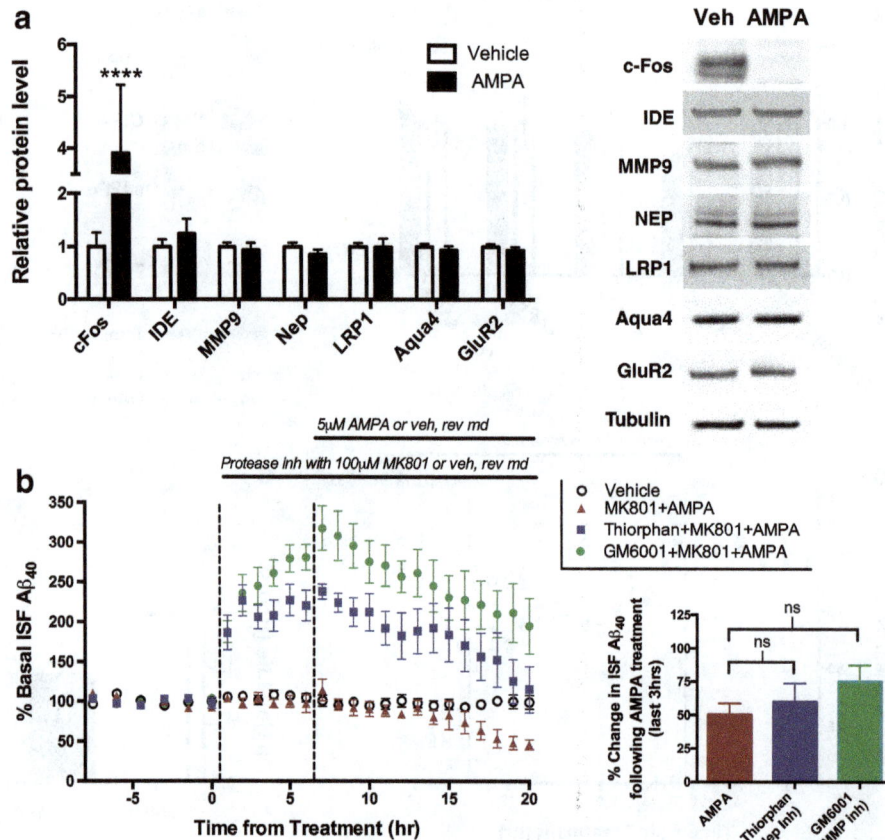

Fig. 6 AMPA-mediated decrease in Aβ not due to changes in clearance-related proteins or proteases. **a** 2–4 month old APP/PS1 mice were treated with either 5 µM AMPA (n = 6) or aCSF (n = 8) via reverse microdialysis for 14 h. Tissue surrounding the microdialysis probe was analyzed via Western blot to determine levels of proteins involved in Aβ elimination and clearance. Bands were normalized to GAPDH and displayed relative to control. Blot images are representative examples. cFos protein expression was increased 2.9 ± 0.4 fold (p < 0.0001, two-way ANOVA, Sidak post hoc test) in the AMPA group compared to the controls. No other proteins showed a significant difference between treatment groups. **b** Reverse microdialysis was used to treat APP/PS1 mice (n = 7) with 10 µM thiorphan (neprilysin inhibitor), 25 µM GM6001 (broad-spectrum MMP inhibitor), or vehicle for 6 h, followed by 14 h of co-treatment with 5 µM AMPA. The Aβ concentrations in the last 3 h of each treatment were averaged and the differences between the end of inhibitor/vehicle treatment and after the addition of AMPA were compared. Inhibiting protease activity with thiorphan or GM6001 did not alter the decrease in ISF Aβ levels observed following AMPA treatment (p = 0.40, one-way ANOVA, Dunnet's post hoc test). Data plotted as mean ± SEM

murine Aβ in the ISF. We treated IL-6$^{-/-}$ and WT mice with MK801 to block NMDA-R signaling for 6 h, then added 7.5 µM AMPA into the perfusion buffer for an extended period (Fig. 8). Because murine Aβ levels are much lower in these mice than in our amyloidosis models, samples were collected every 2.5 h. Similar to our observations in APP/PS1 mice, AMPA treatment led to a decrease in ISF Aβ by approximately 67% in WT mice. Conversely, AMPA failed to produce a significant change in ISF Aβ levels in IL-6$^{-/-}$ mice, suggesting that IL-6 signaling is necessary for AMPA-R regulation of Aβ.

Discussion

In this study, we provide evidence that though steady-state levels of AMPA-Rs encourage heightened ISF Aβ levels, evoked AMPA-R signaling decreases extracellular

Aβ concentration through two different pathways (see Fig. 9 for model). The first of these pathways acts on Aβ through an indirect network effect; AMPA-R stimulation increases glutamatergic transmission, including elevated NMDA-R signaling on the postsynaptic neuron. It has been previously shown that NMDA-Rs regulate Aβ levels by using calcium as a second messenger to activate ERK and increase α-secretase activity. Second, we found that AMPA-Rs can also influence Aβ levels independently of NMDA-Rs. This purely AMPA-R-mediated pathway takes longer to recruit, increases the rate of ISF Aβ clearance, and requires IL-6 signaling. Gene expression and protein levels of many primary clearance-related molecules remain unchanged, possibly indicating cell-type specific changes or alterations in protein function or localization.

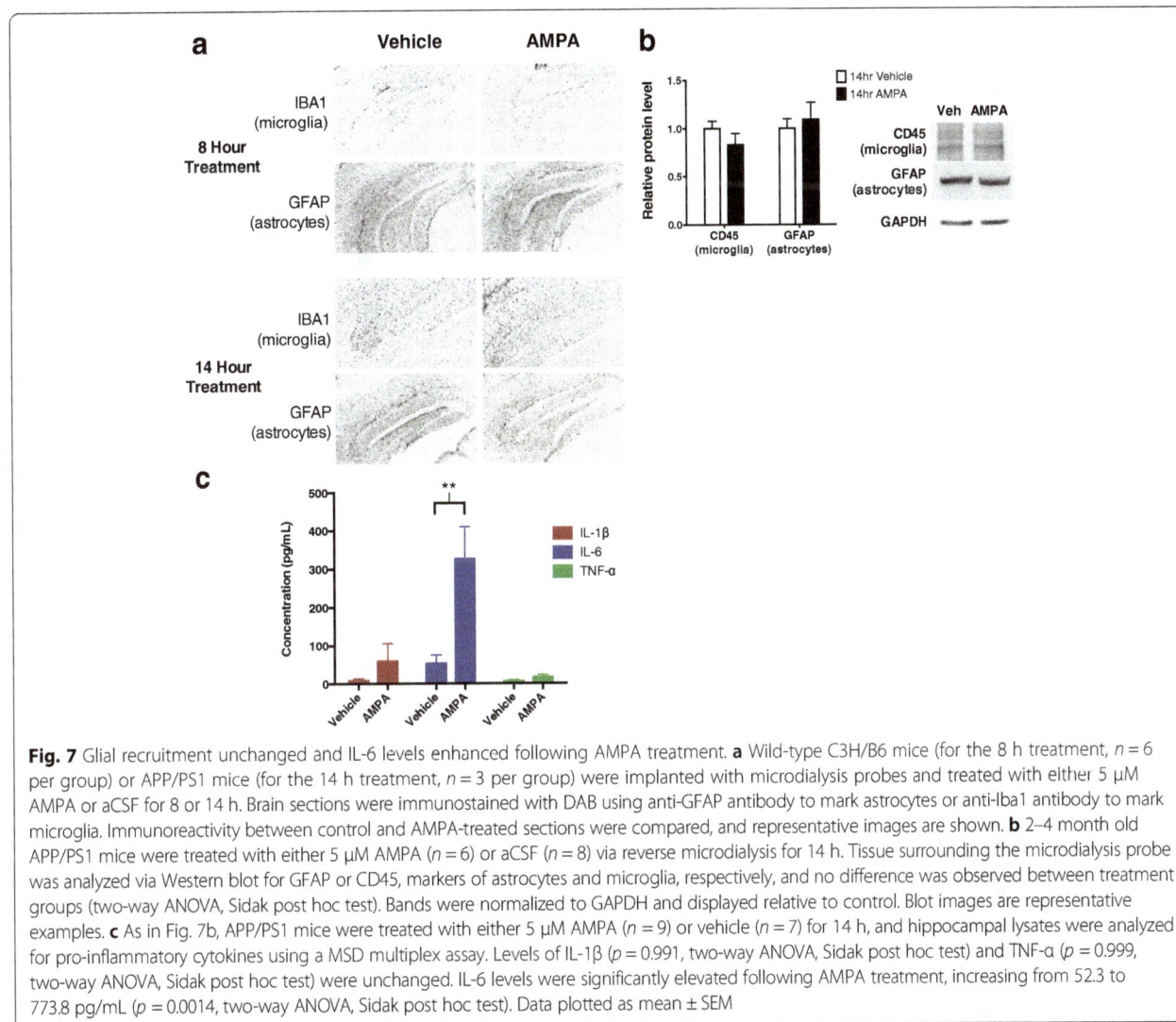

Fig. 7 Glial recruitment unchanged and IL-6 levels enhanced following AMPA treatment. **a** Wild-type C3H/B6 mice (for the 8 h treatment, $n = 6$ per group) or APP/PS1 mice (for the 14 h treatment, $n = 3$ per group) were implanted with microdialysis probes and treated with either 5 μM AMPA or aCSF for 8 or 14 h. Brain sections were immunostained with DAB using anti-GFAP antibody to mark astrocytes or anti-Iba1 antibody to mark microglia. Immunoreactivity between control and AMPA-treated sections were compared, and representative images are shown. **b** 2–4 month old APP/PS1 mice were treated with either 5 μM AMPA ($n = 6$) or aCSF ($n = 8$) via reverse microdialysis for 14 h. Tissue surrounding the microdialysis probe was analyzed via Western blot for GFAP or CD45, markers of astrocytes and microglia, respectively, and no difference was observed between treatment groups (two-way ANOVA, Sidak post hoc test). Bands were normalized to GAPDH and displayed relative to control. Blot images are representative examples. **c** As in Fig. 7b, APP/PS1 mice were treated with either 5 μM AMPA ($n = 9$) or vehicle ($n = 7$) for 14 h, and hippocampal lysates were analyzed for pro-inflammatory cytokines using a MSD multiplex assay. Levels of IL-1β ($p = 0.991$, two-way ANOVA, Sidak post hoc test) and TNF-α ($p = 0.999$, two-way ANOVA, Sidak post hoc test) were unchanged. IL-6 levels were significantly elevated following AMPA treatment, increasing from 52.3 to 773.8 pg/mL ($p = 0.0014$, two-way ANOVA, Sidak post hoc test). Data plotted as mean ± SEM

Exogenous application of AMPA decreases ISF Aβ through postsynaptic signaling

We found that infusion of AMPA directly into the hippocampus of APP/PS1 mice through reverse microdialysis decreases ISF Aβ levels by up to 75% following the maximal dose of 10 μM. Treatment with AMPA induces a potent, long-lasting effect on Aβ levels, with even a brief application initiating a full response. AMPA-Rs, therefore, appear to be significant regulators of Aβ levels in the extracellular space. Factors that influence extracellular levels of Aβ have the potential to directly influence AD pathogenesis by altering the likelihood of Aβ to aggregate [52]. That AMPA increases activity but suppresses Aβ levels is somewhat surprising considering previous reports that synaptic activity drives production of Aβ. Treatment with the GABA$_A$ receptor antagonist picrotoxin, high levels of potassium chloride, or electrical stimulation promotes Aβ secretion into the extracellular space [7–9]. In a more physiological setting, increasing activity within the barrel cortex through vibrissal stimulation results in higher levels of ISF Aβ in APP/PS1 mice [4, 53]. In humans, the highest levels of amyloid deposition are found in brain regions with the highest baseline metabolic activity [10].

Considering these findings, it would be reasonable to hypothesize that AMPA-Rs, as excitatory channels, should increase Aβ levels. Paradoxically, however, we found increasing AMPA-R activation through exogenous AMPA treatment significantly decreases ISF Aβ. Because AMPA-Rs are susceptible to rapid desensitization, we considered the possibility that AMPA-Rs act on Aβ levels through induced synaptic depression [30, 31]. However, when receptor desensitization was blocked with cyclothiazide, the decrease in Aβ in response to AMPA was potentiated. Receptor desensitization only limited Aβ suppression, and receptor activation is directly responsible for the reduction of Aβ levels.

Though general increases in synaptic activity upregulate Aβ production, the activation of certain postsynaptic

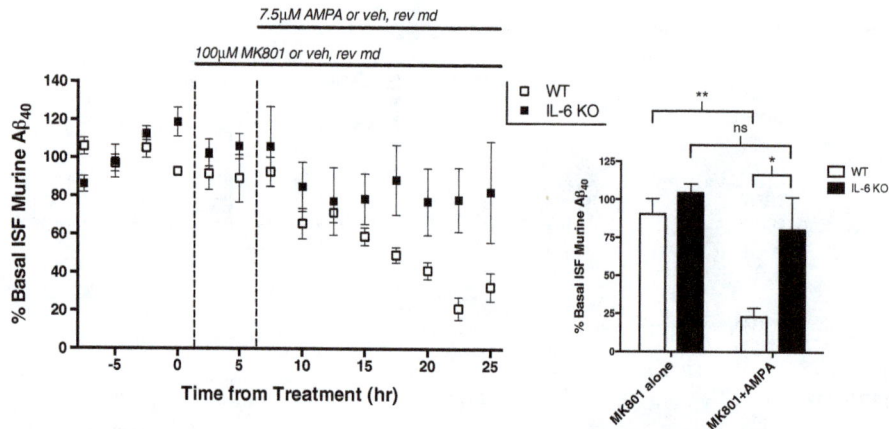

Fig. 8 IL-6 is required for AMPA-R regulation of ISF Aβ levels. Both IL-6$^{-/-}$ mice ($n = 5$) and C3H/B6 WT mice ($n = 6$) were treated with 100 μM MK801 for 6 h via reverse microdialysis, then co-treated with MK801 and 7.5 μM AMPA for an additional 17 h. The last five hours of each treatment (MK801 alone vs MK801 + AMPA) were averaged for each treatment group and compared (two-way ANOVA, Sidak post hoc test). In WT animals, ISF Aβ levels decreased by 67.34% from MK801 alone to MK801 + AMPA ($p = 0.002$). In IL-6$^{-/-}$ animals, the addition of AMPA resulted in a non-significant decrease in ISF Aβ levels of 23.96% ($p = 0.652$). Furthermore, ISF Aβ levels IL-6$^{-/-}$ mice following extended AMPA treatment are significantly higher than observed in WT mice (80.26 and 23.0%, respectively; $p = 0.027$). Data plotted as mean ± SEM

signaling systems can alter APP processing to yield varied effects on Aβ levels, particularly when α-secretase is targeted. As mentioned above, serotonin receptor activation decreases Aβ levels through PKA and ERK activation [12, 13]. The serotonin receptor illustrates the specificity involved in Aβ regulation; only the G_s-linked receptors decrease Aβ whereas the other G-protein coupled serotonin receptors have no effect or increase Aβ [13]. Additionally, M1 muscarinic acetylcholine (mACh) receptor agonists decrease Aβ production, and deleting this receptor leads to increased Aβ and amyloid pathology [54–56]. Within the glutamate receptor family, muscarinic glutamate receptor 5 has been shown

to trigger Aβ production [57, 58], and NMDA-Rs can modulate Aβ levels bidirectionally [32, 33, 59]. Clearly, postsynaptic effects on Aβ are diverse and markedly context-specific.

Spontaneous and evoked AMPA-R activation differentially regulate Aβ levels

In these studies we have shown that AMPA-R regulation of Aβ is multifarious (see model Fig. 9). When basal AMPA-R activity is antagonized, ISF Aβ decreases by 20%. The same decrease occurs even after action potentials are blocked and evoked synaptic transmission is inhibited, indicating that the basal AMPA-R signaling

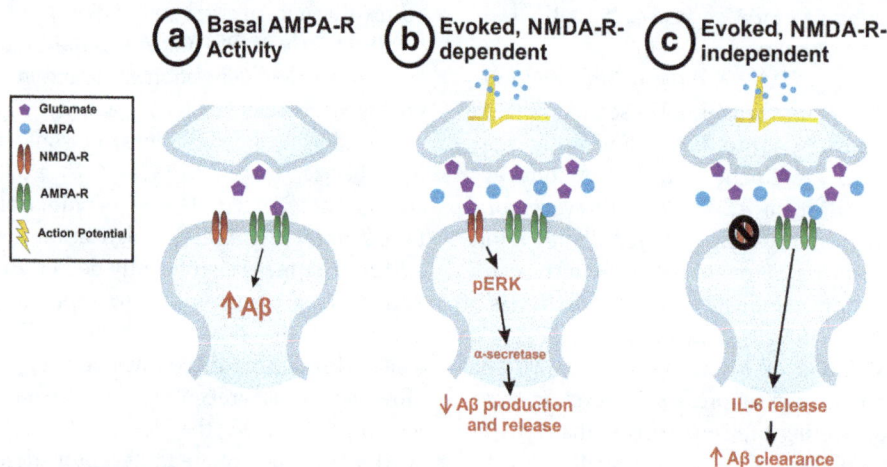

Fig. 9 Model of AMPA-R-mediated Aβ regulation. **a** Tonic, steady-state AMPA-R activity driven by spontaneous neurotransmission increases levels of Aβ in the ISF. **b** Evoked glutamatergic transmission resulting from AMPA treatment initially decreases ISF Aβ through NMDA-R activation. As described in previous studies, NMDA-Rs lead to decreased Aβ production and release into the ISF through ERK phosphorylation and enhanced α-secretase activity. **c** Extended AMPA-R activation, independent of NMDA-Rs, increases IL-6 signaling to stimulate clearance of Aβ from the ISF

that increases Aβ levels is likely due to spontaneous transmission (Fig. 9a). Conversely, application of AMPA via reverse microdialysis causes direct AMPA-R activation as well as stimulates evoked glutamatergic transmission. In this scenario, AMPA-R activation decreases Aβ levels. This dual effect of AMPA-Rs, depending on the mode of transmission, has been seen in various contexts. Sara and colleagues (2011) utilized a use-dependent AMPA-R antagonist to show that spontaneous and evoked transmission activate discrete populations of AMPA-Rs [60]. Additionally, several studies found that receptors that respond differentially to spontaneous and evoked transmission are physically and functionally distinct [61–66]. Intriguingly, spontaneous activity appears to suppress protein synthesis while evoked activity stimulates translation. Another possible explanation is that the effects of AMPA-Rs on Aβ are dependent on relative levels of AMPA-R activation. During basal transmission, a smaller set of AMPA-Rs is active compared to the AMPA-Rs targeted by action potentials or exogenous AMPA treatment. How endogenous AMPA-Rs promote increased levels of ISF Aβ remains unknown, though we speculate that basal AMPA-ergic signaling induces amyloidogenic APP processing through increased endocytosis within or near the presynaptic terminal, as described in previous studies [7–9, 67].

Extended AMPA treatment decreases ISF Aβ half-life

Adding an additional layer of complexity, exogenous AMPA treatment appears to act on Aβ levels through two distinct pathways. Within the first 8 h of treatment, AMPA's ability to modulate Aβ levels depends on NMDA-R signaling (Fig. 9b). This pathway relies on presynaptic activity to increase glutamatergic transmission, thus stimulating NMDA-R activation on downstream neurons to decrease Aβ production in these cells [32, 33]. The reverse is not true, however; AMPA-Rs do not appear to play a role in NMDA-R-mediated decreases in Aβ. Following longer AMPA treatment, a novel pathway by which AMPA-Rs influence Aβ independently of both presynaptic activity and NMDA-Rs emerges.

As detailed above, studies regarding synaptic and postsynaptic regulation of Aβ have primarily addressed the effects of activity on Aβ production. However, we were unable to detect changes in APP processing-related gene expression or in APP fragment levels in hippocampal lysates following either 8 or 14 h of AMPA treatment. Instead, using microdialysis along with a potent γ-secretase inhibitor, we found that treatment with AMPA for 14 h decreased the half-life of ISF Aβ, implying that AMPA-Rs modulate Aβ clearance (Fig. 9c). This does not appear to involve glial recruitment, a broad inflammatory response, or changes in key clearance-related

proteins. We found that one proinflammatory cytokine, IL-6, increased dramatically following AMPA treatment. IL-6 has been shown to have both normal physiological as well as inflammatory, pathological roles in the CNS [49, 51, 68, 69] and has been shown to be secreted in response to neuronal depolarization [47, 48]. Furthermore, IL-6 signaling has been linked to increased Aβ clearance through microglial phagocytosis [50, 51]. Given the substantial increase in IL-6 following AMPA treatment, we propose that AMPA could be causing IL-6 release and enhanced phagocytosis of Aβ. In support of this hypothesis, mice deficient in IL-6 fail to show decreased ISF Aβ levels in response to AMPA treatment, suggesting that IL-6 signaling is involved in AMPA-R regulation of ISF Aβ levels. The IL-6 receptor is expressed on neurons, microglia, and astrocytes [70, 71], so this synaptic activity-dependent clearance pathway could be mediated by multiple cell types. Though we propose a connection between neuronal IL-6 release and microglial clearance, our data do not indicate which cell types are involved. Furthermore, we have only tested a handful of cytokines in response to AMPA treatment thus far, leaving open the possibility that multiple cytokines are involved in this pathway. Future experiments will address the mechanism through which AMPA-Rs affect Aβ clearance.

The finding that AMPA treatment decreases Aβ levels is supported by a previous study by Hoey and colleagues conducted in primary cortical neurons [22]. Unlike our study, however, the authors conclude that Aβ production is decreased when AMPA directly acts to increase non-amyloidogenic APP processing. In contrast, our in vivo studies suggest that AMPA treatment requires an intermediary step of NMDA-R activation in order to increase non-amyloidogenic processing of APP. Additionally, our studies model a second pathway in which AMPA directly acts on Aβ through enhanced clearance. Because this pathway likely involves multiple cell types interacting, experiments using neuronal cultures would not recapitulate the effects we observed. Furthermore, the discrepancies in findings could also be explained by developmental differences between our two systems. Hoey et al. (2013) found that AMPA-mediated alterations in APP processing are at least partially due to calcium-permeable AMPA-Rs. There is evidence that GluA2, the receptor subunit responsible for determining the receptor's calcium permeability, is developmentally regulated [72–75]. Finally, we have found that even slight changes in AMPA concentration can change Aβ's response, and our two studies used very different doses. We administered 5 μM AMPA through the microdialysis probe of which only an estimated 10% diffuses into the extracellular space. In contrast, Hoey et al. (2013) administered 50 μM AMPA, potentially activating a different pathway than we observed.

Though both production and clearance determine the steady state levels of Aβ in the extracellular space, late-onset AD (LOAD) is primarily characterized by dysfunctions in Aβ clearance [38, 76]. In 2003, we found that ISF Aβ half-life as measured by microdialysis is doubled in an aged APP transgenic model compared to young animals [25]. In human studies, metabolic labeling and CNS analysis revealed impaired clearance rates in participants with LOAD, though Aβ production was unaltered [76]. Furthermore, many of the genetic factors associated with LOAD are related to clearance, including *APOE*, *CLU*, *CR1*, and *CD33*. Given the evident prominence of Aβ clearance in AD, our results highlight the importance of understanding the ways in which synaptic activity impinges on previous clearance-related studies.

Conclusions

There are clearly numerous mechanisms that together regulate Aβ levels. Though the confluence of these various synaptic-mediated pathways appears to result in increased Aβ, we propose that certain postsynaptic signaling pathways, such as those described in these studies, act as protective mechanisms that aid in maintaining Aβ homeostasis. The failure of these Aβ-suppressing pathways may contribute to the breakdown of homeostasis that ultimately results in the build-up of pathology. Indeed, glutamatergic transmission is one of the first systems targeted by toxic species of amyloid as the disease progresses [77–80].

As the dominant excitatory ionotropic receptors in the brain, AMPA-Rs have the potential to greatly influence extracellular Aβ levels and amyloid pathology. We have found that activation of AMPA-Rs initiates a varied and complex response in which opposing pathways act concurrently to regulate Aβ levels. Our results link postsynaptic signaling through AMPA-Rs to the increased release of IL-6 and enhanced Aβ clearance. Soluble, monomeric Aβ production is a normal process of every brain. Even those brains destined to develop AD pathology produce Aβ for decades without formation of toxic aggregates. The point at which Aβ becomes pathogenic is likely influenced by a number of factors, including the loss of homeostatic pathways. Identifying and understanding how, early in our lives, Aβ levels are controlled may give us clues to disease etiology or even prevention.

Abbreviations
aCSF: Artificial cerebrospinal fluid; AD: Alzheimer's disease; AMPA-R: AMPA receptors; APP: Amyloid precursor protein; APP/PS1: *APPswe/PS1ΔE9*; Aβ: Amyloid-β; BBB: Blood brain barrier; BSA: Bovine serum albumin; CTZ: Cyclothiazide; ERK: Extracellular regulated kinase; GAPDH: Glyceraldehyde 3-phosphate dehydrogenase; GFAP: Glial fibrillary acidic protein; Iba1: Ionized calcium-binding adaptor molecule 1; IDE: Insulin-degrading enzyme; IL: Interleukin; ISF: Interstitial fluid; LOAD: Late-onset AD; LRP1: Low density lipoprotein receptor-related protein 1; LTP: Long-term potentiation; mACh: Muscarinic acetylcholine; MMP: Matrix metalloproteinase; NMDA-R: NMDA receptor; qPCR: Quantitative real-time

PCR; TNF: Tumor necrosis factor; TTX: Tetrodotoxin; WT: Wild-type; β-CTF: β-C-terminal fragment

Acknowledgements
The authors would like to thank the Mouse Genetics Core at Washington University for maintaining the APP/PS1 mouse colony. We also thank Diane Bender in the Center for Human Immunology and Immunotherapy Programs' (CHiiPs) Immunomonitoring Laboratory (IML) for her help with the MSD cytokine assay.

Funding
This work is supported by National Institute of Health (NIH)/NINDS (P01 NS074969; JRC, DMH, GB), NIH/NIA (R01 AG042513, P50 AG005681; JRC), and the Charles F. and Joanne Knight ADRC at Washington University (JRC).

Authors' contributions
JCH, JRC, DMH, and GB designed the research. JCH and HL performed the research. JCH analyzed the data and JCH and JRC wrote the paper. All authors read and approved the final manuscript.

Ethics approval
All animal studies were performed in accordance with the guidelines of the Association for Assessment and Accreditation of Laboratory Animal Care (AAALAC) and the Institutional Animal Care and Use Committee (IACUC) at Washington University.

Competing interests
The authors declare that they have no competing interests.

Author details
[1]Department of Neurology, Knight Alzheimer's Disease Research Center, Hope Center for Neurological Disorders, Washington University School of Medicine, Campus Box 8111, 660 South Euclid Avenue, St. Louis, MO 63110, USA. [2]Department of Neuroscience, Mayo Clinic, Jacksonville, FL 32224, USA.

References
1. Sperling RA, Aisen PS, Beckett LA, Bennett DA, Craft S, Fagan AM, et al. Toward defining the preclinical stages of Alzheimer's disease: recommendations from the National Institute on Aging and the Alzheimer's association workgroup. Alzheimers Dement. 2011;7:280-92.
2. Hardy JA, Higgins GA. Alzheimer's disease: the amyloid cascade hypothesis. Science. 1992;256:184–5.
3. Musiek ES, Holtzman DM. Three dimensions of the amyloid hypothesis: time, space and "wingmen". Nat Neurosci. 2015;18:800–6. Nature Research
4. Bero AW, Yan P, Roh JH, Cirrito JR, Stewart FR, Raichle ME, et al. Neuronal activity regulates the regional vulnerability to amyloid-β deposition. Nat Neurosci. 2011;14(6):750. Nature Research
5. Meyer-Luehmann M, Stalder M, Herzig MC, Kaeser SA, Kohler E, Pfeifer M, et al. Extracellular amyloid formation and associated pathology in neural grafts. Nat Neurosci. 2003;6:370–7. Nature Publishing Group
6. Yan P, Bero AW, Cirrito JR, Xiao Q, Hu X, Wang Y, et al. Characterizing the appearance and growth of amyloid plaques in APP/PS1 mice. J Neurosci. 2009;29:10706–14.
7. Kamenetz F, Tomita T, Hsieh H, Seabrook G, Borchelt D, Iwatsubo T, et al. APP processing and synaptic function. Neuron. 2003;37:925–37.
8. Cirrito JR, Yamada K a, Finn MB, Sloviter RS, Bales KR, May PC, et al. Synaptic activity regulates interstitial fluid amyloid-beta levels in vivo. Neuron. 2005; 48:913–22.
9. Cirrito JR, Kang J-E, Lee J, Stewart FR, Verges DK, Silverio LM, et al. Endocytosis is required for synaptic activity-dependent release of amyloid-beta in vivo. Neuron. 2008;58:42–51.
10. Buckner RL, Snyder AZ, Shannon BJ, LaRossa G, Sachs R, Fotenos AF, et al. Molecular, structural, and functional characterization of Alzheimer's disease:

evidence for a relationship between default activity, amyloid, and memory. J Neurosci. 2005;25:7709–17. Society for Neuroscience

11. Buckner RL, Sepulcre J, Talukdar T, Krienen FM, Liu H, Hedden T, et al. Cortical hubs revealed by intrinsic functional connectivity: mapping, assessment of stability, and relation to Alzheimer's disease. J Neurosci. 2009; 29:1860–73. Society for Neuroscience

12. Cirrito JR, Disabato BM, Restivo JL, Verges DK, Goebel WD, Sathyan A, et al. Serotonin signaling is associated with lower amyloid-β levels and plaques in transgenic mice and humans. Proc Natl Acad Sci U S A. 2011;108:14968–73.

13. Fisher JR, Wallace CE, Tripoli DL, Sheline YI, Cirrito JR. Redundant Gs-coupled serotonin receptors regulate amyloid-β metabolism in vivo. Mol Neurodegener. 2016;11:45. BioMed Central

14. Hartmann B, Ahmadi S, Heppenstall PA, Lewin GR, Schott C, Borchardt T, et al. The AMPA receptor subunits GluR-A and GluR-B reciprocally modulate spinal synaptic plasticity and inflammatory pain. Neuron. 2004;44:637–50. Elseevier

15. Wang Y, Durkin JP. Alpha-Amino-3-hydroxy-5-methyl-4-isoxazolepropionic acid, but not N-methyl-D-aspartate, activates mitogen-activated protein kinase through G-protein beta subunits in rat cortical neurons. J Biol Chem. 1995;270:22783–7. American Society for Biochemistry and Mol Biol

16. Wang Y, Small DL, Stanimirovic DB, Morley P, Durkin JP. AMPA receptor-mediated regulation of a Gi-protein in cortical neurons. Nature. 1997;389:502–4.

17. Perkinton MS, Sihra TS, Williams RJ. Ca(2+)-permeable AMPA receptors induce phosphorylation of cAMP response element-binding protein through a phosphatidylinositol 3-kinase-dependent stimulation of the mitogen-activated protein kinase signaling cascade in neurons. J Neurosci. 1999;19:5861–74. Society for Neuroscience

18. Rao VR, Finkbeiner S. NMDA and AMPA receptors: old channels, new tricks. Trends Neurosci. 2007;30:284–91. Elsevier

19. Chang EH, Savage MJ, Flood DG, Thomas JM, Levy RB, Mahadomrongkul V, et al. AMPA receptor downscaling at the onset of Alzheimer's disease pathology in double knockin mice. Proc Natl Acad Sci U S A. 2006;103: 3410–5. National Academy of Sciences

20. Shepherd JD, Huganir RL. The cell biology of synaptic plasticity: AMPA receptor trafficking. Annu Rev Cell Dev Biol. 2007;23:613–43. Annual Reviews

21. Hsieh H, Boehm J, Sato C, Iwatsubo T, Tomita T, Sisodia S, et al. AMPAR removal underlies Abeta-induced synaptic depression and dendritic spine loss. Neuron. 2006;52:831–43.

22. Hoey SE, Buonocore F, Cox CJ, Hammond VJ, Perkinton MS, Williams RJ. AMPA receptor activation promotes non- Amyloidogenic amyloid precursor processing and suppresses neuronal amyloid-beta production. PLoS One. 2013;8:e78155.

23. Jankowsky JL, Slunt HH, Ratovitski T, Jenkins NA, Copeland NG, Borchelt DR. Co-expression of multiple transgenes in mouse CNS: a comparison of strategies. Biomol Eng. 2001;17:157–65.

24. Jankowsky JL, Slunt HH, Gonzales V, Jenkins NA, Copeland NG, Borchelt DR. APP processing and amyloid deposition in mice haplo-insufficient for presenilin 1. Neurobiol Aging. 2004;25:885–92.

25. Cirrito JR, May PC, O'Dell MA, Taylor JW, Parsadanian M, Cramer JW, et al. In vivo assessment of brain interstitial fluid with microdialysis reveals plaque-associated changes in amyloid-beta metabolism and half-life. J Neurosci. 2003;23:8844–53.

26. Spandidos A, Wang X, Wang H, Seed B. PrimerBank: a resource of human and mouse PCR primer pairs for gene expression detection and quantification. Nucleic Acids Res. 2010;38:D792–9.

27. Spandidos A, Wang X, Wang H, Dragnev S, Thurber T, Seed B, et al. A comprehensive collection of experimentally validated primers for polymerase chain reaction quantitation of murine transcript abundance. BMC Genomics. 2008;9:633. BioMed Central

28. Wang X, Seed B. A PCR primer bank for quantitative gene expression analysis. Nucleic Acids Res. 2003;31:154e–154. Oxford University Press

29. Kaczmarek L. Glutamate receptor-driven gene expression in learning. Acta Neurobiol Exp (Wars). 1993;53:187–96.

30. Trussell LO, Zhang S, Ramant IM. Desensitization of AMPA receptors upon multiquantal neurotransmitter release. Neuron. 1993;10:1185–96.

31. Yamada KA, Rothman SM. Diazoxide blocks glutamate desensitization and prolongs excitatory postsynaptic currents in rat hippocampal neurons. J Physiol. 1992;458:409–23.

32. Verges DK, Restivo JL, Goebel WD, Holtzman DM, Cirrito JR. Opposing synaptic regulation of amyloid-β metabolism by NMDA receptors in vivo. J Neurosci. 2011;31:11328–37.

33. Hoey SE, Williams RJ, Perkinton MS. Synaptic NMDA receptor activation stimulates alpha-secretase amyloid precursor protein processing and inhibits amyloid-beta production. J Neurosci. 2009;29:4442–60.

34. Plant K, Pelkey KA, Bortolotto ZA, Morita D, Terashima A, McBain CJ, et al. Transient incorporation of native GluR2-lacking AMPA receptors during hippocampal long-term potentiation. Nat Neurosci. 2006;9:602–4. Nature Publishing Group

35. Santos AE, Duarte CB, Iizuka M, Barsoumian EL, Ham J, Lopes MC, et al. Excitotoxicity mediated by Ca2+−permeable GluR4-containing AMPA receptors involves the AP-1 transcription factor. Cell Death Differ. 2006;13: 652–60. Nature Publishing Group

36. Wei W, Nguyen LN, Kessels HW, Hagiwara H, Sisoda S, Malinow R. Amyloid beta from axons and dendrites reduces local spine number and plasticity. Nat Neurosci. 2010;13:190–6. Nature Research

37. Tanzi RE, Moir RD, Wagner SL. Clearance of Alzheimer's Aβ Peptide: the many roads to perdition. Neuron. 2004;43:605–8.

38. Tarasoff-Conway JM, Carare RO, Osorio RS, Glodzik L, Butler T, Fieremans E, et al. Clearance systems in the brain-implications for Alzheimer disease. Nat Rev Neurol. 2015;11:457–70.

39. Holtzman DM, Morris JC, Goate AM. Alzheimer's disease: the challenge of the second century. Sci Transl Med. 2011;3:77sr1.

40. Olney JW, Collins RC, Sloviter RS. Excitotoxic mechanisms of epileptic brain damage. Adv Neurol. 1986;44:857–77.

41. Denes A, Vidyasagar R, Feng J, Narvainen J, McColl BW, Kauppinen RA, et al. Proliferating resident microglia after focal cerebral ischaemia in mice. J Cereb Blood Flow Metab. 2007;27:1941–53.

42. Eng LF, Yu AC, Lee YL. Astrocytic response to injury. Prog Brain Res. 1992;94:353–65.

43. Hanisch U-K, Kettenmann H. Microglia: active sensor and versatile effector cells in the normal and pathologic brain. Nat Neurosci. 2007;10:1387–94. Nature Publishing Group

44. Ito D, Tanaka K, Suzuki S, Dembo T, Fukuuchi Y. Enhanced Expression of Iba1, Ionized Calcium-Binding Adapter Molecule 1, After Transient Focal Cerebral Ischemia In Rat Brain. Stroke. 2001;32:1208–15. Lippincott Williams & Wilkins

45. Bush T, Puvanachandra N, Horner C, Polito A, Ostenfeld T, Svendsen C, et al. Leukocyte infiltration, neuronal degeneration, and Neurite outgrowth after ablation of scar-forming, reactive astrocytes in adult transgenic mice. Neuron. 1999;23:297–308.

46. Bennetta ML, Bennetta C, Liddelowa SA, Ajami B, Zamanian JL, Fernhoff NB, et al. New tools for studying microglia in the mouse and human CNS. PNAS. 2016;113:E1738-46.

47. Juttler E, Tarabin V, Schwaninger M. Interleukin-6 (IL-6): a possible neuromodulator induced by neuronal activity. Neuroscientist. 2002;8:268–75.

48. Sallmann S, Jüttler E, Prinz S, Petersen N, Knopf U, Weiser T, et al. Induction of interleukin-6 by depolarization of neurons. J Neurosci. 2000;20:8637–42.

49. Erta M, Quintana A, Hidalgo J. Interleukin-6, a major cytokine in the central nervous system. Int J Biol Sci. 2012;8:1254–66. Ivyspring International Publisher

50. Chakrabarty P, Jansen-West K, Beccard A, Ceballos-Diaz C, Levites Y, Verbeeck C, et al. Massive gliosis induced by interleukin-6 suppresses a deposition in vivo: evidence against inflammation as a driving force for amyloid deposition. FASEB J. 2010;24:548–59.

51. Wang W-Y, Tan M, Yu J-T, Tan L. Role of pro-inflammatory cytokines released from microglia in Alzheimer's disease. Ann Transl Med. 2015;3:1–15.

52. Lomakin A, Teplow DB, Kirschner DA, Benedek GB. Kinetic theory of fibrillogenesis of amyloid beta-protein. Proc Natl Acad Sci U S A. 1997; 94:7942–7.

53. Tampellini D, Capetillo-Zarate E, Dumont M, Huang Z, Yu F, Lin MT, et al. Effects of synaptic modulation on beta-amyloid, synaptophysin, and memory performance in Alzheimer's disease transgenic mice. J Neurosci. 2010;30:14299–304. NIH Public Access

54. Jones CK, Brady AE, Davis AA, Xiang Z, Bubser M, Tantawy MN, et al. Novel selective allosteric activator of the M1 muscarinic acetylcholine receptor regulates amyloid processing and produces antipsychotic-like activity in rats. J Neurosci. 2008;28:10422–33.

55. Davis AA, Fritz JJ, Wess J, Lah JJ, Levey AI. Deletion of M1 muscarinic acetylcholine receptors increases amyloid pathology in vitro and in vivo. J Neurosci. 2010;30:4190–6.

56. Fisher A. Cholinergic modulation of amyloid precursor protein processing with emphasis on M1 muscarinic receptor: perspectives and challenges in treatment of Alzheimer's disease. J Neurochem. 2012;120:22–33.

57. Hamilton A, Esseltine JL, DeVries RA, Cregan SP, Ferguson SSG. Metabotropic glutamate receptor 5 knockout reduces cognitive impairment and pathogenesis in a mouse model of Alzheimer's disease. Mol Brain. 2014; 7:40. BioMed Central

58. Kim SH, Fraser PE, Westaway D, St George-Hyslop PH, Ehrlich ME, Gandy S. Group II metabotropic glutamate receptor stimulation triggers production and release of Alzheimer's amyloid(beta)42 from isolated intact nerve terminals. J Neurosci. 2010;30:3870–5.

59. Lesné S, Ali C, Gabriel C, Croci N, MacKenzie ET, Glabe CG, et al. NMDA receptor activation inhibits alpha-secretase and promotes neuronal amyloid-beta production. J Neurosci. 2005;25:9367–77.

60. Sara Y, Bal M, Adachi M, Monteggia LM, Kavalali ET. Use-dependent AMPA receptor block reveals segregation of spontaneous and evoked glutamatergic neurotransmission. J Neurosci. 2011;31:5378–82.

61. Sutton MA, Taylor AM, Ito HT, Pham A, Schuman EM. Postsynaptic decoding of neural activity: eEF2 as a biochemical sensor coupling miniature synaptic transmission to local protein synthesis. Neuron. 2007; 55:648–61.

62. Sutton MA, Wall NR, Aakalu GN, Schuman EM. Regulation of dendritic protein synthesis by miniature synaptic events. Science. 2004;304:1979–83. American Association for the Advancement of Science

63. Sutton MA, Ito HT, Cressy P, Kempf C, Woo JC, Schuman EM. Miniature neurotransmission stabilizes synaptic function via tonic suppression of local dendritic protein synthesis. Cell. 2006;125:785–99.

64. Murphy TH, Blatter LA, Bhat RV, Fiore RS, Wier WG, Baraban JM. Differential regulation of calcium/calmodulin-dependent protein kinase II and p42 MAP kinase activity by synaptic transmission. J Neurosci. 1994;14:1320–31.

65. Sutton MA, Schuman EM. Partitioning the synaptic landscape: distinct microdomains for spontaneous and spike-triggered neurotransmission. Sci Signal. 2009;2:pe19. Science Signaling

66. Atasoy D, Ertunc M, Moulder KL, Blackwell J, Chung C, Su J, et al. Spontaneous and evoked glutamate release activates two populations of NMDA receptors with limited overlap. J Neurosci. 2008;28:10151–66.

67. Koo EH, Squazzo SL. Evidence that production and release of amyloid beta-protein involves the endocytic pathway. J Biol Chem. 1994;269: 17386–9.

68. Gruol DL. IL-6 regulation of synaptic function in the CNS. Neuropharmacology. 2015;96:42–54.

69. Gadient R, Otten U. Interleukin-6 - a molecule with both beneficial and destructive potentials. Prog Neurobiol. 1997;52:379–90.

70. Yasukawa K, Hirano T, Watanabe Y, Muratani K, Matsuda T, Nakai S, et al. Structure and expression of human B cell stimulatory factor-2 (BSF-2/IL-6) gene. EMBO J. 1987;6:2939–45. European Molecular Biology Organization

71. Schöbitz B, de Kloet ER, Sutanto W, Holsboer F. Cellular localization of interleukin 6 mRNA and interleukin 6 receptor mRNA in rat brain. Eur J Neurosci. 1993;5:1426–35.

72. Tian X, Feig LA. Age-dependent participation of Ras-GRF proteins in coupling calcium-permeable AMPA glutamate receptors to Ras/Erk signaling in cortical neurons. J Biol Chem. 2006;281:7578–82. American Society for Biochemistry and Molecular Biology

73. Wang H-X, Gao W-J. Development of calcium-permeable AMPA receptors and their correlation with NMDA receptors in fast-spiking interneurons of rat prefrontal cortex. J Physiol. 2010;588:2823–38. Wiley-Blackwell

74. Murphy KM, Tcharnaia L, Beshara SP, Jones DG. Cortical development of AMPA receptor trafficking proteins. Front Mol Neurosci. 2012;5:65. Frontiers Media SA

75. Cantanelli P, Sperduti S, Ciavardelli D, Stuppia L, Gatta V, Sensi SL. Age-dependent modifications of AMPA receptor subunit expression levels and related cognitive effects in 3xTg-AD mice. Front Aging Neurosci. 2014;6:200. Frontiers Media SA

76. Mawuenyega KG, Sigurdson W, Ovod V, Munsell L, Kasten T, Morris JC, et al. Decreased clearance of CNS beta-amyloid in Alzheimer's disease. Science. 2010;330:1774. American Association for the Advancement of Science

77. Olney JW, Wozniak DF, Farber NB. Excitotoxic neurodegeneration in Alzheimer disease. New hypothesis and new therapeutic strategies. Arch Neurol. 1997;54:1234–40.

78. Francis PT. Glutamatergic systems in Alzheimer's disease. Int J Geriatr Psychiatry. 2003;18:S15–21.

79. Lacor PN, Buniel MC, Furlow PW, Clemente AS, Velasco PT, Wood M, et al. Abeta oligomer-induced aberrations in synapse composition, shape, and density provide a molecular basis for loss of connectivity in Alzheimer's disease. J Neurosci. 2007;27:796–807.

80. Marcello E, Epis R, Di Luca M. Amyloid flirting with synaptic failure: towards a comprehensive view of Alzheimer's disease pathogenesis. Eur J Pharmacol. 2008;585:109–18.

Permissions

List of Contributors

Michael C. Pace, Guilian Xu, Susan Fromholt, John Howard, Benoit I. Giasson and Jada Lewis
Department of Neuroscience, Center for Translational Research in Neurodegenerative Disease, McKnight Brain Institute, University of Florida, 1275 Center Drive, BMS Building J-491, Gainesville, FL 32610-0244, USA

David R. Borchelt
Department of Neuroscience, Center for Translational Research in Neurodegenerative Disease, McKnight Brain Institute, University of Florida, 1275 Center Drive, BMS Building J-491, Gainesville, FL 32610-0244, USA
SantaFe Healthcare Alzheimer's Disease Center, Gainesville, FL, USA

Justin Rustenhoven, Leon C. Smyth, Deidre Jansson, Emma L. Scotter, Miranda Aalderink and Mike Dragunow
Department of Pharmacology and Clinical Pharmacology, The University of Auckland, Private Bag 92019, Auckland 1142, New Zealand
Centre for Brain Research, The University of Auckland, Auckland, New Zealand

Thomas I. H. Park
Department of Pharmacology and Clinical Pharmacology, The University of Auckland, Private Bag 92019, Auckland 1142, New Zealand
Centre for Brain Research, The University of Auckland, Auckland, New Zealand
Department of Anatomy and Medical Imaging, The University of Auckland, Auckland, New Zealand

Maurice A. Curtis, Richard L. M. Faull, Natacha Coppieters and Molly E. V. Swanson
Department of Pharmacology and Clinical Pharmacology, The University of Auckland, Private Bag 92019, Auckland 1142, New Zealand
Department of Anatomy and Medical Imaging, The University of Auckland, Auckland, New Zealand

Pritika Narayan and Renee Handley
Centre for Brain Research, The University of Auckland, Auckland, New Zealand
School of Biological Sciences, The University of Auckland, Auckland, New Zealand

Amy M. Smith
Division of Brain Sciences, Department of Medicine, Imperial College London, London, UK

Chris Overall
Center for Brain Immunology and Glia, University of Virginia, Charlottesville, Virginia, USA
Departmemt of Neuroscience, University of Virginia, Charlottesville, Virginia, USA

Patrick Schweder and Peter Heppner
Auckland City Hospital, Auckland, New Zealand

Rebecca Kusko, Jermaine Ross, Yoonjeong Cha, Renan Escalante-Chong and Ben Zeskind
Immuneering Corporation, Cambridge, MA 02142, USA

Jennifer Dreymann, Daphna Laifenfeld, Michael E. Burczynski, Michal Geva and Iris Grossman
Research and Development, Teva Pharmaceutical Industries Ltd, Netanya, Israel

Michael R. Hayden
Research and Development, Teva Pharmaceutical Industries Ltd, Netanya, Israel
Translational Laboratory in Genetic Medicine, Agency for Science, Technology and Research, Singapore (A*STAR), Singapore 138648, Singapore
Centre for Molecular Medicine and Therapeutics, Child and Family Research Institute, University of British Columbia, Vancouver, BC V5Z 4H4, Canada
Department of Medicine, Yong Loo Lin School of Medicine, National University of Singapore, Singapore 117597, Singapore

Marta Garcia-Miralles and Liang Juin Tan
Translational Laboratory in Genetic Medicine, Agency for Science, Technology and Research, Singapore (A*STAR), Singapore 138648, Singapore

Mahmoud Pouladi
Translational Laboratory in Genetic Medicine, Agency for Science, Technology and Research, Singapore (A*STAR), Singapore 138648, Singapore
Department of Medicine, Yong Loo Lin School of Medicine, National University of Singapore, Singapore 117597, Singapore

Tatyana A. Shelkovnikova, Haiyan An, Pasquale Dimasi and Svetlana Alexeeva
School of Biosciences, Cardiff University, Museum Avenue, Cardiff CF10 3AX, UK

Vladimir L. Buchman and Michail S. Kukharsky
School of Biosciences, Cardiff University, Museum Avenue, Cardiff CF10 3AX, UK

Institute of Physiologically Active Compounds Russian Academy of Sciences, 1 Severniy proezd, Chernogolovka, Moscow Region, Russian Federation142432

Osman Shabir and Paul R. Heath
The Sheffield Institute for Translational Neuroscience, 385A Glossop Road, Sheffield S10 2HQ, UK

Giovanni Nardo, Maria Chiara Trolese, Mattia Verderio and Caterina Bendotti
Laboratory of Molecular Neurobiology, Department of Neuroscience, IRCCS - Istituto di Ricerche Farmacologiche Mario Negri, Via La Masa 19, 20156 Milan, Italy

Alessandro Mariani and Massimiliano de Paola
Laboratory of Analytical Biochemistry, Department of Environmental Health Sciences, IRCCS - Istituto di Ricerche Farmacologiche Mario Negri, Via La Masa 19, 20156 Milan, Italy

Nilo Riva, Giorgia Dina and Angelo Quattrini
Neuropathology Unit, Department of Neurology, INSPE- San Raffaele Scientific Institute, Dibit II, Via Olgettina 48, 20132 Milan, Italy

Nicolò Panini and Eugenio Erba
Laboratory of Cancer Pharmacology Department of Oncology, Flow Cytometry Unit, IRCCS – Istituto di Ricerche Farmacologiche Mario Negri, via La Masa 19, 20156 Milan, Italy

Srikant Rangaraju, Syed Ali Raza, Hailian Xiao, Tianwen Gao, James J. Lah, Nicholas T. Seyfried and Allan I. Levey
Department of Neurology, Emory University, Atlanta, GA 30322, USA

Duc M. Duong and Eric B. Dammer
Department of Biochemistry, Emory University, Atlanta, GA 30322, USA

Priyadharshini Rathakrishnan
Emory University, Atlanta, GA 30322, USA

Michael W. Pennington
Peptides International, Louisville, KY 40269, USA

Xianyuan Xiang
Metabolic Biochemistry, Biomedical Center (BMC), Faculty of Medicine, Ludwig-Maximilians-Universität München, Munich, Germany
Graduate School of Systemic Neuroscience, Ludwig-Maximilians- University Munich, Munich, Germany

Christian Haass
Metabolic Biochemistry, Biomedical Center (BMC), Faculty of Medicine, Ludwig-Maximilians-Universität München, Munich, Germany
German Center for Neurodegenerative Diseases (DZNE) Munich, Munich, Germany
Munich Cluster for Systems Neurology (SyNergy), Munich, Germany

Gernot Kleinberger
Metabolic Biochemistry, Biomedical Center (BMC), Faculty of Medicine, Ludwig-Maximilians-Universität München, Munich, Germany
Munich Cluster for Systems Neurology (SyNergy), Munich, Germany

Thomas M. Piers, Anna Mallach and Jennifer M. Pocock
Department of Neuroinflammation, Cell Signalling Lab, University College London Institute of Neurology, WC1N 1PJ, London, UK

Bettina Brunner
German Center for Neurodegenerative Diseases (DZNE) Munich, Munich, Germany

Kaichuan Zhu
German Center for Neurodegencrative Diseases (DZNE) Munich, Munich, Germany
Munich Cluster for Systems Neurology (SyNergy), Munich, Germany

Wolfgang Wurst
German Center for Neurodegenerative Diseases (DZNE) Munich, Munich, Germany
Munich Cluster for Systems Neurology (SyNergy), Munich, Germany
Institute of Developmental Genetics, Helmholtz Zentrum München, German Research Center for Environmental Health, Neuherberg, Germany
Technische Universität München-Weihenstephan, 85764 Neuherberg/ Munich, Germany

Jochen Herms
German Center for Neurodegenerative Diseases (DZNE) Munich, Munich, Germany
Munich Cluster for Systems Neurology (SyNergy), Munich, Germany
Center for Neuropathology and Prion Research, Ludwig-Maximilians-Universität München, Munich, Germany

Benedikt Wefers
German Center for Neurodegenerative Diseases (DZNE) Munich, Munich, Germany

Institute of Developmental Genetics, Helmholtz Zentrum München, German Research Center for Environmental Health, Neuherberg, Germany

Wilbur Song and Marco Colonna
Department of Immunology and Pathology, Washington University in St. Louis, St. Louis, MO, USA

En-Lin Dong, Chong Wang, Shuang Wu, Ying-Qian Lu, Xiao-Hong Lin, Hui-Zhen Su, Miao Zhao, Jin He and Xiang Lin
Department of Neurology and Institute of Neurology, The First Affiliated Hospital of Fujian Medical University, Fuzhou 350005, China

Ning Wang and Wan-Jin Chen
Department of Neurology and Institute of Neurology, The First Affiliated Hospital of Fujian Medical University, Fuzhou 350005, China
Fujian Key Laboratory of Molecular Neurology, Fujian Medical University, Fuzhou 350005, China

Li-Xiang Ma
Department of Anatomy, Histology and Embryology, Shanghai Medical College, Fudan University, Shanghai 200032, China

Zhen Zhao, Abhay P Sagare, Yingxi Wu, Min Wang, Nelly Chuqui Owens and Berislav V Zlokovic
Center for Neurodegeneration and Regeneration, Zilkha Neurogenetic Institute and Department of Physiology and Neuroscience, Keck School of Medicine, University of Southern California, Los Angeles, California 90033, USA

Qingyi Ma
Center for Neurodegeneration and Regeneration, Zilkha Neurogenetic Institute and Department of Physiology and Neuroscience, Keck School of Medicine, University of Southern California, Los Angeles, California 90033, USA
Lawrence D. Longo, MD Center for Neonatal Biology, Division of Pharmacology, Department of Basic Sciences, Loma Linda University School of Medicine, Loma Linda, CA 92350, USA

Philip B Verghese
C2N Diagnostics, LLC, Saint Louis, MO 63110, USA

Joachim Herz
Department of Molecular Genetics, University of Texas Southwestern Medical Center, Dallas, TX, USA
Department of Neuroscience, University of Texas Southwestern Medical Center, Dallas, TX, USA

Department of Neurology and Neurotherapeutics and Center for Translational Neurodegeneration Research, University of Texas Southwestern Medical Center, Dallas, TX, USA

David M Holtzman
Department of Neurology, Hope Center for Neurological Disorders, Knight Alzheimer's Disease Research Center, Washington University School of Medicine, Saint Louis, MO 63110, USA

Lodewijk J. A. Toonen, Maurice Overzier, Kristina M. Hettne and Willeke M. C. van Roon-Mom
Department of Human Genetics, Leiden University Medical Center, 2300 RC Leiden, The Netherlands

Melvin M. Evers
Department of Research and Development, uniQure, Amsterdam, The Netherlands

Leticia G. Leon
Cancer Pharmacology Lab, University of Pisa, Ospedale di Cisanello, Edificio 6 via Paradisa, 2, 56124 Pisa, Italy

Sander A. J. van der Zeeuw and Hailiang Mei
Sequencing Analysis Support Core, Leiden University Medical Center, 2300 RC Leiden, The Netherlands

Szymon M. Kielbasa and Jelle J. Goeman
Department of Biomedical Data Sciences, Leiden University Medical Center, 2300 RC Leiden, The Netherlands

Olafur Th. Magnusson
deCODE genetics/Amgen, Sturlugata 8, 101 Reykjavik, Iceland

Marion Poirel and Alexandre Seyer
MedDAY Pharmaceuticals, Paris, France

Peter A. C. 't Hoen
Department of Human Genetics, Leiden University Medical Center, 2300 RC Leiden, The Netherlands
Centre for Molecular and Biomolecular Informatics, Radboud Institute for Molecular Life Sciences, Radboud University Medical Center, 6500 HB, Nijmegen, The Netherlands

Michael C. Pace, Guilian Xu, Susan Fromholt, John Howard, Benoit I. Giasson and Jada Lewis
Department of Neuroscience, Center for Translational Research in Neurodegenerative Disease, McKnight Brain Institute, University of Florida, 1275 Center Drive, BMS Building J-491, Gainesville, FL 32610-0244, USA

David R. Borchelt
Department of Neuroscience, Center for Translational Research in Neurodegenerative Disease, McKnight Brain Institute, University of Florida, 1275 Center Drive, BMS Building J-491, Gainesville, FL 32610-0244, USA
SantaFe Healthcare Alzheimer's Disease Center, Gainesville, FL, USA

Takae Kiyama, Ping Pan and Chai-An Mao
Ruiz Department of Ophthalmology and Visual Science, McGovern Medical School at The University of Texas Health Science Center at Houston (UTHealth), 6431 Fannin St., MSB 7.024, Houston, TX 77030, USA

Ching-Kang Chen
Department of Ophthalmology, Baylor College of Medicine, 1 Baylor Plaza, Houston, TX 77030, USA

Steven W Wang and William H Klein
Department of Systems Biology, The University of Texas MD Anderson Cancer Center, 1515 Holcombe Blvd, Houston, TX 77030, USA

Zhenlin Ju and Jing Wang
Department of Bioinformatics and Computational Biology, The University of Texas MD Anderson Cancer Center, 1515 Holcombe Blvd, Houston, TX 77030, USA

Shinako Takada
Department of Biochemistry and Molecular Biology, The University of Texas MD Anderson Cancer Center, 1515 Holcombe Blvd, Houston, TX 77030, USA
Present Address: Office of Scientific Review, National Institute of General Medical Sciences, National Institutes of Health, Bethesda, MD 20892, USA

Erin G. Reed-Geaghan, Taylor R. Jay and J. Colleen Karlo
Department of Neurosciences, Case Western Reserve University, School of Medicine, Cleveland, OH 44106, USA

Paul J. Cheng-Hathaway, and Gary E. Landreth and Brad T. Casali
Department of Neurosciences, Case Western Reserve University, School of Medicine, Cleveland, OH 44106, USA
Department of Anatomy and Cell Biology, Indiana University, School of Medicine, Indianapolis, IN 46202, USA
Paul and Carole Stark Neurosciences Research Institute, Indiana University, School of Medicine, Indianapolis, IN 46202, USA

Bruce T. Lamb
Department of Neurosciences, Case Western Reserve University, School of Medicine, Cleveland, OH 44106, USA
Paul and Carole Stark Neurosciences Research Institute, Indiana University, School of Medicine, Indianapolis, IN 46202, USA
Department of Medical and Molecular Genetics, Indiana University, School of Medicine, Indianapolis, IN 46202, USA
Cleveland Clinic Lerner Research Institute, Cleveland, OH 44195, USA

Miguel Moutinho, Victoria E. von Saucken and Roxanne Y. Williams
Department of Anatomy and Cell Biology, Indiana University, School of Medicine, Indianapolis, IN 6202, USA
Paul and Carole Stark Neurosciences Research Institute, Indiana University, School of Medicine, Indianapolis, IN 46202, USA

Guixiang Xu, Shane M. Bemiller and Shweta S. Puntambekar
Paul and Carole Stark Neurosciences Research Institute, Indiana University, School of Medicine, Indianapolis, IN 46202, USA
Department of Medical and Molecular Genetics, Indiana University, School of Medicine, Indianapolis, IN 6202, USA

Richard M. Ransohoff
Cleveland Clinic Lerner Research Institute, Cleveland, OH 44195, USA

Jane C. Hettinger, Hyo Lee, David M. Holtzman and John R. Cirrito
Department of Neurology, Knight Alzheimer's Disease Research Center, Hope Center for Neurological Disorders, Washington University School of Medicine, Campus 660 South Euclid Avenue, St. Louis, MO 63110, USA

Guojun Bu
Department of Neuroscience, Mayo Clinic, Jacksonville, FL 32224, USA

Index